Complications in
Canine Cranial Cruciate Ligament Surgery

Complications in Canine Cranial Cruciate Ligament Surgery

Edited by

Ron Ben-Amotz, DVM, MS, CCRP, DACVS-SA, DECVS
Koret School of Veterinary Medicine
Jerusalem, Israel

David L. Dycus, DVM, MS, CCRP, DACVS-SA
Nexus Veterinary Bone & Joint Center
Baltimore, United States

WILEY Blackwell

AMERICAN COLLEGE of VETERINARY SURGEONS
ACVS® FOUNDATION

This edition first published 2022

This work is a co-publication between the American College of Veterinary Surgeons Foundation and Wiley-Blackwell.

Registered Office
John Wiley & Sons, Inc., 111 River Street, Hoboken, NJ 07030, USA

Editorial Office
111 River Street, Hoboken, NJ 07030, USA

For details of our global editorial offices, customer services, and more information about Wiley products visit us at www.wiley.com.

Wiley also publishes its books in a variety of electronic formats and by print-on-demand. Some content that appears in standard print versions of this book may not be available in other formats.

Library of Congress Cataloging-in-Publication Data

Names: Ben-Amotz, Ron, editor. | Dycus, David L., 1983- editor. | American College of Veterinary Surgeons, issuing body.
Title: Complications in canine cranial cruciate ligament surgery / edited by Ron Ben-Amotz, David L. Dycus.
Other titles: Advances in veterinary surgery
Description: First edition. | Hoboken, NJ : Wiley-Blackwell ; [Germantown, Md.] : American College of Veterinary Surgeons, 2022. | Series: Advances in veterinary surgery | Includes index.
Identifiers: LCCN 2021028940 (print) | LCCN 2021028941 (ebook) | ISBN 9781119654377 (hardback) | ISBN 9781119654391 (Adobe PDF) | ISBN 9781119654346 (epub)
Subjects: MESH: Anterior Cruciate Ligament Injuries–surgery | Dog Diseases–surgery | Intraoperative Complications–veterinary | Anterior Cruciate Ligament Injuries–veterinary | Rupture–surgery | Intraoperative Complications–therapy
Classification: LCC SF991 (print) | LCC SF991 (ebook) | NLM SF 992.J64 | DDC 636.7/089747–dc23
LC record available at https://lccn.loc.gov/2021028940
LC ebook record available at https://lccn.loc.gov/2021028941

Cover Design: Wiley
Cover Image: © Ron Ben-Amotz and David L. Dycus

Set in 9.5/11.5pt Palatino by Straive, Pondicherry, India

Printed in Singapore
M103676_260721

Contents

List of Contributors

Marc H. Balligand, DMedVet, PhD, CertSAO, Diplomate ECVS
Full Professor and Head
Small Animal Surgery Service
Faculty of Veterinary Medicine,
University of Liège
Liège, Belgium

Matthew D. Barnhart, DVM, MS, Diplomate ACVS
Surgery Specialty Leader
MedVet Medical & Cancer Centers for Pets
Worthington, OH, USA

R. Randy Basinger, DVM, Diplomate ACVS
VetSurg LLC
Irmo, SC, USA

Brian S. Beale, DVM, Diplomate ACVS
ACVS Founding Fellow Minimally-Invasive Surgery (Orthopedics)
CEO and Surgeon
Beale's Best LLC
Beale Veterinary Specialists and Emergency
Victoria, TX, USA

Ron Ben-Amotz, DVM, MS, CCRP, Diplomate ACVS, ECVS
Section Head, Small Animal Orthopedics
Koret School of Veterinary Medicine
Lecturer, The Hebrew University of Jerusalem
Jerusalem, Israel

Jeffery Biskup, DVM, Diplomate ACVS
Small Animal Surgeon
Animal Health Partners
North York, ON, Canada

Matthew W. Brunke, DVM, CCRP, CVPP, CVA, Diplomate ACVSMR
Medical Director,
Veterinary Surgical Centers Rehabilitation
Vienna, VA, USA

Steven C. Budsberg, DVM, MS, Diplomate, ACVS
Professor of Orthopedics
College of Veterinary Medicine
University of Georgia
Athens, GA, USA

Michael G. Conzemius, DVM, PhD, Diplomate ACVS
Endowed Professor of Surgery
Veterinary Clinical Sciences
University of Minnesota
St Paul, MN, USA

Matt Corse, DVM, MS, Diplomate, ACVS
Chief of Orthopedic Surgery
Northlake Veterinary Surgery
Clarkston, GA, USA

David L. Dycus, DVM, MS, CCRP, Diplomate ACVS
Chief of Orthopedic Surgery
Nexus Veterinary Bone & Joint Center
Medical Director
Nexus Veterinary Specialists
Co-Founder/Co-Director
Veterinary Sports Medicine and Rehabilitation Institute (VSMRI)
Baltimore, MD, USA

Katie L. Hoddinott, BSc, DVM, DVSc, Diplomate ACVS
Assistant Professor, Small Animal Surgery
Atlantic Veterinary College, University of Prince Edward Island
Charlottetown, PE, Canada

Ian G. Holsworth, BSc, BVSc, MANZCVS (Surgery), Diplomate ACVS
ACVS Founding Fellow Minimally-Invasive Surgery (Orthopedics)
Director
VetSurg
Ventura, CA, USA

Don Hulse, DVM, Diplomate ACVS, ECVS
Professor of Orthopedics
College of Veterinary Medicine
Texas A&M University
College Station, TX, USA

Stephen C. Jones, MVB, MS, Diplomate ACVS, ECVS
Assistant Professor Small Animal Surgery
College of Veterinary Medicine
The Ohio State University
Columbus, OH, USA

Sorrel J. Langley-Hobbs, MA, BVetMed, DSAS(O), Diplomate ECVS, FHEA, FRCVS
Chair in Small Animal Orthopaedic Surgery
RCVS Specialist in Small Animal Surgery (Orthopedics)
EBVS® European Specialist in Small Animal Surgery
Bristol Vet School, University of Bristol
Bristol, UK

David Levine, PT, PhD, DPT, CCRP, FAPTA
Professor and Walter M. Cline Chair of Excellence in Physical Therapy
Department of Physical Therapy
The University of Tennessee at Chattanooga
Chattanooga, TN, USA
Veterinary Care and Specialty Group, Chattanooga, TN, USA

Denis J. Marcellin-Little, DEDV, Diplomate ACVS, ACVSMR
Professor, Orthopedic Surgery
Department of Veterinary Surgical and Radiological Sciences
University of California, Davis
Davis, CA, USA

Bill Oxley, MA, VetMB, DSAS(Orth), MRCVS
Director Vet3D
Billy's Space
Staveley, UK

Eva Schnabl-Feichter, Diplomate ECVS
Team Leader Small Animal Orthopedics
Department for Companion Animals and Horses
University Clinic for Small Animal Surgery
University of Veterinary Medicine
Vienna, Austria

Ameet Singh, DVM, DVSc, Diplomate ACVS
Associate Professor
Ontario Veterinary College
University of Guelph
Guelph, ON, Canada

Selena Tinga, DVM, PhD, Diplomate ACVS
Assistant Professor
Veterinary Clinical Sciences
The Ohio State University
Columbus, OH, USA

Bryan T. Torres, DVM, PhD, Diplomate ACVS, ACVSMR
Assistant Professor
Orthopedic Surgery – Small Animal
Director of the Motion Analysis Laboratory
Department of Veterinary Medicine and Surgery
College of Veterinary Medicine
University of Missouri
Columbia, MO, USA

Aldo Vezzoni, med. vet., S.C.M.P.A., Diplolmate ECVS
EBVS® European Specialist in Small Animal Surgery
Clinica Veterinaria Vezzoni srl
Cremona, Italy

J. Scott Weese, DVM, DVSc, Diplomate ACVIM, FCAHS
Professor, Ontario Veterinary College
Director, Centre for Public Health and Zoonoses
University of Guelph
Guelph, ON, Canada

Joshua S. Zuckerman, VMD, Diplomate ACVS
Staff Surgeon
Cape Cod Veterinary Specialists
Buzzards Bay, MA, USA

Preface

The American College of Veterinary Surgeons Foundation is excited to present *Complications in Cranial Cruciate Ligament Surgery* in the book series entitled *Advances in Veterinary Surgery*. Cranial cruciate ligament repair is likely the most common orthopedic surgery performed on dogs and a book dedicated to the complications of the procedures we use is appropriate. My sage mentors taught me that complications are an unfortunate part of surgery and our duty is to own them, manage them to get the best possible outcome for our patients, and learn from them to minimize the chance of future complications. As one of the key missions of the ACVS Foundation is to promote cutting-edge education for diplomates, this topic is timely and very reflective of the educational mission of the Foundation.

Complications in Cranial Cruciate Ligament Surgery is edited by Drs Ron Ben-Amotz and David L. Dycus. I'd like to congratulate and thank them for taking on this project. They have chosen a group of strong contributing authors to detail the identification, management, and prevention of complications in cranial cruciate surgery. We are sure you will find this reference extremely valuable.

The ACVS Foundation is an independently chartered philanthropic organization devoted to advancing the educational, scientific, and charitable goals of the American College of Veterinary Surgeons. The mission of the ACVS Foundation is to support the advancement of surgical care of all animals through funding of educational and research opportunities for veterinary surgical residents and board-certified veterinary surgeons.

The ACVS Foundation's collaboration with Wiley Blackwell benefits all those who are interested in veterinary surgery by presenting the latest evidence-based information on relevant surgical topics. The ACVS Foundation is proud to partner with Wiley Blackwell in this important series and is honored to present this newest book in the *Advances in Veterinary Surgery* series.

R. Randy Basinger, DVM, ACVS
Chair, Board of Trustees
ACVS Foundation

Foreword

I have tremendous respect and gratitude towards Drs Dycus and Ben-Amotz for taking on the challenge of putting together this book as a vital resource for veterinarians who want to treat patients *and* educate clients in the most optimal and comprehensive way possible. While a book project is always daunting, it is relatively easy to write about "when things go right," but extremely difficult to write about "when things go wrong" as the authors and editors have done for this valuable text. Speaking from experience, the latter is much more important, so I highly recommend that every veterinarian involved in preoperative, intraoperative, and/or postoperative care of dogs being treated for cranial cruciate ligament disease adds this book to their daily-use library.

Acknowledging and understanding complications are the keys to avoiding them, and this all-star line-up of experienced authors communicates these keys in a comprehensive and transparent way that is refreshing and inspiring. Importantly, the editors and authors committed themselves to an evidence-based approach to each and every chapter such that information provided is both reliable and pragmatic. Equally importantly, each chapter answers the question, "What do I do now?" so that readers are provided with decision-making algorithms, tools, and techniques to address complications, both intraoperatively and postoperatively, and to know when and how to revise cases in order to rescue the outcome. This text is well written and well illustrated such that the knowledge provided is readily applied to "real-life" clinical practice.

Again, I sincerely compliment the editors and the authors on their valuable effort, which has resulted in a rich resource for everyone involved in the care of dogs with cranial cruciate ligament disease. I hope that veterinarians of all experience levels will take advantage of this resource by taking it to heart and using the same evidence-based approach put forth in this book in their delivery of care to patients and honest communication with clients.

James L. Cook, DVM, PhD
William and Kathryn Allen Distinguished
Chair of Orthopedic Surgery
Director, Thompson Laboratory for
Regenerative Orthopaedics
University of Missouri

Acknowledgments

To err is human – an existence and experience marred by miscalculation and misjudgment. Errors infiltrate every aspect of our existence, including our professional lives. As surgeons, we carry a greater burden than most, operating daily with the knowledge that our errors may be catastrophic.

The idea for this book arose from an unrewarding reference search. We all know that complications occur, and that countless publications exist in which these complications are described in detail. But my question was this: what happens next? In particular, I noted a surprising lack of answers to this question even with regard to the surgical treatment of canine cruciate ligament disease, one of the most common orthopedic problems we routinely address. It was then that I began to realize that providing these answers in an accessible format would serve not only our residents, novice surgeons, and general practitioners, but the entire surgical community.

As David and I embarked on the mission of editing this book, I was continuously reminded of Benjamin Franklin's quote: "by failing to prepare, you are preparing to fail." Not only must we prepare for every surgery we perform, we must also know how to face our mistakes when things do not go according to plan. Understanding and, more importantly, acknowledging our mistakes is the key to avoiding them in the future. We must have the courage and humility to admit when things go wrong before we can attain the wisdom to correct them.

Without the dedicated support and encouragement of those who have joined me on this journey, I could never have become who I am today. I owe many thanks to former resident-mates, who endured the initial training with me, and to my current and former students and residents who ensure that my knowledge base remains sharp and up to date. Of course, that knowledge wouldn't even be there without the help of my mentors and professors, all of whom contributed in unique and unforgettable ways, and the AO community, who welcomed me as a young faculty member, and whose members tirelessly work to advance our chosen field. In particular, I owe special thanks to Dr Jonathan Dyce, who pushed my boundaries and expected nothing less than excellence and perfection in return, Dr Robert Orsher, who has been invaluable in his support of my professional aspirations, and Dr Joshua Zuckerman, who enthusiastically accompanies me on my writing expeditions.

I would like to express my most sincere thanks to the distinguished authors who contributed an incalculable wealth of knowledge and experience to this textbook. All of your dedication and hard work resonates within these pages. Thank you as well to the ACVS Foundation for their endorsement and belief in this project, and to Merryl Le Roux and Erica Judisch from Wiley Blackwell, without whom it could never have become a reality.

I am indebted to my parents, Gadi and Lia, who have supported me along every step of my education and career. They taught me the importance of hard work, compassion, perseverance, dedication, and honesty. To my sister Dana and my brother Oded, I am grateful for their belief that I can overcome every hurdle encountered along the way.

The true dedication of this book belongs to my beloved wife Shir-Raz, who sacrificed everything so I could fulfill my dreams. She tirelessly supported my goals, traveled the world with me, and never gave up on me. Without her I would not be who I am or where I am today. Finally, to my beautiful children Shai, Yoni, and Gali, who remind me every day what is really important in life.

And of course, to our canine and feline companions, who bring joy to our lives. We owe them our compassion, professional dedication, and love.

Ron Ben-Amotz

We as surgeons always want the best for our patients, and when we put the scalpel to the skin should be prepared to provide that. As Dr Atul Gawande has stated, "No matter what measures are taken, doctors will sometimes falter, and it isn't reasonable to ask that we achieve perfection. What is reasonable is to ask that we never cease to aim for it." I remember back in 2018 when Dr Ben-Amotz approached me about an idea for a book dedicated to complications for a particular disease condition. Recognizing the commonality of cruciate ligament disease in veterinary medicine and the vast array of procedures led to the birth of this textbook. We realized that stabilization techniques are briefly taught in veterinary school, and in-depth training comes in the form of a formal surgical residency. However, the majority of individuals learn these techniques through mentorship in practice or through continuing education. As an instructor for courses that teach stabilization techniques, it became apparent that we were teaching individuals how to perform the procedure but lacking on the preparation for minimizing complications, identifying intraoperative complications, and how to recognize and address postoperative complications. My hope is this textbook serves to fill in those gaps.

Many thanks are due to Erica Judisch, and various editors from Wiley Blackwell, for supporting us in the development of this book. They were supportive from the conception of this book and through the entire process. In addition, a thank you is due to the ACVS Foundation for supporting the book series as well as believing in the need for this book.

I still consider myself a young and developing surgeon and I would not be where I am today without the help of many mentors, colleagues, interns, residents, and general practitioners. It is the collection of everyone that has shaped me and helped me grow. Mentors have pushed me, taught me, and helped me when I was struggling. There are far too many to list here; however, a special thank you to Dr Ron McLaughlin who from my first year in veterinary school to the last day of my surgical residency instilled in me the desire to achieve perfection and laid the groundwork for me to get to where I am today. In addition, the words given to me by Dr Don Hulse to "make it better" have never been truer. His advice to never stop learning and keep thinking outside the box have helped evolve my desire to always keep pushing forward to help our patients.

However, the book is truly dedicated to my wife Brooke and daughter Kennedy. Without both of them I am nothing. My hope is that as my daughter grows older, she understands the work ethic I have tried to instill in her and recognizes the commitment that I have put forth in the veterinary industry. I hope she takes these things to become a successful woman who is able to critically think for herself and is always striving to make the world a better place. For Brooke, who has been with me since day one; she is my rock, best friend, and partner. There is no way I would have survived veterinary school, internship, residency, private practice, performing research, and teaching without her. She has "held the fort" for all the years of me working late at night, traveling, and working through the weekends. For this I owe her a debt of gratitude. In addition, a special thank you to my parents, Don and Vickie, who instilled in me to be the best I can be in whatever I do. While hard at times, I was taught the value of hard work and a strong worth ethic. The principles, values, and morals they taught me set me up to succeed not only as a veterinarian but also as a human.

Finally, no veterinarian would be able to do what we do without our patients and their owners. Recognizing the bond that animals bring to our lives helps inspire all veterinary professionals to do our best. Animals bring out the best in all of us and we certainly don't deserve them, so being able to help them in a time of need is one of the most humbling and wonderful experiences.

David L. Dycus

Disclosures

- Matthew D. Barnhart is a paid lecturer for Securos and Everost (Steris) and receives royalties from the sales of some of their products.
- Matt Corse is a paid consultant for Arthrex Vet Systems.
- David L. Dycus is a paid lecturer for Veterinary Orthopedic Implants.
- Ian G. Holsworth is a paid consultant and receives royalties from IMEX Veterinary Inc., Veterinary Instrumentation~Covetrus, Sontec Instruments, VetSurg Surgical instrumentation, and Arthrex Vet Systems.

Section I

Introduction

1 Pathology, Diagnosis, and Treatment Goals of Cranial Cruciate Ligament Rupture and Defining Complications

David L. Dycus, Jeffery Biskup, Michael G. Conzemius, and Ron Ben-Amotz

1.1 Introduction

The cranial cruciate ligament (CCL) is a robust intraarticular, yet extrasynovial structure responsible for preventing stifle hyperextension, excessive internal rotation, and cranial subluxation of the tibia in relation to the femur. It originates from the caudomedial aspect of the lateral femoral condyle, and travels in a craniomedial direction to insert on the cranial intercondyloid region of the tibia [1]. It is composed of two distinct bands: the craniomedial and caudolateral portions. During stifle extension, both the craniomedial and caudolateral bands are taut, while during flexion the craniomedial band remains taut while the caudolateral band becomes lax [2].

Cranial cruciate ligament disease is considered to be the most common cause of pelvic limb lameness in the canine, affecting approximately 2.55% of the population [3, 4]. It is a broad term that encompasses a variety of different pathological disorders that may affect the ligament. For example, in skeletally immature canines, avulsion of the CCL may occur secondary to a traumatic event. In the skeletally mature canine, traumatic rupture occurs less commonly, although it may still be induced by forced hyperextension with internal tibial rotation [5]. The most likely etiology for rupture of the CCL in mature dogs is progressive degeneration of the ligament. This degenerative process likely explains the high incidence of bilateral and contralateral CCL pathology. Contralateral CCL pathology has been documented in over 50% of canines [6]. Complicating the matter is the fact that the exact cause of degeneration is poorly understood. Various factors have been investigated in the etiology and pathogenesis of CCL degeneration. Tibial plateau angle [7], genetics, age, bony confirmation, body weight, gait, and vascularity of the ligament [8–10] have all been identified as risk factors for CCL rupture. To date, none of these factors has proved definitive and as such, the degeneration of the CCL is considered multifactorial.

Regardless of the cause of CCL damage, rupture results in a cascade of events that causes altered kinetics and kinematics of the stifle. It is these altered dynamics that likely lead to progressive osteoarthritis (OA) and increased likelihood of meniscal pathology. Kinematic analysis of the CCL-deficient stifle has shown that the joint remains in a more flexed position throughout the gait cycle. As a result of the

Complications in Canine Cranial Cruciate Ligament Surgery, First Edition. Edited by Ron Ben-Amotz and David L. Dycus.

increased stifle flexion, the hip and tarsocrural joints compensate by maintaining a greater degree of extension during the stance phase [11]. Kinetic analysis has revealed decreases in peak vertical force (PVF), vertical impulse, braking, and propulsion impulses in dogs with CCL pathology [12]. For example, the PVF in the normal canine pelvic limb was 70% of static body weight; however, when the CCL was transected, the PVF decreased to 25% of static body weight. This was only improved to 32% and 37% at 6 and 12 weeks post transection respectively [13]. Therefore, this demonstrates continued loss of PVF even after periarticular fibrosis has developed. It could be argued that because of this lack of improvement in kinetic function, surgical stabilization of the cruciate-deficient stifle should be considered.

Along with altered weight bearing and joint flexion/extension, there is also evidence to suggest that the CCL-deficient stifle exhibits increased cranial subluxation of the tibia in relation to the femur. Up to 8–12mm of subluxation has been noted during the stance phase of the gait [14].

Long-term changes have been evaluated in the canine following CCL transection. Following initial transection of the CCL, there was 10mm more tibial subluxation compared to patients with an intact CCL. Two months following transection, tibial subluxation was noted only during the stance phase and not during the late swing/early stance phase (paw strike). Two years following transection, 5mm of tibial thrust was noted at the end of the swing phase. It was suggested that the reason for these changes was the presence of an intact medial meniscus. It was theorized that in the CCL-deficient stifle, the meniscus minimizes tibial subluxation by elastically deforming during tibial subluxation and aiding in reduction of the subluxation once the swing phase begins (alternatively, as the load from the stance phase is removed) [15]. Interestingly, tibial subluxation as the result of instability has been called into question as it demonstrated that instability following CCL rupture is actually a caudal slippage of the femur at the beginning of the stance phase. As such, documented continuation of instability in some stifles exists following common osteotomy procedures such as the tibial plateau leveling osteotomy (TPLO) and tibial tuberosity advancement (TTA) [16].

In addition to controlling sagittal joint motion of the stifle, the CCL also aids in limiting internal rotation. To date, no osteotomy modifying procedures effectively eliminate excessive internal rotation. Initially, this was thought to play a minimal role in the CCL-deficient stifle. While significant changes in internal rotation were not noted immediately following transection of the CCL, 2 months following transection the range of abduction and adduction in the stifle was increased. These rotary changes remained increased 2 years following transection [15]. Recognition of the importance of preventing excessive internal rotation has led to the idea and development of augmentation to prevent excessive internal rotation following certain osteotomy procedures such as the TPLO (Figure 1.1).

Interestingly, a population of CCL-deficient canines will exhibit persistent internal rotation following surgical stabilization. This persistent internal rotation likely falls under the umbrella term of "pivot shift." Unfortunately, to date, it is not possible to predict which population of patients will exhibit persistent internal rotation following surgical stabilization. In the authors' opinion, patients with acute CCL rupture, large

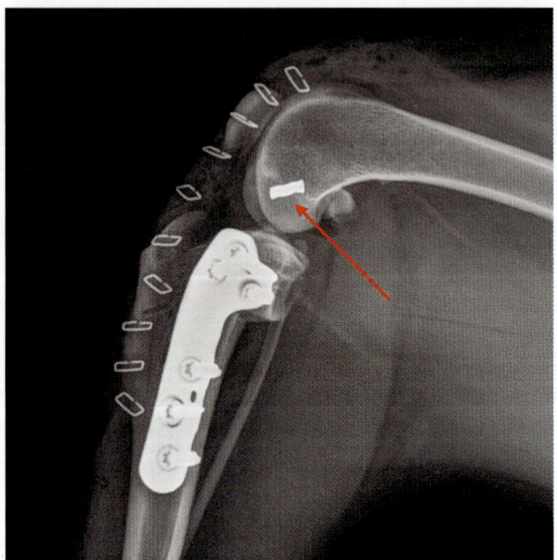

Figure 1.1 An immediate postoperative radiograph of stifle stabilization via a TPLO. Intraoperatively persistent excessive internal rotation was noted so a lateral fabellotibial suture was placed. Note the metallic crimp (red arrow) that has been added.

medial meniscal bucket handle tears, and lack of periarticular fibrosis tend to have persistent internal rotation following certain surgical procedures such as the TPLO. Recently, it was shown that the use of a lateral fabellotibial suture in combination with a TPLO was effective for managing CCL instability in patients with excessive internal rotation identified either preoperatively or intraoperatively [17]. Therefore, the authors recommend the use of adjunct lateral fabellotibial suture in identified patients with excessive internal rotation or "pivot shift" (Figure 1.1).

1.2 Diagnosis

The diagnosis of CCL pathology is made based on signalment, history and clinical signs, orthopedic examination findings, and diagnostic imaging. While the old saying "a hindlimb lameness in a mature dog is cruciate disease until proven otherwise" holds true, it is important to ensure that the lameness is due to CCL pathology and not another underlying pathological condition of the stifle or another anatomical structure of the pelvic limb.

Signalment information in canines with CCL pathology varies, with most affected dogs presenting for evaluation between 2 and 10 years of age. However, the authors have seen dogs as young as 12 weeks (Figure 1.2) and as old as 16 years present for CCL pathology. The authors (DD and RBA) have also observed a high incidence of 9–13-month-old American Pit Bull Terriers and American Staffordshire Terriers presenting with bilateral CCL pathology. The reason for this is unknown but could be due to demographics and possible breeding practices. Virtually any breed can be affected with CCL pathology; one study revealed the highest prevalence in the Rottweiler, Newfoundland, and Staffordshire Terrier [18]. Another study revealed that breeds at risk for suffering CCL rupture before 2 years of age included the Neapolitan Mastiff, Mastiff, St Bernard, Rottweiler, Akita, Newfoundland, Chesapeake Bay Retriever, Labrador Retriever, and American Staffordshire Terrier [19]. Female dogs have an increased prevalence of CCL pathology (similar to human female athletes), as do neutered canines compared to sexually intact canines [19].

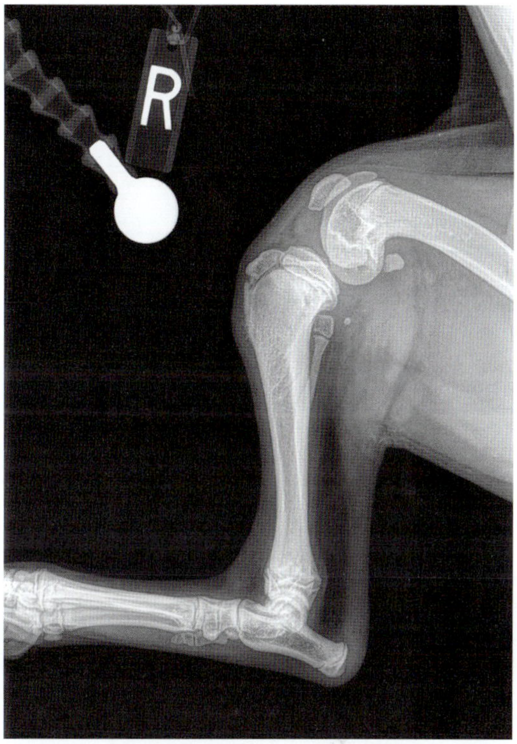

Figure 1.2 Radiograph of a 12-week-old dog that suffered a traumatic CCL injury.

Historical findings of patients with CCL pathology may include an acute or chronic onset of hindlimb lameness that may range in severity from mild to nonweight bearing. Some patients may only exhibit stiffness when rising or after heavy activity or may offload the affected limb at a stance (Figure 1.3). When questioning owners, it is important to obtain a timeline of abnormalities they have noticed even when the lameness appears acute. The authors have found that when questioning owners, many patients have a longer standing history of subtle clinical signs before an acute lameness develops. This further emphasizes the degeneration of the CCL. The common scenario following complete rupture of the CCL is a nonweight-bearing status for several days. As the inflammatory phase starts to subside, patients will begin to toe touch and use the limb with a noticeable weight-bearing lameness. Many owners perceive this as their dog improving, when in reality this is consistent with the normal progression of CCL pathology.

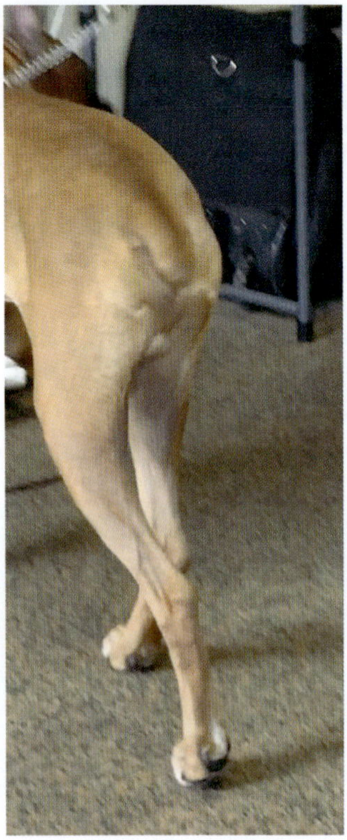

Figure 1.3 Representation of offloading the left pelvic limb at a stance. This patient was diagnosed with a left CCL rupture. Notice when the dog is standing full weight is not applied to the left pelvic limb.

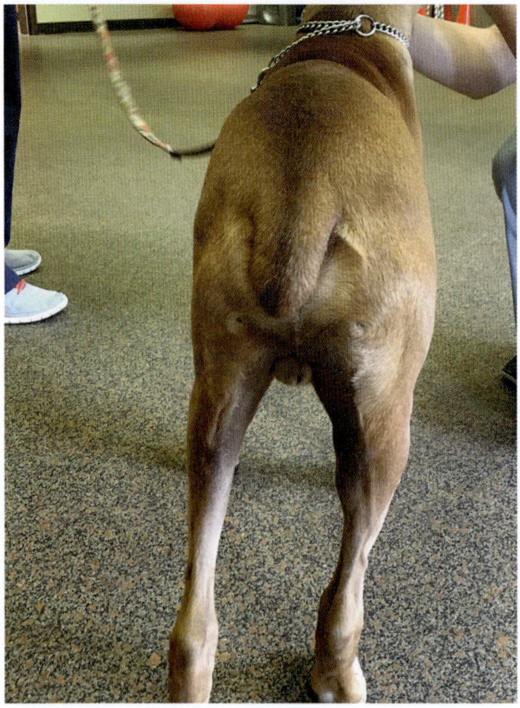

Figure 1.4 A patient with instability of the left pelvic limb secondary to a CCL rupture. Notice the degree of muscle loss on the left hindlimb compared to the right.

The orthopedic examination is aimed at demonstrating stifle instability; however, other aspects of the stifle and pelvic limb should be evaluated. Pending the severity of the condition as well as the timeframe, there may be pain upon flexion and extension of the stifle, in particular with hyperflexion and hyperextension. In chronic cases of CCL pathology, there may be thickening of the proximal medial tibial or the so-called "medial buttress" which is development of periarticular fibrosis. The periarticular fibrosis can limit range of motion in the stifle, which may ultimately result in loss of active range of motion. A loss of active range of motion can translate into loss of limb function [20]. In cases with more advanced OA, crepitus may be noted as range of motion is evaluated, and in cases in which meniscal pathology is present, there may be either a consistent or intermittent clicking ("meniscal click") during range of motion of the stifle. A recent study concluded that a meniscal click in CCL-deficient stifles carries a high specificity for a bucket handle tear of the meniscus. In addition, the presence of a meniscal click during examination is strongly indicative of a meniscal tear being diagnosed at surgery. However, a lack of meniscal click carries a low sensitivity in diagnosing the absence of meniscal tear [21, 22]. This emphasizes the need for meniscal evaluation in every joint undergoing CCL stabilization.

Loss of function of a limb will ultimately lead to loss of muscle strength. Unfortunately, in the canine, loss of muscle strength has never been reported but loss of muscle mass has [23] (Figure 1.4). Therefore, it is important to measure mass at the time of the initial consultation as well as at each follow-up visit. Additional information on measurement of hindlimb muscle mass can be found in Chapter 15. In addition, measurement of joint motion of the stifle should be performed [24] to determine the flexion and extension of both the affected and unaffected limbs not only at the initial consultation but at all follow-up visits. Additional

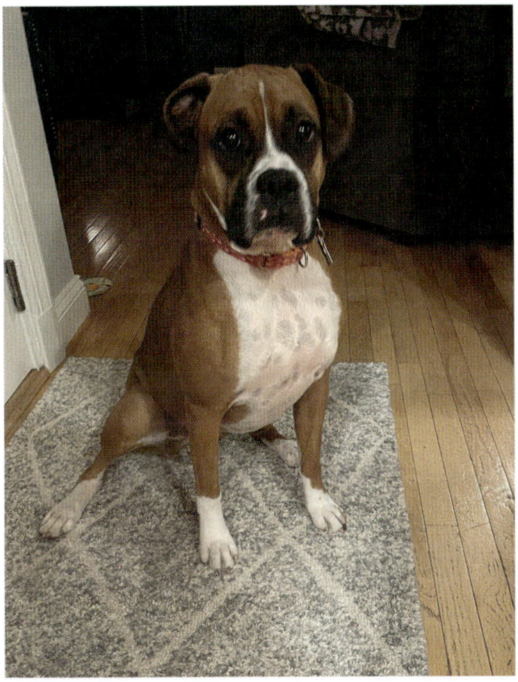

Figure 1.5 An example of a positive sit test in a patient with a right CCL tear. Notice how the right hindlimb is projected outward and the patient is not sitting squarely.

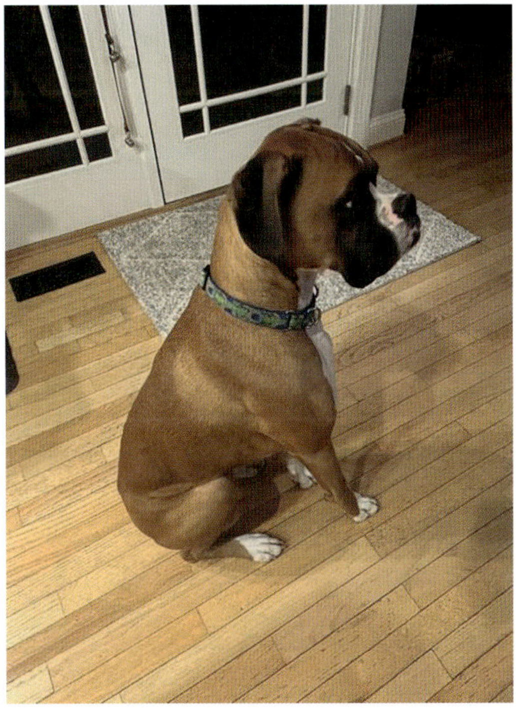

Figure 1.6 An example of a square sit in a patient with no CCL pathology. Notice how both stifles are fully flexed and the patient is sitting square.

information on measurement of joint motion can be found in Chapter 15.

One question that every clinician should ask themselves is: how do you know your patients are truly improving and how can you detect subtle complications? Gathering as much objective information as possible is vital; muscle mass measurements as well as measurement of joint motion of both the affected and unaffected limbs should be part of the objective information gathered (more information on this can be found in Chapter 15). With CCL pathology, there may be an abnormal sit, sometimes referred to as a "positive sit test." This is characterized by patients sitting with the affected limb projecting out to the side or tucked under them (Figure 1.5) rather than sitting square (Figure 1.6). Alternatively, patients may sit with weight shifted off the affected limb (Figure 1.5). The abnormal sitting posture is thought to be due to discomfort associated with hyperflexion of the stifle when forced to sit squarely. Unfortunately, some dogs may still exhibit an abnormal sit test following CCL stabilization. The reason for this is unknown but it could be due to continued stifle discomfort upon full flexion.

Instability of the stifle is commonly demonstrated through the cranial drawer test and tibial compression test. The cranial drawer test (Figure 1.7) is performed most commonly and tends to be the mainstay of testing for stifle instability by general veterinarians. It is performed by applying a force to the tibia while holding the femur stable, thereby creating craniocaudal translation of the tibia. The operator may stand either behind (caudal) the patient or behind and slightly to the side (caudal and lateral). One hand is placed on the distal femur with the thumb on the lateral fabella and the index finger on the patella. The other hand is placed on the proximal tibia with the thumb on the fibular head and the index finger on the tibial tuberosity. The goal is to move the hand on the proximal tibia cranially while holding the hand on the distal femur stable. Commonly, mistakes made by the inexperienced operator

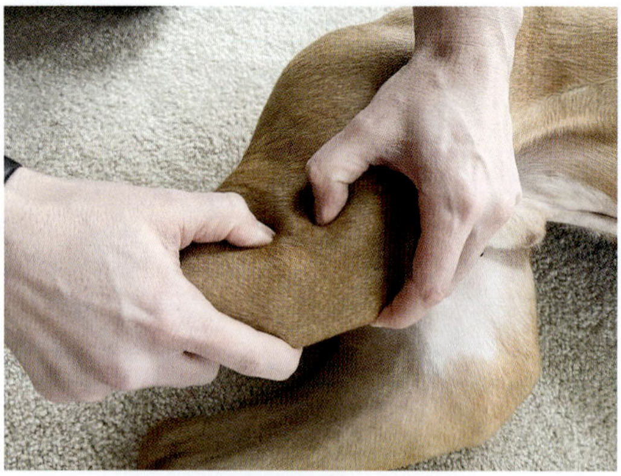

Figure 1.7 Demonstration of the cranial drawer test. One hand is placed on the distal femur with the thumb on the lateral fabella and the index finger on the patella. The other hand is placed on the proximal tibia with the thumb on the fibular head and the index finger on the tibial tuberosity. The goal is to move the hand on the proximal tibia cranially while holding the hand on the distal femur stable.

stem from trying to move both hands simultaneously or trying to grab the tissues (both soft and bony) too firmly. Forcing cranial drawer or grasping the tissues too firmly will cause the patient's muscles to tense, making interpretation difficult. Cranial drawer should first be checked in extension, and if positive is likely indicative of a complete tear (typically greater than 75% tearing of the CCL as subjectively noted by one author, DD). If negative, it should then be checked in flexion. A positive cranial drawer in flexion but negative in extension typically indicates an incompetent (unstable) partial CCL tear (usually 50–75% tearing of the CCL as subjectively noted by one author, DD). If cranial drawer is negative in both extension and flexion, then the stifle should be placed in hyperextension to evaluate for discomfort. Discomfort with joint effusion and negative cranial drawer may indicate a competent (stable) partial CCL tear (usually less than 50% tearing of the CCL as subjectively noted by one author, DD).

The make-up of the craniomedial and caudolateral bands of the CCL can explain why it is possible for the cranial drawer test to be positive in flexion even if it is negative in extension. The craniomedial band is the primary supporter of tibial translation and tends to degenerate first. During range of motion, it is taut in both flexion and extension. The caudolateral band is a secondary supporter of tibial translation and is taut in extension but lax in flexion. Therefore, if the craniomedial band is torn, cranial drawer will be absent in extension but present in flexion. Lack of cranial drawer may indicate tearing of the caudolateral band with an intact craniomedial band or subtle tearing of the craniomedial band or both the craniomedial and caudolateral band. In anxious or nervous patients or those with negative cranial drawer, the authors recommend performing a sedated examination to ensure there is no instability. Unfortunately, when chronic periarticular fibrosis or advanced OA is present, cranial drawer may be negative due to the presence of significant fibrous tissue or permeant translation of the tibia in relation to the femur. Skeletally immature patients often exhibit some physiological cranial drawer ("puppy drawer") of up to about 3–5 mm. However, there should be an abrupt stop point at the end of cranial drawer to differentiate this from pathological cranial drawer.

The tibial compression test (Figure 1.8), while still a passive test, aims to mimic load bearing of the stifle. The operator may stand either behind (caudal) the patient or behind and slightly to the side (caudal and lateral). One hand is placed on the distal femur with the thumb on the lateral fabella and the index finger on the patella. The other hand is used to hold the metatarsals and tarsocrural joint. With the stifle held stable, the tarsocrural joint is flexed and extended. The clinician observes for a cranial-to-caudal motion of the tibial tuberosity indicating pathology of the CCL. Mistakes made by the inexperienced operator stem from trying to flex and extend both the stifle and tarsocrural joint simultaneously. In addition, the stifle should be held in a sagittal plane with no excessive internal or external rotation. Holding the stifle internally rotated can lead to a false positive of tibial thrust.

Diagnostic imaging of the stifle in patients with CCL pathology is usually centered around radiographic evaluation. Radiographic examination is warranted in every case of hindlimb lameness even if surgical intervention is not an option. It should be suggested that good-quality orthogonal views of both the affected and unaffected stifles should be performed

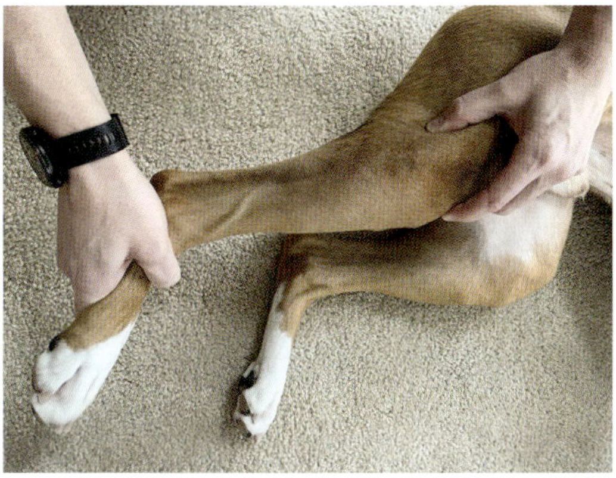

Figure 1.8 Demonstration of the tibial compression test. One hand is placed on the distal femur with the thumb on the lateral fabella and the index finger on the patella. The other hand is used to hold the metatarsals and tarsocrural joint. With the stifle held stable, the tarsocrural joint is flexed and extended. The clinician observes for a cranial-to-caudal motion of the tibial tuberosity indicating pathology of the CCL.

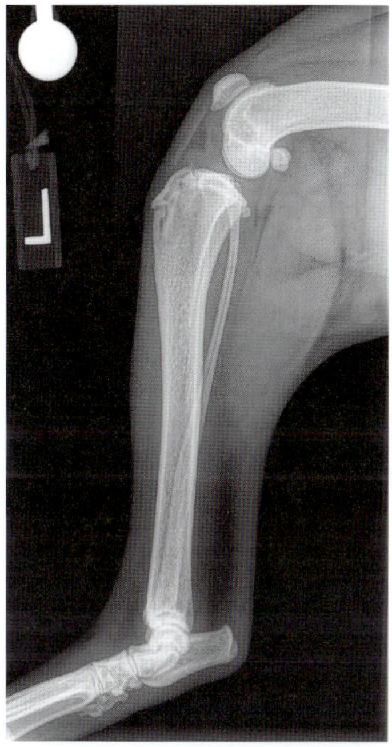

Figure 1.9 A lateral radiograph documenting appropriate positioning of the stifle. Notice there is superimposition of the femoral condyles and the tibial plateau demonstrating a straight view in the sagittal plane.

(Figures 1.9 and 1.10). While the CCL itself is not visible on radiographs (unless associated with an avulsion of the CCL), there are two key findings that can be appreciated: osteoarthritic changes and intraarticular changes (meniscal edema, synovial hyperplasia, and joint effusion).

The earliest finding of CCL pathology is the presence of joint effusion (Figure 1.11). This is noted by cranial displacement of the infrapatellar fat pad on the lateral view. The normal fat pad should be triangular in shape and located adjacent to the cranial margin of the femoral condyles and the cranial aspect of the tibial condyles. In most cases, any displacement from these normal margins is consistent with the presence of joint effusion. In addition, there may be displacement of the caudal joint capsule (Figure 1.11). The degree of joint effusion in some cases can be roughly correlated with the degree of CCL pathology. Generally, patients with competent partial CCL pathology will have less joint effusion than patients with incompetent or complete CCL pathology. Evidence of likely synovitis can be noted as subtle regions of sclerosis noted on the caudal aspect of the trochlear groove as seen on the lateral view.

Degenerative changes can readily be seen in patients with CCL pathology (Figure 1.12). In

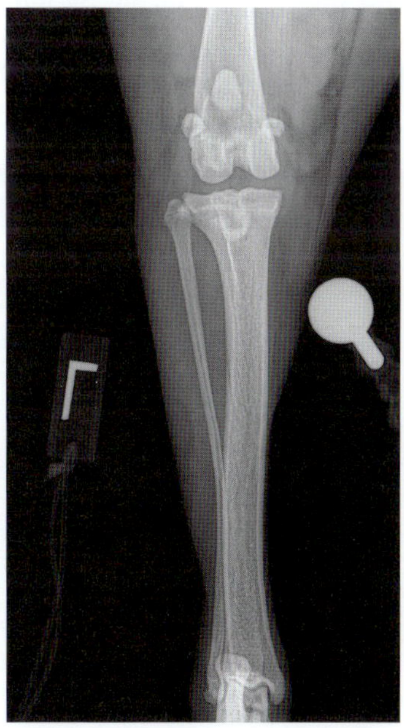

Figure 1.10 A cranial-caudal radiograph documenting appropriate position of the stifle. Notice how the calcaneus intersects the center of the trochlear ridge of the talus demonstrating a straight view in the frontal plane.

particular, changes will be noted at the proximal trochlear groove, lateral and medial femoral trochlea, distal pole of the patella (patella apex), caudal tibial plateau, medial and lateral aspects of the tibial condyle margins, and both fabellae. In some cases, the sesamoid bone of the popliteal muscle can be displaced proximally and/or caudally. The importance of taking contralateral radiographs at the time of initial diagnosis is for the evaluation of OA and joint effusion as well as detection of other pathologies that might exist. If noted on the contralateral stifle (even in the face of joint stability), one should assume there is already CCL pathology present and the likelihood of joint instability developing is high. If this is present, it is important to educate the owner regarding this finding.

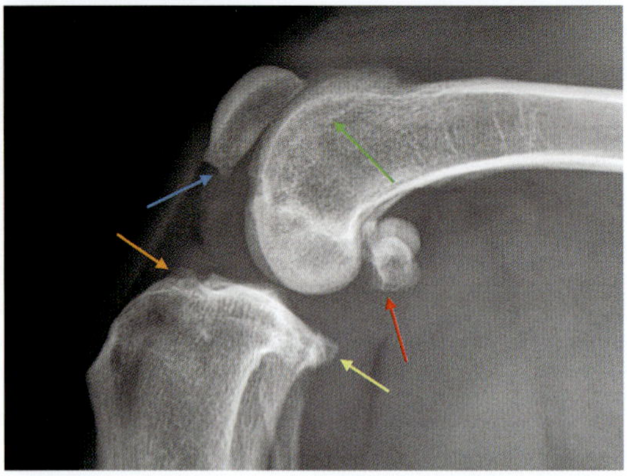

Figure 1.12 Evidence of degenerative changes in the stifle of a patient with CCL pathology. Commonly noted areas are the distal pole of the patella (blue arrow), cranial tibial plateau (orange arrow), caudal tibial plateau (yellow arrow), and fabella (red arrow). In addition, a small area of sclerosis can be seen around the trochlear groove (green arrow) indicative of synovitis or osteophytosis of the medial or lateral femoral trochlea.

1.3 Treatment

A number of methods for stifle stabilization exist. They are commonly characterized as extraarticular stabilization, intraarticular stabilization, and osteotomy modifying procedures. One of the complicating factors of stifle stabilization (and indeed, one of the reasons for the existence of so many surgical procedures) is the lack of definitive guidelines for what constitutes a successful postoperative outcome.

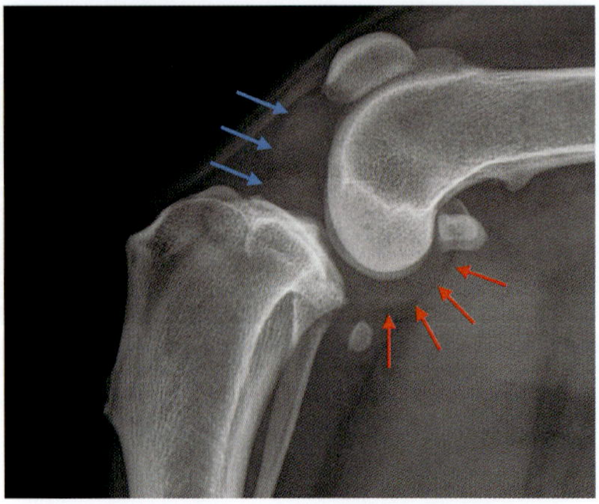

Figure 1.11 Evidence of joint effusion in the stifle of a patient with CCL pathology. In the caudal compartment, there is displacement of the joint capsule as can be noted by the red arrows. The opacity in the cranial compartment (blue arrows) is joint effusion that is displacing the fat pad cranially.

While all correctly executed surgical procedures can stabilize the stifle, not one of these procedures ultimately restores completely normal stifle kinematics or kinetics. In defining a good outcome, should we consider a stable stifle to be the predominant deciding factor? Interestingly, work has been completed that demonstrates ongoing instability following surgical stabilization [16, 25], yet retrospective and client assessment studies have shown high success rates with certain procedures. What about return to function? Success rates among all surgical procedures are in the high 80% to low 90% range when evaluating most retrospective studies. While this suggests that most surgical procedures do a good job of returning canines to "normal" function, probably the best way to tell would be return to sport or work for our canine athletes. Recent data have suggested that following TPLO, agility dogs have a good prognosis for return to sport [26].

Elimination of progression of OA has been stated as a possible determination of outcome and goal of treatment. This is likely not an achievable feat. Once the CCL has become damaged and instability in the stifle is present, there is abnormal joint loading. Thus, damage to the chondrocytes has occurred. Therefore, it is probably better to evaluate surgical stabilization procedures in terms of which are the most capable of slowing down and minimizing progression of OA, rather than which can eliminate it entirely.

1.4 Defining a Complication

The ability to recognize and manage complications should be considered when choosing a surgical procedure. Generally, the complication rate of currently practiced surgical stabilization procedures is low, but individual techniques are associated with their own unique set of potential complications and it is of the utmost importance that the clinician is familiar with the management of these complications prior to undertaking the initial procedure. In the past, much focus has been on the actual surgical procedure and training of how to perform it. Unfortunately, what is missed is how to identify patients that might be at an increased risk of complications, how to identify intraoperative complications, decision making to avoid intraoperative complications, recognition of postoperative complications, and how to revise complications in the postoperative period should they occur.

1.4.1 Assessment of Success and Complications

Although a high success rate (intended outcome) is important when deciding to perform a surgery, the risk of an unintended outcome, severity of potential adverse events, and owner financial burden need to be considered and communicated to the owner. Avoiding iatrogenic harm should be an emphasis of all practicing veterinarians. In veterinary orthopedics, standardized definitions of complications have been suggested in an attempt to improve consistency and comparability in veterinary orthopedic research [27]. For example, a method to classify catastrophic, major and minor complications has been published so results between studies can be accurately translated and to allow the clinician to decide if an intervention causes unacceptable morbidity.

One method to quantify success and harm factors is a ratio between the number of patients needed to treat (NNT) and number needed to harm (NNH). NNT is defined as:

$$\text{NNT} = 1/\text{Attributable risk}$$

where attributable risk is the difference between the frequencies of a successful outcome between two interventions. The NNT assesses how many patients would have to be treated with one treatment compared to another before there would be one additional positive outcome. For example, if surgery A had a success rate of 75% and surgery B had a success rate of 67%, the NNT would be 13 (1/(0.75–0.65) = 12.5); the result of 12.5 was rounded up to the nearest whole number to make the result more clinically relevant and prevent overestimating the benefit of surgery A. This means that surgery A would have to be performed on 13 patients before one additional beneficial outcome would be seen. In human medicine, a single-digit result is generally considered a good NNT [28].

Conversely, NNH assesses how many patients need to be treated with one treatment compared to another before you would see one additional complication. NNH is calculated similar to NNT but with complication frequencies. When calculating NNH, a specific complication(s) needs to be selected. For example, if surgery A had an infection rate of 10% and surgery B had an infection rate of 0%, the NNH would be 10. This means that one more infection would be seen for surgery A after completing 10 surgeries. A target NNH depends on the severity of the complication being assessed. A single-digit NNH may be acceptable for a minor complication such as incisional redness compared to a NNH of 100 for a major complication like implant infection.

For both NNT and NNH, it is also important to evaluate the overall frequency of success, or a complication, to direct clinical decision making. For example, if the NNH is 10 but the overall frequency of infection is 90% vs 80%, a clinician may conclude neither procedure should be used.

Finally, likelihood to be helped or harmed (LHH) can be calculated (NNH:NNT). A number >1 tells us that the treatment is that many times more likely to help than to harm. Using the above example, surgery A has a LHH of 10/13 = 0.77. When the LHH is <1, the treatment is more likely to harm than to help. A LHH <1 is usually only acceptable when the complication assessed is minor or transient. The more serious the complication assessed, the higher the desired LHH.

Other considerations when discussing complications include the effect of duration of follow-up and unique complications to the procedure. Time after an intervention can influence success and complication rate; a longer follow-up period may allow for an improved treatment response but also allows for a greater opportunity for an unintended outcome, like OA. In veterinary orthopedics, 12 months has been defined as the length of "long-term" follow-up; this terminology is reasonable but has been inconsistently followed [27].

It is important that statistical and clinical significance is considered when designing a study and interpreting results. Statistical significance is an important scientific evaluation of a dataset, but it is important to remember that it may be of little or no value when considering the care of an individual patient [29, 30]. One consideration is that investigations that include large sample sizes can result in clinically unimportant variables gaining statistical significance.

Although a p value is a common method to inform us of a statistical difference between groups, effect size and minimal clinically important difference (MCID) should also be investigated. Effect size helps quantify the magnitude of the difference observed and is not influenced by sample size. It is calculated by finding the difference between the means of two groups and dividing the result by the standard deviation [31]. Cohen suggested 0.2 is a small effect size, 0.5 is an average effect size, and 0.8 is a large effect size. For perspective, when there is an effect size of 0.8, 79% of the treatment group will be above the mean of the control group (a reference chart can provide this information for all effect size values).

Minimal clinically important difference was defined as "the smallest difference in score in the domain of interest which patients perceive as beneficial and which would mandate, in the absence of troublesome side effects and excessive cost, a change in the patient's management" [32] which was later simplified to "the smallest change that is important to patients" [33]. Although many human studies use patient-reported outcomes to define MCID, it is often compared to objective data. The major limitations of MCID include inconsistent definitions or values for MCID, cost of treatment not being taken into consideration, and MCID often varies depending on the baseline (more severely affected patients often need a smaller improvement to be pleased with the outcome). Alternative methods to put datasets into context include utilizing confidence intervals and probability. Regardless of the statistical methods used, they should be considered prior to the onset of a study so investigators remain unbiased. Unfortunately, most veterinary journals, reviewers, and investigators rely solely on the p value to determine significance, limiting thorough evaluation of different interventions.

References

1. Arnoczky, S.P. and Marshall, J.L. (1977). The cruciate ligaments of the canine stifle: an anatomical and functional analysis. *Am. J. Vet. Res.* 38: 1807–1814.
2. Tanegashima, K., Edamura, K., Akita, Y. et al. (2019). Functional anatomy of the craniomedial and caudolateral bundles of the cranial cruciate ligament in beagle dogs. *Vet. Comp. Orthop. Traumatol.* 32: 182–191.
3. Wilke, V.L., Robinson, A., Evans, R.B. et al. (2005). Estimate of the annual economic impact of treatment of the cranial cruciate ligament injury in dogs in the United States. *J. Am. Vet. Med. Assoc.* 227: 1604–1607.
4. Witsberger, T.H., Villamil, J.A., Schultz, L.G. et al. (2008). Prevalence of and risk factors for hip dysplasia and cranial cruciate ligament deficiency in dogs. *J. Am. Vet. Med. Assoc.* 232: 1818–1824.
5. Vezzoni, A., Bohorquez Vanelli, A., Modenato, M. et al. (2008). Proximal tibial epiphysiodesis to reduce tibial plateau slope in young dogs with cranial cruciate ligament deficient stifle. *Vet. Comp. Orthop. Traumatol.* 21: 343–348.
6. Muir, P., Schwartz, Z., Malek, S. et al. (2001). Contralateral cruciate survival in dogs with unilateral non-contact cranial cruciate ligament rupture. *PLoS One* 10: e25331.
7. Morris, E. and Lipowitz, A.J. (2001). Comparison of tibial plateau angles in dogs with and without cranial cruciate ligament injuries. *J. Am. Vet. Med. Assoc.* 218: 363–366.
8. Cook, J.L. (2010). Cranial cruciate ligament. Disease in dogs: biology versus biomechanics. *Vet. Surg.* 39: 270–277.

9. Hayashi, K., Manley, P.A., and Muir, P. (2004). Cranial cruciate ligament pathophysiology in dogs with cruciate ligament disease: a review. *J. Am. Anim. Hosp. Assoc.* 40: 385–390.
10. Kuroki, K., Williams, N., Ikeda, H. et al. (2019). Histologic assessment of ligament vascularity and synovitis in dogs with cranial cruciate ligament disease. *Am. J. Vet. Res.* 80: 152–158.
11. DeCamp, C.E., Riggs, C.M., Olivier, N.B. et al. (1996). Kinematic evaluation of gait in dogs with cranial cruciate ligament rupture. *Am. J. Vet. Res.* 57: 120–126.
12. Budsberg, S.C., Verstraete, M.C., Soutas-Little, R.W. et al. (1988). Force plate analysis before and after stabilization of canine stifles for cruciate injury. *Am. J. Vet. Res.* 46: 1522–1524.
13. O'Connor, B.L., Visco, D.M., Heck, D.A. et al. (1989). Gait alterations in dogs after transection of the anterior cruciate ligament. *Arthritis Rheum.* 32: 1142–1147.
14. Korvick, D.L., Pijanowski, G.J., and Schaeffer, D.J. (1994). Three-dimensional kinematics of the intact and cranial cruciate ligament-deficient stifle of dogs. *J. Biomech.* 27: 77–87.
15. Tashman, S., Aderst, W., Kolowich, P. et al. (2004). Kinematics of the ACL-deficint canine knee during gait: serial changes over two years. *J. Orthop. Res.* 22: 931–941.
16. Rey, J., Fischer, M.S., and Bottcher, P. (2014). Sagittal joint instability in the cranial cruciate ligament insufficient canine stifle. Caudal slippage of the femur and not cranial tibial subluxation. *Tierarztl. Prax. Ausg. K. Kleintiere Heimtiere* 42: 151–156.
17. Schaible, M., Shani, J., Ben-Amotz, R. et al. (2017). Combined tibial plateau leveling osteotomy and lateral fabellotibial suture for cranial cruciate ligament rupture with severe rotational instability. *J. Small Anim. Pract.* 58 (4): 219–226.
18. Whitehair, J.G., Vasseur, P.B., and Willits, N.H. (1993). Epidemiology of cranial cruciate ligament rupture in dogs. *J. Am. Vet. Med. Assoc.* 203: 1016–1019.
19. Duval, J.M., Budsberg, S.C., Flo, G.L. et al. (1999). Breed, sex, and body weight as risk factors for rupture of the cranial cruciate ligament in young dogs. *J. Am. Vet. Med. Assoc.* 215: 811–814.
20. Marcellin-Little, D.J. and Levine, D. (2015). Principles and application of range of motion and stretching in companion animals. *Vet. Clin. North Am. Small Anim. Pract.* 45: 57–72.
21. Neal, B., Ting, D., Bonczynski, J. et al. (2015). Evaluation of meniscal click for detecting meniscal tears in stifles with cranial cruciate ligament disease. *Vet. Surg.* 44: 191–194.
22. Gleason, H., Hudson, C., and Cerroni, B. (2020). Meniscal click in cranial cruciate deficient stifles as a predictor of specific meniscal pathology. *Vet. Surg.* 49: 155–159.
23. Dycus, D.L., Levine, D., and Marcellin-Little, D.J. (2017). Physical rehabilitation for the management of canine hip dysplasia. *Vet. Clin. North Am. Small Anim. Pract.* 47: 823–850.
24. Jaegger, G., Marcellin-Little, D.J., and Levine, D. (2002). Reliability of goniometry in Labrador retrievers. *Am. J. Vet. Res.* 63: 979–986.
25. Kim, S.E., Lewis, D.D., and Pozzi, A. (2012). Effect of tibial plateau leveling osteotomy on femorotibial subluxation: in vivo analysis during standing. *Vet. Surg.* 41: 465–470.
26. Heidorn, S.N., Canapp, S.O., Zink, C.M. et al. (2018). Rate of return to agility competition for dogs with cranial cruciate ligament tears treated with tibial plateau leveling osteotomy. *J. Am. Vet. Med. Assoc.* 253: 1439–1444.
27. Cook, J.L., Evans, R., Conzemius, M.G. et al. (2010). Proposed definitions and criteria for reporting time frame, outcome, and complications for clinical orthopedic studies in veterinary medicine. *Vet. Surg.* 39: 905–908.
28. Citrome, L. and Ketter, T.A. (2013). When does a difference make a difference? Interpretation of number needed to treat, number needed to harm, and likelihood to be helped or harmed. *Int. J. Clin. Pract.* 67: 407–411.
29. Copay, A.G., Subach, B.R., Glassman, S.D. et al. (2007). Understanding the minimum clinically important difference: a review of concepts and methods. *Spine J.* 7: 541–546.
30. Lascelles, B.D.X., Brown, D.C., Conzemius, M. et al. (2019). Measurement of chronic pain in companion animals: priorities for future research and development based on discussions from the Pain in Animals Workshop (PAW) 2017. *Vet. J.* 252: 105370. https://doi.org/10.1016/j.tvjl.2019.105370.
31. Kim, H.Y. (2015). Statistical notes for clinical researchers: effect size. *Restor. Dent. Endod.* 40: 328–331.
32. Jaeschke, R., Singer, J., and Guyatt, G.H. (1989). Measurement of health status. Ascertaining the minimal clinically important difference. *Control. Clin. Trials* 10: 407–415.
33. Stratford, P.W., Binkley, J.M., Riddle, D.L. et al. (1998). Sensitivity to change of the Roland-Morris Back Pain Questionnaire: part 1. *Phys. Ther.* 78: 1186–1196.

2 Surgeon and Patient Preparation to Minimize Surgical Site Complications and Infection Surveillance Programs

Katie L. Hoddinott, J. Scott Weese, and Ameet Singh

2.1 Introduction

The reported incidence of surgical site infections (SSIs) in companion animal veterinary medicine ranges from 3% to 18.1%, with increasing risk of SSI development associated with increasing classification of the surgical procedure (Table 2.1) [1–7]. Orthopedic surgeries are most commonly classified as clean procedures; however, SSI rates are often higher in clean orthopedic surgeries (3.54–12.9%) when compared to other clean surgical procedures (2.5–4.8%) [5, 7–9]. Furthermore, SSI rates vary amongst surgical stabilization techniques for treatment of cranial cruciate ligament ruptures. Extracapsular repair techniques, including the lateral fabellotibial suture and Arthrex Canine Cruciate Ligament Repair Anchor System™, have reported SSI rates ranging from 3.9% to 21% [6, 10–12] while proximal tibial osteotomy procedures, including tibial plateau leveling osteotomy (TPLO), tibial tuberosity advancement (TTA), triple tibial osteotomy, and cranial closing wedge osteotomies, have reported SSI rates ranging from 4.7% to 25.9% [13–26].

Many risk factors have been associated with development of SSIs following surgical stabilization of the cranial cruciate-deficient stifle. These risk factors may be associated with the host, the environment, details surrounding the surgical procedure and the use of antimicrobials. Host factors include breed, sex, body weight, American Society of Anesthesiologists (ASA) status, methicillin-resistant *Staphylococcus pseudintermedius* (MRSP) carrier status, and skin microbiome. Environmental factors include the number of personnel in the surgical suite and potential for bacterial contamination from surrounding surfaces. Surgical procedure factors include the method of stifle stabilization, length of general anesthesia, length of surgical procedure, surgeon preparation, intraoperative contamination, adherence to Halstead's principles (Table 2.2), and choice of implant and wound closure materials. Finally, the use of antimicrobials in the preoperative, perioperative, and postoperative periods has been documented as a risk factor for SSI.

2.2 Host Factors

2.2.1 Breed, Sex, and Body Weight

Several host factors identified as risk factors for SSI development are beyond the control of the veterinary team, such as breed, sex, and body

Complications in Canine Cranial Cruciate Ligament Surgery, First Edition. Edited by Ron Ben-Amotz and David L. Dycus.

Table 2.1 Surgical procedure classification.

Clean	No infection No break in aseptic technique Nontraumatic
Clean-contaminated	Controlled access to a hollow viscus Minor break in aseptic technique
Contaminated	Entry through nonseptic, yet inflamed tissues Spillage from a hollow viscus – localized, controlled Major break in aseptic technique Fresh, traumatic wounds (<4 h)
Dirty	Perforated hollow viscus Septic purulent discharge encountered Chronic, traumatic wounds (>4 h)

Source: Based on Turk et al. [1], Eugster et al. [2], Nicholson et al. [3], Fitzpatrick and Solano [4], Beal et al. [5], Frey et al. [6], and Vasseur et al. [7].

Table 2.2 Halstead's principles.

Gentle tissue handling
Meticulous hemostasis
Strict aseptic technique
Preservation of blood supply
Elimination of dead space
Accurate apposition of tissues while minimizing tension

weight. Bulldogs and German Shepherds have been identified as having an increased risk for development of SSI following TPLO surgery [21, 27]. Labrador Retrievers and mixed-breed dogs have been identified as having a lower SSI development risk following TPLO surgery [4, 3]. Both Fitzpatrick and Solano and Nicholson et al. identified intact male dogs to be at higher risk of SSI; however, sex was not identified as a risk factor in other studies [3, 4, 17, 28]. Increased body weight has been significantly associated with an increased SSI risk in several studies [2, 4, 10, 15, 28–30]. In one study, each 1 kg increase in body weight resulted in 1.03 times increased odds of developing an SSI, while a second study noted that for each 1 kg increase in body weight, the odds of developing an SSI increased by 4.7% [28, 29]. As these factors are inherent to the patient and cannot be specifically controlled, this information can be utilized to distinguish those animals at higher risk of developing an SSI and thus requiring greater preventive measures.

2.2.2 ASA Status and Endocrinopathies

Preoperative ASA score (Table 2.3) has been correlated with risk for developing an SSI, such that the risk for SSI increases with each increment in ASA score [2]. As ASA scores take into consideration the overall health status of a patient, the higher the ASA score, the more systemically ill the patient. Animals with endocrinopathies have also been identified to be 8.2 times more likely to develop an SSI, likely due to alterations in immune function [3]. Logically, if an animal has a chronic illness, such as an unmanaged or poorly controlled endocrinopathy, postponement of elective orthopedic procedures until these illnesses are adequately addressed should be considered, when possible.

2.2.3 MRSP Carrier Status

As *Staphylococcus* spp. have been identified as one of the most common bacteria contributing to the development of SSIs following TPLO, and MRSP SSIs are increasing in frequency, monitoring for carriers of MRSP has been investigated [4, 13, 21, 31–34]. In one study, 4.4% of animals were identified to be MRSP carriers preoperatively and carriers were 6.72 times more likely to develop an SSI. While screening for MRSP may help to determine those animals at higher risk for SSI, current screening tests are time-consuming and not practical for routine implementation as this would result in

Table 2.3 American society of anesthesiologists (ASA) scores.

ASA I	Normal, healthy patients
ASA II	Patients with mild systemic disease
ASA III	Patients with severe systemic disease
ASA IV	Patients with severe systemic disease that is life-threatening
ASA V	Patients that will not survive 24 h without surgical intervention

Source: Based on Eugster et al. [2].

delaying surgery [21]. Additionally, in human medicine, the goals of methicillin-resistant *Staphylococcus aureus* (MRSA) screening are to allow for decolonization preoperatively [35–38]. In veterinary medicine, preoperative decolonization of MRSP is a challenge, due to not only the limited number of effective antimicrobials against MRSP, but also the inherent challenges of topical treatment of the sites most commonly colonized – the nasal passages, pharynx, and rectum [21].

While decolonization may not be feasible, it is reasonable to alter perioperative antimicrobial prophylaxis in MRSP carriers undergoing higher risk procedures like TPLO. This may include measures such as adding a single dose of amikacin preoperatively to the typical (e.g., cefazolin) antimicrobial regime, assuming renal health has been evaluated.

2.2.4 Dermatitis, Clipping, and Skin Preparation

As mentioned, *Staphylococcus* spp. are amongst the most common bacteria causing SSIs. *S. pseudintermedius* is a commensal bacteria within the normal microbiome of dogs [39]. Assessment of the animal's skin for evidence of local or distant dermatitis is recommended, to reduce the risk of contamination of the surgical site (Figure 2.1). Despite this logical recommendation, 17.5% of all animals undergoing TPLO in one study had evidence of active local or distant dermatitis. Of those with local dermatitis, 16.7% developed an SSI and 10.2% with distant dermatitis developed an SSI [27]. As there was no significant difference identified between local and distant dermatitis resulting in SSI, the risk for SSI development should not be considered lower for animals with dermatitis not affecting the direct surgical site, as anecdotally thought, and postponement of elective orthopedic surgeries with local or distant dermatitis should be considered [27].

Identifying the underlying cause of the skin disease is paramount for improving the skin barrier and reducing the risk for SSI development. Depending on the type and severity of the dermatitis, cleansing with medicated shampoos, application of topical antimicrobials or antifungals and/or systemic antimicrobials or antifungals may be required. When managing bacterial dermatitis, local to or distant from the surgical site, culture and susceptibility testing is recommended to guide antimicrobial therapy and determine if MRSP is present. While awaiting these results, empirical treatment is recommended with cephalexin (22–30 mg/kg, PO q8h) or clindamycin (11 mg/kg, PO q12h). Antimicrobials should be continued for 1 week beyond resolution of clinical signs.

Ideally, the surgical site should be free of skin lesions prior to considering surgery. In circumstances where postponing surgery is not possible, topical treatment is recommended, along with the addition of amikacin to the routine perioperative antimicrobials. When lesions are located at sites other than the surgical site, topical treatment is recommended ± systemic medications as determined by the extent of the disease process. Bathing these patients with a chlorhexidine shampoo the night prior to surgery can also be considered [40].

Before skin preparation can occur, hair is clipped from the proposed surgical field to facilitate direct skin preparation and the limb is suspended (Figure 2.2). Clipping should be performed following induction of general anesthesia and not sooner due to the increased risk for SSI development [41, 42]. This risk is likely associated with the greater potential for direct skin trauma that may occur when attempting to clip hair on a conscious patient. Any microtrauma caused by rough clipping or poorly maintained clipper blades may also play a role in increasing the risk for SSI development.

Skin preparation (Figure 2.3) begins with the removal of surface dirt and oils using a neutral, nonmedicated soap as antiseptic agents are not active in the presence of organic material. Antiseptic agents are subsequently applied to reduce the bacterial load present on the skin at the time of surgery. Antiseptic agents commonly used in veterinary medicine include povidone-iodine and chlorhexidine gluconate (Figure 2.4). These antiseptic solutions are applied to the skin using a scrub technique or a paint or spray technique. Ultimately, contact time, meaning the time the antiseptic solution is in direct contact with the skin, is the most important aspect of skin preparation. Both the World Health Organization and the Centers for

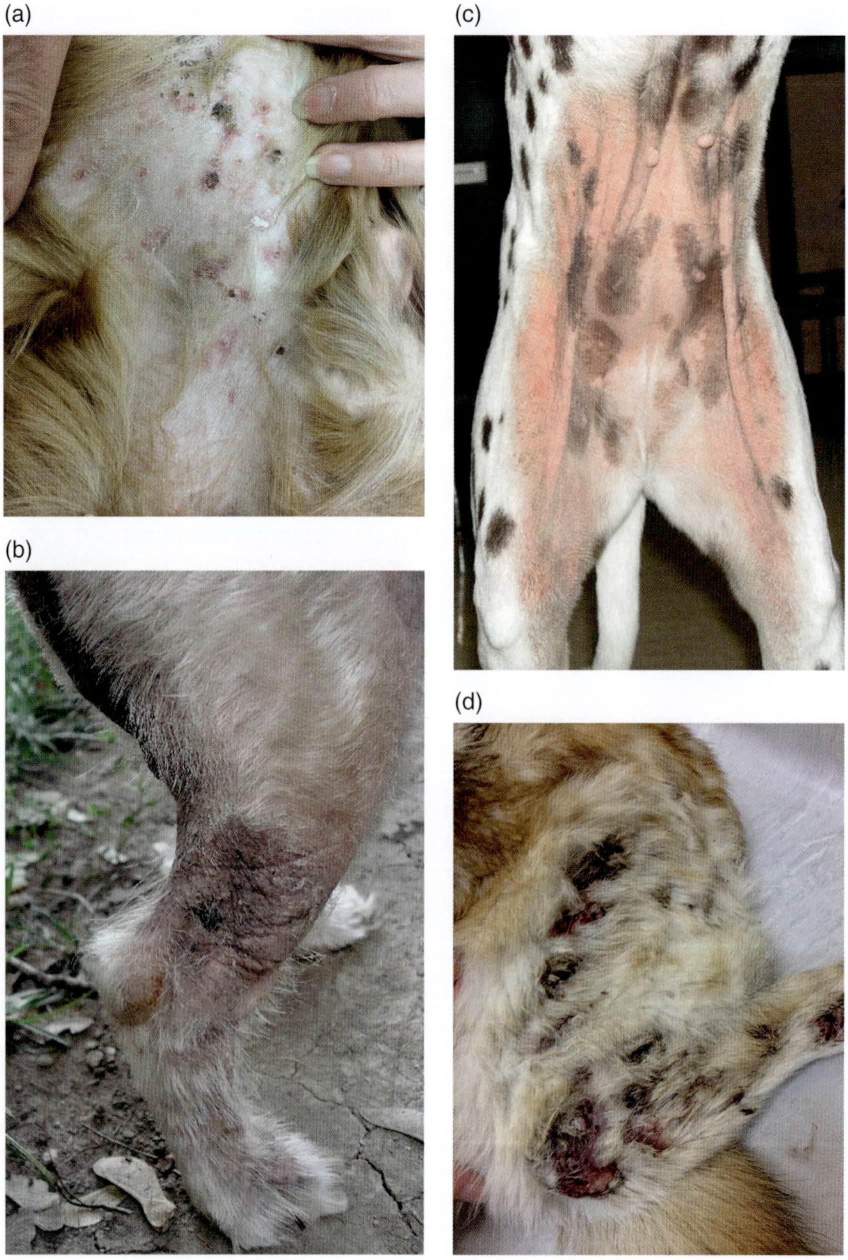

Figure 2.1 (a) Mild bacterial dermatitis with pustules and plaques. (b) Mild to moderate localized dermatitis without pustules or plaques. (c) Moderate generalized dermatitis. (d) Severe generalized dermatitis over the medial aspect of the pelvic limb. Source: All photos courtesy of Dr Charlotte Pye, DACVD.

Disease Control and Prevention recommend the use of alcohol-based solutions for surgical skin preparation [43, 44]. However, in veterinary medicine, aqueous solutions of povidone-iodine and alcohol solutions of chlorhexidine gluconate have been proven to be equally effective in reducing bacterial colony-forming units on canine skin [45, 46]. As many different antiseptic skin preparation solutions exist, following the instructions for your chosen

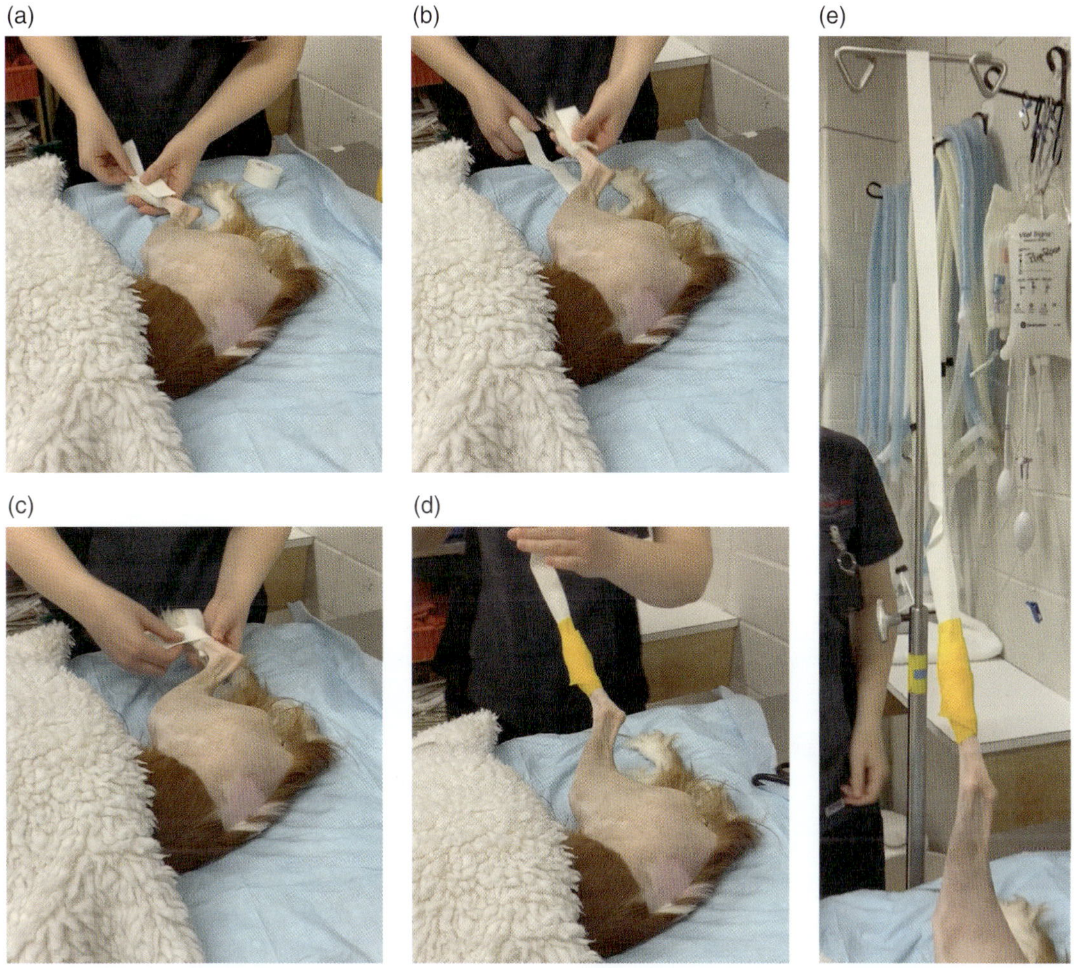

Figure 2.2 Hanging leg technique for limb suspension. (a) A piece of 2 in. tape is applied to the lateral aspect of the unclipped distal limb, with an equal amount of tape contacting the limb and extending beyond the distal aspect of the limb. (b) Using the 2 in. tape roll, a second piece of tape is placed on the medial aspect of the unclipped distal limb, mimicking the lateral aspect. The two sticky surfaces of tape are adhered together distally, with the entire tape roll remaining attached (for later use). (c) A third piece of 2 in. tape is wrapped from proximal to distal around the circumference of the unclipped distal limb. (d) The taped distal limb is covered in nonsterile Vetrap™. (e) Using the 2 in. tape roll that remains attached to the medial aspect of the limb, the limb is suspended from an IV pole.

product to ensure adequate contact time is key for appropriate skin preparation.

The initial skin preparation is carried out using nonsterile gloves and gauze. This initial preparation is performed by alternating antiseptic soap and alcohol, three times, ensuring an appropriate total contact time. A final application of an alcohol-based antiseptic paint may also be performed. Protection of the prepared surgical site with sterile drapes is recommended prior to transport to the operating room (OR), to decrease the risk of inadvertent contamination.

A final sterile skin preparation is subsequently performed in the OR using sterile gloves and sterile gauze. This final preparation may be performed by a nonsterile assistant wearing sterile gloves or by a sterile assistant or surgeon. The final skin preparation is performed by alternating between the antiseptic solution (Figure 2.4) and alcohol, performed three times, or using an alcohol-based antiseptic paint alone.

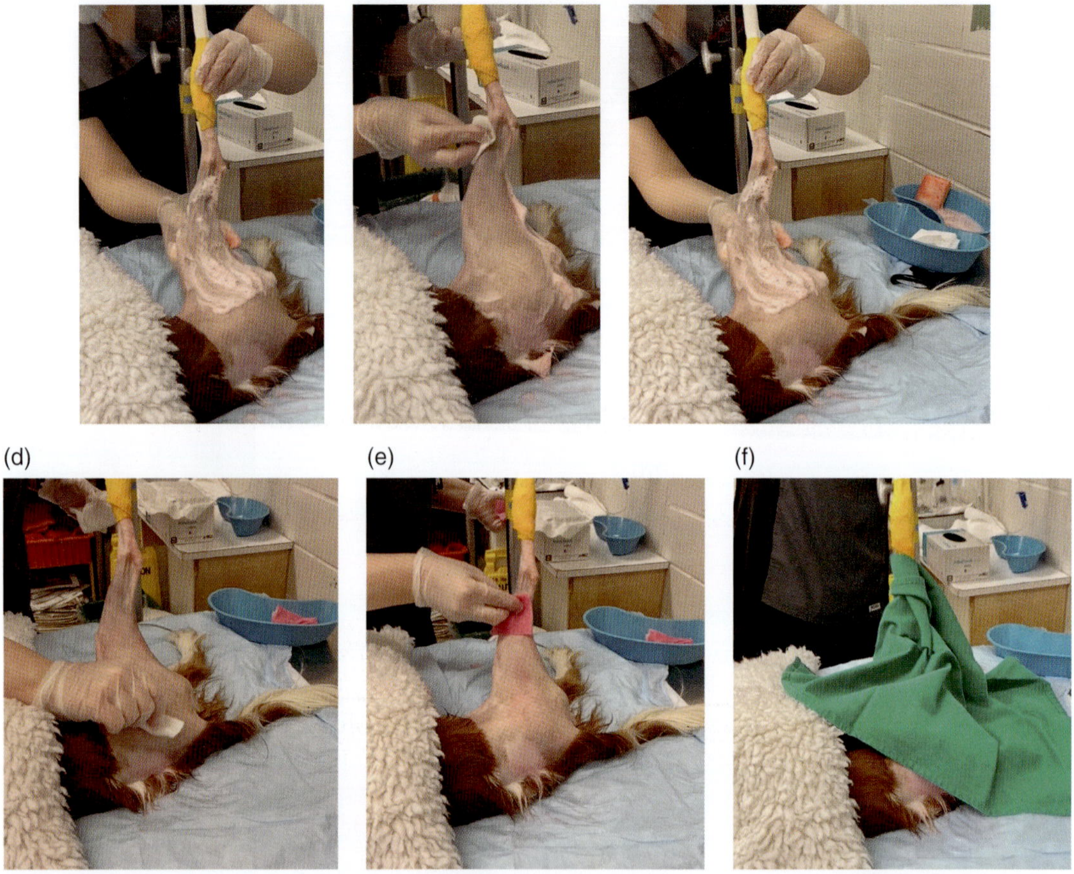

Figure 2.3 Skin preparation steps. Note the assistant is wearing nonsterile gloves for the initial skin preparation. (a) Using a nonmedicated neutral soap, the skin is cleansed to remove oils and debris. (b) The soap suds are removed using dry nonsterile gauze squares, working from the proposed surgical site outwards. (c) Using a chlorhexidine scrub brush (or antiseptic soap of choice on nonsterile gauze), the skin is scrubbed, working from the proposed surgical site outwards. (d) The soap suds are removed using nonsterile, alcohol-soaked gauze squares working from the proposed surgical site outwards. Steps (c) ad (d) are repeated three times, until all soap suds are removed. (e) Finally, an alcohol-based chlorhexidine paint is applied to the skin using nonsterile gauze squares, working from the proposed surgical site outwards until the entire field has been painted*. (f) A sterile drape is applied over the field prior to transport into the OR. Steps (c) (using an aqueous or alcohol-based antiseptic solution in place of an antiseptic soap) and (d) (or alternatively step (e) alone) are repeated in the OR using sterile gauze and sterile gloves for the final skin preparation. *Note step (e) is optional during the initial skin preparation.

Whichever antiseptic soap is used for the initial skin preparation must be the same antiseptic solution used in the final skin preparation.

2.3 Environmental Factors

2.3.1 Sources of Contamination

The perisurgical environment, including the anesthesia prep area, patient transportation, the OR, the radiology suite and surrounding personnel, plays a role as a source of possible bacterial contamination. Bacteria most commonly identified in surgical sites at the time of closure during orthopedic surgeries arise from aersol transmission [47]. One study identified 81% of elective orthopedic procedures as experiencing some form of bacterial contamination [47]. Possible sources identified included surgeon hands, surgeon gloves, animal skin, patient footwrap, sink faucet, transportation gurney, radiology

(a) (b)

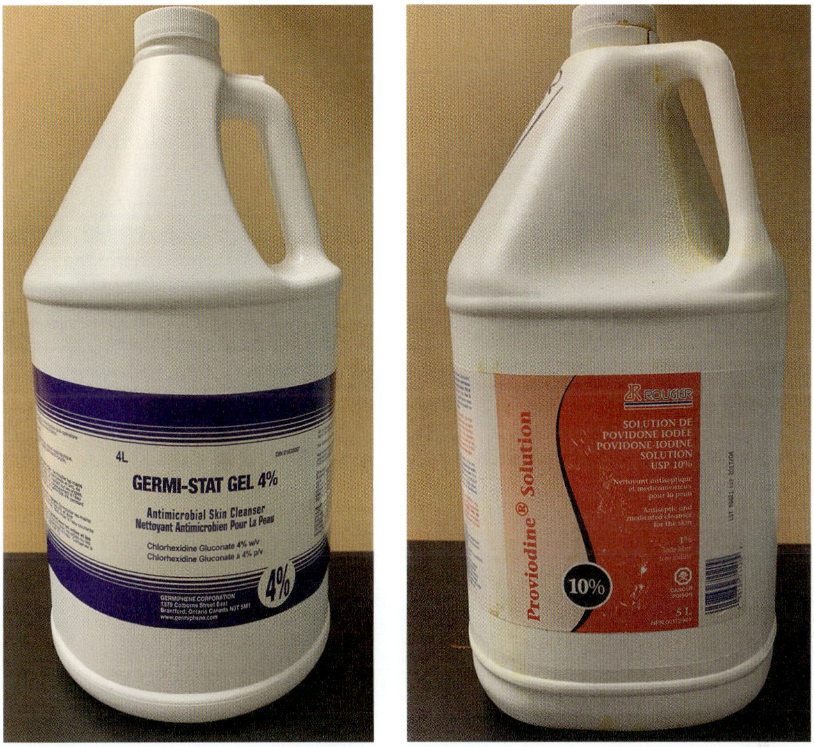

Figure 2.4 (a) Chlorhexidine gluconate 4% soap solution. (b) Povidone-iodine 10% solution, with 1% free iodine.

table, and OR computers [47]. Despite this high number of reported contamination events and numerous sources identified, a correlation with SSI could not be made [47]. Historically, scalpel blades have been suspected to be a source of increased bacterial contamination into deeper tissues when the same blade is used for skin incisions and deeper tissue incision; this remains unclear at this time, as conflicting data exist [48–50]. However, with documented potential for bacterial transmission from the skin blade, use of a second surgical blade for deeper tissues is advised. Suction tips have also been identified as sources of contamination in clean surgical procedures. In one study, a positive culture rate of 92% was identified at the end of clean surgical procedures, with a second study identifying a 42% positive culture rate at the end of clean orthopedic procedures [51, 52]. While these sources of contamination cannot necessarily be avoided, hospital surveillance of these known sources of contamination is recommended.

2.3.2 Personnel

As the majority of bacteria identified in contamination of surgical sites with and without SSIs arise from the microbiome of humans and animals within the OR, it is no surprise that an increasing number of OR personnel has been correlated with an increased SSI rate [2]. Reducing traffic in and out of the OR during clean orthopedic procedures may therefore reduce the amount of aerosolized bacterial contaminants and decrease contamination rates [53]. In academic settings, traffic in and out of the OR can anecdotally be higher, therefore in animals with inherent risk factors for SSI, attempts to reduce traffic in the OR are recommended. Both MRSA and MRSP have been identified in small animal hospital environments and among small animal employees [54]. It is possible that hospital personnel carrying MRSA and MRSP may cause direct or indirect transmission to animals [54].

2.4 Surgical Procedure

2.4.1 Surgeon Factors – Hand Hygiene, Glove Perforation, Surgical Technique

Surgeon microbiome contributes to bacterial contamination of surgical sites and therefore surgeon hand and forearm preparation is recommended to reduce the microbial burden prior to donning sterile surgical gowns and gloves.

Two main options exist for hand and forearm preparation – surgical scrub versus alcohol-based rubs (ABRs) (Figure 2.5). Chlorhexidine and povidone-iodine are the surgical scrubs most commonly used in veterinary medicine and are equally effective at reducing bacterial colony-forming units [55]. ABRs, however, provide a faster and more effective sustained reduction in bacteria counts [1, 56]. The use of ABRs, preceded by hand washing using non-medicated soaps to remove gross debris and oils, results in increased compliance likely due to the reduced time required to apply an ABR than to perform a traditional scrub [57]. A traditional scrub requires a minimum of 3-minute contact time to be effective, whereas ABRs may be applied in under 2 minutes [58]. A traditional scrub is not required for the first case of the day prior to use of ABRs, as has been previously recommended. Use of ABRs as sole hand and forearm preparation is appropriate as pre-scrubbing with disinfecting soaps may decrease the effect of ABRs [59, 60]. ABRs are now considered superior for presurgical hand asepsis due to their improved dermal tolerance, along with their reduction in water usage, carbon waste, and potential chances for recontamination on sink fixtures compared to standard scrubs [61].

The incidence of intraoperative contamination reported to occur secondary to glove perforations ranges between 18% and 43% [46, 62, 63]. An increased number of glove perforations are associated with orthopedic surgery, likely in part due to the use of power equipment, screws, pins, and wire [62, 63]. Use of thicker orthopedic gloves was not associated with a reduced rate of glove perforation [63]. However, a hospital-wide policy change to the use of orthopedic gloves for TPLO surgeries, in addition to other protocol changes, lead to a reduction in

(a) (b)

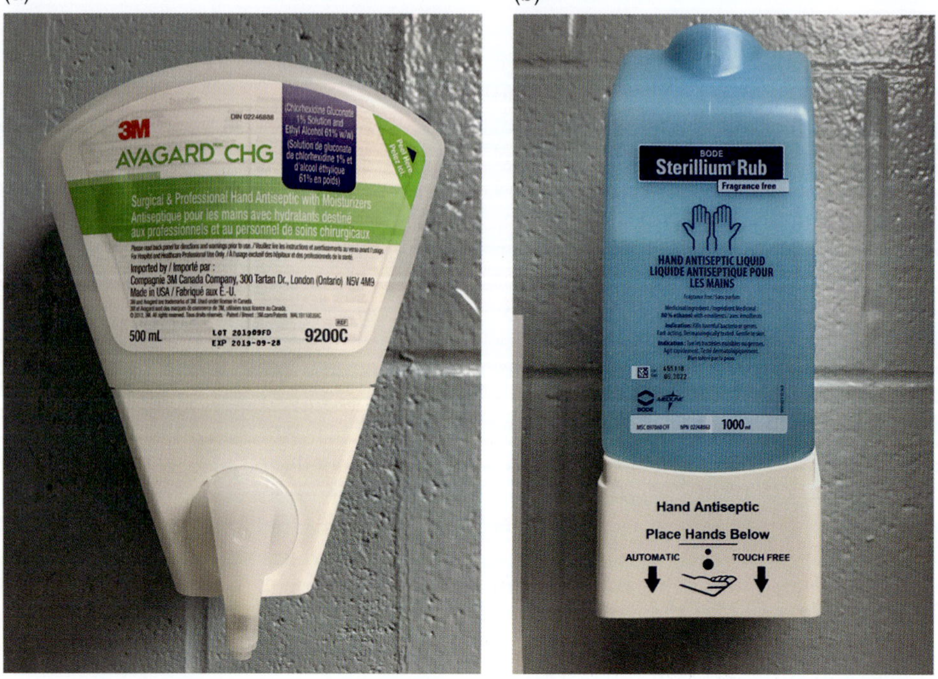

Figure 2.5 (a) Avagard™ chlorhexidine gluconate 1% + ethyl alcohol 61%. (b) Sterillium™ ethyl alcohol 80%.

SSI rate in one hospital [64]. Identification of glove perforations was poor, but the addition of color indicator undergloves increased the identification rate [62, 63]. The primary surgeon is at highest risk for glove perforation [62, 63].

Evidence exists that SSI rates may differ between surgeons within an institution and may be associated with surgeon experience [14, 27]. Surgeons performing >20 TPLO procedures had reduced SSI rates compared to novice surgeons in one study [27]. While this may not be true in all institutions, two factors that may contribute to a novice surgeon having increased SSI rates include prolonged surgery times and inferior surgical techniques. Excellent surgical technique following Halstead's principles of surgery may aid in reduction of SSI development due to reduced tissue trauma, preservation of blood supply, limited hemorrhage, reduction of dead space, tissue apposition under minimal tension, and adherence to strict aseptic technique [65].

2.4.2 Anesthesia and Surgery Time

Both prolonged anesthesia and surgery times have been associated with increased SSI rates [2, 5, 9, 14, 16, 40, 41]. The risk for SSI has been reported to increase between 0.5% and 4% per minute of anesthesia and 7% per minute of surgery [5, 9, 16]. Theories that lead to this increased SSI rate have included hypotension, hypothermia, and tissue hypoxia but no correlation has been made between these factors [5]. One study that correlated prolonged anesthesia and surgery times with the development of SSI also identified that with prolonged anesthesia and surgery times, more antimicrobial resistance developed [14].

Reducing anesthesia and surgery times requires a concerted effort between members of the surgical team, anesthetists, and diagnostic imaging. Ensuring all equipment is available and all involved personnel are prepared before inducing anesthesia may aid in efficiency and therefore reduce anesthesia and surgery times. In an academic setting where student teaching occurs, it may not be possible to reduce these times, especially when novice surgeons (i.e., surgical interns and residents) are performing portions of the surgical procedure. For animals with known inherent risk factors for SSI, reducing these times may aid in lowering their SSI risk. Introducing surgical checklists (Figure 2.6) is one way to improve communication between the surgery and anesthesia team and reduce complications that can lead to increased patient morbidity and mortality [66, 67].

2.4.3 Draping

Draping of the surgical site (Figure 2.7) is advised to minimize contamination and use of impervious single-use disposable drapes is considered best practice [68]. While there are limited studies investigating the use of incise films, noniodonated incise films have been shown to increase bacterial growth beneath the drape, thus increasing the risk for SSI [68]. Despite a lack of evidence for iodinated incise films to reduce the SSI rate, there have been no reports of increased bacterial growth beneath iodinated drapes, which makes an iodinated incise film a superior choice to a noniodinated incise film, if elected for use [30, 68]. When applying incise films, appropriate application without lifting the edges following application is recommended to reduce the risk of bacterial contamination. Implementation of an iodinated incise film, in addition to other protocol changes, lead to the reduction of SSI rate in one hospital following TPLO [64].

2.4.4 Implant Choices

As a variety of surgical procedures exist for stabilization of the CCL-deficient stifle, a wide variety of implants also exist. Implants themselves have been significantly associated with the risk of developing a SSI [1]. When considering extracapsular stabilization techniques, suture types have included nylon fishing line, nylon leader line, ultra high molecular weight polyethylene (UHMWPE), and other multifilamented nonabsorbable suture materials [11, 12, 69]. Nylon has been shown to have reduced bacterial adherence compared to UHMWPE with variation in bacterial colonization of nylon between methods of sterilization [69]. In 1981, multifilamented nonabsorbable suture material used for extracapsular stabilization was reported

Date:
Clinicians:
Procedure:
Surgery Start Time:
Surgery End Time:

Patient Sticker

Pre-Operative
To Be Completed Out Loud Before Skin Incision

- ☐ Introduction of the surgical team
- ☐ **Anesthesia:** Confirm the patient's name
- ☐ **Surgeon:** Confirm procedure and site(s).
- ☐ Radiographs in OR **Y / N**

To Surgeon

- ☐ What are the critical or non-routine steps?
- ☐ Expected duration of procedure? ________
- ☐ Anticipated blood loss

♦ Minimal < 5% ♦ Moderate 5–10% ♦ Severe > 10%

If Moderate or Severe, ask:

- ☐ Has the patient been blood typed?
- ☐ Are blood products available?
- ☐ Are biopsies or samples being collected? **Y / N**

Y – Is the sample being inked **Y / N**

To Anesthesia

- ☐ Has antibiotic prophylaxis been given with in the last 45 minutes? **Y / N**
- ☐ Can this patient receive an NSAID? **Y / N**
- ☐ Do you have any patient specific concerns?

To OR Tech

- ☐ Is all the equipment present in the room?
- ☐ Are there any equipment concerns?
- ☐ **Pre-Operative Sponge Count**

Lap Sponges:________
Gauze Squares:________

Post Operative
To Be Completed Out Loud Before Patient Leaves the OR

- ☐ Planned procedures have been completed
- ☐ Sharps have been placed in the green tray
- ☐ Is post operative imaging needed? **Y / NA**

Y– Has Radiology been notified? **Y / N**

- ☐ Is bandaging required **Y / N**
- ☐ Equipment concerns have been reported
- ☐ Purse string has been removed ? **Y / NA**
- ☐ Is a urinary catheter required? **Y / N**

Y – Have supplies been gathered? **Y / N**

To Surgeon

- ☐ Person to contact the owner has been identified

To Anesthesia

- ☐ Recovery location? **ICU / IMC / Wards**
- ☐ Any recovery concerns

To OR Tech

- ☐ **Post Op Sponge Count**

Lap Sponges:________
Gauze Squares:________

Figure 2.6 Example of a surgical safety checklist, based on the World Health Organization template found at www.who.int/patientsafety/topics/safe-surgery/checklist/en/.

to have an SSI rate of >21% [11]. In a more recent study using multifilamented UHMWPE, an SSI rate of 1.8% was reported [12]. The discrepancy in SSI rates may be due to improved sterilization and aseptic surgical techniques. Anecdotally, additional protective measures such as applying new sterile gloves prior to handling these materials may reduce the chances of bacterial colonization from skin contamination.

When considering proximal tibial osteotomy procedures, a variety of plates exist for stabilization of the osteotomy. Several studies have identified increased SSI risk associated with a variety of plates used specifically for TPLOs. Savicky et al. noted an increased SSI rate with Synthes plates whereas Thompson identified an increased SSI risk with Slocum implants [31, 34]. Solano et al. identified an increased risk associated with nonlocking plates compared to locking plates, whereas Giannetto found no significant difference in SSI rates between locking and nonlocking implants [28, 70]. Another study found no significant difference in SSI rates when comparing nonlocking plates, standard locking plates, and double locking plates used in animals >50 kg [19]. As many other factors contribute to the risk of developing an SSI, no one implant associated with TPLO has been shown to be superior at reducing this risk.

The majority of *S. pseudintermedius* isolates have been identified to be strong to moderate biofilm producers, with no difference between methicillin-resistant and methicillin-susceptible forms [71]. A biofilm is a sessile community of bacteria embedded in a self-produced matrix which is adhered to a surface [72]. With the inherent ability to produce a biofilm, *S. pseudintermedius* can create an implant-associated biofilm, making it more difficult for targeted antimicrobial treatment as minimum inhibitory concentrations are much higher for biofilm bacteria than planktonic bacteria [73]. As such, implant coatings such as silver have been assessed for their ability to resist biofilm formation. Silver-coated implants are excellent

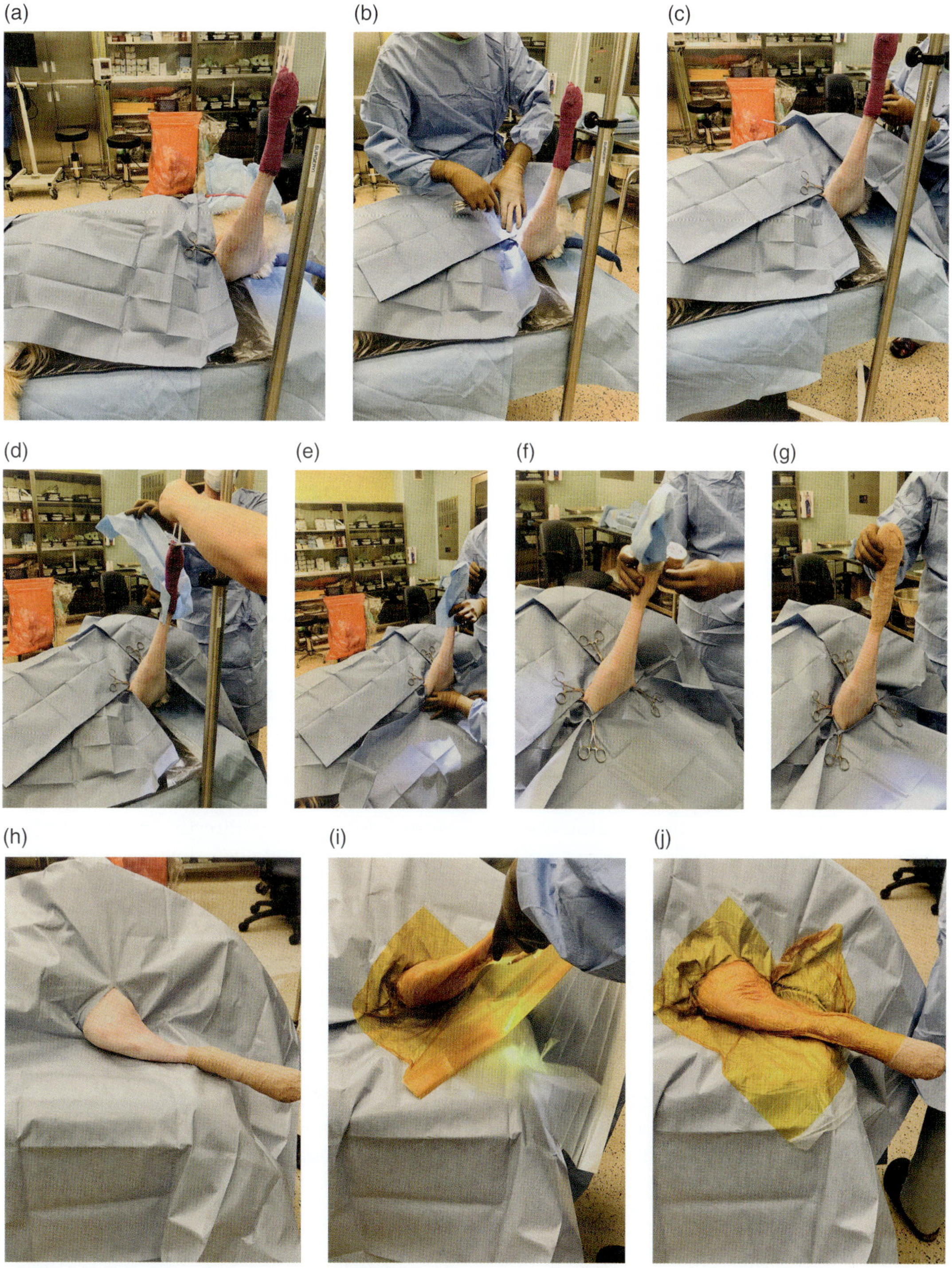

Figure 2.7 Following final skin preparation in the OR with the limb suspended, draping is performed by the sterile surgical team using a four-quarter technique and top drape, with an optional iodinated incise film. (a) The cranial quarter drape is applied first. (b) A lateral quarter drape applied second. (c) The caudal quarter drape is applied next. (d) A sterile, nonpermeable dressing is used to grasp the nonsterile Vetrapped distal limb, while a nonsterile assistant cuts the tape suspending the limb. (e) While the sterile dressing is applied to the nonsterile distal limb, the final quarter drape is applied. (f) Sterile Vetrap is applied from proximal to distal around the sterile covered distal limb to adhere the sterile dressing in place. (g) Final sterile covering of the distal limb. (h) A top drape is applied over the four-quarter drapes. (i) An iodinated incise film is applied to the skin. This step is optional. (j) Final appearance of draping.

at resisting MRSP biofilm formation *in vitro*, but *in vivo* evidence is not yet available in veterinary medicine [74]. Other implant coatings for biofilm prevention include heparin as an anti-adhesive, chitosan as an antimicrobial, and hydroxyapatite which inhibits biofilm formation while encouraging bone growth [75]. None of these coated implants is used widely in veterinary medicine, nor are there reports of clinical use. Therefore, this may be an avenue for further clinical research as antimicrobial resistance becomes increasingly prevalent.

2.4.5 Wound Closure and Protection

Surgical wound closure and protection play a controversial role in SSI development. Surgical staples in comparison to intradermal skin closures have been reported to increase, decrease or not have any effect on surgical site inflammation and/or SSI development [6, 30, 32]. Skin closure using absorbable skin staples has shown no benefit over stainless steel surgical staples in reducing SSI development [20]. With inconclusive evidence to suggest superiority of one closure method over another, considerations such as time for closure, associated tissue trauma, and potential irritation to the patient must play a role in decision making. While staples may reduce the closure time and thus overall surgery time, this is likely to be negligible for an experienced surgeon. Tissue trauma may also be reduced with skin staples due to minimal manipulation required for placement, but increased inflammation has been noted when surgical staples are used compared to intradermal sutures [6]. Finally, the noncompliant nature of skin staples may lead to increased local irritation and thus potential for self-trauma from licking or chewing at the surgical site, if not adequately protected from access.

Suture has the proven propensity for biofilm formation and as such may act as a nidus for SSI development [76]. Antimicrobial-coated suture, specifically triclosan-coated suture, has been assessed *in vitro* and *in vivo* for its ability to resist or reduce SSI development. *In vitro*, triclosan-coated monofilament suture had the least bacterial adherence compared to other monofilament and braided suture materials and had greater inhibition for *S. pseudintermedius*, including MRSP, than *Escherichia coli* [77, 78]. *In vivo*, the use of triclosan-coated monofilament suture was not shown to significantly reduce the risk of SSI in one hospital, while its use contributed to a reduction in SSI rates in another hospital [32, 64]. Further investigation of the use of antimicrobial-coated suture is warranted. While a true benefit to antimicrobial-coated suture remains unclear, the only limitation to its use is its increased cost, and as such, use of antimicrobial-coated sutures should be considered.

Postoperative fibrin formation to create a complete seal of a surgical wound takes 3–5 hours and therefore protection of the fresh surgical wound from its environment is recommended [79]. Considering evidence for environmental contamination from the anesthesia transportation gurney and radiology table used for postoperative radiographs, immediate protection with a sterile dressing is recommended [46]. Despite these recommendations, direct comparison of a topical adhesive applied to the incision, an adhesive antimicrobial barrier dressing, and no dressing following TPLO surgery found no significant difference in SSI rates amongst the dressing options [28]. In another study involving significant protocol changes for animals undergoing TPLO surgery, the addition of a soft padded bandage with mupirocin ointment directly on the surgical wound, use of single-use gloves for all postoperative patient interactions, and placement of an Elizabethan collar for additional barrier protection resulted in an 88% reduction in the odds ratio for developing an SSI [64]. While many factors likely contributed to this SSI reduction, simple incisional protective measures are easy to implement into routine postoperative care. Additionally, while the use of gloves does not replace appropriate hand hygiene, sterile gloves are recommended to be worn during examination of clean surgical wounds to prevent transmission of bacteria to the surgical site [80].

2.5 Antimicrobial Use

The overall goal of antimicrobial therapy in orthopedic surgery is to reduce the bacterial load present at the time of surgery. The bacteria of concern are skin commensals, most commonly *Staphylococcus* spp., and are most susceptible to cefazolin. The administration of antimicrobials for this purpose is required only during the period of risk (i.e., the surgical procedure) and is not required preoperatively and rarely required postoperatively.

2.5.1 Preoperative

The use of preoperative antimicrobials is most often associated with a distant active infection, most commonly associated with wound and skin infections [70]. The use of preoperative antimicrobials has been associated with an increased risk for SSI and as such, postponement of elective orthopedic cases requiring preoperative antimicrobials is recommended [2]. Misuse and overuse of antimicrobials are known to contribute to antimicrobial resistance, therefore avoiding the potential for SSI development by postponing surgery in the face of active antimicrobial use should limit the animal's risk of developing a multidrug-resistant SSI.

2.5.2 Perioperative

The use of perioperative antimicrobials for reduction of SSI is widely practiced in veterinary medicine. Few studies exist in veterinary medicine that provide insight into the appropriate timing for administration of perioperative antimicrobials. Therefore, guidelines followed for perioperative antimicrobial prophylaxis are largely adapted from human medicine. Current guidelines in human medicine state that an appropriate antimicrobial should be administered at least 60 minutes before the first surgical incision to allow time to achieve high serum levels, readministration of said antimicrobial should be performed every two half-lives, and antimicrobial administration should be discontinued within 24 hours of surgery [81]. A few older veterinary studies provide evidence for perioperative antimicrobial prophylaxis as a protective factor against SSI development. These studies suggest that administration of antimicrobials should be limited to procedures longer than 90 minutes, the first dose of antimicrobial should be administered within 30 minutes of the first surgical incision, and if used appropriately, perioperative antimicrobial prophylaxis can reduce the SSI rate by 6–7 times [2, 7, 82].

Recently, appropriate perioperative antimicrobial administration has been documented to be received by 42.5–85% of animals [13, 83, 84]. Generally, more animals receive an appropriately timed first dose than those requiring additional dosing over the course of surgery. However, in one study, the previously recommended initial dosing of perioperative antimicrobial administration 30 minutes before incision was challenged, as antimicrobial administration 60 minutes or more before incision was protective against development of SSI in a cohort of animals undergoing TPLO procedures [84]. In another study, inappropriate timing of perioperative administration was not significantly associated with the development of an SSI [13]. As this is a single finding, further supportive evidence is required before considering this association to be true and thus alter perioperative antimicrobial prophylaxis recommendations.

At this time, evidence suggests that there is major room for improvement regarding compliance of perioperative antimicrobial prophylaxis, and implementation of a preoperative surgical safety checklist may improve compliance rates [67]. This lack of compliance may be leading to increased SSI rates being reported. Current recommendations for orthopedic antimicrobial prophylaxis include the use of cefazolin (22 mg/kg), administered 30 minutes before the first surgical incision, readministration every 90 minutes intraoperatively until skin closure, and discontinuation of antimicrobial therapy within 24 hours of surgery.

2.5.3 Postoperative

While perioperative antimicrobial prophylaxis is recommended to be discontinued within 24 hours of surgery, a definition of when perioperative prophylaxis ends and postoperative antimicrobial therapy begins remains unknown. In human medicine, it is rare for antimicrobials to be continued beyond 24–48 hours postoperatively, even in the case of transplanted organs. Despite this knowledge, the increased incidence of SSI in clean elective orthopedic procedures has led to an increased use of postoperative antimicrobials. This is a controversial topic amongst veterinary surgeons, with evidence to both support and refute its use. Several studies including mainly TPLO surgeries, fewer TTA surgeries and some broad clean orthopedic procedures have identified a protective effect against SSI when postoperative antimicrobials are used [4, 9, 13, 21, 22, 30, 70, 83]. Fewer studies have identified a lack of effect on alteration of the SSI rate when postoperative antimicrobials are administered [8, 14, 16, 27, 29]. Additional studies identify postoperative antimicrobial use in clean orthopedic procedures including TPLO and the Arthrex Canine Cruciate Ligament Repair Anchor System™, without evaluating their effect on SSI rates [12, 19, 28, 52].

At this time, there are a greater number of studies to support the use of postoperative antimicrobial use following TPLO surgery; however, the duration of treatment has been variable and specific recommendations cannot be made, although short courses of 3–5 days' duration are likely sufficient. Further prospective evaluation of postoperative antimicrobial protocols should be considered. Many factors can contribute to an individual's estimated risk for developing an SSI and these should be considered together before deciding to use postoperative antimicrobials. Postoperative antimicrobials should never be used as a surrogate for aseptic technique and good surgical practices.

2.6 Surveillance

Infection control in veterinary medicine tends to be reactive instead of proactive. SSIs are often identified only when animals present for clinical signs associated with SSIs or when incidentally identified during a routine follow-up examination. This is considered to be a form of passive surveillance, where no specific effort is made to identify SSIs [68]. Alternatively, active surveillance occurs when specific outcomes or indicators are sought to increase the rate of detection [85].

The goals of an active SSI surveillance program are to create a monitoring system that will determine the baseline level of expected SSI within a facility. By determining the baseline, a critical limit (a value beyond the expected SSI rate) can be established to determine when interventions should be employed to reduce the risk of SSI [84]. For active surveillance to be universal, definitions of outcomes must be provided. This would require defining what constitutes an SSI (see Chapter 3 for further details) as well as defining clinical signs that may be associated with an SSI and thus warrant further direct investigation of the patient. In relation to postoperative SSIs, active surveillance can be achieved through scheduled owner contact using telephone interviews or electronic questionnaires or by communication with referring veterinarians [1, 86]. During this contact, questions can be posed with regard to incisional healing, local tissue recovery, limb use, as well as if medical interventions have been required. Ideally, these forms of communication would be performed more than once during the patient's recovery period, encompassing timeframes associated with early development (within 30 days of surgery) and late development of SSI (within 90 days of surgery) [87].

In veterinary medicine, two prospective studies using active postdischarge surveillance for assessment of SSIs identified that 27.8–35% of all SSIs would have been missed without active surveillance [1, 86]. This is not an insignificant finding and therefore should encourage the development of active surveillance practices for SSI assessment.

2.7 Conclusion

Overall, TPLO has higher reported rates of SSI than other methods of stifle stabilization for cranial cruciate ligament ruptures (6,10,12–20,22,24,25). This may be due to the increased soft tissue dissection, thermal necrosis of the bone, and increased surgical times compared to extracapsular repairs. When compared to other tibial osteotomies, the overall higher incidence of SSIs may only be due to the increased frequency with which TPLOs are performed and thus reported.

As SSIs lead to further medical or surgical interventions, they have been identified to cause an increased financial burden for owners, along with increased morbidity for our veterinary patients [28, 88]. Despite the increased costs, protracted recoveries and increased patient morbidities, owner assessment of long-term outcome was not significantly affected [23]. While not all risk factors can be controlled, many risk factors can be addressed with diligent surgeon and patient preoperative preparation. Additionally, active surveillance may help to improve the rate of identification of SSIs, which may lead to earlier interventions.

References

1. Turk, R., Singh, A., and Weese, J.S. (2015). Prospective surgical site infection surveillance in dogs. *Vet. Surg.* 44: 2–8.
2. Eugster, S., Schawalder, P., Gaschen, F., and Boerlin, P. (2004). A prospective study of postoperative surgical site infections in dogs and cats. *Vet. Surg.* 33: 542–550.
3. Nicholson, M., Beal, M., Shofer, F., and Brown, D.C. (2002). Epidemiologic evaluation of postoperative wound infection in clean-contaminated wounds: a retrospective study of 239 dogs and cats. *Vet. Surg.* 31: 577–581.
4. Fitzpatrick, N. and Solano, M.A. (2010). Predictive variables for complications after TPLO with stifle inspection by arthrotomy in 1000 consecutive dogs. *Vet. Surg.* 39: 460–474.
5. Beal, M.W., Brown, D.C., and Shofer, F. (2000). The effects of perioperative hypothermia and the duration of anesthesia on postoperative wound infection rate in clean wounds: a retrospective study. *Vet. Surg.* 29: 123–127.
6. Frey, T.N., Hoelzler, M.G., Scavelli, T.D. et al. (2010). Risk factors for surgical site infection-inflammation in dogs undergoing surgery for rupture of the cranial cruciate ligament: 902 cases (2005–2006). *J. Am. Vet. Med. Assoc.* 236 (1): 88–94.
7. Vasseur, P.B., Levy, J., Dowd, E., and Eliot, J. (1988). Surgical wound infection rates in dogs and cats: data from a teaching hospital. *Vet. Surg.* 17 (2): 60–64.
8. Aiken, M.J., Hughes, T.K., Abercromby, R.H. et al. (2015). Prospective, randomized comparison of the effect of two antimicrobial regimes on surgical site infection rate in dogs undergoing orthopedic implant surgery. *Vet. Surg.* 44: 661–667.
9. Pratesi, A., Moores, A.P., Downes, C. et al. (2015). Efficacy of postoperative antimicrobial use for clean orthopedic implant surgery in dogs: a prospective randomized study in 100 consecutive cases. *Vet. Surg.* 44: 653–660.
10. Casale, S.A. and McCarthy, R.J. (2009). Complications associated with lateral fabellotibial suture surgery for cranial cruciate ligament injury in dogs: 363 cases (1997-2005). *J. Am. Vet. Med. Assoc.* 234: 229–235.
11. Dulisch, M. (1981). Suture reaction following extra-articular stabilization in the dog. Part II: a prospective study of 66 stifles. *J. Am. Anim. Hosp. Assoc.* 17: 572–574.
12. Rappa, N.S. and Radasch, R.M. (2016). Postoperative complications associated with the Arthrex Canine Cranial Cruciate Ligament Repair Anchor System in small- to medium-sized dogs: a retrospective analysis (2009–2012). *Can. J. Vet. Res.* 57: 847–852.
13. Nazarali, A., Singh, A., and Weese, J.S. (2014). Perioperative administration of antimicrobials during tibial plateau leveling osteotomy. *Vet. Surg.* 43: 966–971.
14. Clark, A.C., Greco, J.J., and Bergman, P.J. (2020). Influence of administration of antimicrobial medications after tibial plateau leveling osteotomy on surgical site infections: a retrospective study of 308 dogs. *Vet. Surg.* 49: 106–113.
15. Wolf, R.E., Scavelli, T.D., Hoelzler, M.G. et al. (2012). Surgical and postoperative complications associated with tibial tuberosity advancement for cranial cruciate ligament rupture in dogs: 458 cases (2007–2009). *J. Am. Vet. Med. Assoc.* 240 (12): 1481–1487.
16. Yap, F.W., Calvo, I., Smith, K.D., and Parkin, T. (2015). Perioperative risk factors for surgical site infection in tibial tuberosity advancement: 224 stifles. *Vet. Comp. Orthop. Traumatol.* 28: 199–206.
17. Costa, M., Craig, D., Cambridge, T. et al. (2017). Major complications of tibial tuberosity advancement in 1613 dogs. *Vet. Surg.* 46: 494–500.
18. Serratore, V.R. and Barnhart, M.D. (2018). Results and complications after removal of tibial tuberosity advancement cage for treatment of surgical site infections: a retrospective study. *Vet. Surg.* 47: 768–773.
19. Tuan, J., Solano, M.A., and Danielski, A. (2019). Risk of infection after double locking plate and screw fixation of tibial plateau leveling osteotomies in dogs weighing greater than 50 kilograms. *Vet. Surg.* 48: 1211–1217.
20. Watson, F.C., McMullan, W., Jordan, C.J. et al. (2019). The use of absorbable staples for skin closure after tibial plateau leveling osteotomy. *Vet. Surg.* 48: 35–41.
21. Nazarali, A., Singh, A., Moens, N.M.M. et al. (2015). Association between methicillin-resistant *Staphylococcus pseudintermedius* carriage and the development of surgical site infections following tibial plateau leveling osteotomy in dogs. *J. Am. Vet. Med. Assoc.* 247 (8): 909–916.
22. Hans, E.C., Barnhart, M.D., Kennedy, S.C., and Naber, S.J. (2017). Comparison of complications following tibial tuberosity advancement and tibial plateau levelling osteotomy in very large and giant dogs 50 kg or more in body weight. *Vet. Comp. Orthop. Traumatol.* 30: 299–305.
23. Brown, G., Maddox, T., and Siles, M.M.B. (2016). Client-assessed long-term outcome in dogs with surgical site infection following tibial plateau levelling osteotomy. *Vet. Rec.* 179: 409.

24. Livet, V., Taroni, M., Ferrand, F.-X. et al. (2019). Modified triple tibial osteotomy for combined cranial cruciate ligament rupture, tibial deformities, or patellar luxation. *J. Am. Anim. Hosp. Assoc.* 55: 291–300.
25. Frederick, S.W. and Cross, A.R. (2017). Modified cranial closing wedge osteotomy for treatment of cranial cruciate ligament insufficiency in dogs with excessive tibial plateau angles: technique and complications in 19 cases. *Vet. Surg.* 46: 403–411.
26. De Sousa, R., Egan, P., Parsons, K. et al. (2017). Treatment of tibial diaphyseal fractures following plateless tibial tuberosity advancement to manage cranial cruciate disease. *J. Small Anim. Pract.* 58: 372–379.
27. Lopez, D.J., VanDeventer, G.M., Krotscheck, U. et al. (2018). Retrospective study of factors associated with surgical site infection in dogs following tibial plateau leveling osteotomy. *J. Am. Vet. Med. Assoc.* 253 (3): 315–321.
28. Giannetto, J.J. and Aktay, S.A. (2019). Prospective evaluation of surgical wound dressings and the incidence of surgical site infections in dogs undergoing a tibial plateau levelling osteotomy. *Vet. Comp. Orthop. Traumatol.* 32: 18–25.
29. Spencer, D.D. and Daye, R.M. (2018). A prospective, randomized, double-blinded, placebo-controlled clinical study on postoperative antibiotherapy in 150 arthroscopy-assisted tibial plateau leveling osteotomies in dogs. *Vet. Surg.* 47: E79–E87.
30. Atwood, C., Maxwell, M., Butler, R., and Wills, R. (2015). Effects of incision closure method on infection prevalence following tibial plateau leveling osteotomy in dogs. *Can. Vet. J.* 56: 375–381.
31. Savicky, R., Beale, B., Murtaugh, R. et al. (2013). Outcome following removal of TPLO implants with surgical site infection. *Vet. Comp. Orthop. Traumatol.* 26: 260–265.
32. Etter, S.W., Ragetly, G.R., Bennett, R.A., and Schaeffer, D.J. (2013). Effect of using triclosan-impregnated suture for incisional closure on surgical site infection and inflammation following tibial plateau leveling osteotomy in dogs. *J. Am. Vet. Med. Assoc.* 242: 355–358.
33. Gallagher, A.D. and Mertens, W.D. (2012). Implant removal rate from infection after tibial plateau leveling osteotomy in dogs. *Vet. Surg.* 41: 705–711.
34. Thompson, A.M., Bergh, M.S., Wang, C., and Wells, K. (2011). Tibial plateau levelling osteotomy implant removal: a retrospective analysis of 129 cases. *Vet. Comp. Orthop. Traumatol.* 24: 450–456.
35. van Rijen, M., Bonten, M., Wenzel, R., and Kluytmans, J. (2008). Intranasal mupirocin for reduction of *Staphylococcus aureus* infections in surgical patients with nasal carriage: a systematic review. *J. Antimicrob. Chemother.* 61 (2): 254–261.
36. Thompson, P. and Houston, S. (2013). Decreasing methicillin-resistant *Staphylococcus aureus* surgical site infections with chlorhexidine and mupirocin. *Am. J. Infect. Control.* 41 (7): 629–633.
37. Rao, N., Cannella, B., Crossett, L. et al. (2011). Preoperative screening/decolonization for *Staphylococcus aureus* to prevent orthopedic surgical site infection: prospective cohort study with 2-year follow-up. *J. Arthroplasty* 26 (8): 1501–1507.
38. Courville, X., Tomek, I., Kirkland, K. et al. (2012). Cost-effectiveness of preoperative nasal mupirocin treatment in preventing surgical site infection in patients undergoing total hip and knee arthroplasty: a cost-effectiveness analysis. *Infect. Control Hosp. Epidemiol.* 33 (2): 152–159.
39. Diribe, O., Thomas, S., AbuOun, M. et al. (2015). Genotypic relatedness and characterization of *Staphylococcus pseudintermedius* associated with post-operative surgical infections in dogs. *J. Med. Microbiol.* 64: 1074–1081.
40. Borio, S., Colombo, S., La Rosa, G. et al. (2015). Effectiveness of a combined (4% chlorhexidine digluconate shampoo and solution) protocol in MRS and non-MRS canine superficial pyoderma: a randomized, blinded, antibiotic-controlled study. *Vet. Dermatol.* 26: 339–e72.
41. Mayhew, P.D., Freeman, L., Kwan, T., and Brown, D.C. (2012). Comparison of surgical site infection rates in clean and clean-contaminated wounds in dogs and cats after minimally invasive versus open surgery: 179 cases (2007–2008). *J. Am. Vet. Med. Assoc.* 240 (2): 193–198.
42. Brown, D.C., Conzemius, M., Shofer, F., and Swann, H. (1997). Epidemiologic evaluation of postoperative wound infections in dogs and cats. *J. Am. Vet. Med. Assoc.* 210 (9): 1302–1306.
43. Berrios-Torres, S., Umscheid, C., Bratzler, D. et al. (2017). Centers for Disease Control and Prevention guideline for the prevention of surgical site infection. *J. Am. Med. Assoc. Surg.* 152 (8): 784–791.
44. World Health Organization (2016). Global Guidelines for the Prevention of Surgical Site Infection. Geneva: WHO.
45. Belo, L., Serrano, I., Cunha, E. et al. (2018). Skin asepsis protocols as a preventive measure of surgical site infections in dogs: chlorhexidine – alcohol versus povidone-iodine. *BMC Vet. Res.* 14 (95): 1–6.
46. Melekwe, G.O., Uwagie-Ero, E.A., Zoaka, H.A., and Odigie, E.A. (2018). Comparative clinical effectiveness of preoperative skin antiseptic preparations of chlorhexidine gluconate and povidone iodine for preventing surgical site infections in dogs. *Int. J. Vet. Sci. Med.* 6 (1): 113–116.
47. Andrade, N., Schmiedt, C.W., Cornell, K. et al. (2016). Survey of intraoperative bacterial

contamination in dogs undergoing elective orthopedic surgery. *Vet. Surg.* 45: 214–222.

48. Straw, R.C., Tomlinson, J.L., and Fales, W.H. (1987). Scalpel blade contamination with skin bacteria during orthopedic and neurosurgical procedures in dogs. *Vet. Surg.* 16: 25–30.
49. Lioce, C.G., Davis, E.C., Bennett, J.W. et al. (2019). Scalpel blade contamination and risk of postoperative surgical site infection following abdominal incisions in dogs. *BMC Res. Notes* 12: 459.
50. Belo, L., Serrano, I., Cunha, E. et al. (2020). Surgical blades as bacteria dissemination vehicles in dogs undergoing surgery–a pilot study. *Biomed. Eng. Int.* 2 (1): 25–29.
51. Sturgeon, C., Lamport, A.I., Lloyd, D.H., and Muir, P. (2000). Bacterial contamination of suction tips used during surgical procedures performed on dogs and cats. *Am. J. Vet. Res.* 61 (7): 779–783.
52. Medl, N., Guerrero, T.G., Holzle, L. et al. (2012). Intraoperative contamination of the suction tip in clean orthopedic surgeries in dogs and cats. *Vet. Surg.* 41: 254–260.
53. Weese, J.S. (2008). A review of post-operative infections in veterinary orthopaedic surgery. *Vet. Comp. Orthop. Traumatol.* 21: 99–105.
54. Feßler, A.T., Schuenemann, R., Kadlec, K. et al. (2018). Methicillin-resistant *Staphylococcus aureus* (MRSA) and methicillin-resistant *Staphylococcus pseudintermedius* (MRSP) among employees and in the environment of a small animal hospital. *Vet. Microbiol.* 221: 153–158.
55. Larson, E. (1995). APIC guidelines for handwashing and hand antisepsis in health care settings. *Am. J. Infect. Control* 23 (4): 251–269.
56. Verwilghen, D.R., Mainil, J., Mastrocicco, E. et al. (2011). Surgical hand antisepsis in veterinary practice: evaluation of soap scrubs and alcohol based rub techniques. *Vet. J.* 190 (3): 372–377.
57. Parienti, J.J., Thibon, P., Heller, R. et al. (2002). Hand-rubbing with an aqueous alcoholic solution vs traditional surgical hand-scrubbing and 30-day surgical site infection rates. *J. Am. Med. Assoc.* 288 (6): 722–727.
58. Hingst, V., Juditzki, I., Heeg, P., and Sonntag, H.-G. (1992). Evaluation of the efficacy of surgical hand disinfection following a reduced application time of 3 instead of 5 minutes. *J. Hosp. Infect.* 20 (2): 79–86.
59. Verwilghen, D. and Kampf, G. (2016). Letter to the editor: antibacterial efficacy of several surgical hand preparation products used by veterinary students. *Vet. Surg.* 45: 1118–1119.
60. Hübner, N., Kampf, G., Kamp, P. et al. (2006). Does a preceding hand wash and drying time after surgical hand disinfection influence the efficacy of a propanol-based hand rub? *BMC Microbiol.* 6: 57.
61. Widmer, A.F., Rotter, M., Voss, A. et al. (2010). Surgical hand preparation: state-of-the-art. *J. Hosp. Infect.* 74 (2): 112–122.
62. Meakin, L.B., Gilman, O.P., Parsons, K.J. et al. (2016). Colored indicator undergloves increase the detection of glove perforations by surgeons during small animal orthopedic surgery: a randomized controlled trial. *Vet. Surg.* 45: 709–714.
63. Hayes, G.M., Reynolds, D., Moens, N.M.M. et al. (2014). Investigation of incidence and risk factors for surgical glove perforation in small animal surgery. *Vet. Surg.* 43: 400–404.
64. Stine, S.L., Odum, S.M., and Daniel Mertens, W. (2018). Protocol changes to reduce implant-associated infection rate after tibial plateau leveling osteotomy: 703 dogs, 811 TPLO (2006–2014). *Vet. Surg.* 47: 481–489.
65. Boothe, H.W. (2017). Instrument and tissue handling techniques. In: *Veterinary Surgery*, 2e (eds. S.A. Johnston and K.M. Tobias), 733. St Louis, MO: Elsevier.
66. Cadman, C. (2016). The impact of surgical safety checklists on theatre departments: a critical review of the literature. *J. Perioper. Pract.* 26 (4): 62–71.
67. Haynes, A., Weiser, T., Berry, W. et al. (2009). A surgical safety checklist to reduce morbidity and mortality in a global population. *N. Engl. J. Med.* 360: 491–499.
68. Verwilghen, D. and Singh, A. (2015). Fighting surgical site infections in small animals: are we getting anywhere? *Vet. Clin. North Am. Small Anim. Pract.* 45 (2): 243–276.
69. Gatineau, M., El-warrak, A.O., Bolliger, C. et al. (2012). Effects of sterilization with hydrogen peroxide gas plasma, ethylene oxide, and steam on bioadhesive properties of nylon and polyethylene lines used for stabilization of canine stifle joints. *Am. J. Vet. Res.* 73: 1665–1659.
70. Solano, M.A., Danielski, A., Kovach, K. et al. (2015). Locking plate and screw fixation after tibial plateau leveling osteotomy reduces postoperative infection rate in dogs over 50 kg. *Vet. Surg.* 44: 59–64.
71. Singh, A., Walker, M., Rousseau, J., and Weese, J.S. (2013). Characterization of the biofilm forming ability of *Staphylococcus pseudintermedius* from dogs. *BMC Vet. Res.* 9: 93.
72. Donlan, R.M. (2001). Biofilm formation: a clinically relevant microbiological process. *Clin. Infect. Dis.* 33: 1387–1392.
73. Walker, M., Singh, A., Nazarali, A. et al. (2016). Evaluation of the impact of methicillin-resistant *Staphylococcus pseudintermedius* biofilm formation on antimicrobial susceptibility. *Vet. Surg.* 45: 968–971.
74. Azab, M.A., Allen, M.J., and Daniels, J.B. (2016). Evaluation of a silver-impregnated coating to inhibit colonization of orthopaedic

implants by biofilm forming methicillin-resistant Staphylococcus pseudintermedius. *Vet. Comp. Orthop. Traumatol.* 29 (6): 347–350.
75. Arciola, C.R., Campoccia, D., Speziale, P. et al. (2012). Biofilm formation in *Staphylococcus* implant infections. A review of molecular mechanisms and implications for biofilm-resistant materials. *Biomaterials* 33 (26): 5967–5982.
76. Konig, L., Klopfleisch, R., Kershaw, O., and Gruber, A.D. (2015). Prevalence of biofilms on surgical suture segments in wounds of dogs, cats, and horses. *Vet. Pathol.* 52 (2): 295–297.
77. McCagherty, J., Yool, D.A., Paterson, G.K. et al. (2020). Investigation of the in vitro antimicrobial activity of triclosan-coated suture material on bacteria commonly isolated from wounds in dogs. *Am. J. Vet. Res.* 81 (1): 84–90.
78. Morrison, S., Singh, A., Rousseau, J. et al. (2015). Impact of polymethylmethacrylate additives on methicillin-resistant *Staphylococcus pseudintermedius* biofilm formation in vitro. *Am. J. Vet. Res.* 76 (5): 395–401.
79. Boothe, D.M. and Boothe, H.W. Jr. (2015). Antimicrobial considerations in the perioperative patient. *Vet. Clin. North Am. Small Anim. Pract.* 45 (3): 585–608.
80. Anderson, M.E.C. (2015). Contact precautions and hand hygiene in veterinary clinics. *Vet. Clin. North Am. Small Anim. Pract.* 45 (2): 343–360.
81. Bratzler, D. (2005). Antimicrobial prophylaxis for surgery: an advisory statement from the National Surgery Infection Prevention Project. *Am. J. Surg.* 189: 395–404.
82. Whittem, T.L., Johnson, A.L., Smith, C. et al. (1999). Effect of perioperative prophylactic antimicrobial treatment in dogs undergoing elective orthopedic surgery. *J. Am. Vet. Med. Assoc.* 215: 212–216.
83. Weese, J.S. and Halling, K.B. (2006). Perioperative administration of antimicrobials associated with elective surgery in dogs: 83 cases (2003–2005). *J. Am. Vet. Med. Assoc.* 229 (1): 92–95.
84. Hagen, C.R.M., Singh, A., Weese, J.S. et al. (2020). Contributing factors to surgical site infection after tibial plateau leveling osteotomy: a follow-up retrospective study. *Vet. Surg.* 49: 930–939.
85. Burgess, B.A. (2019). Prevention and surveillance of surgical infections: a review. *Vet. Surg.* 48: 284–290.
86. Stickney, D.N.G. and Mankin, K.M.T. (2018). The impact of postdischarge surveillance on surgical site infection diagnosis. *Vet. Surg.* 47: 66–73.
87. Centers for Disease Control and Prevention (2020). *Surgical Site Infection (Event)*. Atlanta, GA: CDC.
88. Nicoll, C., Singh, A., and Weese, J.S. (2014). Economic impact of tibial plateau leveling osteotomy surgical site infection in dogs. *Vet. Surg.* 43: 899–902.

3 Identification, Addressing, and Following Up on Surgical Site Infection After Cranial Cruciate Ligament Stabilization

Katie L. Hoddinott, J. Scott Weese, and Ameet Singh

3.1 Introduction

Prompt and accurate diagnosis of surgical site infections (SSIs) is important for patient management and facility infection control. Identifying infections promptly allows for early intervention. Differentiation of SSI from inflammation helps avoid unnecessary treatment. A good understanding of infection rates and early identification of increases in infection rates can allow for an earlier investigation and intervention. Therefore, SSI surveillance is a critical area for any surgeon, surgical team, and facility.

3.2 Identification of Surgical Site Infections

A superficial incisional SSI is confined to the skin and subcutaneous tissues of the incision and must be differentiated from cellulitis. The Centers for Disease Control and Prevention (CDC) defines cellulitis as localized redness, heat, and swelling, without purulent discharge or identification of microorganisms [1]. The clinical features associated with cellulitis are often identified in postoperative wounds and presumed to indicate SSI without performing diagnostic testing to identify a causative organism, thus confirming an active SSI [2, 3]. Subsequently, when reviewing the literature, a category such as "infection-inflammation" may be reported, making it difficult to accurately detect and report SSI rates based on CDC definitions [2, 3]. One such study including the infection-inflammation category defines infection-inflammation as the presence of purulent discharge, a localized abscess or fistulous tract associated with the incision or the presence of three or more of the following: redness, swelling, heat, pain, serous discharge, and dehiscence [3]. While some of the cases collected in this category may appropriately represent an SSI, it does not distinguish SSI from cellulitis and as such may be falsely increasing the reported SSI rates. Other studies have reported SSI rates based on CDC definitions including positive culture results, while also reporting an infection-inflammation rate to encompass those patients presenting with abnormal incisions [4].

Early detection and intervention for SSIs is critical. Löfqvist et al. identified marked elevations of serum C-reactive protein (CRP) and serum amylase A (SAA) 6 days following tibial plateau leveling osteotomy (TPLO) [5].

Complications in Canine Cranial Cruciate Ligament Surgery, First Edition. Edited by Ron Ben-Amotz and David L. Dycus.

Table 3.1 Swabbing techniques.

Swabbing technique	Collection method
Levine technique	The swab is rotated over 1 cm^2 for 5 sec with sufficient pressure to exude fluid from the tissues
Z-technique	The swab is rotated as it is moved from margin to margin, without touching the skin edges, in a 10-point fashion

The cut-off values reported (CRP>43.9 mg/L, SAA >63.8 mg/L) may be used for patients both with and without clinical evidence of an active SSI and may therefore lead to earlier detection of subclinical SSIs [5]. While these serum markers may be able to identify subclinical SSIs, the clinical utility of this test is low as there are no clinical criteria that can be monitored to determine which patients to test. Following discharge from the hospital, owners should be advised to monitor the surgical site for evidence of localized swelling, pain, heat, or erythema. If any of these signs are detected, evaluation by a veterinarian should be sought.

Clinically, identification of SSIs will require gross reassessment of the surgical site to differentiate between cellulitis and infection as defined above and allow for collection of aseptic samples to identify microorganisms via cytology or bacterial culture. This may include direct swabbing of the wound or deep fine needle local aspirates. Before collecting a direct swab, the wound should be lavaged with sterile saline and any devitalized tissues debrided. The swab should be collected from the healthiest appearing portion of the wound bed. Two direct swabbing techniques have been described and are recommended to improve the chances of collecting a representative sample (Table 3.1). Of the two, the Levine technique (Figure 3.1) is considered superior [6]. When collecting a deep local fine needle aspirate, known regions of contamination should be avoided and the skin should be cleaned with alcohol to reduce the risk of skin contaminants. If microorganisms are identified cytologically from your sample, a bacterial culture and susceptibility test is recommended to further guide therapy. Radiographic assessment for evidence of lucency surrounding implants or evidence of osteomyelitis should also be considered to determine the extent of the suspected SSI. Radiographic evidence to support a deep SSI causing osteomyelitis may include periosteal reaction and bone lysis surrounding the implants (Figure 3.2).

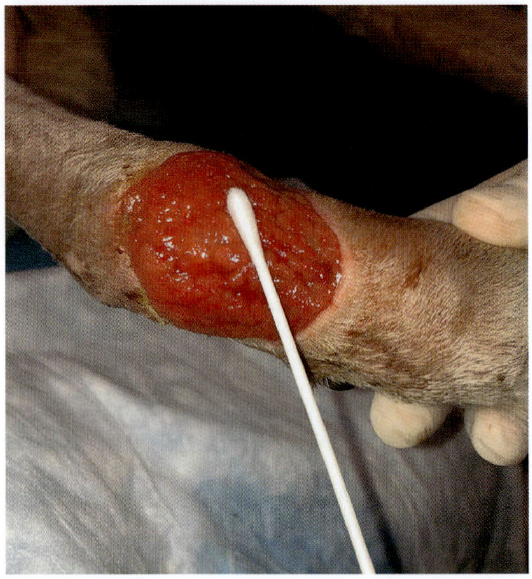

Figure 3.1 For the Levine technique, the swab is contacting the wound bed only, with sufficient application of pressure to result in exudation of fluid from the underlying tissues. Source: Adapted from Weese JS. Wound sampling for culture and cytology. Clinician's Brief, March 2020. www.cliniciansbrief.com/article/wound-sampling-culture-cytology.

As not all owners will seek veterinary care for perceived minor changes at the surgical site, another tool in our arsenal to improve detection of SSI is utilization of surveillance programs. Lack of communication between the surgical facility and primary care veterinarian can also result in underidentification of SSI rates, particularly when owners may return to their primary care veterinarian for minor complications as these may not be reported to the surgeon. Further, deficiencies in medical record quality can impact retrospective identification of SSIs.

Two recent prospective veterinary studies on postdischarge surveillance programs reported that 28–35% of identified SSIs were not documented in the medical record, leading to falsely lower SSI rates when retrospectively evaluated using medical records alone [4, 7]. Both studies carried out owner questionnaires at 30 days postoperatively and one study repeated the

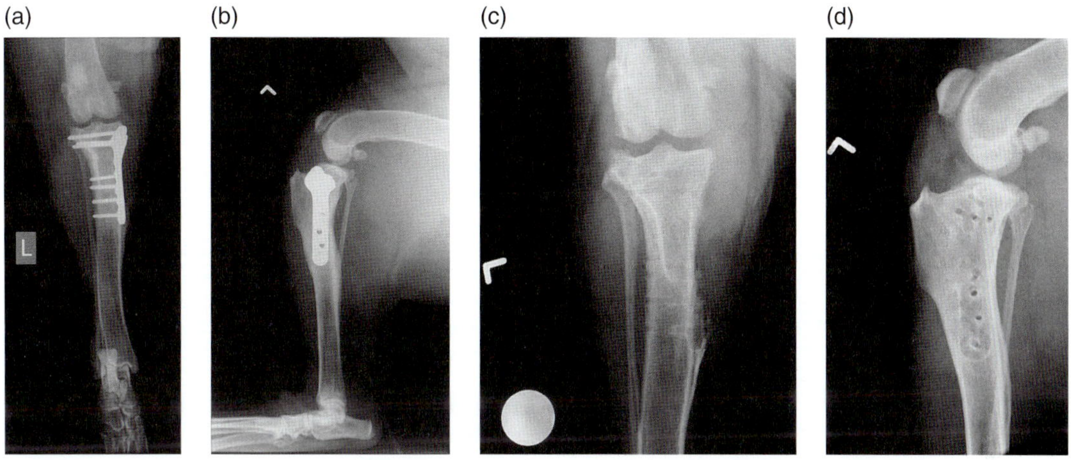

Figure 3.2 (a) A craniocaudal (CC) view of a TPLO with periosteal reaction evident at the distal aspect of the implant. (b) A lateral view of a TPLO with periosteal reaction evident at the cranial aspect of the implant, as evidenced by the increased bone density in this region corresponding to the location of periosteal reaction on the CC view. (c) A CC view following implant removal, highlighting the previously identified periosteal reaction. (d) A lateral view following implant removal, highlighting the periosteal reaction outlining the previous implant.

questionnaire at 90 days for patients having a surgical implant [4, 7]. This active surveillance approach will yield more accurate SSI information; however, these types of active surveillance approaches require time, effort, and corresponding personnel costs.

Developing an active surveillance protocol is an important quality control tool, but it can be challenging to achieve due to the time commitment involved [4]. However, empowering a member of the surgical team to champion an active surveillance program is highly recommended to ensure uptake and quality control. Alternatively, improving passive surveillance methods, beyond routine examination at the time of suture removal, may also be beneficial. Emphasizing the importance of SSI reporting from referring veterinarians and clients, along with defined measures of surgical site assessment to report, may help to improve the accuracy of SSI rates within your hospital [4].

More recently, electronic approaches to surveillance have been investigated. The proliferation of smartphones and email access creates the potential for easy, cost-effective monitoring and data collection. In the future, it is likely that approaches using personal devices will become common SSI surveillance tools.

For SSIs to be appropriately identified, the use of specific criteria to define SSIs must be employed. The CDC has categorized SSIs as superficial incisional SSI, deep incisional SSI (Figure 3.3), and organ/space SSI based on

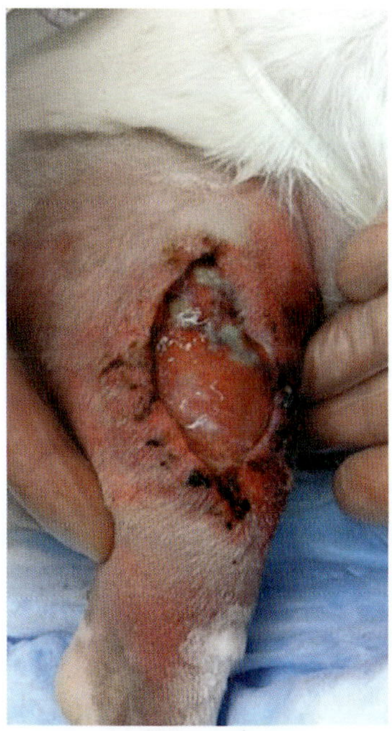

Figure 3.3 A dehisced lateral stifle incision with local erythema and purulent material present at the skin edges and present on the underlying muscle belly. This is considered to be a deep SSI.

Table 3.2 Surgical site infection (SSI) definitions.

Surgical site infection category	Criteria
Superficial SSI	MUST: 1. Occur within **30 days** of surgery 2. Involve only the **skin or subcutaneous tissues** of the incision 3. Must have AT LEAST one of the following: a. **Purulent discharge** from the incision b. **Organism(s)** identified from an aseptically collected sample c. **Incision is reopened with purpose** and organisms are identified from an aseptically collected sample AND the patient exhibits localized swelling, pain, erythema, or heat d. Diagnosed as an SSI by a physician
Deep SSI	MUST: 1. Occur within **30 days (no implant)** or **90 days (implant)** 2. Involves tissues **deep to the subcutaneous tissues** 3. Must have AT LEAST one of the following: a. **Purulent discharge** from the incision b. **Incision spontaneously dehisces or is reopened with purpose** AND **organisms** are identified from an aseptically collected sample AND the patient exhibits **localized pain or pyrexia** c. Local **abscess** formation
Organ/space	MUST: 1. Occur within **30 days (no implant)** or **90 days (implant)** 2. Involves any tissues **deep to the fascia/muscle that was opened during surgery** 3. Must have AT LEAST one of the following: a. **Purulent discharge** from a drain within the organ/space b. **Organisms** are identified from an aseptically collected sample from fluid or tissue within the organ/space c. Local **abscess** formation

specific criteria (Table 3.2). Recently, these categories have been redefined with regard to implant-associated SSI, such that an implant-associated SSI must occur within 90 days of surgery [1].

3.3 Addressing Surgical Site Infections

The vast majority of SSIs occur secondary to contamination of the surgical site by commensal or pathogenic organisms arising from the patient's own microbiome [8]. The most common microorganism identified in SSIs is *Staphylococcus pseudintermedius*. Other common microorganisms identified include *Streptococcus* spp., *Pseudomonas aeruginosa*, and *Escherichia coli*. *Staphylococcus pseudintermedius* is an opportunistic pathogen with an ability to create a biofilm, leading to its increased virulence [9]. The ability to create a biofilm is important as it makes eradication of these SSIs more challenging. Additionally, resistance of *S. pseudintermedius* is on the rise, creating an even greater challenge for management of patients with SSIs [9].

Following the diagnosis of a SSI, several factors must be considered prior to determining a treatment protocol. These include the patient's overall clinical status, category of SSI (superficial, deep, organ/space), susceptibility of inciting microorganisms, presence of biofilm formation, stage of healing, availability of treatment options, and client considerations such as emotional and financial strain associated with treatment.

The vast majority of SSIs reported by category in the veterinary literature are limited to superficial or deep tissue layers, with an organ/space SSI occurring in <1% of infections [4, 10].

For superficial incisional SSIs, topical or systemic antimicrobial therapy may be sufficient. Topical therapies may include antiseptic agents such as chlorhexidine or povidone-iodine or antimicrobial therapies such as medical-grade honey or silver compounds. When the SSI is relatively focal or has minimal purulent discharge, topical antiseptic solutions may be used to clean the site several times daily and may result in resolution of the SSI. However, when a large portion of the wound appears to be affected or when there are large volumes of purulent discharge, topical antimicrobial therapies are best employed if the wound is reopened and explored. This allows for greater source control by lavaging the wound and removing the large microbial burden and allows topical therapies to be in direct contact with the affected tissues. Medical-grade honey and silver ointments are often used in these scenarios. There is no evidence for antimicrobial resistance for honey, but resistance may exist for silver compounds [11]. This resistance has been demonstrated *in vitro* and may not be clinically applicable.

Regardless of the potential for resistance, response to topical therapy should be monitored and treatments altered if there is a lack of response. Ideally, a bacterial culture should be submitted from the onset of clinical signs, so that an appropriate systemic antimicrobial can be added to the treatment regime, should topical therapy fail to resolve the SSI.

Systemic antimicrobial therapies should be employed in the face of an intact incision and direct identification of microorganisms. Initially, systemic antimicrobials will be chosen empirically until the results of culture and susceptibility testing are available to guide specific therapy. It is important to collect and submit a bacterial culture when an SSI is suspected, to ensure appropriate antimicrobial stewardship is followed and reduce the risk of potentiating antimicrobial resistance.

Initial empirical recommendations will vary based on hospital known infectious agents and their resistance patterns. Appropriate duration of therapy is a topic of debate and varies between prescribers, with reported treatment lengths ranging from 1 to 6 weeks of antimicrobial therapy [12, 13]. While extended durations of antimicrobial therapy are reported, these prolonged courses of antimicrobials are not likely required unless implanted materials are involved. Most uncomplicated, superficial SSIs will resolve with a systemic course of antimicrobials for 3–5 days. Ultimately, when antimicrobial therapy is discontinued and there is recurrence of clinical signs, involvement of implanted materials should be considered and prolonged antimicrobial therapy based on culture and susceptibility results will be required until implanted materials can be removed or local therapies can be employed [12].

Deep SSIs involving implanted materials can be more challenging to manage, due to the risk for biofilm formation. A biofilm is a community of sessile bacteria embedded in a self-produced matrix that has adhered to a surface (Figure 3.4) [14]. The most commonly implicated bacterium in veterinary SSIs is *S. pseudintermedius* which has a propensity for biofilm formation and multidrug resistance [9, 15, 16]. The self-produced matrix protects the bacteria from antimicrobial penetration and makes treatment more complex as minimum inhibitory concentrations are much higher for bacteria in a biofilm than planktonic bacteria [17].

Because of this increased challenge of eradicating a biofilm-associated infection, implant removal is often recommended. However, if the SSI is identified early postoperatively and insufficient healing has occurred, methods other than implant removal must be considered. Antimicrobials are often used in situations like this to try to control the SSI, with a realization that the goal is most likely to allow

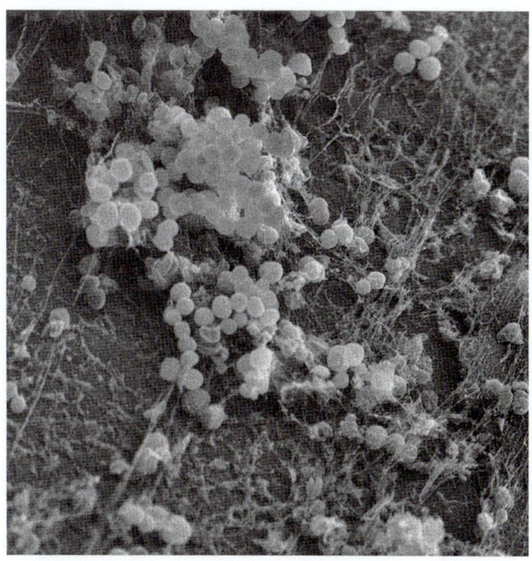

Figure 3.4 Scanning electron microscopy image of a biofilm. Source: Adapted from Singh et al. [9].

for bone healing, at which point implant removal would be indicated. In the face of a completely healed osteotomy or adequately stabilized extracapsular repair, implant removal, and thus biofilm eradication, are often recommended. Several studies have reported implant removal rates for TPLO, tibial tuberosity advancement (TTA), cranial closing wedge osteotomy, triple tibial osteotomy, and lateral fabellar suture extracapsular repairs [12, 13, 18–23]. Explant rates for management of an SSI ranged from 1.3% to 71%, with TPLO and lateral fabellar sutures being the highest rate of explanted materials [12, 13, 18–20, 22, 23].

Additional approaches to biofilm infections are currently limited. Two enzymes have been identified as being able to prevent biofilm formation; deoxyribonuclease I and dispersin B. While both are capable of inhibiting biofilm formation, only dispersin B has been proven to be able to disrupt an established biofilm [24]. A recent *in vitro* study has identified that the combination of dispersin B and amikacin in a biodegradable gel allows for rapid elution of dispersin B with a gradual reduction in concentrations over a period of 10 days [25]. While this is a promising avenue, clinical application has not yet been assessed.

When implant removal cannot yet be performed, local antimicrobial therapies (Table 3.3) may be employed. The main goal of these therapies is to allow higher antimicrobial concentrations to be achieved locally than could be tolerated systemically, with limited systemic exposure [26]. Alternative local therapies may include antimicrobial-eluting bone cement, gel polymer, or collagen sponges, with the most common antimicrobials used being gentamicin, amikacin, and clindamycin.

Bone cement consisting of a calcium base or polymethylmethacrylate (PMMA) may be formed into beads containing various antimicrobials and may be placed locally at the surgical site (Figure 3.5). The antimicrobial powder or liquid solution is added to the PMMA powder before the addition of the methylmethacrylate liquid. It is important that the antimicrobial of choice will remain stable during the exothermic reaction that takes place when the PMMA powder and methylmethacrylate liquid are combined [26]. Once combined, beads can be formed around a small gauge cerclage wire, to create a string of beads. *In vitro* evaluation identified that gentamicin-susceptible methicillin-resistant *S. pseudintermedius* (MRSP) was effectively treated with gentamicin-impregnated beads, whereas gentamicin-resistant MRSP was not effectively treated and silver-impregnated beads had no effect on MRSP biofilms [11]. PMMA beads, however, are not biodegradable and require removal at a later date, whereas calcium-based beads can be degraded locally, thus not requiring removal [27]. Therefore, when considering antimicrobial-impregnated beads, one must determine the susceptibility of the microorganisms to effectively choose an antimicrobial and

Table 3.3 Pros and cons of implantable antimicrobial elution products.

Product	Pros	Cons
PMMA beads	Readily available (especially if used for other orthopedic procedures in your facility)	Nonbiodegradable Must be removed Surgical implantation
Calcium-based beads	Biodegradable – no removal required	Surgical implantation
Polymer gel	Can combine with dispersin B to break down biofilm Minimally invasive application – injectable Biodegradable – no removal required	Cannot flush surgical site to dilute microbial burden Location of application less precise
Collagen sponge	Biodegradable – no removal required	Surgical implantation Incites inflammation Causes lameness with IA application Causes renal impairment

IA, intraarticular; PMMA, polymethylmethacrylate.

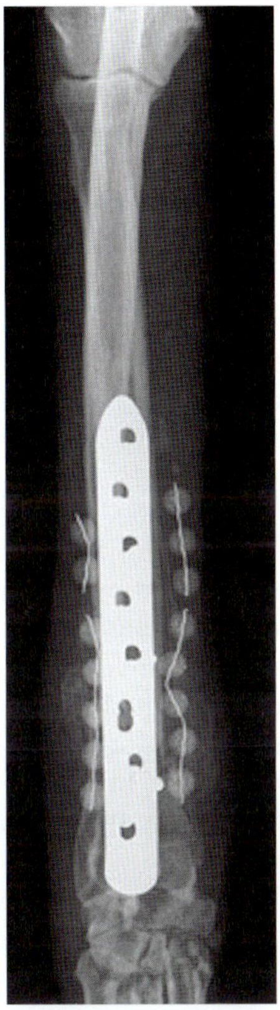

Figure 3.5 In this craniocaudal view of the antebrachium, two discontinuous strands of antimicrobial-impregnated PMMA beads can be seen on the lateral and medial aspects of the bone.

take into consideration the potential requirement for removal of beads if PMMA is chosen.

Antimicrobial-impregnated dextran polymer gel has been proven *in vitro* to elute high concentrations of antimicrobials that maintain their bioactivity after elution [28]. Gels can be injected locally, without requiring a surgical approach, and do not require removal as they are naturally resorbed [28]. A single case series of an amikacin and clindamycin-impregnated dextran polymer gel used in combination with explantation of TPLO plates resulted in excellent clinical outcomes after 12 weeks [29]. Despite limited data existing at this time, this may be a promising option for the future and application without implant removal should be further evaluated.

Commercially available gentamicin-impregnated collagen sponges have been placed intraarticularly in a study population of dogs with sterilely induced synovitis. A rapid elution rate was identified, resulting in a rapid rise of intraarticular gentamicin concentrations, but a rapid decline was also observed. This rapid decline may not be clinically relevant, as gentamicin is a concentration-dependent antimicrobial and thus the high concentrations achieved may be sufficient to result in bactericidal activity.

The gentamicin-impregnated sponge was found to incite joint inflammation, lameness, and renal impairment and was thus not recommended for clinical use [30]. However, one case report exists of its use in a clinical incidence of septic arthritis following an extracapsular stifle stabilization procedure. This case reports clinical resolution of the septic arthritis but systemic gentamicin was administered simultaneously, making it hard to determine the role of the intraarticular gentamicin [31]. A separate case series combined implant removal with an amikacin-impregnated collagen sponge being placed at the site of implant removal for treatment of TPLO SSI, which resulted in a 96.8% long-term resolution rate [32]. The benefit of an antimicrobial collagen sponge is its absorbable nature, thus precluding the requirement for retrieval following SSI resolution.

While all of these local antimicrobial-eluting options provide increased levels of local therapy, differences in biodegradability may play a role in clinical decision making. If these local therapies are being employed in the face of an incompletely healed osteotomy or incomplete stabilization of an extracapsular repair, implant removal cannot be performed concurrently. Two sides of the coin can therefore be considered following complete healing of the osteotomy or adequate stifle stabilization. On the one hand, a biodegradable option does not require further surgical extraction and if the SSI is clinically resolved, the implant may not require removal. However, on the other hand, a nonbiodegradable option must be surgically removed and allows the opportunity for concurrent implant removal. With the major concern of biofilm formation on implanted materials, locally applied antimicrobial therapy may not be sufficient to eradicate the SSI and recurrence may result in further treatment and possible implant removal at a later date.

In the case of implant removal, the major microorganism burden is removed with the implant, assuming that most of these SSIs are biofilm related and as such systemic or local therapies may not be required (Figure 3.6). Of the various studies reporting treatment of SSIs with implant removal, few indicate whether postoperative systemic antimicrobial therapy was continued empirically and/or altered pending culture and susceptibility testing results. While all these studies encourage culture and susceptibility testing of implants that are removed, how this information is applied clinically is unknown. As such, evidence-based recommendations for postoperative systemic antimicrobial use following implant removal for management of an SSI remain unclear. Logically, if the major burden of disease has been removed, monitoring for clinical recurrence of SSI signs is recommended. Thus, patients without active evidence of an SSI at the time of implant removal do not require systemic antimicrobial therapy and results of culture and susceptibility testing should be employed only in the face of recurrent signs of SSI.

Though few studies exist, when local antimicrobial therapy is combined with implant removal, such as implantation of an amikacin-impregnated collagen sponge or amikacin and clindamycin polymer gel, SSI resolution rates ranged from 95% to 96.8%, without the concurrent use of systemic antimicrobials [29, 32].

Regardless of local or systemic therapies used in conjunction with implant removal, bacterial culture and susceptibility testing is recommended following implant removal. While a positive culture may not indicate the need for antimicrobial treatment, it allows for proper selection of the antimicrobial if treatment is determined to be clinically indicated. A positive culture result has been reported following implant removal in 72–80% of cases [18, 23]. However, sonication of implants may aid in improved bacterial recovery when considering culture and susceptibility testing [33]. As sonication is not likely to be performed routinely for culture and susceptibility testing, this may play a role in identification of negative culture results following implant removal for SSI. Alternatively, preoperative treatment with antimicrobial therapy targeted at the known microorganisms may be sufficient to eradicate or significantly reduce the microbial burden, such that a negative culture result is achieved post implant removal [13, 18, 23].

3.4 Follow-Up

Following diagnosis of an SSI, continued frequent communication is necessary to ensure response to therapy. If empirical therapy is instituted without improvement of clinical signs, bacterial culture and susceptibility testing

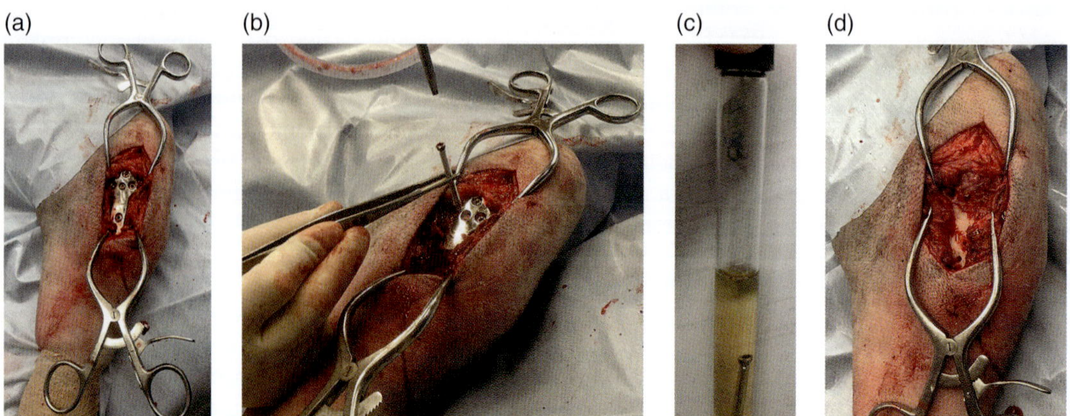

Figure 3.6 (a) Exposed TPLO plate. (b) Screw removed. When removing screws to submit for culture, use a pair of forceps that have not touched the skin to stabilize the screw while it is being removed. Do not allow the screw to contact the skin to avoid growth of skin contaminants on your bacterial culture. (c) Screw placed in broth medium for bacterial culture submission. (d) Surgical site following implant removal.

is recommended to guide therapy, if this is not already under way. Duration of antimicrobial therapy is controversial but should reflect the level of the infection, such that a superficial SSI receives a shorter course of antimicrobial therapy than a deep or organ/space SSI. At any time that antimicrobial therapy has been discontinued and clinical signs of SSI recur, implant removal should be considered to remove the largest burden of disease associated with a likely biofilm-associated implant infection. Following discontinuation of antimicrobial therapy or implant removal, active surveillance protocols to acquire follow-up information regarding resolution or recurrence of clinical signs should be implemented. Setting in place an infection control plan in your hospital to determine annual SSI rates in general, but specifically associated with surgically implanted devices, will be beneficial to document and monitor trends, thus allowing earlier interventions when SSI rates are increasing.

References

1. Centers for Disease Control and Prevention (2020). Centers for disease control and prevention: surgical site infection (SSI) event.
2. Wolf, R.E., Scavelli, T.D., Hoelzler, M.G. et al. (2012). Surgical and postoperative complications associated with tibial tuberosity advancement for cranial cruciate ligament rupture in dogs: 458 cases (2007–2009). *J. Am. Vet. Med. Assoc.* 240 (12): 1481–1487.
3. Frey, T.N., Hoelzler, M.G., Scavelli, T.D. et al. (2010). Risk factors for surgical site infection-inflammation in dogs undergoing surgery for rupture of the cranial cruciate ligament: 902 cases (2005–2006). *J. Am. Vet. Med. Assoc.* 236 (1): 88–94.
4. Turk, R., Singh, A., and Weese, J.S. (2015). Prospective surgical site infection surveillance in dogs. *Vet. Surg.* 44: 2–8.
5. Löfqvist, K., Kjelgaard-Hansen, M., and Nielsen, M.B.M. (2018). Usefulness of C-reactive protein and serum amyloid a in early detection of postoperative infectious complications to tibial plateau leveling osteotomy in dogs. *Acta Vet. Scand.* 60 (30): 1–8.
6. Bonham, P.A. (2009). Swab cultures for diagnosing wound. *J. Wound Osto. Cont. Nurses. Soc.* 36 (August): 389–395.
7. Stickney, D.N.G. and Mankin, K.M.T. (2018). The impact of postdischarge surveillance on surgical site infection diagnosis. *Vet. Surg.* 47: 66–73.
8. Belo, L., Serrano, I., Cunha, E. et al. (2018). Skin asepsis protocols as a preventive measure of surgical site infections in dogs: chlorhexidine – alcohol versus povidone-iodine. *BMC Vet. Res.* 14 (95): 1–6.
9. Singh, A., Walker, M., Rousseau, J., and Weese, J.S. (2013). Characterization of the biofilm forming ability of Staphylococcus pseudintermedius from dogs. *BMC Vet. Res.* 9: 93.
10. Costa, M., Craig, D., Cambridge, T. et al. (2017). Major complications of tibial tuberosity advancement in 1613 dogs. *Vet. Surg.* 46: 494–500.
11. Morrison, S., Singh, A., Rousseau, J. et al. (2015). Impact of polymethylmethacrylate additives on methicillin-resistant *Staphylococcus pseudintermedius* biofilm formation in vitro. *Am. J. Vet. Res.* 76 (5): 395–401.
12. Gallagher, A.D. and Mertens, W.D. (2012). Implant removal rate from infection after tibial plateau leveling osteotomy in dogs. *Vet. Surg.* 41: 705–711.
13. Brown, G., Maddox, T., and Siles, M.M.B. (2016). Client-assessed long-term outcome in dogs with surgical site infection following tibial plateau levelling osteotomy. *Vet. Rec.* 179: 409.
14. Donlan, R.M. (2001). Biofilm formation: a clinically relevant microbiological process. *Clin. Infect. Dis.* 33: 1387–1392.
15. Nazarali, A., Singh, A., and Weese, J.S. (2014). Perioperative administration of antimicrobials during tibial plateau leveling osteotomy. *Vet. Surg.* 43: 966–971.
16. Stull, J.W. (2015). Hospital-associated infections in small animal practice. *Vet. Clin. North Am. Small Anim. Pract.* 45 (2): 217–233.
17. Walker, M., Singh, A., Nazarali, A. et al. (2016). Evaluation of the impact of methicillin-resistant *Staphylococcus pseudintermedius* biofilm formation on antimicrobial susceptibility. *Vet. Surg.* 45: 968–971.
18. Thompson, A.M., Bergh, M.S., Wang, C., and Wells, K. (2011). Tibial plateau levelling osteotomy implant removal: a retrospective analysis of 129 cases. *Vet. Comp. Orthop. Traumatol.* 24: 450–456.
19. Casale, S.A. and McCarthy, R.J. (2009). Complications associated with lateral fabellotibial suture surgery for cranial cruciate ligament injury in dogs: 363 cases (1997–2005). *J. Am. Vet. Med. Assoc.* 234: 229–235.
20. Yap, F.W., Calvo, I., Smith, K.D., and Parkin, T. (2015). Perioperative risk factors for surgical site infection in tibial tuberosity advancement: 224 stifles. *Vet. Comp. Orthop. Traumatol.* 28: 199–206.
21. Serratore, V.R. and Barnhart, M.D. (2018). Results and complications after removal of tibial tuberosity advancement cage for treatment of surgical site infections: a retrospective study. *Vet. Surg.* 47: 768–773.

22. Frederick, S.W. and Cross, A.R. (2017). Modified cranial closing wedge osteotomy for treatment of cranial cruciate ligament insufficiency in dogs with excessive tibial plateau angles: technique and complications in 19 cases. *Vet. Surg.* 46: 403–411.
23. Nicoll, C., Singh, A., and Weese, J.S. (2014). Economic impact of tibial plateau leveling osteotomy surgical site infection in dogs. *Vet. Surg.* 43: 899–902.
24. Kaplan, J.B. (2009). Therapeutic potential of biofilm-dispersing enzymes. *Int. J. Artif. Organs* 32 (9): 545–554.
25. Hagen, C., Singh, A., Weese, J.S. et al. (2020). in vitro elution of amikacin and dispersin B from a polymer hydrogel. *Vet. Surg.* 49: 1035–1042.
26. Hayes, G., Moens, N., and Gibson, T. (2013). A review of local antibiotic implants and applications to veterinary orthopaedic surgery. *Vet. Comp. Orthop. Traumatol.* 26: 251–259.
27. Boothe, D.M. and Boothe, H.W. Jr. (2015). Antimicrobial considerations in the perioperative patient. *Vet. Clin. North Am. Small Anim. Pract.* 45 (3): 585–608.
28. Thomas, L.A., Bizikova, T., and Minihan, A.C. (2011). in vitro elution and antibacterial activity of clindamycin, amikacin, and vancomycin from R-gel polymer. *Vet. Surg.* 40: 774–780.
29. Reed, T.P., Thomas, L.A., Weeren, F.R. et al. (2016). A novel dextran polymer hydrogel local antimicrobial therapy in dogs: a pilot study. *Can. J. Vet. Res.* 57: 189–195.
30. Hayes, G., Gibson, T., Moens, N.M.M. et al. (2016). Intra-articular implantation of gentamicin impregnated collagen sponge causes joint inflammation and impaired renal function in dogs. *Vet. Comp. Orthop. Traumatol.* 29: 159–163.
31. Owen, M.R., Moores, A.P., and Coe, R.J. (2004). Management of MRSA septic arthritis in a dog using a gentamicin-impregnated collagen sponge. *J. Small Anim. Pract.* 45: 609–612.
32. Lee, S.J., Frederick, S.W., and Cross, A.R. (2019). Use of an amikacin-infused collagen sponge concurrent with implant removal for treatment of tibial plateau leveling osteotomy surgical site infection in 31 cases. *Vet. Surg.* 48: 700–706.
33. Keeshen, T.P., Case, J.B., Wellehan, J.F., and Dujowich, M. (2017). Bacterial recovery using sonication versus swabbing of titanium and stainless steel implants inoculated with *Staphylococcus pseudintermedius* or *Pseudomonas aeruginosa*. *Vet. Comp. Orthop. Traumatol.* 30: 346–350.

Section II

Intraarticular Repair Techniques

4 Complications Associated with Intraarticular Repair Techniques

Jeffery Biskup and Michael G. Conzemius

4.1 An Introduction to Intraarticular Repair in Veterinary Medicine

Despite its present unpopularity, intraarticular (IA) repair has been researched and performed clinically since the mid-twentieth century. A more in-depth description of the history of IA repair can be found elsewhere, although it is interesting to note that 30 years ago, IA repairs were more common in veterinary medicine and often the preferred repair technique for certain demographics of dogs [1–4].

In 1952, an IA repair was described utilizing a lateral fascia lateral graft placed through tibial and femoral bone tunnels and anchored with suture to the soft tissue external to the tunnels [5, 6]. This original repair was modified throughout the years until the "over the top" and "under and over" techniques were developed [5, 7–9]. The decline of IA repairs was likely a combination of personal observation of outcomes of IA repair compared to current extraarticular repairs (including tibial osteotomies and extraarticular sutures), papers with objective outcomes showing superior results with extraarticular repairs [10, 11], and studies demonstrating continued stifle instability, progressive cartilage degeneration, and donor site morbidity with IA repairs [10–17]. These findings are not surprising given the limited mechanical properties of the fascia lata and suture [18].

Despite these limitations, it is possible that the concept of an IA repair was abandoned too quickly and can better mimic the mechanical function of the native cranial cruciate ligament (CCL) compared to tibial osteotomies and extracapsular sutures. By assessing the complications of these previously described techniques, we can hopefully learn and improve future IA repairs techniques.

4.2 Intraarticular Repair Complications in Humans

An extensive review of human anterior cruciate ligament (ACL) repair techniques and complications is beyond the scope of this chapter but a brief review is important to help understand complications in human knee repair and what we may observe on the veterinary side.

In humans, surgery continues to be considered the gold standard for high-performance athletes and adolescent patients, with persistent instability in 75% of patients who do not undergo surgery [19]. The gold standard ACL

Complications in Canine Cranial Cruciate Ligament Surgery, First Edition. Edited by Ron Ben-Amotz and David L. Dycus.

repair technique in humans is reconstruction of an ACL by IA placement of a graft at the origin and insertion of the ACL. Currently, there is no consensus on the ideal graft nor on the method of fixation [20, 21] and new methods of ACL reconstruction, like bridge-enhanced ACL repair, continue to be investigated. To help demonstrate the variety of repair combinations, common grafts include a variety of autografts such as the central third of the patella ligament (bone-ligament-bone graft), hamstring graft, quadriceps graft, allografts from similar donor sites, and prosthetic grafts. Furthermore, it is debated if the grafts should be single, double or quadruple bundled or twisted. Similarly, debate exists among surgeons regarding exact bone tunnel location, graft fixation, graft preconditioning, and graft tensioning. Last, meniscus status can play a large role in outcome, with 50.4% of patients who had a partial or total meniscectomy having osteoarthritis compared to 16.4% without a meniscectomy [22].

Due to this variety, a blanket summary about ideal repair, complication rate, and complication types in human medicine cannot be made. This section rather aims to give an overview of complication rate ranges and the common complications seen in human medicine. This may allow veterinary medicine to better anticipate possible complications after IA techniques and set goals to equal or exceed human success rates.

Complications in human medicine are often characterized into donor site complications during autograft harvesting or repair complications. Donor site complications include pain or numbness (7–57%), patella fracture (7%), and patella tendon rupture (7%) [23]. Repair complications included loss of range of motion of the knee (2–50%), infection (1–2%), hardware removal (5–12%), postoperative meniscal tears (6–10%), and pain during kneeling (44%).

Three recent human systemic reviews have assessed success and complications. A study by de Sa et al. compared an "all-inside technique" and found that autografts (73.8%) continue to be more commonly used compared to an allograft (26.2%) [24]. The complication rate was 5.89% over the 13 studies assessed but the mean follow-up time was limited to only 18 months. Complications included graft rupture (2.47%), loss of knee extension between 1° and 10° (1.14%), and cartilage or meniscal injuries (0.76%). A second recent systematic review compared an "over the top" human technique to placing the graft at the footprints of the ACL [25]. No difference was found between the two techniques, with 94% returning to sports and 69% returning to preinjury level. Another review of 20 studies compared the success of surgery for children and adults [26]. Overall, 92% of people returned to sports, with 78.6% reaching preinjury performance and no difference between groups. The major complication was graft rupture with a high rate of 14%. In high-performance athletes, 83% were able to return to their sport 6–13 months after surgery [27]. Although some athletes did not return to preinjury level, many performed as well as athletes without an injury. A second paper with a 10.5-year follow-up found 98% of amateur athletes returned to sport, with 71.6% returning to their preinjury level [28]. As a comparison, after a tibial plateau leveling osteotomy (TPLO), 65–68% of agility dogs are able to return to activity, although one study found close to 50% of dogs that returned to agility competed at a lower level [29, 30].

Revision surgery is an important area of research in human medicine. Potentially relevant to veterinary medicine, high tibial osteotomies to correct posterior tibial slope during placement of a graft are becoming more common for revision surgery and contemplated for the primary surgery. In humans, an excessive tibial slope is considered to be >12° and is commonly corrected to <5° [31]. Other studies suggest that decreasing the posterior slope helps improve anterior instability and patients who undergo primary repair and have their posterior slope decreased by >5° have a better functional outcome than patients who do not have their slope lessened [32, 33]. In a systematic review of 60 revision surgeries with high tibial osteotomies, no graft rerupture was reported, with the only complication being stiffness in the knee in one case [34]. Fifty-eight percent of these patients had osteoarthritis at follow-up, although 51% had osteoarthritis before the revision surgery.

Besides correcting tibial slope, surgeons can concurrently correct varus. A study used high tibial osteotomies on patients undergoing primary ACL repair who also had medial compartment osteoarthritis [35]. A correction from

7° varus to 1.2° valgus resulted in improved side-to-side instability and improvements of functional outcome measures. It may be necessary to perform similar corrections in dogs for IA repair to be consistently successful. While this may be ideal, it may also result in a procedure with an enormous financial burden to the owner and excessive surgical risks to the patient.

4.3 Intraarticular Repair Complications in Canines

Assessing complications of IA repair in dogs is even more difficult than assessing effectiveness as many studies were performed on a small number of research dogs where CCL transection was performed. This model does not fully reproduce the naturally occurring disease because of patient predisposition to joint disease, duration of disease prior to surgery, postoperative management, etc. Also, there is great variation in graft selection and fixation technique between studies. In addition, for an IA repair to have a chance of being successful, the graft/implant and graft fixation technique need to be strong enough to counteract forces transferred through the stifle during recovery (leash walks, sitting, standing, etc.). Very few studies assess the initial strength of the graft or fixation technique, raising the question whether the technique investigated had little chance of success. Certainly, the biology of any graft repair is important but if the graft cannot survive the mechanical environment it is in, the biology becomes irrelevant. That being said, some studies have objective outcomes such as histopathology and mechanical testing that have greatly aided our understanding of IA repairs. The most common complication reported is graft failure, with progression of osteoarthritis, infection, meniscal injury, and continued instability also described. In the following section, relevant literature will be used to further discuss the frequency of these complications.

A study by Thorson et al. placed bone-ligament-bone auto- and allografts in dogs that had their CCL transected 1 month previously. In the allograft group, 3/11 dogs developed infections and an additional two dogs had no visible graft at the completion of the study (four months postoperatively) [36]. In contrast, autografts (n = 4) were reported as viable at the completion of the study. The allografts caused more inflammatory reaction on the outside of the graft than the autografts. In a study that utilized bone-ligament-bone auto- or allografts in nine dogs, 67% of the grafts survived (9 month follow up) [37]. Despite a easonable graft survival rate, mechanical strengths of the grafts were <14% of the contralateral normal CCL. Neither of these studies reported the mechanical strength of the repair used and the results suggest that mechanical overload and a lack of biological ligamentization played a role in failure. In contrast, a study placing allograft ligaments to replace the CCL gained 90% of CCL strength by 36 weeks [38]. Additional studies have found both positive and negative ability of the graft to heal [12, 39, 40].

The effectiveness of the "over the top" and "under and over" techniques is difficult to assess as most reported outcomes were subjective, retrospective or *ex vivo* mechanical evaluations and did not directly compare these procedures to current repairs, although some papers had some promising results [41–43]. Unfortunately, most available clinical studies assessing the "over the top" and "under and over" techniques look at clinical outcome and success rate and not specific types or reasons for complications [11, 44]. A long-term study looked at dogs with naturally occurring CCL disease repaired with a fascial "over the -top" graft and assessed outcome with an owner questionnaire and force platform analysis. With almost 1.5-year follow-up, owner satisfaction was very high, although gait analysis revealed significantly decreased peak vertical force [45]. Osteoarthritis appears to continue to progress in spite of surgical repair in other studies [13]. Similar results were found in 21 dogs with patella tendon/fascia lata grafts where all owners felt their dog showed significant improvement, although instability and progressive osteoarthritis were commonly documented [46]. Ongoing instability or lengthening of grafts also appeared to be a common complication [12, 47]. A study with 50-month follow-up of the "over the top" technique showed a trend of declining function after improved function over the first year postoperatively [3]. The same researcher found that 60% of dogs had progressive osteoarthritis after IA repair [10]. Other complications less commonly reported include excessive scar tissue at the incision and decreased range of motion [48].

Recently, a number of prospective research studies have been published, looking to learn from past mistakes and overcome the weaknesses of previous repairs. One study looked at placement of IA synthetic grafts [49, 50]. A multifilamentous ultra-high molecular weight polyethylene terephthalate core contained within a braided porous nonexpanded polytetrafluoroethylene sheath ligament was placed through 4.5mm femoral and tibial tunnels and secured with an interference screw and a spiked washer and screw on both the femoral and tibial tunnels. The repairs immediately eliminated cranial drawer but *in vivo* placement had an unacceptably high complication rate. Reported major complications included fixation failure, implant failure, infection, medial luxating patella, meniscal tear, and recurrent instability. All dogs with complications achieved satisfactory results, often with a staged explantation of the implants and a tibial tuberosity advancement.

Work by Lopez et al. evaluated a hamstring autograft that was twisted to a diameter of 4.5mm and secured on the tibia and femur with bone staples [51]. Although the study investigated only four dogs with induced CCL injury, the animals had positive outcomes using subjective and objective outcome measures.

Similarly, two clinical trials evaluated an allograft technique that placed IA allografts secured with a femoral cross pin and tibial spiked washer and screw and separate interference screw in the tibial tunnel, referred to as the TransFix® technique (Arthrex Inc., Naples, FL) (Figure 4.1). Before moving forward with clinical cases, *in vitro* mechanical testing showed graft decellularization minimally affected graft mechanics [52] and initial graft and fixation strength was comparable to a native CCL of a similarly sized dog [53, 54]. When patients had an intact graft at 1 year, they had an excellent clinical outcome. Unfortunately, the technique had a 58% graft failure rate, combining the two studies [55, 56], which lead to a conclusion that although IA grafts can succeed, the technique described was not the solution. Given the high failure rate, it is tempting to abandon IA repairs but understanding the reason for the complications may lead to improvement. Furthermore, major complications of current osteotomy repairs

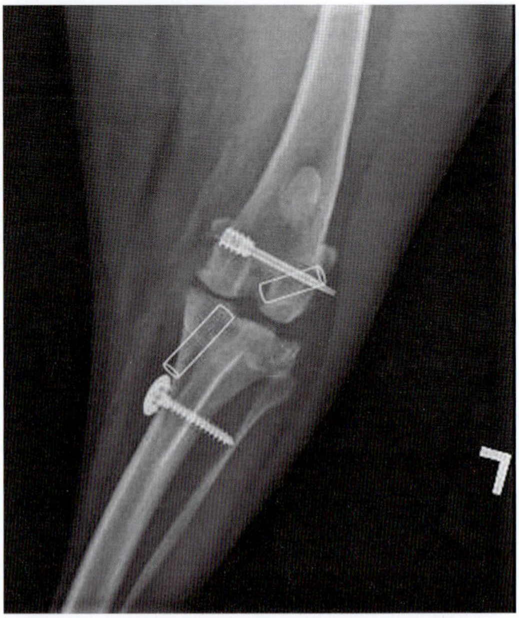

Figure 4.1 Radiograph of a stifle joint with a DDFT allograft secured by use of transverse femoral fixation (allograft looped around a femoral cross pin) and stabilized with a tibial interference screw and two spiked washers on the tibia (DDFT-TF).The tunnels are highlighted with the white outline.

can be upwards of 30%, suggesting that both techniques need improvement [57, 58]. It is suspected that failure with the TransFix® technique was mechanical, as some dogs had femoral-tibial instability as early as the 8-week recheck and no overt signs of graft inflammation were visualized during arthroscopy 1 year postoperatively. If the graft was rejected, it was suspected the remaining graft ends would likely cause continued inflammation. It was hypothesized that graft failure was due to surgeon error (graft damage during placement or improper fixation) or overloading during the early postoperative period. For example, in one dog, the passing wire that was used to pull the looped graft through the bone tunnel twisted and broke. On postoperative radiographs, a 5 mm piece of the wire was identified at the most proximal aspect of the bone tunnel. In humans, it has been shown that a graft weakens during the ligamentization process before regaining strength as native cells repopulate the graft. This highlights the importance of postoperative activity restriction or secondary protection of the graft.

In three other dogs, infections at the tibial bone tunnel exit occurred during the study period, all before the 6-month recheck. Two cases developed draining tracts that could be controlled with antibiotics but when antibiotics were stopped, the draining recurred. Surgical explantation of the screw, washer, and any braided, nonabsorbable suture resolved the infection but the graft was not present on arthroscopy. The third case had radiographs performed that revealed bone lysis at the tibial post site and a minimally displaced tibial fracture. The patient was managed nonsurgically with a splint for 4 weeks, exercise restriction for an additional 8 weeks and antibiotics. Surgical explantation of the screw, washer, and any nonabsorbable suture was performed after the fracture had healed.

Smith et al. assessed a patella bone-tendon-bone ligament autograft and a quadriceps tendon allograft soaked in platelet-rich plasma with a nonabsorbable internal brace in a CCL transection model [59]. At the conclusion of the study 6 months postoperatively, all grafts were intact. The five dogs that received quadricep grafts with an internal brace had similar outcome measures to the control limbs with intact CCLs. Complications seen, more often in the patella group, included residual lameness, pain, effusion, and decreased range of motion of the stifle. Also, the patella graft group saw progression of osteoarthritis and mild fibrillation on arthroscopy. Unique to the quadriceps group, the internal brace was visible in two dogs. Both graft types showed good healing as assessed by histopathology and had similar mechanical strength to the intact CCL during biomechanical testing. This study raises the possibility that biologics, such as platelet-rich plasma or stem cells, may enhance healing of the graft during ligamentization.

4.4 Graft Selection

Based on the available evidence, the ideal graft, graft size, graft length, and graft placement (for example, twisting the graft) are unknown. Furthermore, the ideal initial graft strength, fixation strength, and tension at the time of placement have not been determined in dogs. It is logical to assume that if the graft has similar strength to the native CCL, the strength is adequate. Certainly, that was the goal in more recent studies. However, grafts weaken during healing and ligamentization, a process that takes many months, before regaining strength. In dogs, exercise restriction after surgery for a 4-month period can be challenging, so it may be that initial strength has to be greater than CCL strength.

Initial strength has to be balanced with graft size limitations. In many studies, the maximum size graft that could be safely harvested (autograft) is placed. It is suspected that many autograft techniques have failed because the largest graft possible does not have adequate strength or was not protected (such as internal brace, osteotomy) during healing. In veterinary medicine, using a portion of the straight patella ligament or a strip of the fascia lata is the most commonly reported autograft, although skin, peroneus longus, flexor digitalis pedis longus, long digital extension, periosteum, and semitendinosus/gracilis autografts have all been described [5, 14, 51, 60–64]. Some of these grafts were harvested and used as free grafts, others maintained an original attachment that may have preserved some vascular supply.

For example, patella tendon autograft use, a technique modified from human medicine, allows for either bone or ligament anchor points. The distal end of the graft maintained attachment to the tibia, while the free proximal end was passed through a femoral tunnel and sutured to the gastrocnemius. Very few studies have assessed graft strength or reported dimensions. Tensile testing of the medial third, central third, and lateral third in combination with the fascia lata revealed that no graft was able to mimic the strength or stiffness of the native CCL. Although the central and lateral thirds were stronger than the medial third, it is likely that no partial patella ligament graft has the mechanical properties necessary for recovery in the dog [12, 65]. In fact, it has been reported that the entire patellar tendon is needed to reproduce the mechanical properties of the CCL [53].

The "under and over" technique utilizes the lateral third of the patella tendon and the fascia lata. Described techniques maintain the distal attachment making the graft 15–25 mm wide and 2–3 times the length of the patella-tibial tuberosity length, depending on the method of fixation [47]. Similarly, the "over the top" technique utilizes the medial third of the patella ligament before crossing the patella (harvesting nonarticular bone in the process) and continuing into the fascia lata [66]. The fixation of these grafts varied from suturing to the gastrocnemius to securing them around a screw. *Ex vivo* mechanical testing of these methods suggests their mechanical characteristics are far below those of the intact CCL [18]. Again, this is not only because of the strength of the graft but because of limitations in graft fixation techniques.

Harvesting a hamstring graft has been described by Lopez et al. [51]. A medial skin incision is made over the medial tibia, starting from the patella and heading distally down two-thirds of the tibia. The insertions of the gracilis and semitendinosus muscles are protected while the tendons are dissected free of their muscular origins. The attached dense connective tissue and muscle fascia of the medial aspect of the cranial tibialis muscle are freed to two-thirds the distance of the tibia.

The benefits of using allografts include a natural extracellular matrix (ECM) scaffold with no donor site morbidity, the ability to use entire ligaments (e.g., using the entire patella ligament rather than a third of it), having the donor ligament readily available (no intraoperative collection), and increasing the options of ligaments (e.g., use of the CCL as an allograft). Although allografts have these advantages, they raise concerns about disease transmission, immunological reaction, and alteration of ingrowth characteristics.

Use of allografts has been described in veterinary medicine [39, 67], with studies looking at the ideal graft size, mechanical strength, histology, and clinical outcome [68]. Proper harvesting of allografts requires an understanding of anatomy, asepsis, quality control, and quality assurance. Graft size is often chosen based on the largest tunnel that can be safely drilled in the femur and tibia. In the authors' experience, dogs <32 kg can receive 6 mm tunnels, dogs ≥32 kg and <40 kg can have 6.5 mm tunnels, and dogs ≥40 kg can have 7 mm tunnels created. Of course, individual variability exists beyond body weight. Graft length depends on the fixation technique. For example, for the TransFix® technique, a graft has to be much longer ([length of tibia tunnel + length of femoral tunnel + native CCL length] × 2 + 2 cm for fixation) than a technique that uses a single-strand graft secured in the tunnels.

4.5 Tunnel Creation

The CCL is not a simple band and the fan-like attachment to the axial aspect of the lateral condyle and craniomedial tibia, underneath the intermeniscal ligament, makes placement of bone tunnels challenging. In humans, it has been shown that bone tunnel placement at the footprints of the ACL may not be perfectly isometric points. In dogs, it is suggested that the isometric location may be caudal to the origin of the CCL on the femur and cranial to the footprint on the tibia. Given the complexity of movement in the stifle during range of motion, it was decided to place the origin of the bone tunnels at the footprints for the TransFix® procedure. The authors found it quite straightforward to identify the footprint, measure its size, and drill a guide pin at the desired angle through the center of the footprint. However, the angle of the guide pin often had to be adjusted so the selected drill bit could be used without causing iatrogenic damage to the femoral condyle.

4.6 Graft Fixation

The optimal method of graft fixation is not known in human medicine and likely depends on the type of graft utilized. Multiple techniques for securing bone-ligament and ligamentous grafts have been described, including interference screws, pinning, suture anchors, spiked washers, and suture [69].

Interference screws are easy to use, size can be changed according to size of the graft/tunnel ratio, and they improve contact between the bone tunnel and graft. When using grafts that are folded to double the graft, such as the hamstring tendon or deep digital flexor tendon (DDFT), a cross pin technique can be used. Cross pin transfixation techniques pass a pin through the loop created at the fold in the graft (Figure 4.2). The remaining graft ends can be secured with one of the previously

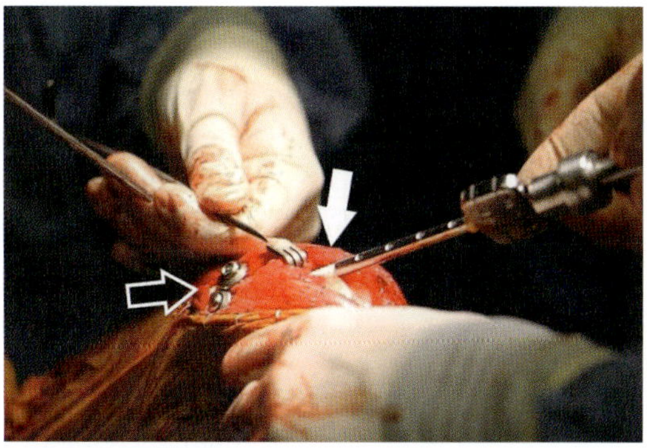

Figure 4.2 Intraoperative photograph of a DDFT allograft repair using the TransFix® system to secure the looped ligament on the femoral side and spiked washers (open arrow) and interference screw (closed arrow) to secure the ligament on the tibial side.

mentioned techniques. Suture and anchors appear to be gaining popularity for human graft fixation given the ease of use and versatility. Often a braided suture is incorporated into the graft, exited out the bone tunnel and secured to a bone anchor or similar fixation system. The main concern with this fixation is having braided material in the joint and bone tunnels.

Empirically, IA cases that mechanically fail tend to fail early in the recovery process. Failure at the fixation site is a concern due to inappropriate initial strength. A unique challenge in the dog is that initial fixation strength has to overcome daily forces generated by the patient. Often a gradual increase in weight bearing is not possible as it is in humans. For example, in cadaver canine stifles, it was shown that an entire patella ligament secured with interference screws or bone anchors was likely not strong enough to withstand daily physiological loads, although these fixation techniques are used in humans [54]. Before attempting any IA repair, it is important that the mechanical strength of the graft–fixation technique combination is determined.

If there is fixation failure, it is likely that the graft is damaged and needs to be replaced. If an autograft was utilized, an allograft may need to be considered on revision. Similarly, damage to local anatomy has to be assessed to determine if a similar fixation technique can be used. The authors suspect that with a failed IA repair, an extracapsular suture or tibial osteotomy could be pursued after explantation of implants and graft. More specifically, a CORA-based leveling osteotomy (CBLO) might be a better tibial osteotomy technique because the osteotomy site could be made below any existing proximal tunnel sites.

4.7 Intraarticular Repair Assessment and Revision

Recheck examinations are important to assess IA graft repair as the presence of stifle instability documents that the graft is no longer functional. Nonweight-bearing radiographs can help assess implants and bone tunnels although bone tunnels cannot be clearly identified in all cases. Similarly, weight-bearing radiographs may help document elongation/failure of a graft. Subluxation measurements can be compared to the contralateral limb, assuming there are no abnormalities in that stifle [55, 70]. Palpation and radiographs may still miss some graft failures as direct palpation and the patient standing induce loads below physiological forces required for walking, running or jumping on the limb.

Currently there are no guidelines for the acceptable amount of cranial drawer or subluxation on weight-bearing radiographs. A normal CCL allows 2–3 mm of femoral-tibial translation and, while patients can have good long-term outcomes (i.e., owner survey, gait analysis) with some instability, it has been reported that after IA repair dogs without palpable instability and an intact graft generally have an excellent outcome [56]. Empirically, after IA reconstruction, patients that developed femoral-tibial instability greater than 10 mm had lameness on a consistent basis; palpable instability less than that was not correlated to patient function. For this reason, the actual complication rate of an IA technique likely cannot be determined without documentation of graft survival. The TransFix® technique demonstrated an excellent outcome on owner questionnaire (close to 100% satisfaction), a good outcome with force plate analysis (similar to slightly better outcomes compared to TPLO results) but a poor outcome with second-look arthroscopy for IA repair. The authors recommended that IA repairs be assessed by visualization or advanced imaging

6–12 months postoperatively to document survival. Even with these imaging modalities, true health of the graft cannot be assessed and biopsy would likely be needed (not necessarily recommended by the authors due to damage to the graft).

If graft failure is detected, the correct course of action depends upon the patient, owner, and surgeon. In our experience, if we palpated femoral-tibial instability but the dog had limb asymmetry <15% on force platform analysis and the owners had no complaints about limb function, we recommended to continue monitoring with no action taken. Practically, the goal is to resolve pain and lameness; we have not made a recommendation for surgery simply because there was palpable femoral-tibial translation. In cases where lameness persists and/or infection is detected, complete explantation of all implants and graft is recommended. In our experience, once the graft has failed, the implants were easy to remove as the grafts tend to fail early in the recovery period before healing has occurred. A stifle stabilizing surgery after implant removal depended upon the cause (e.g., infection, lameness, and joint pain with graft failure) and the amount of femoral-tibial instability.

4.8 Conclusion

The experience from previous studies provides a small but important insight into IA repair failure in veterinary medicine. First, IA grafts can survive and result in an excellent patient outcome [51, 56, 59]. A remaining question is whether successful results can be obtained consistently. Second, graft survival appears to be higher when a CCL transection model is used compared to naturally occurring CCL disease. Caution should be exercised when determining the success and complications of IA repair when using an induced CCL model. Third, given the limited studies on naturally occurring CCL disease with IA repair, lack of studies using surgical techniques and/or implants that have been fully vetted and inconsistency in study designs, definitive rates and recommendations about complications are not possible. Finally, with IA repair it is important to note that the actual complication rate of a technique likely cannot be determined without documentation of graft survival. For example, an IA allograft repair demonstrated an excellent outcome on owner questionnaire, a good outcome with force plate analysis, and a poor outcome with second-look arthroscopy [56]. This and many other studies document the importance of objective outcome measures for gauging both success and specific complications.

Based on lessons learned, the authors recommend the following when evaluating IA repairs: (i) the initial biomechanical properties of the graft and fixation technique are documented, (ii) follow-up time of at least 12 months to allow ligamentization, and (iii) graft survival is evaluated by second-look arthroscopy (or advanced imaging as technology advances).

4.9 Clinical Examples

In the following section, the authors use examples to illustrate complications, clinical consequences, and success of revision therapy.

Clinical Example 4.1 Allograft or Autograft Harvesting

Graft harvesting can result in complications for both auto- and allografts. Autograft donor site morbidity has been well documented in both human and veterinary medicine and may explain the inferior outcomes of a bone-patella-bone autograft compared to an allograft [59]. For both auto- and allografts, damage to the graft during harvest (Figure 4.3), storage or preparation (Figure 4.4) may predispose to failure. After allograft harvesting, the ligaments are wrapped in sterile gauze, soaked in phosphate-buffered saline (PBS), and frozen at −80 °C. They are shipped in Styrofoam™ shipping containers on dry ice that will last 48 hours. Upon receipt of the graft, it should be placed in a −80 °C freezer until use. Grafts can be removed from the freezer 1–2 hours before surgery and stored at room temperature. In the operating room, the inner sterile package can be placed in warm sterile saline to finish the thawing process (~30–60 minutes).

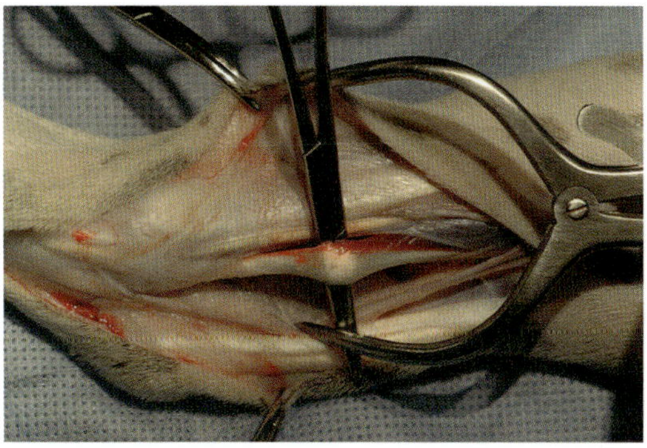

Figure 4.3 Harvesting a DDFT allograft for use in an IA repair. Damaging tendon fibers is possible during dissection, if care is not taken.

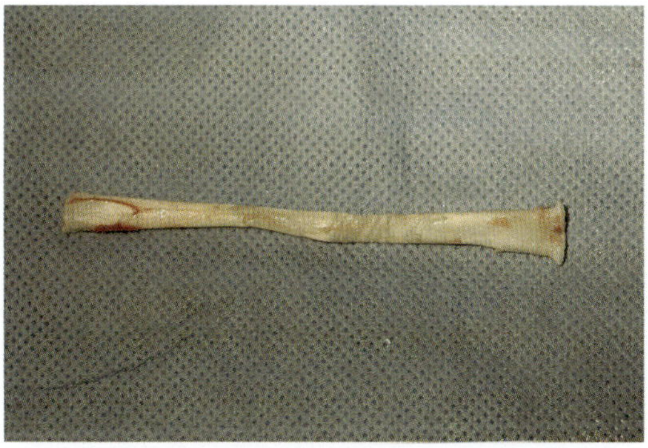

Figure 4.4 A DDFT allograft after harvest. Due to the inconsistent circumference, the tendon has to be trimmed proximally and distally. A graft prep-board aids in accurate trimming but damage is possible as trimming is performed by hand.

Clinical Example 4.2 Tunnel Creation

Most IA repairs use tunnels (Figures 4.5 and 4.6) that are created in the femur and tibia. Precise location of these tunnels is important although the ideal entry point into the joint and angle of the tunnel are debated. In humans, it has been shown that bone tunnel placement at the footprints of the ACL may not be perfectly isometric points [71]. In dogs, it is suggested that the isometric location may be caudal to the origin of the CCL [72]. Improper placement can lead to impingement of the graft or wear and tear leading to failure. Empirically, a graft or implant that has a large enough diameter to reproduce the mechanics of the patients CCL has limited drilling angle options without iatrogenic injury.

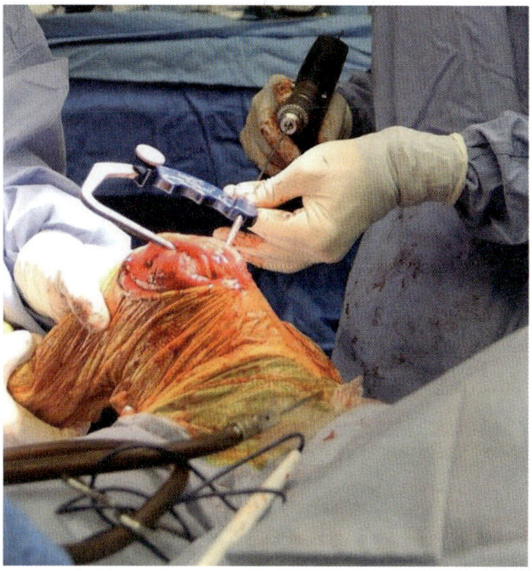

Figure 4.5 Placement of bone tunnels can be aided by use of an aiming guide. Drilling a guide pin initially can help document correct location and orientation of a bone tunnel before overdrilling to the final tunnel diameter.

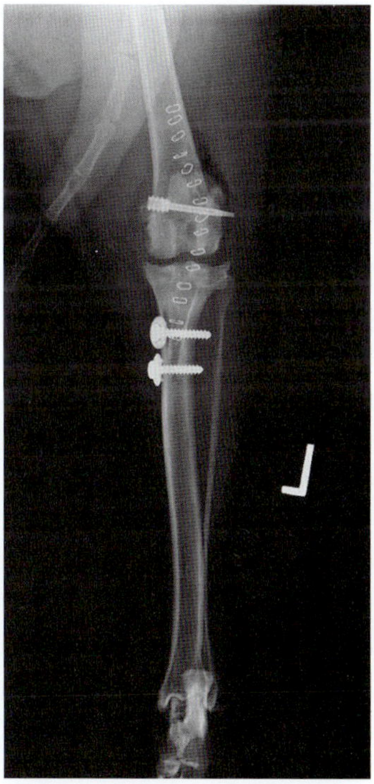

Figure 4.6 Bone tunnels are often difficult to visualize on postoperative radiographs, making assessment difficult. This radiograph is immediately postoperative after an IA repair with a DDFT secured with a cross pin and spiked washer and screw.

Clinical Example 4.3 Graft Placement

A second step common to IA repair is placement of the graft. Most procedures rely on a snug fit of the graft in a bone tunnel which can require substantial force to pull the graft into position. This is often carried out with suture or wire (Figure 4.7), both of which can potentially damage the graft. Finally, a graft can be damaged during fixation. Some techniques purposely deform or pierce the graft, such as an interference screw or spike washer. Other techniques anchor suture that is attached to the graft. The difficulty with any IA repair utilizing a natural graft is that graft damage is often microscopic.

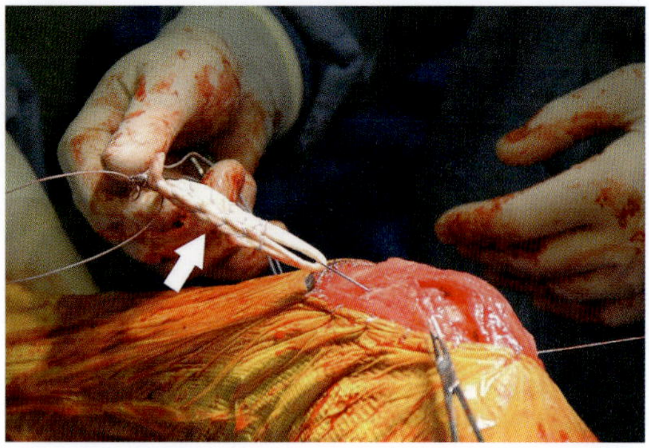

Figure 4.7 A challenge of IA repair can be passing the graft through the bone tunnels. This technique loops the graft over a wire to pull it into the tibial and femoral bone tunnels. Intraoperative damage to the graft was noted in multiple cases and a new allograft had to be placed. Note the braided suture in the ends of the graft to help with tensioning (arrow).

Clinical Example 4.4 Graft Fixation

Consistent execution of the surgery depends on the difficulty of the technique and experience of the surgeon, among many other variables. Each technique will have its own unique challenges but intraoperative and postoperative assessment will continue to be important. Complications seen when using a spiked washer to secure the graft include improper purchase of the graft with the teeth of the washer, breaking the cis or trans cortex during screw tightening, and monocortical purchase of the screw. When using a cross pin to capture a looped graft, complications can include damage to the graft, missing the graft with the implant, and breaking the looping wire (Figure 4.8).

Clinical Example 4.5 Graft Failure

Graft failure (Figures 4.9–4.11) is a common complication in human medicine (~5–10%) and will likely be a common complication in veterinary medicine. It is difficult to confirm the rate of graft rupture in veterinary medicine as follow-up magnetic resonance imaging (MRI) is uncommon and no objective method to document femoral-tibial translation is commonly used. In research models of induced CCL disease in dogs, auto- and allograft survival tends to be excellent. These results may not perfectly translate to the clinical setting.

(a) (b) (c)

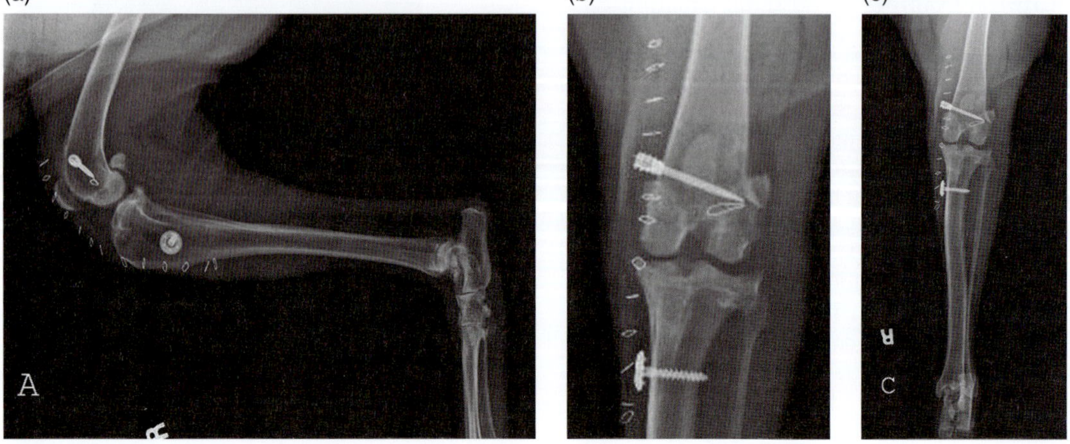

Figure 4.8 **(a–c)** A 6.8-year-old male neutered Labrador Retriever (33 kg) had the cross pin wire break during the procedure. The immediate postoperative radiographs show the broken wire and that the cross pin was not fully seated (a: mediolateral, b: enlarged caudocranial, c: caudocranial). It was elected to not revise the surgery because the stifle palpated stable. At 12 months, the graft was intact and the dog had a net ground reaction force that was 94.5% of normal.

In 19 dogs with CCL disease that had second-look arthroscopy, 10 had graft failure although 68% of the dogs had an excellent outcome on force plate analysis. From this experience, it is suggested that graft assessment (Figures 4.8 and 4.9) at follow-up is necessary to accurately comment on the success of an IA technique.

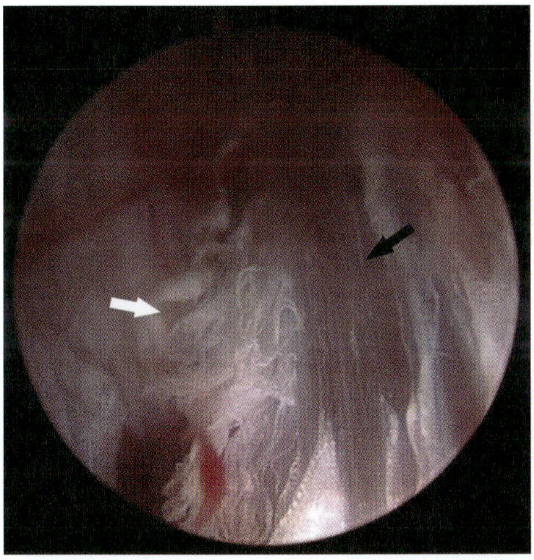

Figure 4.9 A 4.5-year-old male neutered Boxer (35 kg) presented for second-look arthroscopy (scheduled) 12 months after surgery. The dog was not visibly lame and had returned to preinjury activity. Net ground reaction force was within 93% of normal. The arthroscopy image shows a partially torn allograft (torn fibers: white arrow; intact fibers: black arrow).

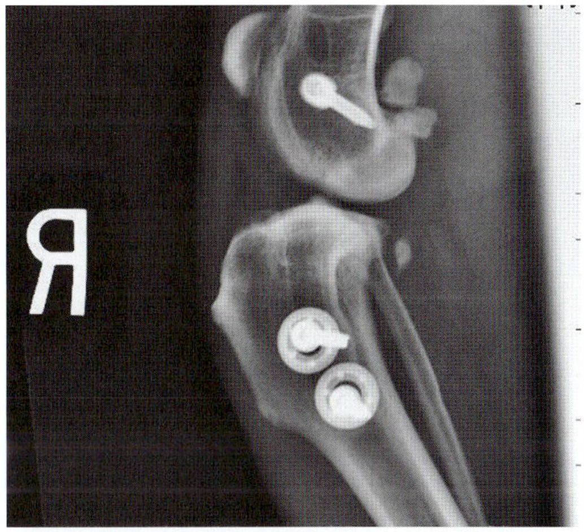

Figure 4.10 This radiograph was taken while the patient was weight bearing. The image demonstrates cranial tibial subluxation, suggesting that the graft had failed.

(a) (b)

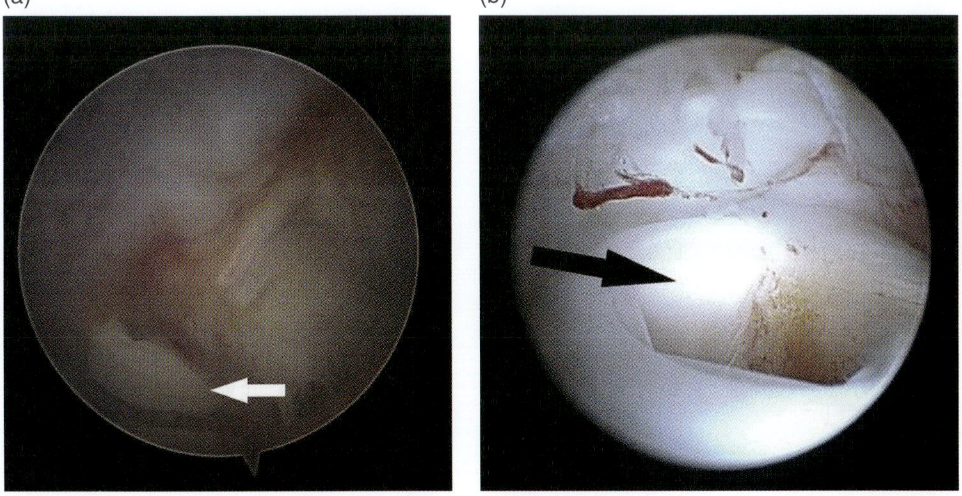

Figure 4.11 **(a)** A 4.5-year-old female spayed Labrador Retriever (33 kg) presented for a 12-month second-look arthroscopy (scheduled). The owners were pleased with the patient's improvement and exercise ability. Net ground reaction force was 86% of normal. The arthroscopy image shows a completely torn graft and an interference screw that has partially migrated into the joint (arrow). **(b)** The insert shows a close-up of the interference screw (screw head: black arrow).

Clinical Example 4.6 Infection

Infection is an uncommon complication described in humans with IA repair although a 10% infection rate is described for allograft repair with a DDFT in dogs (Figures 4.12 and 4.13) [55, 56].

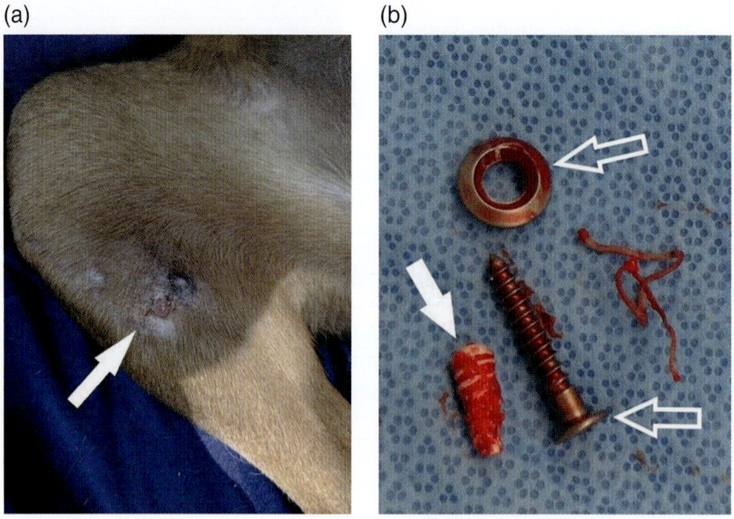

Figure 4.12 (a) A 2.5-year-old male neutered mixed-breed dog (23 kg) presented for a draining tract (arrow) 3 months after IA repair secured to the tibia with a spiked washer and screw (open arrows) and interference screw (closed arrow). (b) Braided material was present to help tension the graft under the washer and may have contributed to the chronic infection.

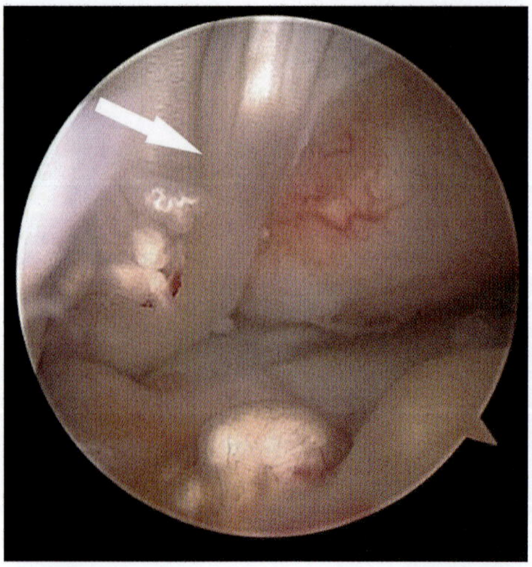

Figure 4.13 The arthroscopy image shows the remnants of the graft (white arrow) taken at the time of implant removal (from the previous case). It is suspected that the tibial implants are more likely to become infected because there is very little soft tissue coverage over the medial tibia. Also, braided, nonabsorbable suture is secured to the ligament in this area. The infections were controlled with oral antibiotics but clinical signs returned when treatment was stopped. Implant removal was necessary along with oral antibiotics to resolve the infection. It is suspected that the infection caused loosening of the graft fixation, leading to mechanical failure.

Clinical Example 4.7 Progressive Osteoarthritis

An important complication is progressive osteoarthritis (Figure 4.14). Nearly all dogs with currently performed tibial osteotomy repairs have documented osteoarthritis after surgical treatment, affecting long-term success [13, 43, 73]. IA repairs have minimal data showing the long-term rate of osteoarthritis. In a small study of 10 dogs receiving IA repairs, there was no significant progression of the osteoarthritis score over 12 months [55]. Further work will have to be done to find the true rate of progressive osteoarthritis after IA repair.

(a) (b)

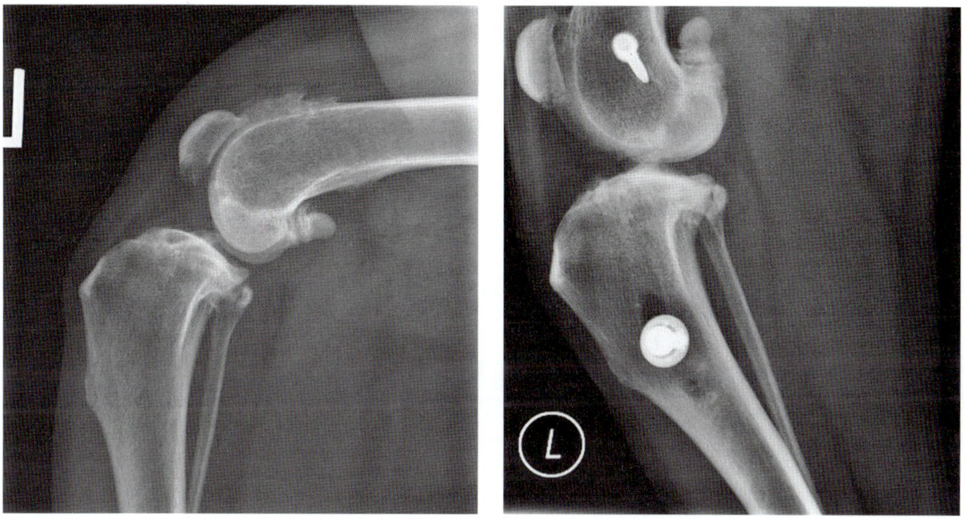

Figure 4.14 (a) Preoperative and (b) 12-month follow-up radiographs from a dog that has undergone an IA repair with a DDFT allograft. The 12-month radiograph was taken with the dog weight bearing. Progression of osteoarthritis can be appreciated at the proximal patella and cranial tibial plateau. Subluxation of the tibia is also apparent, suggesting graft failure.

Clinical Example 4.8 Fracture of the Femur or Tibia

In order to maximize the initial strength of the graft and fixation, very large tunnels have to be created in the tibia and femur. A safe bone tunnel to bone diameter size has not been determined (Figure 4.15).

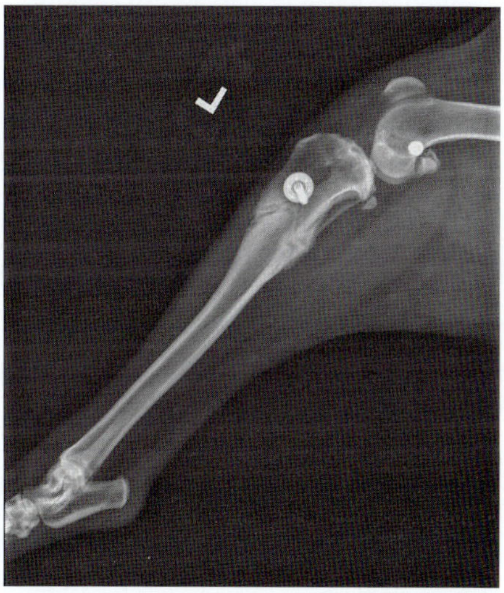

Figure 4.15 A 6.5-year-old female spayed Labrador presented with an acute nonweight-bearing lameness on the operated leg 4 months after surgery. Radiographs revealed bone lysis at the tibial screw site and a minimally displaced tibial fracture. The patient was managed nonsurgically with a splint for 4 weeks, exercise restriction for an additional 8 weeks, and antibiotics. At 7 months after surgery, the fracture had bridging osteosynthesis but lysis was still present around the tibial implants. Surgical explantation of the screw, washer, and any nonabsorbable suture was recommended and performed without complication. Second-look arthroscopy showed complete resorption of the allograft ligament. This dog had residual lameness at the time of second-look arthroscopy and was considered to have an unsuccessful outcome.

References

1. Korvick, D.L., Johnson, A.L., and Schaeffer, D.J. (1994). Surgeons' preferences in treating cranial cruciate ligament ruptures in dogs. *J. Am. Vet. Med. Assoc.* 205: 1318–1324.
2. Moore, K.W. and Read, R.A. (1995). Cranial cruciate ligament rupture in the dog – a retrospective study comparing surgical techniques. *Aust. Vet. J.* 72: 281–285.
3. Innes, J.F., Bacon, D., Lynch, C., and Pollard, A. (2000). Long-term outcome of surgery for dogs with cranial cruciate ligament deficiency. *Vet. Rec.* 147: 325–328.
4. Garcia, É.F.V., Schossler, J.E.W., and Pinheiro, M. (2012). Cranial cruciate ligament rupture in a cat: reconstitution with fascia lata. *Ciênc. Rural* 42: 1446–1449.
5. Knecht, C.D. (1976). Evolution of surgical techniques for cruciate ligament rupture in animals. *J. Am. Anim. Hosp. Assoc.* 12: 717–726.
6. Burnett, Q.M. and Fowler, P.J. (1985). Reconstruction of the anterior cruciate: historical review. *Orthop. Clin. North Am.* 16: 143–157.
7. Singleton, W.B. (1969). Observations based upon the surgical repair of 106 cases of anterior cruciate ligament rupture. *J. Small Anim. Pract.* 10: 269–278.
8. Hulse, D.A., Michaelson, F., Johnson, C. et al. (1980). A technique for reconstruction of the anterior cruciate ligament in the dog: preliminary report. *Vet. Surg.* 4: 135–140.
9. Shires, P.K., Hulse, D.A., and Liu, W. (1984). The under-and-over fascial replacement technique for anterior cruciate ligament rupture in the dog: a retrospective study. *J. Am. Anim. Hosp. Assoc.* 20: 69–77.
10. Innes, J.F., Costello, M., Barr, F.J. et al. (2004). Radiographic progression of osteoarthritis of the canine stifle joint: a prospective study. *Vet. Radiol. Ultrasound* 45: 143–148.
11. Conzemius, M.G., Evans, R.B., Besancon, M.F. et al. (2005). Effect of surgical technique on limb function after surgery for rupture of the cranial cruciate ligament in dogs. *J. Am. Vet. Med. Assoc.* 226: 232–236.
12. Butler, D.L., Hulse, D.A., Kay, M.D. et al. (1983). Biomechanics of cranial cruciate ligament reconstruction in the dog II. Mechanical properties. *Vet. Surg.* 12: 112–118.
13. Elkins, A.D., Pechman, R., Kearney, M.T., and Heron, M. (1991). A retrospective study evaluating the degree of degenerative joint disease in the stifle joint of dogs following surgical repair of anterior cruciate ligament rupture. *J. Am. Anim. Hosp. Assoc.* 27: 533–540.
14. Innes, J.F., Barr, A.R., and Sharif, M. (2000). Efficacy of oral calcium pentosan polysulphate for the treatment of osteoarthritis of the canine stifle joint secondary to cranial cruciate ligament deficiency. *Vet. Rec.* 146: 433–437.
15. Johnson, K.A., Hart, R.C., Chu, Q. et al. (2001). Concentrations of chondroitin sulfate epitopes 3B3 and 7D4 in synovial fluid after intra-articular and extracapsular reconstruction of the cranial cruciate ligament in dogs. *Am. J. Vet. Res.* 62: 581–587.
16. Snow, L.A., White, R., Gustafson, S. et al. (2010). Ex vivo comparison of three surgical techniques to stabilize canine cranial cruciate ligament deficient stifles. *Vet. Surg.* 39: 195–207.
17. Mölsä, S.H., Hielm-Björkman, A.K., and Laitinen-Vapaavuori, O.M. (2013). Use of an owner questionnaire to evaluate long-term surgical outcome and chronic pain after cranial cruciate ligament repair in dogs: 253 cases (2004–2006). *J. Am. Vet. Med. Assoc.* 243: 689–695.
18. Patterson, R.H., Smith, G.K., Gregor, T.P. et al. (1991). Biomechanical stability of four cranial cruciate ligament repair techniques in the dog. *Vet. Surg.* 20: 85–90.
19. Dunn, K.L., Lam, K.C., and Valovich McLeod, T.C. (2016). Early operative versus delayed or nonoperative treatment of anterior cruciate ligament injuries in pediatric patients. *J. Athl. Train.* 51: 425–427.
20. Murray, M.M. (2009). Current status and potential of primary ACL repair. *Clin. Sports Med.* 28: 51–61.
21. Shaerf, D.A., Pastides, P.S., Sarraf, K.M. et al. (2014). Anterior cruciate ligament reconstruction best practice: a review of graft choice. *World J. Orthop.* 5: 23–29.
22. Ruano, J.S., Sitler, M.R., and Driban, J.B. (2017). Prevalence of radiographic knee osteoarthritis after anterior cruciate ligament reconstruction, with or without meniscectomy: an evidence-based practice article. *J. Athl. Train.* 52: 606–609.
23. Grassi, A., Kim, C., Marcheggiani Muccioli, G.M. et al. (2017). What is the mid-term failure rate of revision ACL reconstruction? A systematic review. *Clin. Orthop. Relat. Res.* 475: 2484–2499.
24. de Sa, D., Shanmugaraj, A., Weidman, M. et al. (2018). All-inside anterior cruciate ligament reconstruction – a systematic review of techniques, outcomes, and complications. *J. Knee Surg.* 31: 895–904.
25. Sarraj, M., de Sa, D., Shanmugaraj, A. et al. (2019). Over-the-top ACL reconstruction yields comparable outcomes to traditional ACL reconstruction in primary and revision settings: a systematic review. *Knee Surg. Sports Traumatol. Arthrosc.* 27: 427–444.
26. Kay, J., Memon, M., Marx, R.G. et al. (2018). Over 90% of children and adolescents return to sport after anterior cruciate ligament reconstruction: a systematic review and meta-analysis. *Knee Surg. Sports Traumatol. Arthrosc.* 26: 1019–1036.

27. Lai, C.C.H., Ardern, C.L., Feller, J.A. et al. (2018). Eighty-three per cent of elite athletes return to preinjury sport after anterior cruciate ligament reconstruction: a systematic review with meta-analysis of return to sport rates, graft rupture rates and performance outcomes. *Br. J. Sports Med.* 52: 128–138.
28. Legnani, C., Peretti, G.M., Del Re, M. et al. (2019). Return to sports and re-rupture rate following anterior cruciate ligament reconstruction in amateur sportsman: long-term outcomes. *J. Sports Med. Phys. Fitness* 59: 1902–1907.
29. Heidorn, S.N., Canapp, S.O., Zink, C.M. et al. (2018). Rate of return to agility competition for dogs with cranial cruciate ligament tears treated with tibial plateau leveling osteotomy. *J. Am. Vet. Med. Assoc.* 253: 1439–1444.
30. Tomlinson, J.E. and Manfredi, J.M. (2018). Return to sport after injury: a web-based survey of owners and handlers of agility dogs. *Vet. Comp. Orthop. Traumatol.* 31: 473–478.
31. Dejour, D., Saffarini, M., Demey, G. et al. (2015). Tibial slope correction combined with second revision ACL produces good knee stability and prevents graft rupture. *Knee Surg. Sports Traumatol. Arthrosc.* 23: 2846–2852.
32. Sonnery-Cottet, B., Mogos, S., Thaunat, M. et al. (2014). Proximal tibial anterior closing wedge osteotomy in repeat revision of anterior cruciate ligament reconstruction. *Am. J. Sports Med.* 42: 1873–1880.
33. Arun, G.R., Kumaraswamy, V., Rajan, D. et al. (2016). Long-term follow up of single-stage anterior cruciate ligament reconstruction and high tibial osteotomy and its relation with posterior tibial slope. *Arch. Orthop. Trauma Surg.* 136: 505–511.
34. Gupta, A., Tejpal, T., Shanmugaraj, A. et al. (2019). Surgical techniques, outcomes, indications, and complications of simultaneous high tibial osteotomy and anterior cruciate ligament revision surgery: a systematic review. *HSS J.* 15: 176–184.
35. Jin, C., Song, E.K., Jin, Q.H. et al. (2018). Outcomes of simultaneous high tibial osteotomy and anterior cruciate ligament reconstruction in anterior cruciate ligament deficient knee with osteoarthritis. *BMC Musculoskelet. Disord.* 19: 228–233.
36. Thorson, E., Rodrigo, J.J., Vasseur, P. et al. (1989). Replacement of the anterior cruciate ligament. A comparison of autografts and allografts in dogs. *Acta Orthop. Scand.* 60: 555–560.
37. Vasseur, P.B., Rodrigo, J.J., Stevenson, S. et al. (1987). Replacement of the anterior cruciate ligament with a bone-ligament-bone anterior cruciate ligament allograft in dogs. *Clin. Orthop. Relat. Res.* 219: 268–277.
38. Nikolaou, P.K., Seaber, A.V., Glisson, R.R. et al. (1986). Anterior cruciate ligament allograft transplantation. Long-term function, histology, revascularization, and operative technique. *Am. J. Sports Med.* 14: 348–360.
39. Shino, K., Kawasaki, T., Hirose, H. et al. (1984). Replacement of the anterior cruciate ligament by an allogeneic tendon graft. An experimental study in the dog. *J. Bone Joint Surg. Br.* 66: 672–681.
40. Arnoczky, S.P., Tarvin, G.P., and Marshall, J.L. (1982). Anterior cruciate ligament replacement using patella tendon. *J. Bone Joint Surg.* 64: 217–224.
41. Pichler, M.E., Bacon, J.P., and Evans, J.A. (1982). The fascia lata as a replacement for the cranial cruciate ligament: two new surgical techniques. *J. Am. Anim. Hosp. Assoc.* 18: 779.
42. Denny, H.R. and Barr, A.R.S. (1987). A further evaluation of the "over-the-top" technique for anterior cruciate ligament replacement in the dog. *J. Small Anim. Pract.* 28: 681–686.
43. Innes, J.F. and Barr, A.R. (1998). Clinical natural history of the postsurgical cruciate deficient canine stifle joint: year 1. *J. Small Anim. Pract.* 39: 325–332.
44. Bacon, J.P., Pichler, M.E., Lynd, F.T., and Evans, J.A. (1984). Histopathological examination of two cranial cruciate ligament reconstructions. *J. Am. Anim. Hosp. Assoc.* 20: 65–68.
45. Geels, J.J., Roush, J.K., Hoskinson, J.J. et al. (2000). Evaluation of an intracapsular technique for the treatment of cranial cruciate ligament rupture. *Vet. Comp. Orthop. Traumatol.* 13: 197–203.
46. Vasseur, P.B. and Berry, C.R. (1991). Progression of stifle osteoarthrosis following reconstruction of the cranial cruciate ligament in 21 dogs. *J. Am. Anim. Hosp. Assoc.* 28: 129–136.
47. Coetzee, G.L. and Lubbe, A.M. (1995). A prospective study comparing two fascial reconstruction techniques to stabilise the cranial cruciate deficient stifle in the dog. *Vet. Comp. Orthop. Traumatol.* 8: 82–90.
48. Mölsä, S.H., Hyytiäinen, H.K., Hielm-Björkman, A.K. et al. (2014). Long-term functional outcome after surgical repair of cranial cruciate ligament disease in dogs. *BMC Vet. Res.* 10: 266.
49. Barnhart, M.D., Maritato, K., Schankereli, K. et al. (2016). Evaluation of an intra-articular synthetic ligament for treatment of cranial cruciate ligament disease in dogs: a six-month prospective clinical trial. *Vet. Comp. Orthop. Traumatol.* 29: 491–498.
50. Barnhart, M.D., Bufkin, B.W., and Litsky, A.S. (2019). Biomechanical comparison of four methods of fixation of a polymeric cranial cruciate ligament in the canine femur and tibia. *Vet. Comp. Orthop. Traumatol.* 32: 112–116.
51. Lopez, M.J., Markel, M.M., Kalsheur, V.L. et al. (2003). Hamstring graft technique for stabilization of canine cranial cruciate ligament deficient stifles. *Vet. Surg.* 32: 390–401.

52. Balogh, D.G., Biskup, J.J., O'Sullivan, M.G. et al. (2016). Biochemical, histologic, and biomechanical characterization of native and decellularized flexor tendons specimens harvested from the pelvic limbs of orthopedically normal dogs. *Am. J. Vet. Res.* 77: 388–394.
53. Biskup, J., Freeman, A., Camisa, W. et al. (2014). Mechanical properties of canine patella-ligament-tibia segment. *Vet. Surg.* 43: 136–141.
54. Biskup, J.J., Balogh, D.G., Haynes, K.H. et al. (2015). Mechanical strength of four allograft fixation techniques for ruptured cranial cruciate ligament repair in dogs. *Am. J. Vet. Res.* 76: 411–419.
55. Biskup, J.J., Balogh, D.G., Scott, R.M., and Conzemius, M.G. (2017). Long-term outcome of an intra-articular allograft technique for treatment of spontaneous cranial cruciate ligament rupture in the dog. *Vet. Surg.* 46: 691–699.
56. Biskup, J.J. and Conzemius, M.G. (2020). Long-term arthroscopic assessment of intra-articular allografts for treatment of spontaneous cranial cruciate ligament rupture in the dog. *Vet. Surg.* 49: 764–771.
57. Cappelle, K.K. and Barnhart, M.D. (2019). Short-term complications following single-session versus staged bilateral tibial plateau levelling osteotomies stabilized with locking plates for treatment of bilateral cranial cruciate ligament disease: a retrospective study. *Vet. Comp. Orthop. Traumatol.* 32: 460–466.
58. Ferrell, C.L., Barnhart, M.D., and Herman, E. (2019). Impact of postoperative antibiotics on rates of infection and implant removal after tibial tuberosity advancement in 1,768 canine stifles. *Vet. Surg.* 48: 694–699.
59. Smith, P.A., Stannard, J.P., Bozynski, C.C. et al. (2019). Patellar bone-tendon-bone autografts versus quadriceps tendon allograft with synthetic augmentation in a canine model. *J. Knee Surg.* 33: 1256–1266.
60. Chiroff, R.T. (1975). Experimental replacement of the anterior cruciate ligament. *J. Bone Joint Surg.* 57A: 1124–1127.
61. Arnoczky, S.P., Tarvin, G.P., Marshall, J.L., and Saltzman, B. (1978). The over-the-top procedure: a technique for anterior cruciate ligament substitution in the dog. *J. Am. Anim. Hosp. Assoc.* 15: 283–290.
62. Ramanaiah, C.V., Ramakrishna, O., and Sreeraman, P.K. (1990). Chondrogenic potential of free intra-articular periosteal autografts in dogs. *Indian Vet. J.* 67: 844–847.
63. Veena, P., Ramakrishna, O., Bharathi, S., and Rao, T.C.S. (2003). Reconstruction of ruptured cranial cruciate ligament using whole thickness skin and patellar ligament as a graft in canines. *Indian Vet. J.* 80: 432–434.
64. Penha, E.M., Rezende, C.M.F., Melo, E.G. et al. (2007). Late postoperative of cranial cruciate ligament replacement in dog. *Arq. Bras. Med. Vet. Zootec.* 59: 1184–1193.
65. Johnson, S.G., Hulse, D.A., Hogan, H.A. et al. (1989). System behavior of commonly used cranial cruciate ligament reconstruction autografts. *Vet. Surg.* 18: 459–465.
66. Piermattei, D.L., Flo, G.L., and DeCamp, C.E. (2006). *Handbook of Small Animal Orthopedics and Fracture Repair*, 4e, 599–601. St Louis, MO: Elsevier.
67. Vasseur, P.B., Stevenson, S., Gregory, C.R. et al. (1991). Anterior cruciate ligament allograft transplantation in dogs. *Clin. Orthop. Relat. Res.* 269: 295–304.
68. Qu, J., Thoreson, A.R., An, K.N., and Amadio, P.C. (2015). What is the best candidate allograft for ACL reconstruction? An in vitro mechanical and histologic study in a canine model. *J. Biomech.* 48: 1811–1816.
69. Hill, C., An, Y.H., and Young, F.A. (2005). Tendon and ligament fixation to bone. In: *Repair of Ligament and Tendons* (ed. W. Walsh), 257–278. Totowa, NJ: Humana Press.
70. Kim, S.E., Lewis, D.D., and Pozzi, A. (2012). Effect of tibial plateau leveling osteotomy on femorotibial subluxation: in vivo analysis during standing. *Vet. Surg.* 4: 465–470.
71. Austin, J.C., Phornphutkul, C., and Wojtys, E.M. (2007). Loss of knee extension after anterior cruciate ligament reconstruction: effects of knee position and graft tensioning. *J. Bone Joint Surg. Am.* 89: 1565–1574.
72. Palmisano, M.P., Andrish, J.T., Olmstead, M.L. et al. (2000). A comparative study of the length patterns of anterior cruciate ligament reconstructions in the dog and man. *Vet. Comp. Orthop. Traumatol.* 13: 73–77.
73. Lazar, T.P., Berry, C.R., deHaan, J.J. et al. (2005). Long-term radiographic comparison of tibial plateau leveling osteotomy versus extracapsular stabilization for cranial cruciate ligament rupture in the dog. *Vet. Surg.* 34: 133–141.

5 Complications Associated with Proximal Tibial Epiphysiodesis

Aldo Vezzoni, Joshua S. Zuckerman, and Ron Ben-Amotz

5.1 Introduction

Cranial cruciate ligament (CCL) injuries can occur at any age. In immature dogs, avulsion of the femoral origin from the lateral condyle or more commonly the tibial insertion may be seen. In cases of acute avulsion, internal fixation may be used to reattach the avulsed fragment, but in more chronic cases, contracture of the ligament fibers makes anatomical reduction and stabilization impossible.

The positive effects of tibial plateau leveling osteotomy (TPLO) in the CCL-deficient stifle have been demonstrated [1–7], but this procedure is not appropriate in skeletally immature dogs due to the presence of an open proximal tibial physis. Tibial wedge osteotomy (TWO) or CORA-based leveling osteotomy (CBLO) may be performed distal to the open physis in these dogs in an effort to reduce the tibial plateau angle (TPA), but both procedures require osteotomies [8].

Proximal tibial epiphysiodesis (PTE) was devised by Barclay Slocum in 1997 and described in a posthumously published case report in 2003 [9], in which a screw was inserted in the center of the cranial aspect of the tibial plateau of a 5-month-old Akita Inu with CCL failure in an attempt to restrict progressive increase in TPA as growth proceeds, thereby achieving the same effect of the TPLO without the need for an osteotomy (Figure 5.1). The cranial location of the screw (at the insertion site of the CCL) results in arrested growth in the cranial portion of the proximal tibia while the caudal portion proceeds normally, resulting in a significant decrease in TPA as growth progresses.

The author (AV) has performed PTE in 22 stifles, the results of which were reported in 2008 [10]. Since that time, an additional 24 stifles in 21 dogs have been treated (Table 5.1). The amount of leveling achieved at skeletal maturity was related to the age at which the procedure was performed, with greater correction achieved in dogs 4–5 months of age and less correction noted at 6 months of age. When the procedure was performed in dogs aged 7 months or greater, the degree of correction achieved was usually not enough to counteract the cranial tibial thrust. In a study published in 2010 to determine growth of the proximal tibial physis in the Labrador Retriever, a breed at risk for CCL rupture, PTE performed at 18 weeks of age should achieve the desired TPA target of 5° [11]. Although growth and the effect of PTE

Complications in Canine Cranial Cruciate Ligament Surgery, First Edition. Edited by Ron Ben-Amotz and David L. Dycus.

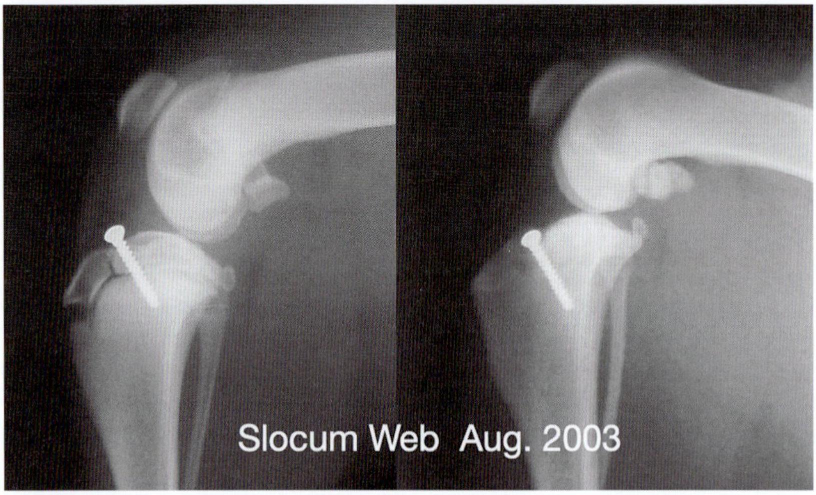

Figure 5.1 Original case published on the Slocum Enterprises website in August 2003. Immediate postoperative (left image) and 1-year (right image) follow-up radiographs of a proximal tibial epiphysiodesis procedure performed on a 5-month-old Akita. Note the change in the tibia plateau angle (TPA, right image). The cranial drawer and tibial compression tests were normal.

on a month-to-month basis are somewhat unpredictable because growth of individual dogs follows a model of saltation and stasis, the end effect was relatively consistent.

In clinical cases, 65% of the total correction achieved at skeletal maturity was obtained during the first month after surgery (Figures 5.2 and 5.3). Therefore, it appears that the rapid growth phase that occurs between 4 and 6 months of age is the timeframe during which PTE has the greatest chance of success. PTE has also been used as treatment for a proximal physeal tibial fracture in a dog [12].

5.2 Identification of Potential Complications

Complications specific to PTE may be mitigated by ensuring appropriate case selection and thorough understanding of proper surgical technique. As previously discussed, the outcome of the procedure is closely related to patient age at the time of surgery. Patients undergoing PTE at >6.5 months of age may be at risk for insufficient TPA leveling, resulting in failure to neutralize cranial tibial thrust and potentially requiring an osteotomy procedure for further correction when maturity is reached. Conversely, performing the procedure in dogs <5 months of age may result in overcorrection of the TPA.

The surgeon must also be aware of the potential for complications secondary to inappropriate screw placement. These include the development of a varus or valgus deformity resulting from eccentric screw placement and/or an insufficient leveling effect resulting from an excessively cranial screw placement or failure of the screw head to engage the tibial plateau (e.g., screw placement is either too superficial or too deep).

5.3 Preoperative Planning Strategies

Appropriately positioned stifle radiographs are required prior to performing surgery. These should include a mediolateral projection of the stifle in a neutral position for preoperative TPA measurement and determination of required screw length (Figure 5.4), an additional mediolateral projection with the stifle moderately flexed while undergoing the tibial compression test (TCT) for confirmation of cranial tibial subluxation when loaded (Figure 5.5), and a craniocaudal projection with the x-ray beam centered on the tibial plateau for measurement of the mechanical medial proximal tibial angle (mMPTA) (Figure 5.6).

Table 5.1 Demographic data from 24 cases of PTE by one author (AV) showing the age at surgery, as well as the original and final TPA and mMPTA.

Breed	Sex	Age at surgery (mo)	Starting TPA	Final TPA	Change in TPA	Starting mMPTA	Final mMPTA	Change in nMPTA	Further surgeries
Newfoundland	M	5.5	35°	13°	22°	96°	101°	5°	
Pug	F	6.5	22°	18°	4°	92°	92°	0°	TPLO 3 mo after
Boxer	M	6.2	25°	Lost for FU	Lost for FU	92°	Lost for FU	Lost for FU	
Labrador	F	5.5	30°	18°	12°	101°	101°	0°	Screw removal 2 mo p.o. + staple
Labrador	M	5.5	26°	2°	24°	98°	99°	1°	Straw removal 2 mo after.
Labrador	F	5.5	23°	10°	13°	96°	99°	3°	
Afgan Hound	M	5.5	32°	−4°	36°	94°	86°	−8°	
Bernese	F	4.5	35°	5°	30°	95°	86°	9°	
Bernese	F	5	34°	−1°	35°	95°	93°	−2°	Screw removal 3 mo after
Russian Terrier	M	6.8	24°	10°	14°	95°	94°	−1°	
Akita	F	5.5	20°	−2°	22°	97°	99°	2°	
Labrador	M	6	20°	3°	17°	93°	96°	3°	
Weimaraner	F	6	28°	27°	1°	94°	95°	1°	TPLO 5 mo after
Golden	F	5.5	27°	9°	18°	90°	98°	8°	
Labrador	M	6.5	24°	14°	10°	97°	97°	0°	
Labrador	M	6.5	28°	16°	12°	98°	98°	0°	
Golden	F	5.2	26°	4°	22°	92°	95°	3°	
Boxer	F	4	22°	5°	17°	94°	95°	1°	
Boxer	F	4	22°	6°	16°	95°	93°	−2°	
Labrador	M	5	27°	7°	20°	96°	97°	1°	
Maremma Shepherd	M	5.5	20°	Lost for FU	Lost for FU	94°	Lost for FU	Lost for FU	
Border Collie	M	4.5	25°	−2°	27°	95°	98°	3°	Screw removal 2 mo post op.
Golden	F	5	41°	In progress	In progress	94°	In progress	In progress	
Labrador	M	6	25°	In progress	In progress	95°	In progress	In progress	

FU, follow-up; mMPTA, mechanical medial proximal tibial angle; TPA, tibial plateau angle.

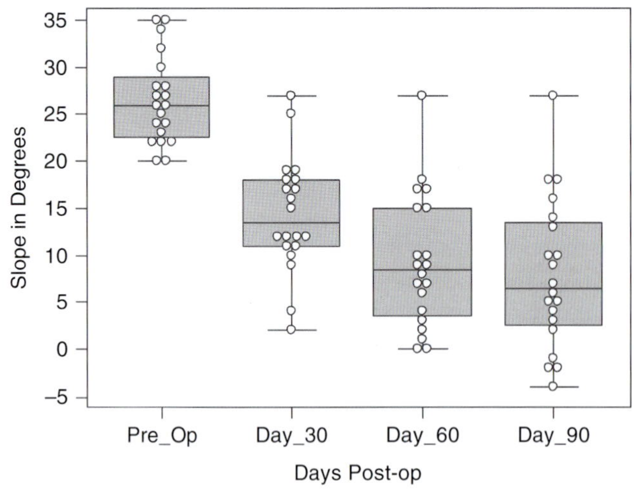

Figure 5.2 Variation of the slope after partial epiphysiodesis in dogs from Table 5.1. Values are reported in the preoperative period (first box) and in the other boxes respectively 1, 2, and 3 months postoperatively.

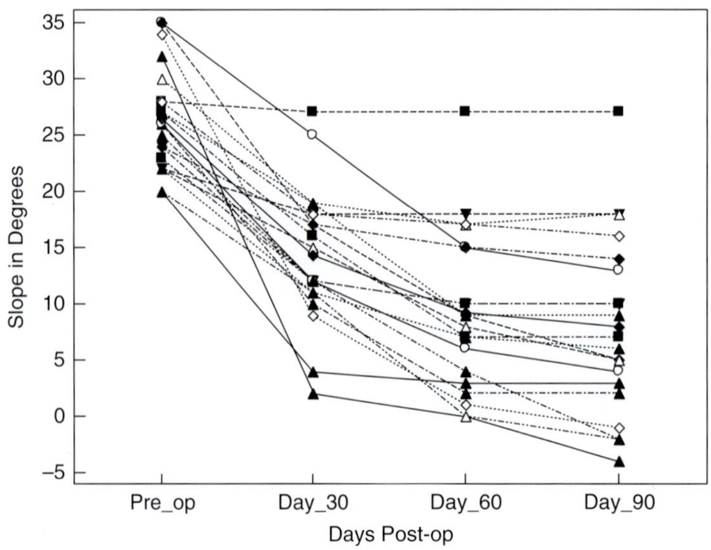

Figure 5.3 Decreasing of the TPA of all dogs after partial epiphysiodesis 30, 60, and 90 days postoperative. Each line represents a single dog from Table 5.1, The thick solid line represents the mean change of the slope.

In addition to their use in preoperative planning, the radiographs may also be used to diagnose CCL avulsion, as evidenced by the presence of an intraarticular bone fragment and a radiolucency at either the origin or insertion of the CCL (Figures 5.7 and 5.8). Even if this is not present, it is imperative to ensure that a complete orthopedic examination has been performed to fully assess the integrity of the CCL. Diagnosis of a partial tear is based upon the presence of a slightly positive cranial drawer sign and TCT with the knee held in moderate flexion, even if these tests are negative when the knee is in extension (Figure 5.5). The presence of a complete CCL tear is confirmed by a positive cranial drawer sign and TCT with the knee in extension (Figure 5.9). These diagnoses may be further confirmed by evaluating the radiographs for cranial displacement of the infrapatellar fat pad (on the mediolateral view),

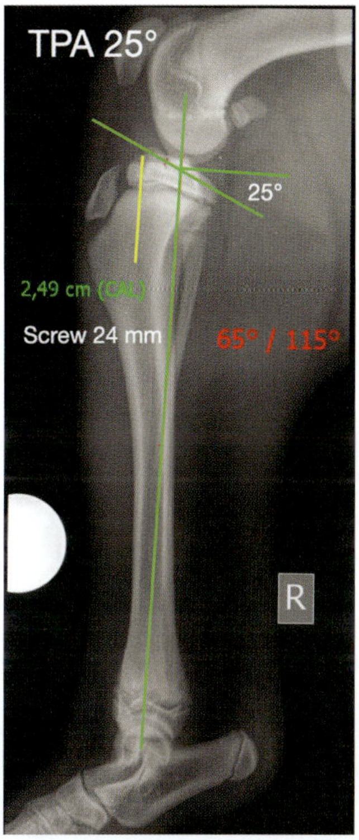

Figure 5.4 Mediolateral radiographic view of the tibia. Both the tibial and the femoral condyles are superimposed for TPA measurement and screw placement templating (size and location).

increased intraarticular density of the caudal aspect of the joint, and the presence of cranial tibial subluxation.

When the stifle is examined both orthopedically and radiographically, it is important to keep other, less common differential diagnoses in mind. These include tearing of the caudal cruciate ligament, in which femoral avulsion of the ligament results in some degree of caudal tibial subluxation together with a caudal drawer sign (Figure 5.10); osteochondrosis/osteochondritis dissecans (OC/OCD) lesions of the medial or lateral femoral condyle (Figure 5.11); and avulsion of the long digital extensor (LDE) tendon (Figure 5.12).

5.4 Surgical Technique

Due to the importance of accurate screw placement, access to fluoroscopy should be considered a mandatory prerequisite for PTE. The detailed use and safety precautions specific to this imaging modality are beyond the scope of the present chapter, but surgeons should familiarize themselves with this information prior to proceeding.

The patient should be placed under general anesthesia in dorsal recumbency and the leg clipped, aseptically prepped, and draped. A

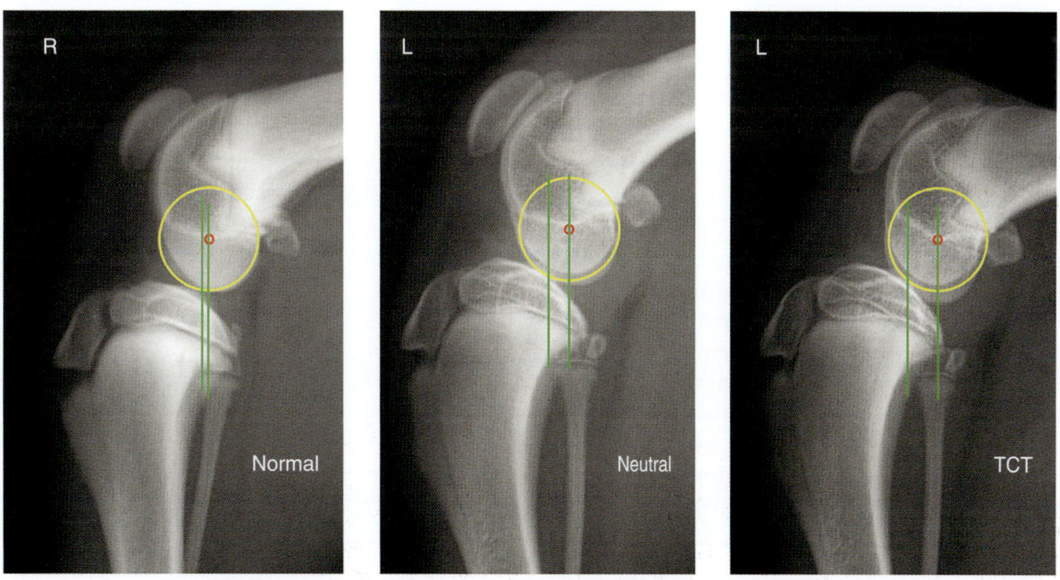

Figure 5.5 Partial CCL rupture in the left stifle of a 5.5-month-old Maremma Shepherd. The neutral and the TCT view show a moderate cranial tibial subluxation and joint effusion (right image). Comparison with normal opposite stifle (right stifle, left image).

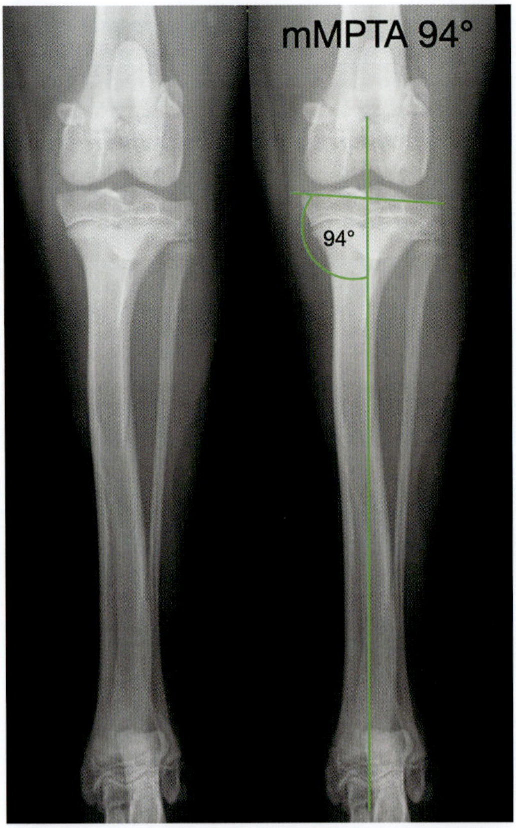

Figure 5.6 Caudocranial radiographic view of the tibia. Mechanical medial proximal tibial angle measurement (mMPTA). Landmarks for the proximal joint orientation line in the frontal plane: the most distal points of the medial and lateral tibial condyles. The proximal landmark for the mechanical axis of the tibia: center of the proximal-most aspect of the intercondylar fossa of the femur. The distal landmark for the mechanical axis of the tibia is the distal intermediate ridge of the tibia.

~3–4 cm skin incision is made medial to the patellar tendon with its center at the level of the patella. Dissection continues until an incision through the fascia and joint capsule allows for the insertion of a Gelpi retractor, facilitating inspection of the CCL. If a recent CCL avulsion is confirmed, the surgical approach may be slightly extended to allow for reduction and stabilization of the fragment using a screw and washer. In cases of femoral avulsion, the fixation of the fragment to the medial side of the lateral femoral condyle is performed (Figures 5.13 and 5.14). In cases of tibial avulsion, the fragment is reattached to the tibial plateau. In the latter case, the same screw used for fixation may also be used for PTE (Figure 5.15).

Insertion of the screw across the tibial plateau is performed by creating a stab incision medial or lateral to the insertion of the patellar tendon into the infrapatellar fat pad. The patellar tendon is then retracted medially or laterally with a small Gelpi retractor, and a 1.4–1.6 mm Kirschner wire is directed toward the tibial shaft and driven into the cranial center of the tibial plateau for use as a guide (Figure 5.16). The desired insertion point for the guide and subsequent screw is in the most proximal part of the tibial plateau, exactly in its center, as determined by visual evaluation of tibial width and palpation of the proximal tibia (Figure 5.17) or with arthroscopy. When directing the insertion, care must be taken to avoid the growth plate of the tibial tuberosity. The position of the K-wire should then be confirmed with fluoroscopy or intraoperative radiographs in both frontal and sagittal planes and must be adjusted if not seated properly (Figure 5.18).

If the K-wire is confirmed to be appropriately seated, a cancellous screw is then inserted, maintaining the same position and orientation as the guide wire (Figure 5.19). As an alternative to cancellous screws, 4.0 malleolar cannulated screws (self-drilling and self-tapping) may be inserted over the guide wire and tightened with a cannulated screwdriver (Figures 5.20 and 5.21). Fluoroscopy or radiographs should then be used once more to confirm that the screw is well positioned, and the screw head is against the cranial tibial plateau. Closure of the arthrotomy and overlying soft tissue is routine. Orthogonal postoperative radiographs should then be taken for final confirmation of adequate implant positioning (Figure 5.22).

5.5 Identification and Correction of Intraoperative Complications

For cases in which avulsion of the origin or insertion of the CCL has been identified, it is important to determine whether the injury is acute or chronic. If the avulsion occurred more than 1 week prior to surgery, contracture of the ligament could make reduction and fixation impossible.

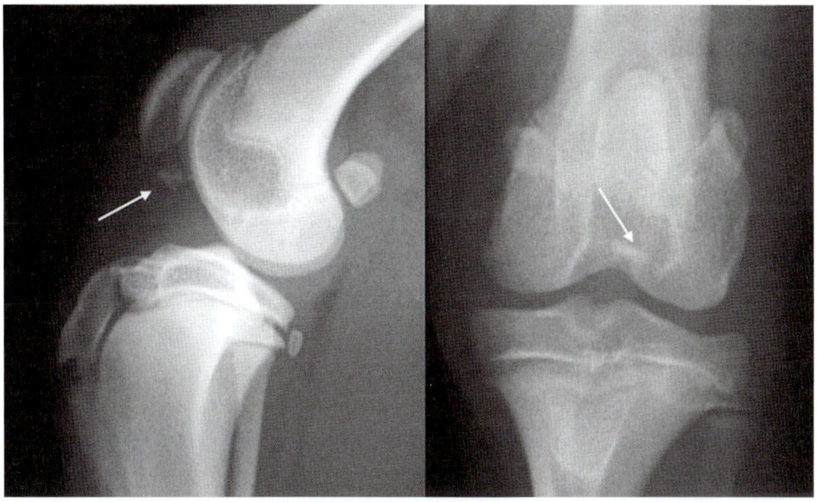

Figure 5.7 Femoral avulsion of the origin of the CCL in a 6-month-old Labrador Retriever. The arrows indicate the avulsed bony fragment.

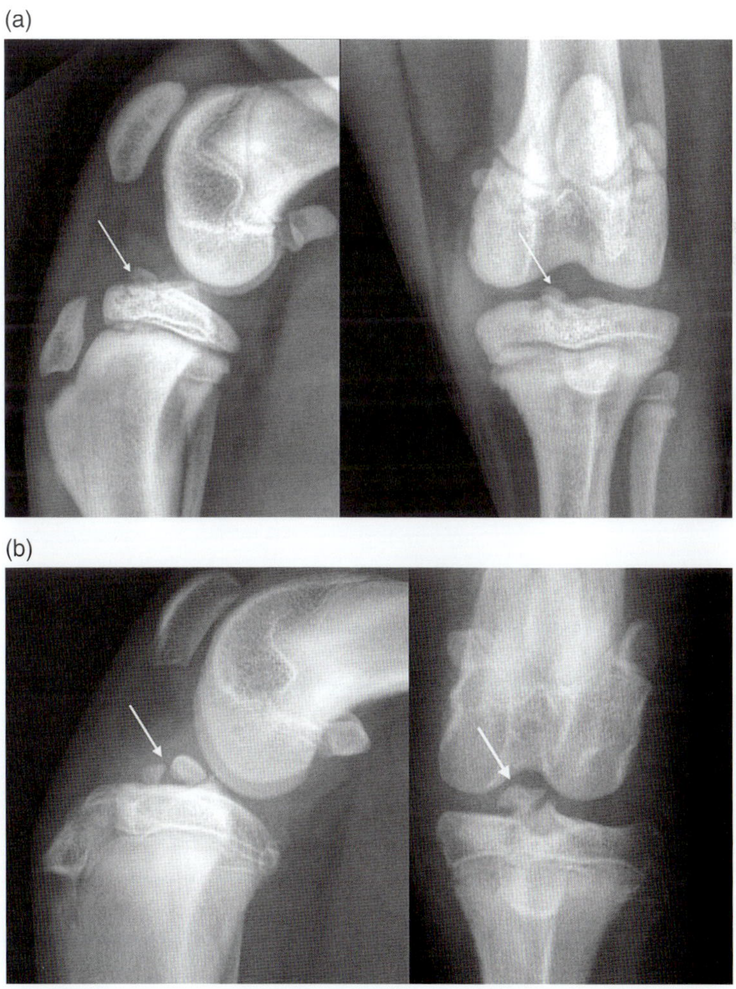

Figure 5.8 Tibial avulsion of the insertion of the CCL in (a) a 5-month-old Labrador Retriever and (b) a 6.5-month-old Border Collie. The arrows indicate the avulsed bony fragments.

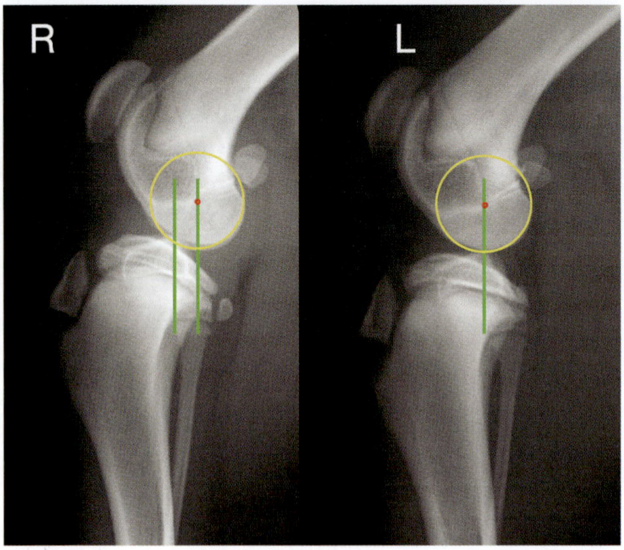

Figure 5.9 Complete rupture of the CCL in the right stifle of a 4.5-month-old Border Collie, with marked cranial tibial subluxation and joint effusion compared to the normal left stifle; neutral views.

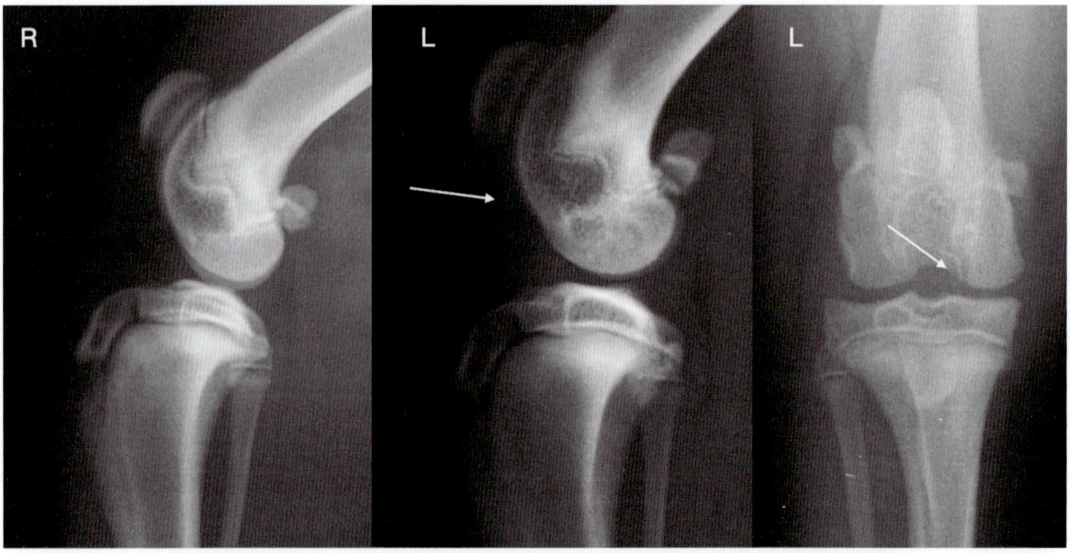

Figure 5.10 Femoral avulsion of the caudal cruciate ligament in the left stifle of a 5.5-month-old Labrador Retriever (white arrows point at the avulsed bony fragment), with caudal tibial subluxation compared to the normal right stifle.

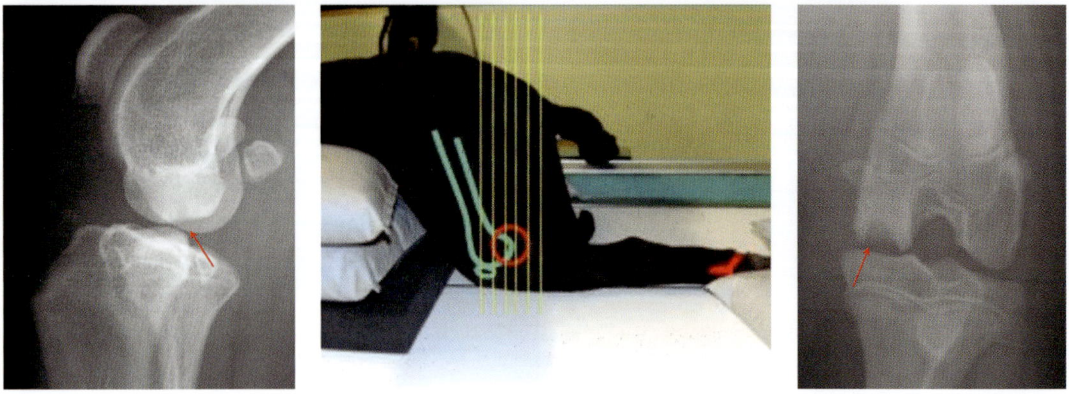

Figure 5.11 A medial femoral condylar osteochondrosis lesion in a 7-month-old Labrador Retriever (red arrow). Caudo-cranial view of the stifle with the femur at 110° to the table. The x-ray beam is tangent to the caudal surface of the femoral condyles.

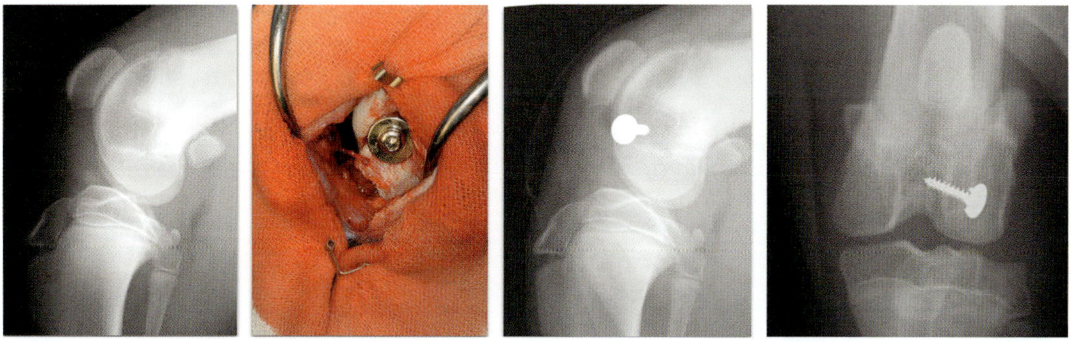

Figure 5.12 Seven-month-old Great Dane with avulsion of the origin of the long digital extensor tendon from the lateral femoral condyle. The ligament was reattached to the femoral fossa with a screw and a spiked washer.

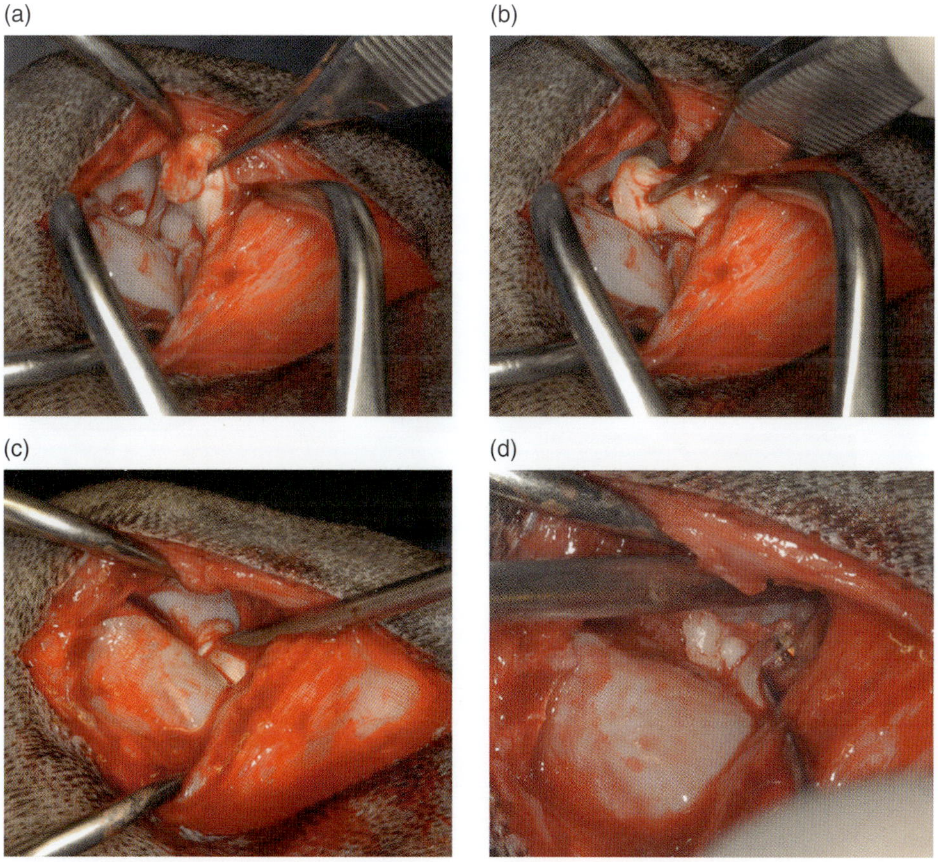

Figure 5.13 (a–d) Intraoperative pictures of an acute femoral avulsion of the CCL in a 5.5-month-old Labrador Retriever. The ligament was secured with a screw and washer.

In these cases, the ligament should be resected along with the bony fragment (Figure 5.23).

During placement of the guide wire and screw, impingement by the patellar tendon may make it more challenging to achieve good alignment along the tibial axis when drilling from the medial side of the joint. Because the lateral cortex of the proximal tibia curves medially, alignment may be more easily achieved when drilling from the lateral side of the joint.

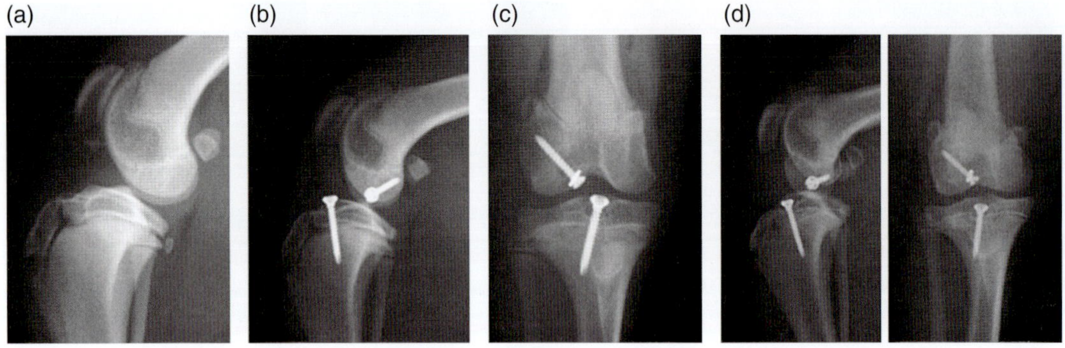

Figure 5.14 Radiographic views of the case shown in Figure 5.13. **(a)** Preoperative view showing a fragment of the avulsed CCL. **(b,c)** Postoperative view showing two screws; one screw is seen in the lateral femoral condyle where the avulsed fragment was reattached to the condyle. The second screw is placed in the tibia as a means for epiphysiodesis. **(d)** Follow-up 2 months postoperative. Note the change in the TPA.

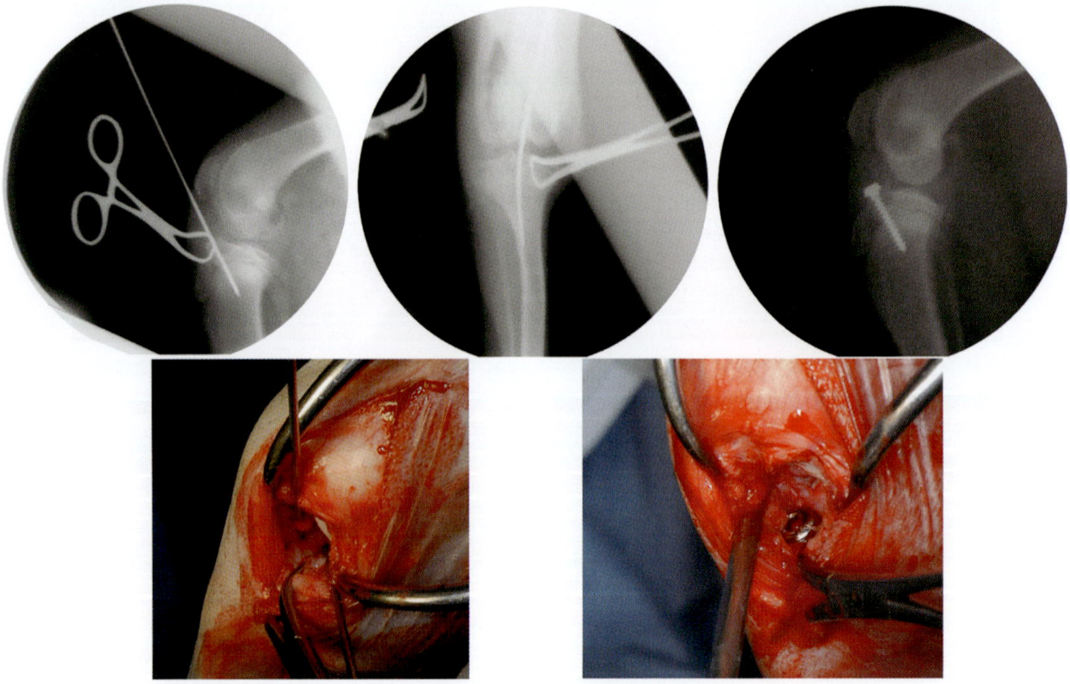

Figure 5.15 Tibial avulsion of the insertion of the CCL in a 5.5-month-old Afghan Hound. Reduction of the bony fragment was achieved using a pointed reduction forceps under fluoroscopic guidance. A screw was used to secure the ligament at its insertion and to provide proximal tibia epiphysiodesis.

Regardless of which side the surgeon drills from, the guide wire must be exactly in the center of the tibial plateau when viewed from the sagittal plane. It should be superimposed on the intercondylar eminences and directed along the long axis of the tibia. When drilling, the caudal cortex is avoided by holding the stifle in flexion and aiming along the tibial shaft. If intraoperative imaging reveals an inappropriately placed implant, it must be removed and reinserted in the correct direction and location (Figure 5.18). This holds true for suboptimal positioning noted on the postoperative radiographs as well (Figure 5.24).

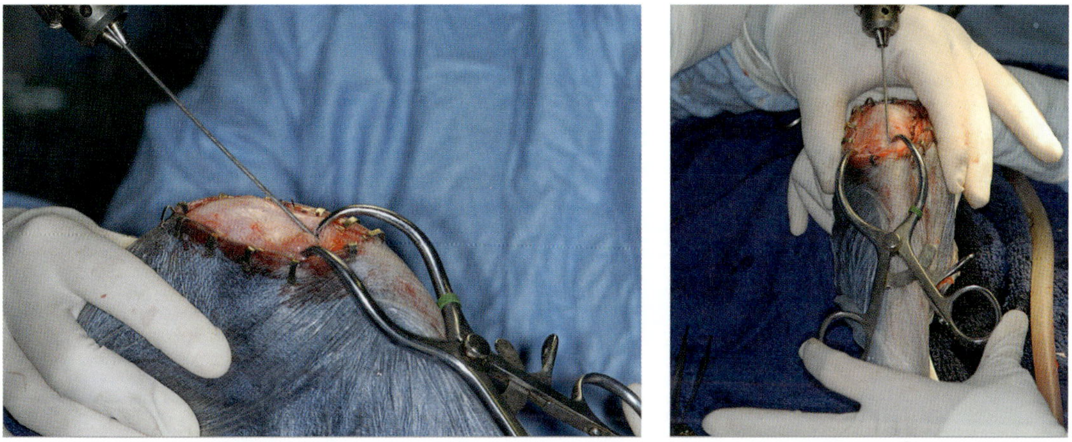

Figure 5.16 Insertion of guide wire: a stab incision is made medial or lateral to the insertion of the patellar tendon. The infrapatellar fat pad is identified. The patellar ligament is retracted medially or laterally using a retractor (Gelpi). A 1.4–1.6 mm K-wire is driven into the cranial center of the tibia plateau, aiming into the tibial shaft. Palpation of the tibia (as seen in the right image) together with visual evaluation of the proximal tibial width aid in correct pin placement.

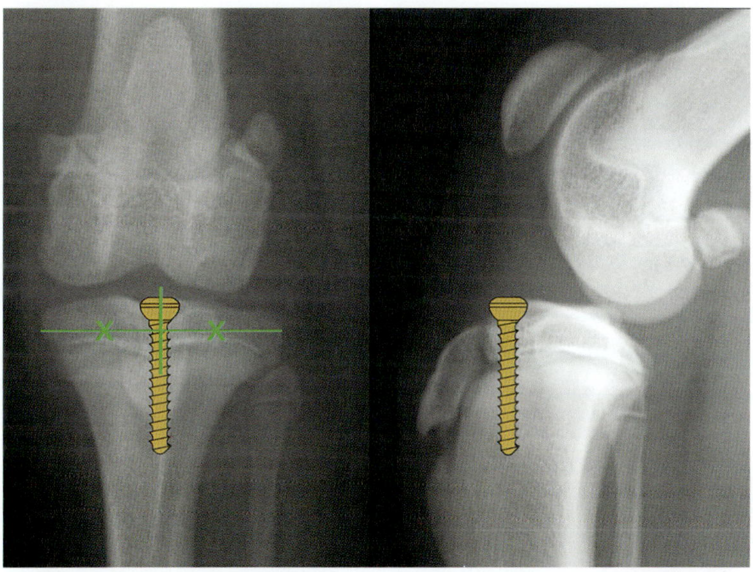

Figure 5.17 Correct screw position at the most proximal part of the tibial plateau, avoiding the growth plate of the tibial tuberosity (right image) with the screw in the center of the tibial plateau (left image).

5.6 Evaluation and Identification of Postoperative Complications

Dogs are evaluated with physical and radiographic exams after 4 weeks, 8 weeks, at skeletal maturity (12–15 months of age), and yearly when possible. The TPA and the mMPTA are measured and the radiographic signs of joint OA are recorded, as is the presence of any observed complications (Figures 5.25 and 5.26).

Ideally, at the 4-week recheck, the TPA should be reduced to 10–20°, though this is dependent on the preoperative TPA and the age of the dog at the time of surgery. At this time, the mMPTA should be unchanged, though a variation up to 4° is acceptable. Any deviation of the screw

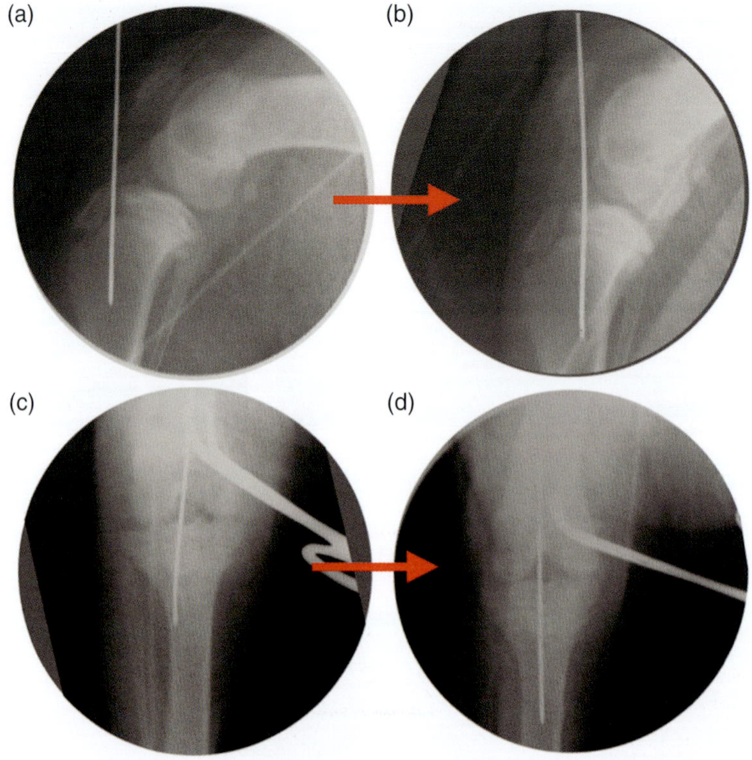

Figure 5.18 The position of the K-wire is confirmed with fluoroscopy, in both the sagittal and frontal planes. **(a,b)** Sagittal projections. **(a)** Incorrect cranial K-wire placement. **(b)** Appropriate K-wire placement. **(c,d)** Frontal plane wire placement. **(c)** Laterally positioned K-wire. **(d)** Appropriately centered K-wire.

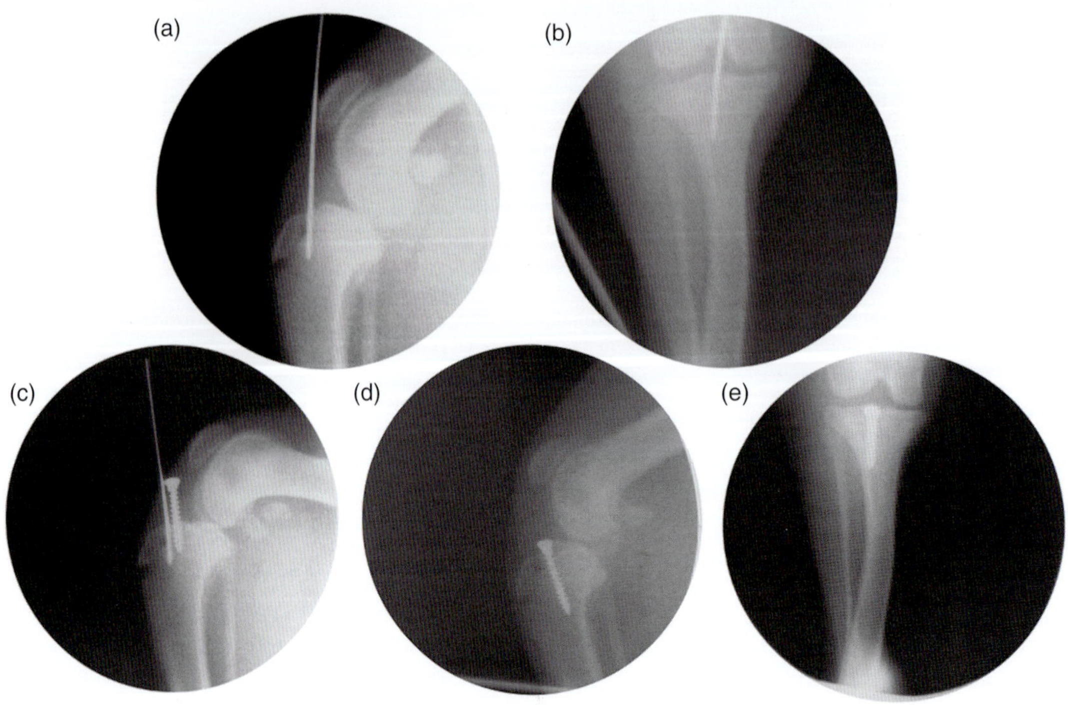

Figure 5.19 **(a–e)** A cancellous screw of a planned length is then inserted using the same position and orientation as the guide K-wire. The screw depth and its head position are confirmed with fluoroscopy.

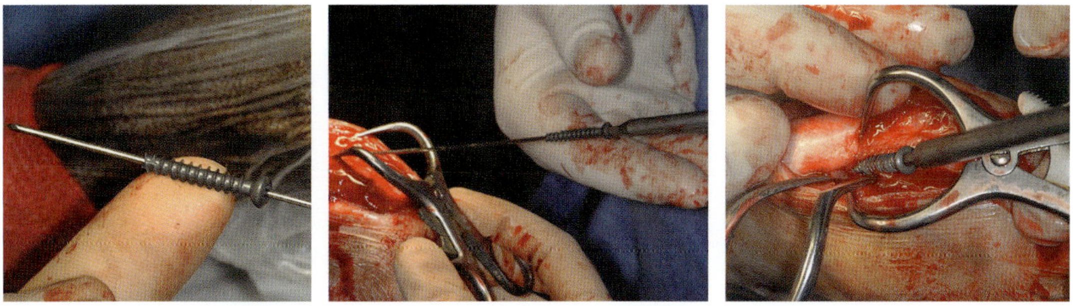

Figure 5.20 Cannulated screw used over a guide wire. Predrilling and tapping are unnecessary.

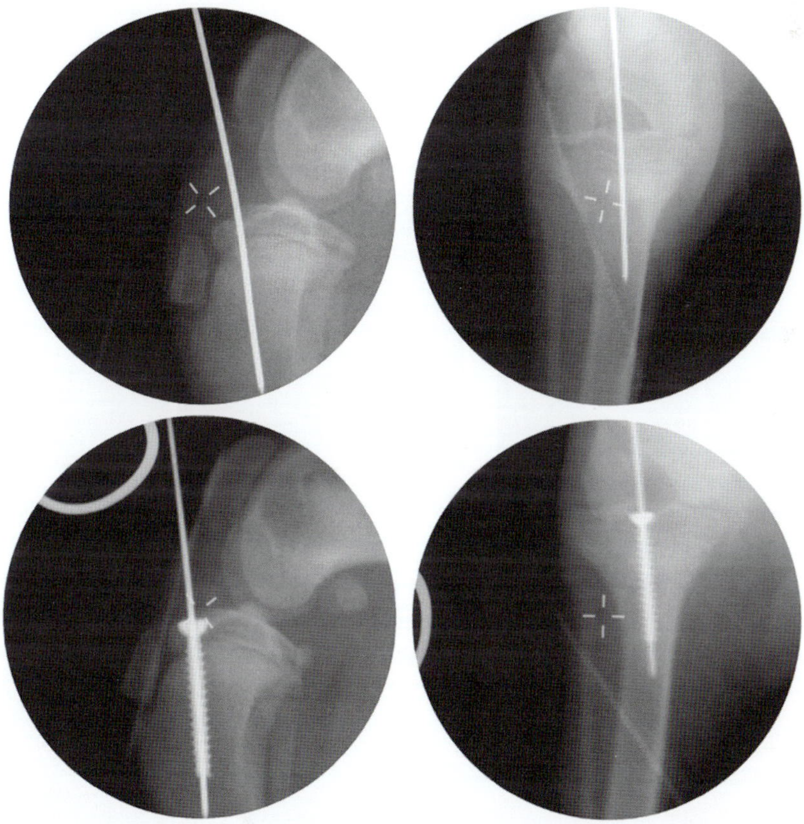

Figure 5.21 Insertion of a cannulated screw over a guide wire is performed once the K-wire position is confirmed.

from the center of the plateau (eccentrically placed) – even a few millimeters – risks the development of a varus (medial screw placement; Figures 5.27 and 5.28) or valgus (lateral screw placement; Figure 5.29) deformity. The extent to which these deformities may develop is also related to the age of the dog at the time of surgery, with younger dogs at risk for more significant deformities. When the screw is perfectly placed in the center of the plateau, no varus or valgus deformities will develop as the dog matures (Figure 5.30).

At the 8-week recheck, the TPA should be reduced to 5–10° (again, depending on the preoperative TPA and age of the dog). If the TPA is close to 0°, removal of the screw may be necessary in dogs that are <7 months of age. At this time, the mMPTA should remain unchanged.

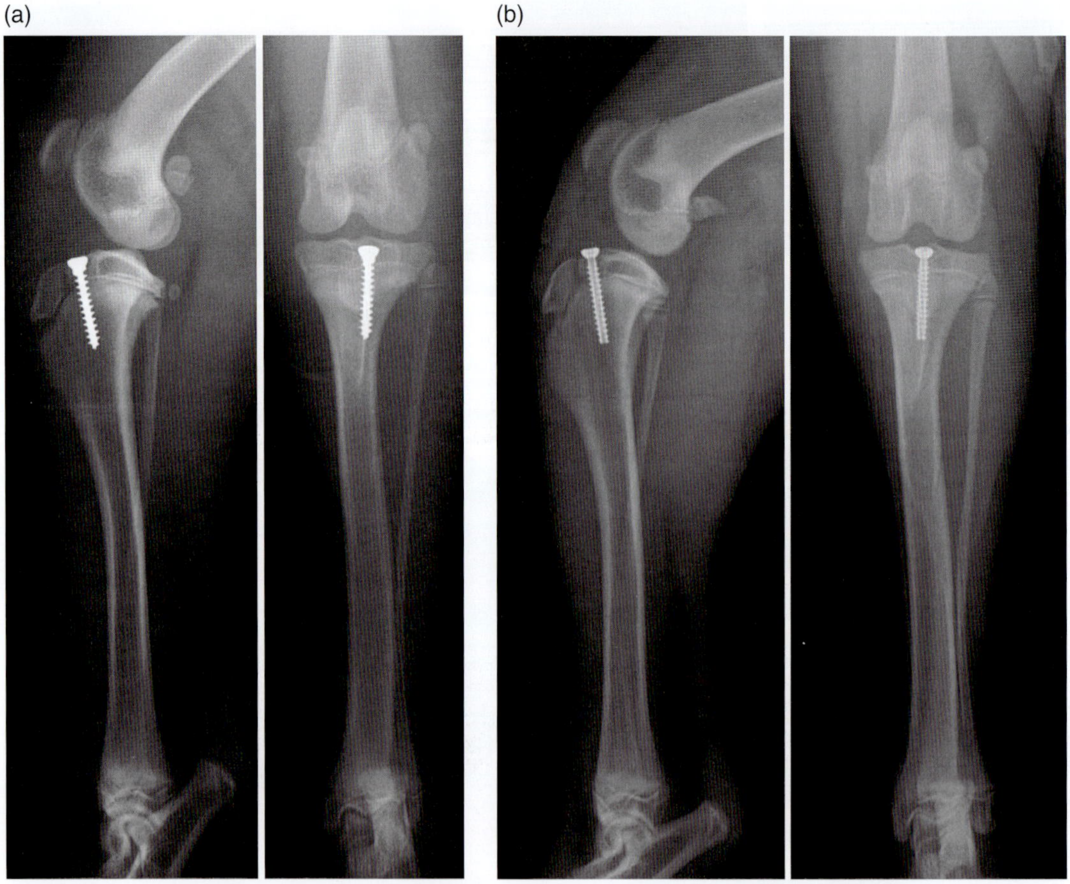

Figure 5.22 (a) Postoperative radiographs (medio-lateral and caudo-cranial) used to evaluate the cancellous screw position. (b) Postoperative radiographs (medio-lateral and caudo-cranial) used to evaluate the cannulated screw.

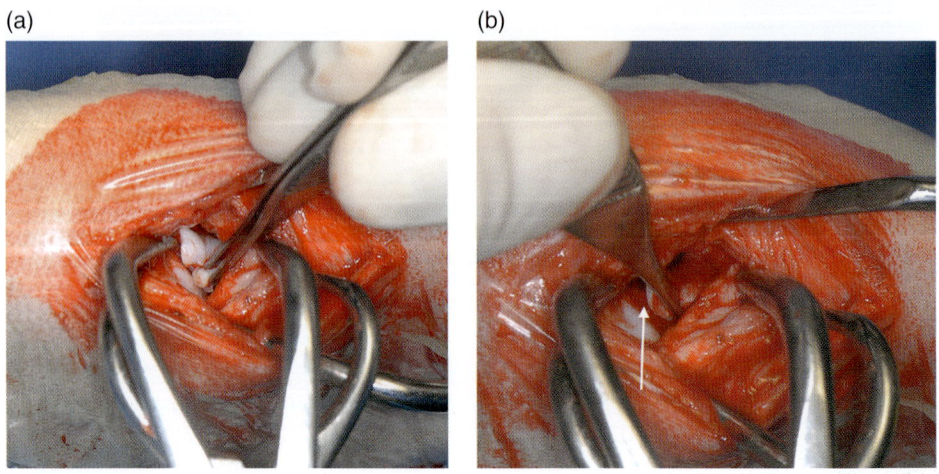

Figure 5.23 (a) Intraoperative image of a 5-month-old Golden Retriever with a chronic femoral avulsion of the CCL. (b) Note the remaining gap (arrow) between the ligament and the bone. In this case the ligament and small bone attachment were excised.

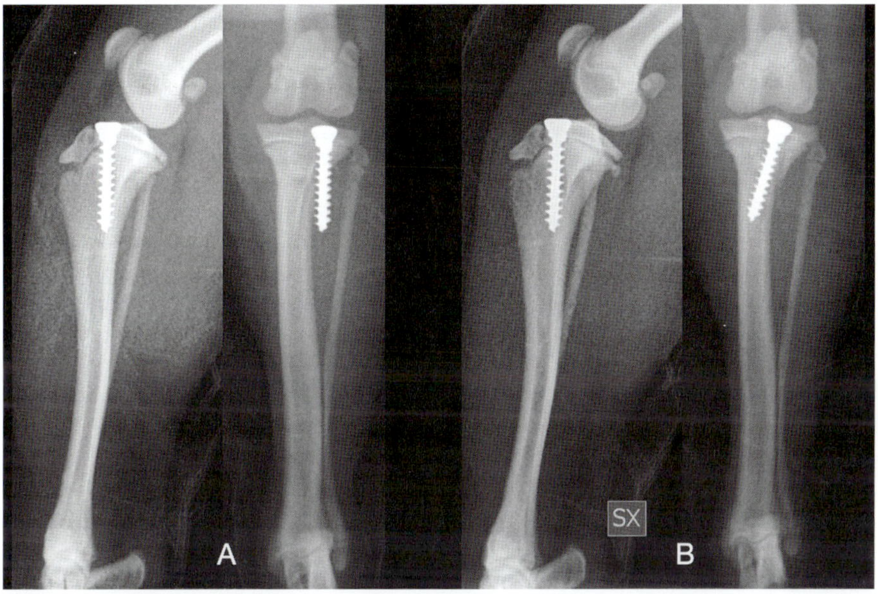

Figure 5.24 (a) Immediate postoperative screw position for PTE. Note the lateral screw position on the frontal plane. (b) Immediate revision screw placement.

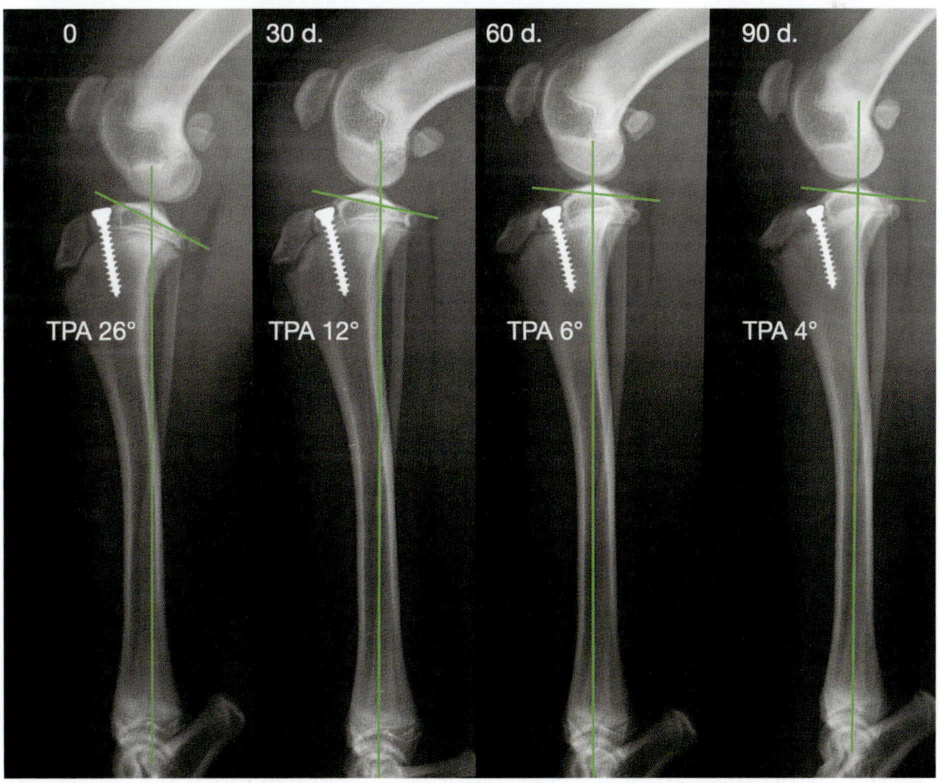

Figure 5.25 Lateral radiographic projection of a 5-month-old Golden Retriever following a PTE procedure. Note the gradual change in the TPA from 26° at day 0 to 4° at 90 days postoperatively.

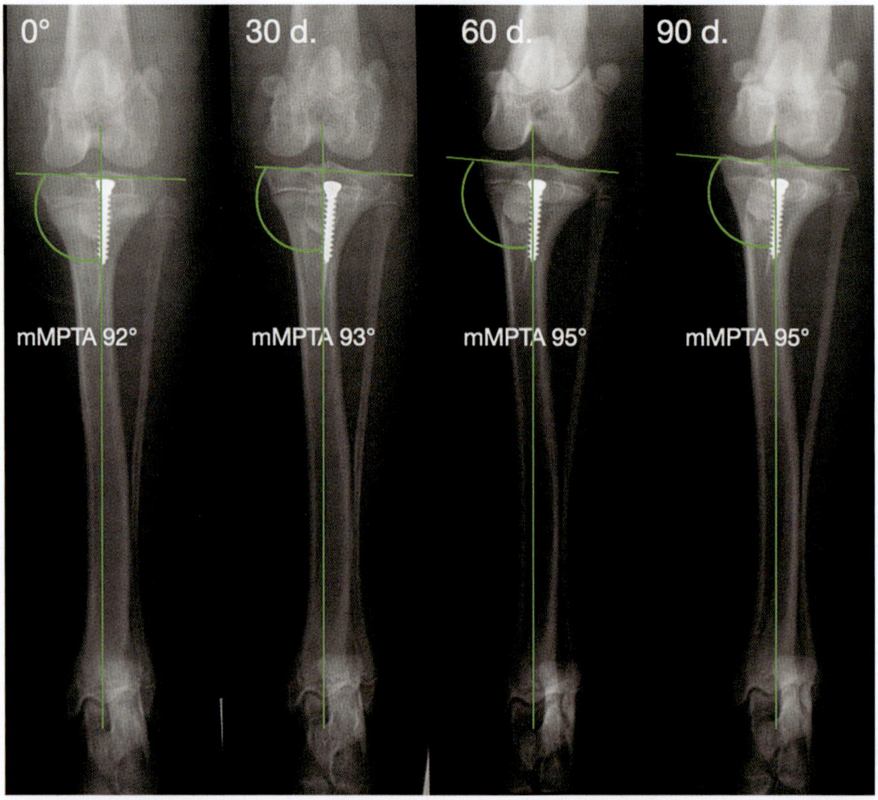

Figure 5.26 Cranio-caudal radiographic views measuring the mMPTA of the same dog in Figure 5.23. Note the change in the medial mechanical proximal tibia angle from 92° at day 0 to 95° at 90 days postoperatively (3° valgus change) due to minimal lateral offset of a screw in the frontal plane.

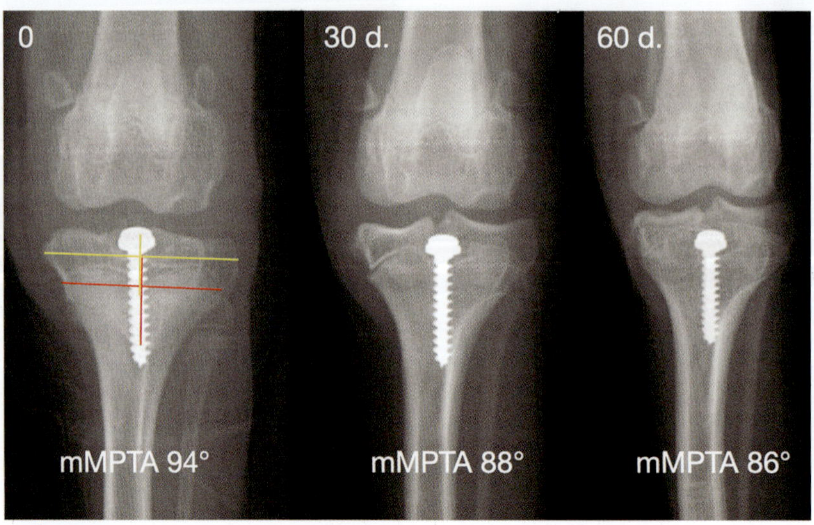

Figure 5.27 A minimal medial offset of a screw (frontal plane) resulted in 8° of tibial varus angulation at 60 days recheck. Note the change in the screw head position at 30 days.

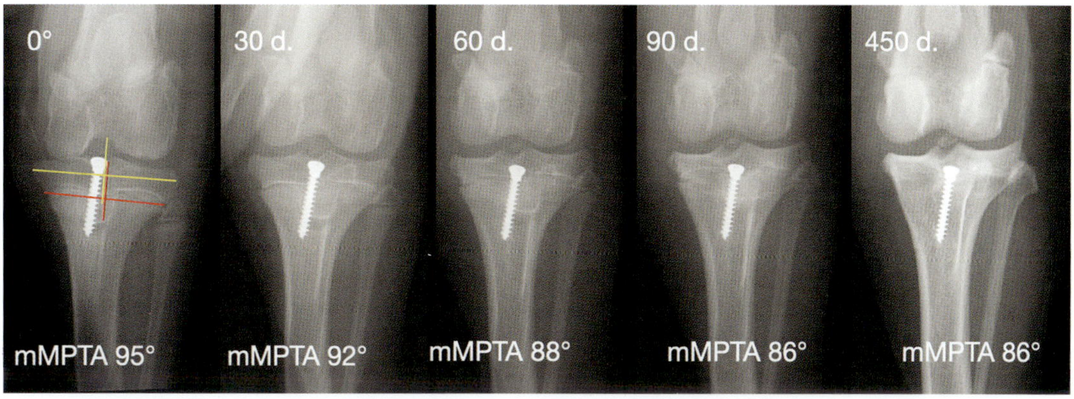

Figure 5.28 A marked medial offset of a screw (frontal plane) resulted in 9° of tibial varus angulation at 90 days postoperatively.

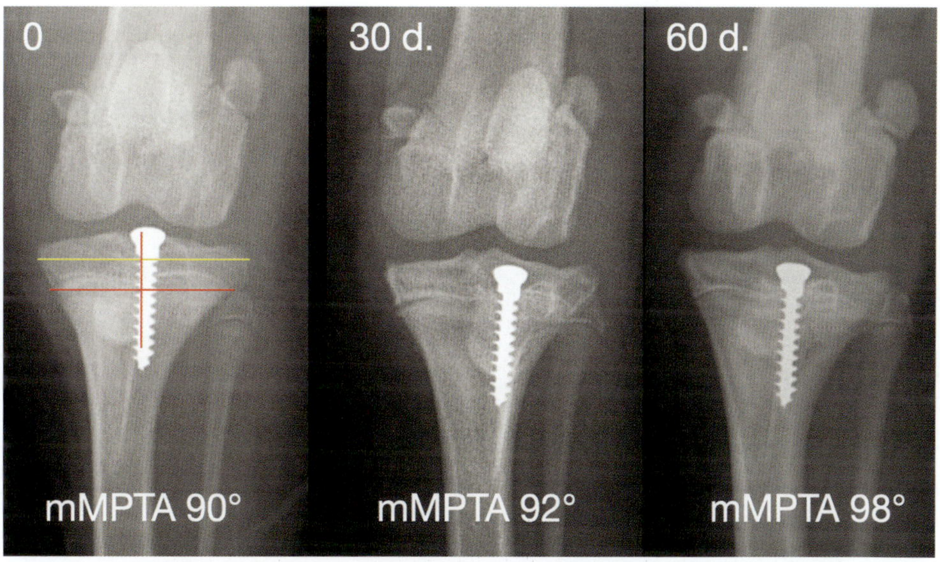

Figure 5.29 Moderate lateral offset of a screw (frontal plane) resulted in 8° tibial valgus angulation at day 60.

At skeletal maturity, the TPA should be between 0° and 8° and the mMPTA should be unchanged relative to the measurements obtained at the 8-week recheck.

Recheck examinations that reveal insufficient leveling of the tibial plateau may be the result of a screw that was not placed in full contact with the tibial plateau (Figure 5.31) or from a screw that was inserted too deeply in a very immature dog with softer bone (Figure 5.32). Insufficient leveling at skeletal maturity could also be due to late surgical timing (over 6 months of age).

5.7 Decision Making for Postoperative Complications

Insufficient leveling apparent on radiographs must be interpreted in conjunction with gait evaluation and physical examination. If, after 3 months, the TPA remains greater than 15° and there is persistent tibial thrust and lameness present, the screw should be removed and TPLO should be performed when the dog has reached skeletal maturity (Figures 5.33 and 5.34). If, after 3 months, leveling is insufficient but the TPA is *less* than 14°, lameness is

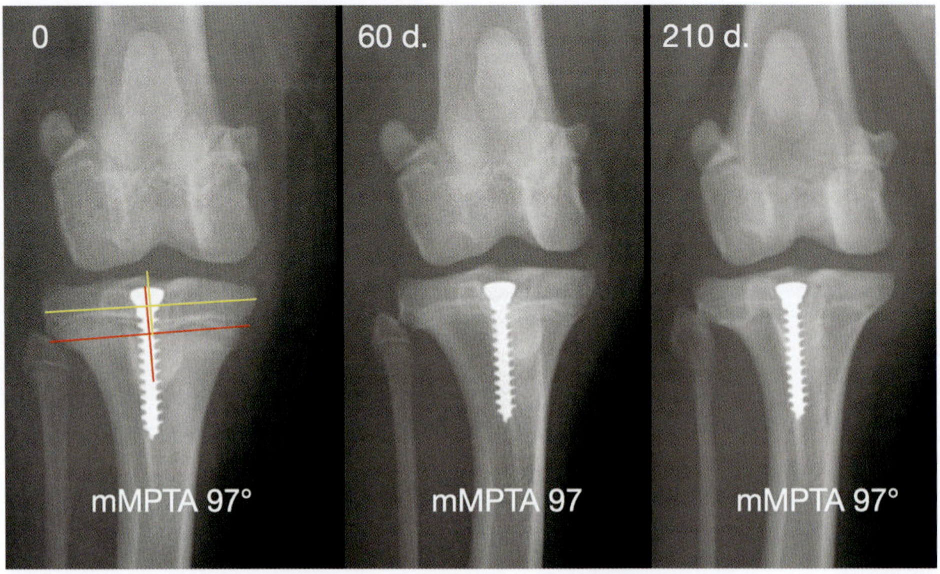

Figure 5.30 Centrally positioned screw (frontal plane) resulted in no change in the mMPTA at 210 days postoperatively.

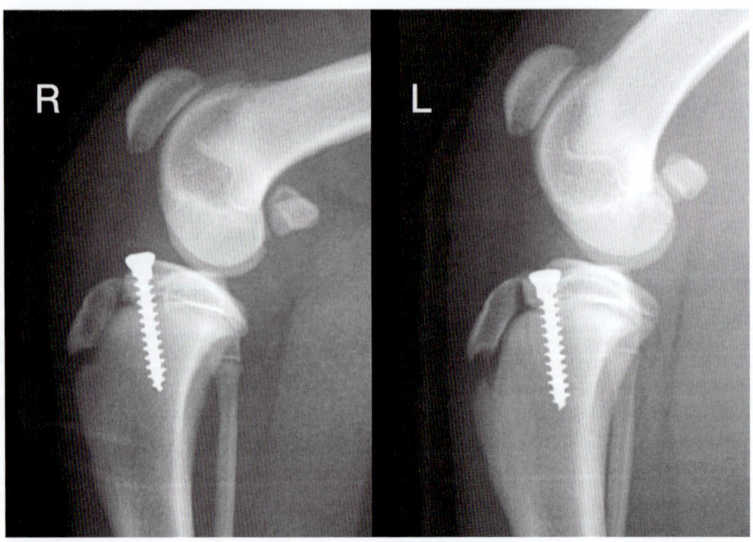

Figure 5.31 Right stifle: a malpositioned screw head can result in an insufficient leveling of the tibia plateau. Left stifle: appropriately positioned screw head as an example.

usually not noticed and TPLO is not necessary [13] (Figures 5.35 and 5.36).

If recheck radiographs reveal excessive leveling of the tibial plateau, with a TPA of 0–2° or less and the growth plate remains fertile, the screw should be removed to prevent further reduction of the TPA (Figure 5.37).

In one author's opinion (AV), varus or valgus deformities of the proximal tibia up to 8° are well tolerated. However, if a dog develops a greater degree of varus or valgus angulation, the screw should be removed and a recheck should be performed at skeletal maturity to determine whether a corrective tibial osteotomy is necessary. Although this outcome is theoretically possible, it has not been observed by the authors.

In specific cases, if a valgus deformity is observed developing as early as the 4-week

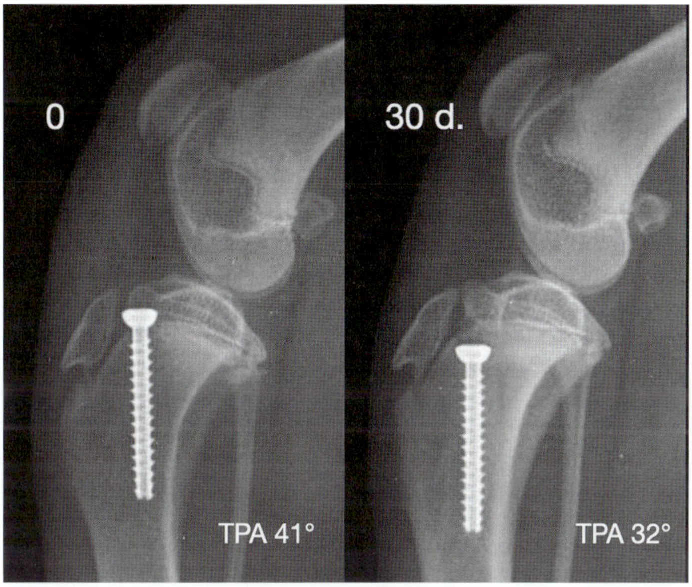

Figure 5.32 Immediate postoperative radiograph showing a screw placed too deep in a 5-month-old Golden Retriever. This can result in an insufficient TPA change (from 41° to 32°). In this case, where PTE was performed to reduce the excessive TPA caused by malunion of a tibial shaft fracture, a future corrective osteotomy procedure might be indicated.

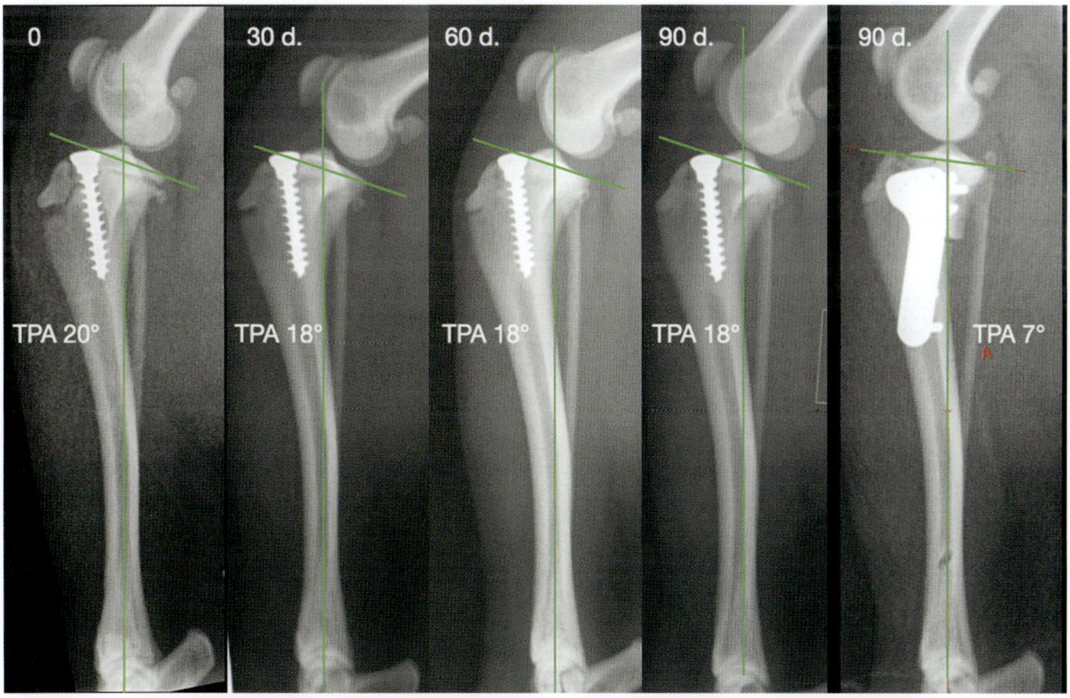

Figure 5.33 An insufficient reduction of a TPA at 3 months postoperatively in a Pug, resulting in an 18° TPA at 90 days post surgery. There was a persistent stifle instability with cranial tibial subluxation. The screw was removed and a TPLO procedure was performed. This resulted in a stable stifle (7° TPA).

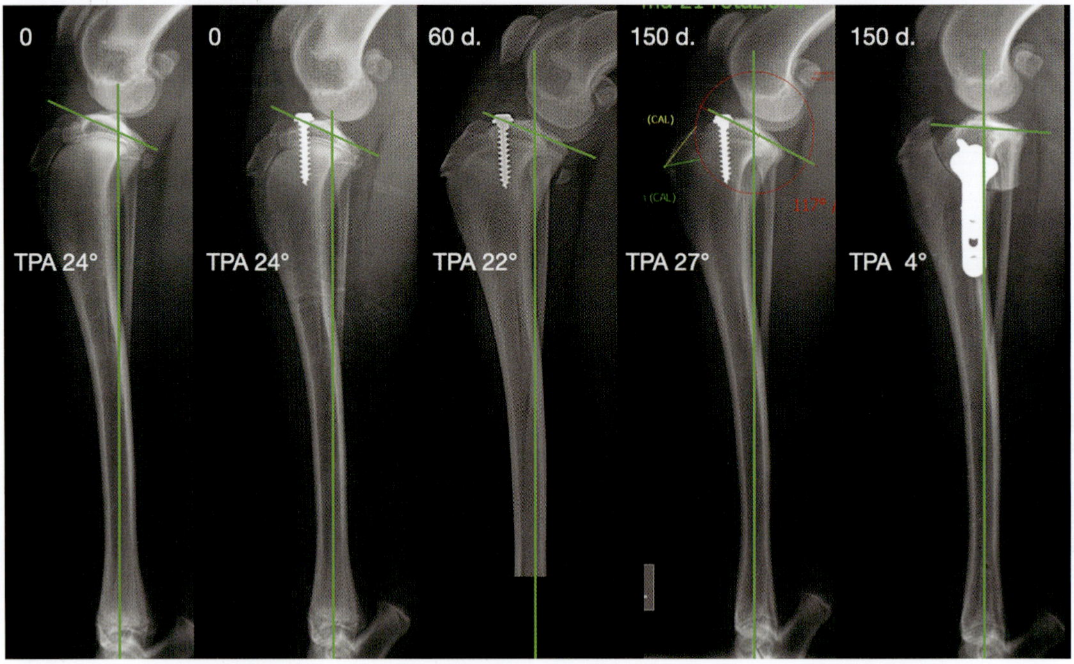

Figure 5.34 PTE performed in a 6-month-old Weimaraner resulted in an insufficient reduction of the TPA (at 150 days). Due to persistent cranial tibial subluxation, the screw was removed and a TPLO procedure was performed (achieving a 4° TPA).

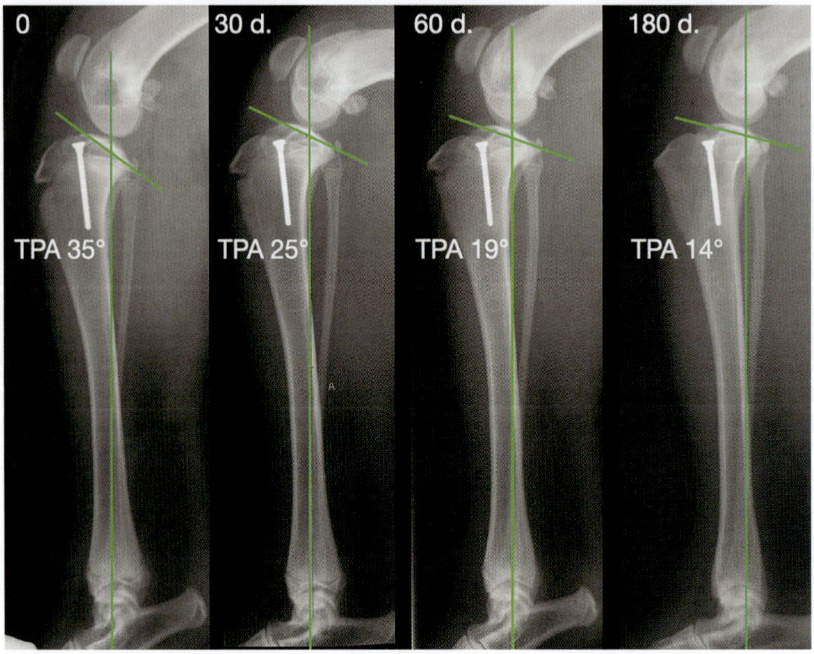

Figure 5.35 PTE performed in a 6-month-old Newfoundland. At 6 months postoperatively the TPA was 14°. Since the stifle palpated stable, no further surgical action was needed.

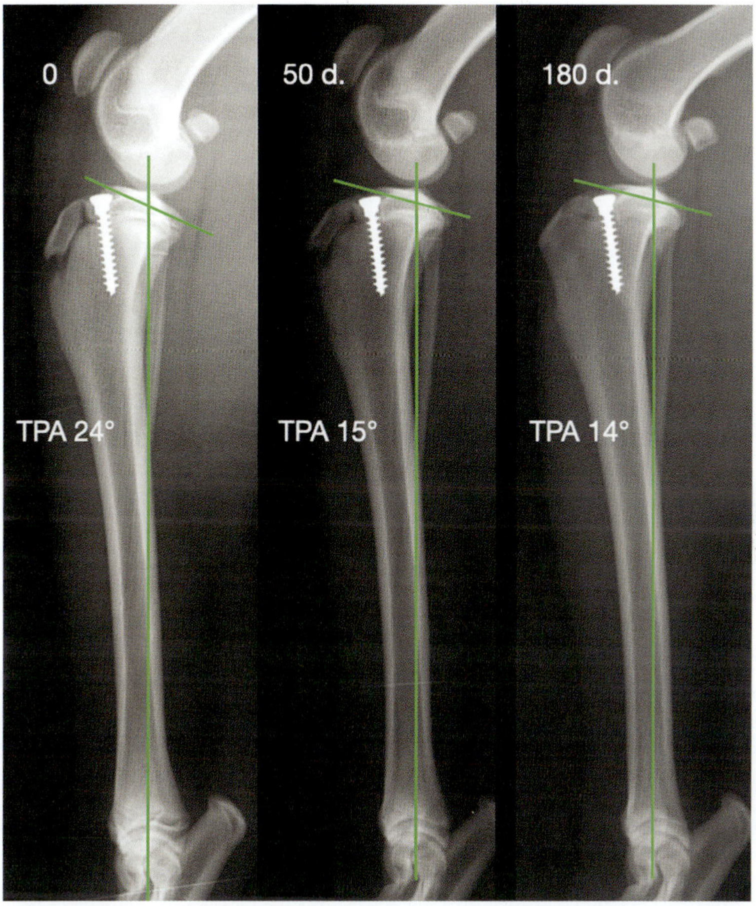

Figure 5.36 PTE performed in a 6-month-old Labrador Retriever. At 6 months postoperatively the TPA was 14°. Since the stifle palpated stable, no further surgical action was needed.

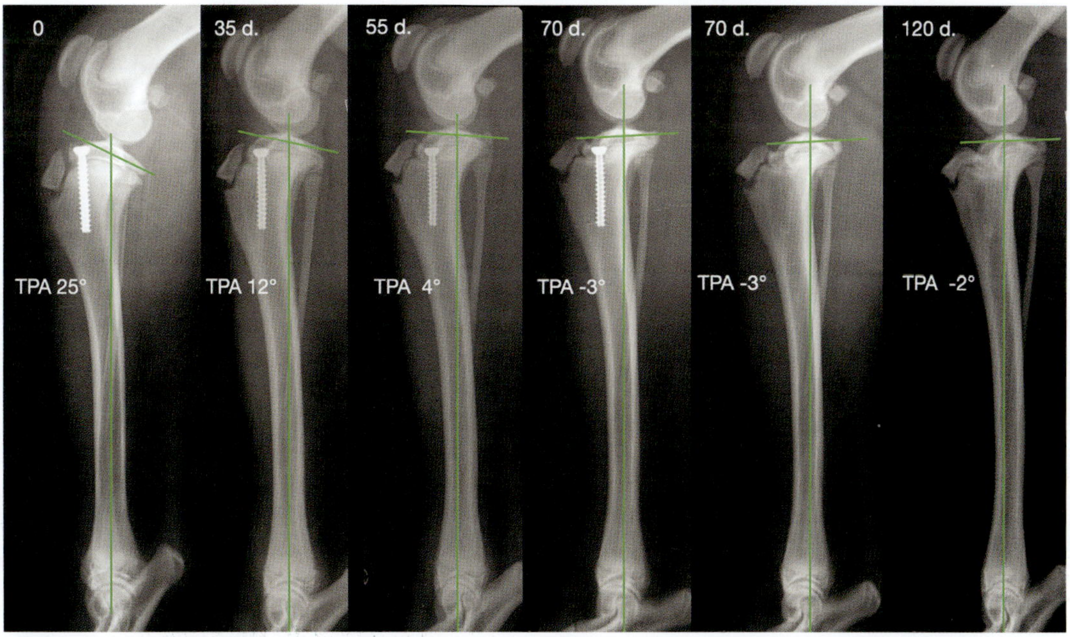

Figure 5.37 PTE performed in a 4.5-month-old Border Collie. At day 70, the TPA was measured at −3°. At this stage, the screw was removed in order to prevent further excessive rotation. At 120 days after surgery this resulted in a TPA of −2°.

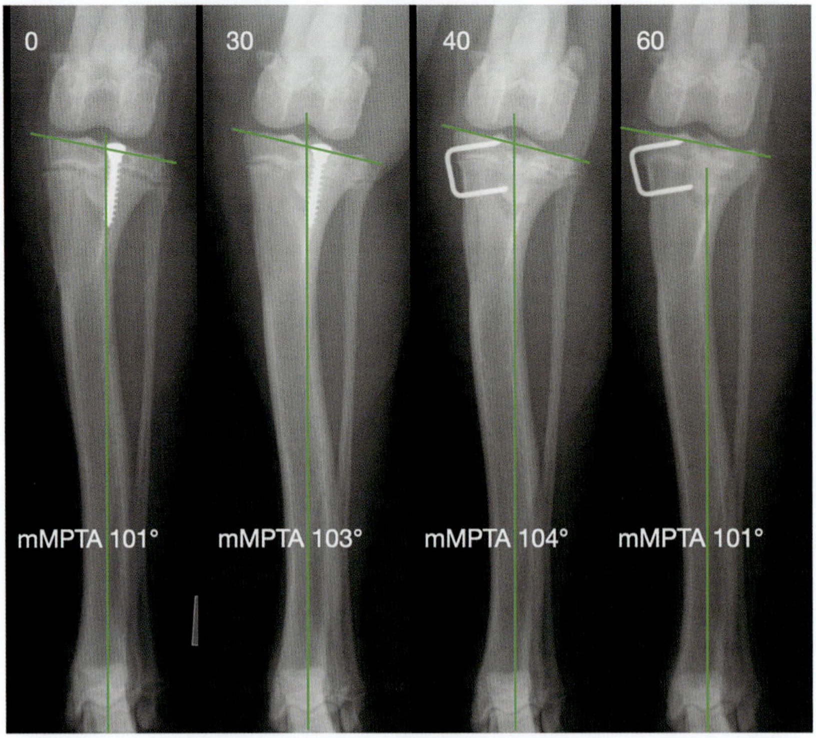

Figure 5.38 PTE performed in a 5.5-month-old Labrador Retriever with a Salter-Harris type I proximal tibia fracture. At day 30, valgus deformity was noted. It was suspected that the screw used resulted in a partial physeal closure leading to a valgus angulation. The screw was removed and a metal staple was placed across the medial physis (allowing lateral physeal growth compensation). Note the valgus correction at day 60.

recheck, a staple applied across the medial aspect of the growth plate could be used to delay medial growth (Figure 5.38).

5.8 Revision Strategies for Postoperative Complications

For cases in which removal of the screw is deemed necessary (excessive leveling with an active growth plate), a small stab incision is made medial to the patellar tendon at the level of its insertion. The screw head may then be identified through the use of fluoroscopy and gentle probing with a K-wire. Once identified, the implant may then be removed with a screwdriver (Figure 5.39). The screw must also be removed if a TPLO is to be performed. This may be most easily accomplished during inspection of the joint while evaluating for meniscal tears.

Application of a medial staple to combat excessive valgus deformity requires identification of the proximal tibial physis and the medial joint surface. The staple, which may be custom made using a 1.4 mm K-wire or a commercially available staple, is inserted into the tibial plateau just cranial to the medial collateral ligament with the proximal arm located between the joint surface and the physis, and the distal arm inserted into the metaphysis. (Figure 5.38).

5.9 Key Points

- Proximal tibial epiphysiodesis in immature dogs with CCL injuries is a procedure designed to decrease the TPA, effectively neutralizing the forces acting on the CCL-deficient knee. If effective, it may be possible to avoid more invasive osteotomy procedures as the dog matures.

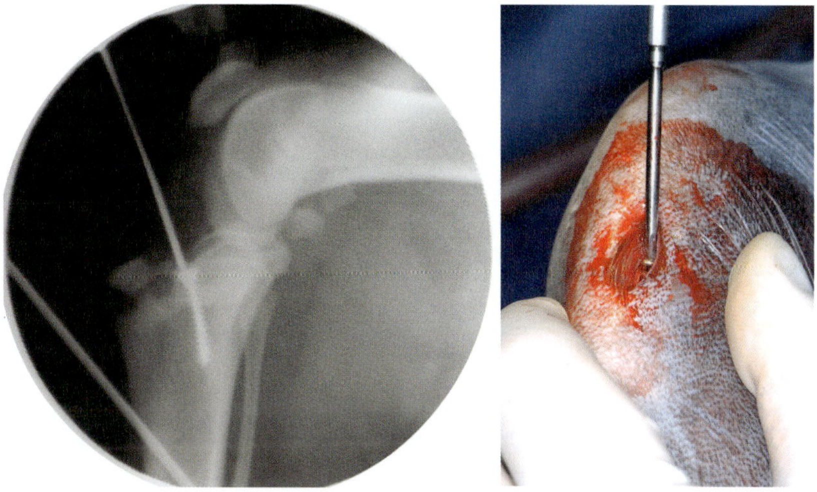

Figure 5.39 Excessive TPA necessitated the removal of the screw. A small incision was made medial to the patellar tendon insertion. Fluoroscopy-assisted K-wire probing to locate the screw head was followed by screw removal with a screwdriver.

- The achievable amount of leveling is related to the age of the dog at the time of treatment, with a greater degree of leveling possible in younger dogs. Consistent and effective leveling of the plateau is usually obtained when performed between 4 and 6 months of age. The maximum age at which the slope can be significantly altered by PTE may be affected by breed variation [12]; however, this was not noted in cases by one author (AV).
- The most challenging part of the surgical procedure is the insertion of the screw in the precise position, perfectly centered in the frontal plane of the tibial plateau. While the insertion of the screw in the tibial plateau can be performed from both sides of the patellar tendon, precise centering in the midpoint of the plateau is essential in both cases.
- In younger puppies (4–5 months of age) removal of the screw prior to complete fusion of the growth plate may be required to avoid excessive leveling of the tibial plateau. Because of this, monitoring the leveling effect in the postoperative period with regular rechecks every 3–4 weeks until closure of the growth plate is mandatory to evaluate the achieved slope and the remaining growth potential.
- Fixation of femoral or tibial avulsions of the CCL is possible in acute cases and may be done in combination with PTE which will promote healing of the fragment by reducing the cranial tibial thrust in the following weeks.
- The technique is minimally invasive, and complications can be avoided by paying meticulous attention to screw placement and by the use of intraoperative fluoroscopy.

References

1. Henderson, R. and Milton, J. (1978). Tibial compression mechanism – a diagnostic aid in stifle surgeries. *J. Am. Anim. Hosp. Assoc.* 14: 474–479.
2. Slocum, B. and Devine, T. (1983). Cranial tibial thrust: a primary force in the canine stifle. *J. Am. Vet. Med. Assoc.* 183: 456–459.
3. Slocum, B. and Devine, T. (1984). Cranial tibial wedge osteotomy: a technique for eliminating cranial tibial thrust in cranial cruciate ligament repair. *J. Am. Vet. Med. Assoc.* 184: 564–569.
4. Slocum, B. and Slocum, T.D. (1993). Tibial plateau leveling osteotomy for repair of cranial cruciate ligament rupture in the canine. *Vet. Clin. North Am. Small Anim. Pract.* 23: 777–795.
5. Warzee, C.C., Dejardin, L.M., Arnoczky, S.P. et al. (2001). Effect of tibial plateau leveling on cranial and caudal tibial thrusts in canine cranial cruciate-deficient stifles: an in vitro experimental study. *Vet. Surg.* 30: 278–286.

6. Reif, U., Hulse, D.A., and Hauptman, J.G. (2002). Effect of tibial plateau leveling on stability of the canine cranial cruciate-deficient stifle joint: an in vitro study. *Vet. Surg.* 31: 147–154.
7. Krotscheck, U., Nelson, S.A., Todhunter, R.J. et al. (2016). Long term functional outcome of tibial tuberosity advancement vs. tibial plateau levelling osteotomy and extracapsular repair in a heterogeneous population of dogs. *Vet. Surg.* 45 (02): 261–268.
8. Kim, S.E., Pozzi, A., and Kowaleski, M.P. (2008). Tibial osteotomies for cranial cruciate ligament insufficiency in dogs. *Vet. Surg.* 37: 111–125.
9. Case of the month: cranial cruciate ligament rupture, immature dog – screw fixation of growth plate for tibial plateau leveling. (2003) www.slocumenterprises.com (accessed 26 March 2021).
10. Vezzoni, A., Bohorquez-Vanelli, A., Modenato, M. et al. (2008). Proximal tibial epiphysiodesis to reduce tibial plateau slope in young dogs with cranial cruciate ligament deficient stifle. *Vet. Comp. Orthop. Traumatol.* 21: 343–348.
11. CS, M.B. Jr., Vezzoni, A., and Conzemius, M.G. (2011). Growth dynamics of the canine proximal tibial physis. *Vet. Surg.* 40: 389–394.
12. Picavet, P.P., Bouvy, B., Lefebvre, H.M., and Balligand, M. (2019). Use of epiphysiodesis as treatment for a proximal physeal tibial fracture in a dog. *VCOT Open* 2: e55–e59.
13. Robinson, D.A., Mason, D.R., Evans, R., and Conzemius, M.G. (2006). The effect of tibial plateau angle on ground reaction forces 4–17 months after tibial plateau leveling osteotomy in labrador retrievers. *Vet. Surg.* 35: 294–299.

Section III

Extraarticular Repair Techniques

6 Extracapsular Stabilization Using Synthetic Material

Ian G. Holsworth

6.1 Introduction

The use of an extracapsular suture (ECS) system for the attempted stabilization of the canine cranial cruciate ligament (CCL)-deficient stifle is the oldest, most widespread stifle stabilization technique and most commonly used canine orthopedic joint procedure in the world. First introduced in the 1950s, the procedure has endured many changes in technique and materials [1, 2]. The procedure's aim is to replace or augment the function of the native CCL that has been damaged and no longer provides sufficient stifle stability to the affected patient. This hopefully allows a return to acceptable function. Although the synthetic material used for the suture is varied and the location of suture placement has expanded over time, the procedural aim is the same.

The primary challenge that all ECS procedures face is true restoration of native stability. There is no definitive scientific evidence that this is possible. In fact, the scientific evidence points to a perceived improvement in patient function without true resolution of stifle instability. The attainment of *functional* stability is therefore the challenge that surgeons face when they elect to offer and perform an ECS procedure. It is very important that when discussing the ECS option with clients prior to performing the procedure, it is made very clear what the aim of the procedure is, what the possible end-result will be for the patient and what the potential operative, immediate post-operative, delayed post-operative, and long-term complications may be. Informed consent must be sought and without a frank and open discussion with clients regarding possible outcomes and complications, surgeons may find themselves in some difficulty during the patient recovery process. The recommendation to clients to perform ECS stabilization by many veterinarians has diminished significantly over time as other stabilization techniques have been developed and more research has been undertaken into the ECS effect and patient response [3–6].

The most common and significant complications encountered in ECS patients fall into four main categories:

- persistent stifle laxity
- infection
- subsequent meniscal tear
- progressive osteoarthritis.

While all these complications are possible and occur not infrequently, the most common

Complications in Canine Cranial Cruciate Ligament Surgery, First Edition. Edited by Ron Ben-Amotz and David L. Dycus.

complication is persistent post-operative laxity. The causes of persistent stifle laxity include inherent issues with the ECS technique, the structural characteristics of the material used, including the technique of securing the material to itself or to the periarticular tissues, and technical errors during implantation.

A body of scientific research has been performed to investigate ECS construct stability *in vitro* and *in vivo* and much has been learned about the shortfalls of this technique [7–13]. There is currently a discrepancy between the objective investigational findings and perception of surgical success when owners and veterinarians are asked to evaluate the post-operative patient's subjective clinical progress. It appears that the correlation between objective post-operative laxity and patient's subjective function is not linear and is nonpredictive [14–17]. The use of objective gait analysis to determine the degree of return of normal limb function in post-operative ECS patients has mostly shown a failure to achieve normal limb function [18–23]. In the small number of studies that did demonstrate objectively normal limb function post-operatively, experimental, not clinical patients were measured [24] and some study conclusions were debatable [25]. When radiographic analysis of progressive osteoarthritis is used to determine ECS success in slowing or stopping degenerative joint disease, the ECS patients examined showed significant visible osteoarthritis progression over time [26–28]. In light of the published scientific data currently available, it is wise that the veterinarian presenting stifle ECS to clients does not state that normal stifle stability or limb function will be restored, and that degenerative osteoarthritis of the affected joint will progress over time.

6.2 Preoperative Patient Classification and Suitability for Extracapsular Suture Procedure

Prior to the decision to proceed with ECS stabilization, it is important to evaluate and understand relevant patient characteristics that may influence the veterinarian to choose ECS as a viable option. The patient factors that may play a role are age, size, activity level, and concurrent medical issues.

As the degree of post-operative stability that is possible with the ECS technique is subnormal and continued instability can affect the patient's ability to exercise comfortably, care should be taken to avoid selecting young, active, and large-breed dogs as ideal ECS patients. As load to the postsurgical joint increases with more intense exercise, more prolonged exercise, larger patient size and weight, the inherent issue of post-operative instability may increase and patient function may be compromised. Use of the ECS technique in older, smaller, and less active patients may be more appropriate.

In patients with concurrent immune-mediated arthropathy, care must be taken when placing an intraarticular implant. The presence of monofilament or multifilament suture material within the joint capsule or exposed to the joint fluid could exacerbate the underlying condition and potentially lead to worsening of the joint inflammation present.

6.3 Preoperative Planning Strategies to Minimize Complications both Intra-operatively and Post-operatively

It is important that all patients scheduled for ECS stabilization undergo a detailed whole-body orthopedic examination with particular care to examine and categorize the salient clinical features of the affected stifle joint. The presence and severity of clinical lameness, the presence of a partial versus complete CCL tear, the degree of palpable laxity (mild, moderate, or severe), the presence and severity of preexisting degenerative joint disease (mild, moderate, or severe) and the presence of concurrent patellar instability should all be determined and recorded in the medical record for future reference.

Radiographic examination of the affected stifle and contralateral stifle prior to surgery is also essential (See Chapter 1 for more information on the radiographic examination). The presence of primary bone or joint pathology (infection, neoplasia, immune-mediated arthropathy) must be ruled out, the presence of bony abnormalities that may affect the surgical plan must be quantified, and the measurement of tibial plateau angle to avoid ECS performance in patients with excessive tibial plateau angle (eTPA) is paramount. Unfortunately, the TPA angle's effect on ECS success has not been investigated closely enough to determine at what tibial plateau angle the ECS becomes an inappropriate choice for the patient. Below a measured TPA of 35° there were no significant correlations with objective or subjective outcome measures when ECS was compared to tibial plateau leveling osteotomy (TPLO) [29]. In the author's opinion, a TPA above 35° is a criterion to move to a plateau leveling osteotomy procedure and above 30°, clients should be advised that concern exists about the ability of the ECS technique to control laxity sufficiently.

6.4 Operative Features of Extracapsular Suture

As the published techniques for ECS surgery have evolved over the past 50 years from the lateral retinacular imbrication technique to the knotless, interference anchor fixation [30–35], a corresponding evolution of surgical site preparation has occurred. As surgical site infection (SSI) has become more widely examined and the presence of antibiotic-resistant bacterial strains with their concomitant biofilm has increased in the community, it has become increasingly important that patients and their surgical fields are prepared carefully and completely to minimize preoperative and intraoperative surgery site contamination. More detailed information on patient preparation to minimize SSI can be found in Chapter 2; the following is pertinent to the ECS procedure.

The choice of skin disinfectant [36–38], the type and arrangement of surgical draping [39], and the routine use of an antimicrobial-impregnated incision drape [40–44] can all affect the inadvertent bacterial contamination of the surgical site during the ECS procedure. These protocol choices should be closely scrutinized and controlled by the primary surgeon. Evidence-based guidelines continue to evolve in the veterinary patient, the surgical team, and for surgical site preparation. Because of this, definitive recommendations are not possible at this stage for many of these areas for the ECS procedure. Surgical teams must review current guidelines, adapt current protocols as new information in these areas becomes available, and continue to evolve surgical preparation protocols to limit surgical site contamination.

Skin sterilization agents have evolved from the universal use of aqueous povidone-iodine-based scrubs and solutions to the adoption by some surgical teams of chlorhexidine-based products. Although experimental findings vary in the human surgical field, chlorhexidine-based products appear somewhat superior in the prevention of post-operative SSI [38].

The other significant change in skin antisepsis protocols has been the introduction of combination products. Applicators with a combination of povidone-iodine or chlorhexidine and 70% plus isopropyl alcohol (Duraprep™, 3M, Chloraprep™, BD) are now readily available. The development of a film-forming iodine acrylate copolymer, povacrylex (Duraprep™) has enhanced water resistance to iodine removal and improved adhesive drape adherence. The combined use of both product types also more effectively reduced the contamination of human surgical wounds [45].

Once the patient's leg skin has been effectively cleaned and prepared for surgery, the draping procedure is initiated. For more information on step-by-step draping for CCL surgery, please refer to Chapter 2. Briefly, placement of four corner drapes to isolate the patient leg and effective, water-resistant, sterile foot covering is recommended for the ECS procedure. A larger fenestrated patient drape can then be placed over the foot to cover the four corner drapes and the rest of the patient's body. Some human and veterinary surgeons use a single fenestrated drape or "key sheet." This drape has a central elastic insert section that is fenestrated and forms a tight, sealed cuff around the thigh. Although this drape type is convenient, its use must not compromise an effective barrier between the patient's aseptic and contaminated skin areas. Migration of the central cuff during surgery can lead to surgical site contamination.

Although an absolute consensus on the value of adhesive drapes in reducing surgical wound contamination and subsequent SSI rates is not possible in either the human or veterinary surgical arenas, it is thought that maintaining an occlusive barrier between the skin surrounding the surgical incision and the surgeon may allow less contamination of the surgical team's gloves during procedural limb manipulation. As part of an asepsis protocol in canine stifle surgery, there is a documented decrease in SSI rates [46] although the many variables involved make it impossible to definitively state that impregnated adhesive drapes should be used for all canine stifle surgery.

6.5 Placement of Implant: Femoral and Tibial Insertion Sites and Options

Extracapsular suture implantation technique and materials have been examined extensively over the past decade and different combinations of the anatomical site, implant type, and means of securing the implant to the patient have been investigated [34, 47–55]. The major technical decisions made by the surgeon include the choice of attachment sites, synthetic material used, the preimplantation material protocol, how the implant is tensioned prior to securement (Figure 6.1), the method of securing the implant to itself and the patient, and the protocol to minimize intraoperative implant contamination.

The choice of femoral and tibial attachment sites is surgeon dependent but should be guided by the underlying research. There are no true isometric extraarticular anatomical locations that effectively replicate the intraarticular origin and insertion of the native CCL. The described sites on the lateral aspect of the stifle differ between different studies and are better termed *quasiisometric* as they approximate rather than accurately mimic the native sites in biomechanical testing. The femoral attachment site is either a soft tissue anchor site at the lateral femorofabellar ligament, with the ECS being looped around the fabella during implantation to capture the ligament (circumfabellar placement), or the identification of a site on the lateral femoral condyle distal to the fabellar articulation and caudal to the lateral collateral ligament where a bone anchor or femoral tunnel can be placed (femoral condyle tunnel). Tibial bone tunnels are utilized distally in all techniques.

The two methods of femoral attachment, circumfabellar or femoral condyle bone tunnel (FCBT), are inherently different and should be considered independently when assessing technique, efficacy, and complications. The circumfabellar lateral fabellotibial suture (LFTS) has a soft tissue-based attachment proximally. Please refer to Chapter 7 for more information on the circumfabellar technique for ECS using nylon leader line. The femoral condyle bone tunnel technique (FCBT) includes both tunnel and the techniques that utilize bone anchors placed at the femoral tunnel origin site. The most well-recognized form of the FCBT in the surgical literature is the Tightrope® CCL. Detailed information regarding complications associated with using multifilament material can be found in Chapter 8.

The tibial insertion sites for bone tunnels have been investigated and vary between surgeons. The long digital extensor tendon groove is abutted cranially by Gerdy's tubercle. Placement of the tibial fixation site 2 mm below the tibial joint line and either cranial, within or caudal to the extensor groove are all options that have been evaluated. There is no definitive evidence for the superiority of any of these sites and different ECS techniques utilize different points. The surgeon must become familiar with the proximal lateral tibial anatomy, be able to consistently localize the chosen landmark for tunnel initiation, and be able to consistently create an accurate, well-formed tunnel for ECS material introduction.

6.6 Choice of Synthetic Material (Monofilament, Multifilament)

The major delineation between implant materials used is the choice of monofilament versus multifilament. Monofilament nylon has been investigated extensively in terms of its mechanical characteristics [56–58]. Multifilament polyblend polyethylene sutures are stronger and stiffer, and elongate less than nylon leader in direct mechanical comparisons [59, 60]. Choice of material between multi- and monofilament affects the method that can be used to secure the material. Monofilament material does not interact with bone anchors as the suture is prone to breakage where it is passed through an anchor eyelet and has too much volume to be pushed into a tunnel alongside a bone interference anchor. Nylon monofilaments are not used routinely in the FCBT technique. For more information on the ECS procedure using nylon monofilament, please refer to Chapter 7.

Biomechanical comparison of traditional round core suture multifilament with a circular cross-section to an ovoid cross-section suture tape showed suture tape had greater knot security, ultimate load to failure, and tensile stiffness [61]. Direct comparison of the two material types in a short-term LFTS outcome study found a higher failure rate with knotted polyethylene multifilament LFTS versus knotted monofilament nylon LFTS; importantly, all multifilament failures were due to suture pull-through of the fabellofemoral ligament, not failure of the suture material itself [62]. Replacing the circular cross-section multifilament suture with an ovoid cross-section tape suture may decrease the propensity for the multifilament material to saw through soft tissue attachments under tension. In human tendon repair, polyblend tape performs more favorably than circular polyblend round suture, with a greater mean load before suture pull-through [63]. Immature bone tunnel damage from multifilament sutures within the FCBT tunnel is recorded and care must be taken to allow bone tunnel maturation prior to excessive stifle motion to allow the tunnel maturation to occur post surgery.

6.7 Prefatigue and Tensioning of Material

Prior to placement of ECS implants, many surgeons prefatigue the ECS suture implants and remove early elastic deformability present. Prefatiguing is particularly relevant for monofilament nylon sutures. The idea of prestretching ECS implants is followed by many surgeons using nylon leader line as monofilament nylon has high memory and it is proposed that early elongation of suture length occurs. How effective pretensioning is at minimizing early postoperative suture loosening has not been examined scientifically. The tensioning of lateral ECS sutures has also been investigated [64, 65] along with its effect on lateral stifle compartment pressure and contact area [66]. Large variability exists between different methods of tensioning and securing LFTS. The use of a mechanical tensioning device increases LFTS construct tension. However, this creates high tension within the lateral compartment which alters contact pressures

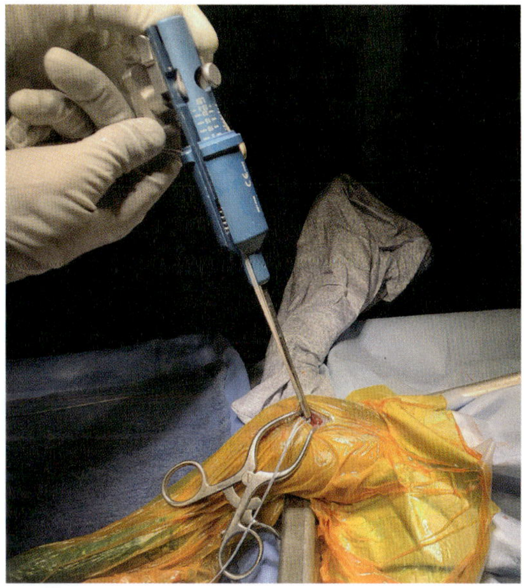

Figure 6.1 Tensioning device being utilized Intra-operatively to set a FCBT Tightrope® CCL implant tension before knotting.

within the joint in cadaver models [66]. A tensioning device is routinely recommended for the FCBT Tightrope® CCL technique (Figure 6.1) with recommended tension limits adjusted dependent on patient size.

Ideal ECS suture tension provides maximum stability without significant increases in joint contact pressures and without limitation to stifle range of motion. Appropriate tension is assessed clinically by testing drawer, thrust, and stifle flexion/extension after securing the suture. If the suture allows cranio-caudal instability, the tension is too low. If the suture restricts flexion/extension, the tension is too high or anchor locations are suboptimal.

6.8 Method of Securing the Material

There is conflicting published peer-reviewed literature utilizing cadaver limb testing regarding whether the strength, resistance to cyclical loading, and overall stability of a knotted multifilament, polyblend polyethylene implant with bone tunnel fixation (FCBT Tightrope® CCL) are superior to a knotted or crimped monofilament nylon or polyethylene multifilament LFTS construct [10, 14, 34]. As experimental load increases and cyclic loading is performed, both construct types failed to control cranial translation (caudal femoral subluxation/cranial tibial subluxation) completely, although the Tightrope® CCL (TR) construct resisted cyclic loading for more cycles in one experimental design [34]. The native CCL was five times stronger than either construct type [10]. Internal rotation is better controlled than cranial translation with all constructs although it does not reliably restore normal rotational stability [12–14].

There is considerable discussion about the type of knot employed (for example, square vs slip knot) to secure sutures with wide variation between knot types and individual surgeon's results in achieving optimal knot security [66–68]. The use of suture crimp clamps to secure nylon LFTS sutures is common and demonstrates an appreciable biomechanical advantage over knotted LFTS sutures [57, 69–73]. Additionally, the use of bone anchors has expanded over the past decade with biocompatible interference anchors placed into FCBT bone sockets to decrease complications with traditional eyed anchor suture interface damage and allow knotless fixation of FCBT constructs to the patient bone [74–76]. Cadaver biomechanical testing of the knotless interference anchor construct showed a trend toward increased resistance to cranio-caudal instability with dynamic cyclical testing when compared to a crimped nylon FTS construct [34].

6.9 Intraoperative Contamination and Avoidance Strategies

Of significant ongoing concern with ECS using multifilament material, and a real focus for surgeons, is the issue of intraoperative bacterial contamination of surgical sites and implants. There is considerable investigation of intraoperative interventions in human surgery with mixed evidence of efficacy [43]. It is well established that up to 80% of SSIs involve the presence of a bacteria-produced biofilm. This biofilm-mediated resistance to treatment of SSIs associated with biomedical implants is termed *antimicrobial recalcitrance* and allows persistent bacterial organisms to survive on the surface of implants in the face of patient immune-mediated defenses and the administration of antibiotics [77]. If biofilm is present, it is frequently necessary to remove colonized implants to allow infection resolution; in the context of ECS, early removal of the implants negates any stabilizing effects of the surgery, highlighting the importance of prevention of infection.

Evidence-based strategies for prevention of microbial biofilm development include weight-based antibiotic prophylaxis, skin antisepsis at the surgery site, maintenance of normothermia, glycemic control, antimicrobial sutures, and the use of surgical site irrigation. The use of intraoperative irrigation solutions is strongly recommended [78] but both bactericidal and patient cytotoxic responses have to be considered [79, 80]. The simplest fluid to irrigate with is an isotonic solution such as normal saline, but of growing interest is the use of aqueous dilute 0.05% chlorhexidine gluconate as an antiseptic irrigation agent in human surgery, with reported favorable responses in both human and animal studies [78, 81–83]. Surgeons should carefully examine the scientific evidence and the pros and cons of implementing antiseptic solution lavage before implementing a change to their surgical protocol. Antiseptic lavage solutions must be prepared immediately prior to surgical use, maintained in sterile form, and used judiciously with thought to what tissue is exposed to them and their potential cytotoxic effects on those patient tissues.

Additional strategies that may be used for prevention of surgical site contamination include double gloving, use of thicker orthopedic surgical gloves, glove changes, and use of paper impervious gowns instead of reusable gowns [84–86]. Outer glove exchange or placement of an overglove immediately before handling implants is recommended to minimize intraoperative contamination (Figure 6.2).

Another strategy to reduce the rate of implant contamination is to keep all implants in a sterile condition until immediately before implantation. By avoiding implants being exposed to surgical operating room airflow and premature handling by operative staff, the rate of preimplantation contamination can also be reduced. Informing operating room staff of implant exposure and handling protocols is vital in implementing surgical protocol success

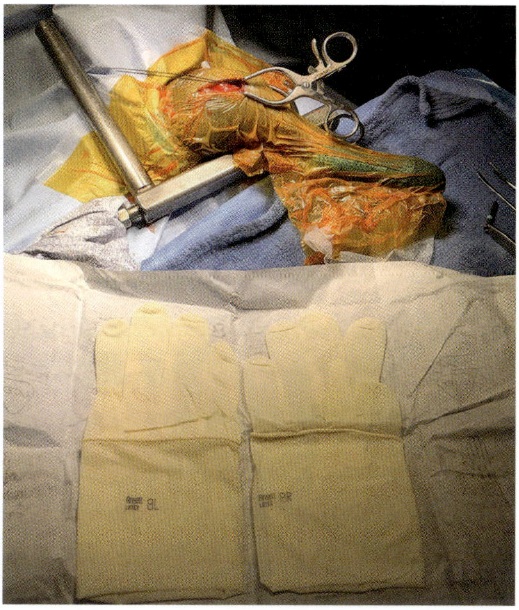

Figure 6.2 Second pair of gloves prepared for overgloving process prior to implant handling.

and achieving a decreased rate of implant contamination and subsequent SSI. The primary surgeon is responsible for initiating and maintaining intraoperative protocols and should direct implant handling in a clear and thorough fashion to minimize confusion and error amongst all personnel.

6.10 Soft Tissue Plane(s) Closure and Material Used

Following ECS implantation, closure of the surgical site should be performed in an efficient and timely fashion. With multiple layer closure necessary for all major procedures, the selection of suture material and closure pattern should reflect the tissue type, its rate of healing, and the tissue plane closure strength required. The use of antibacterial sutures (triclosan-coated) has been investigated in human surgery and a significant reduction in SSI rate has been found when triclosan-coated sutures are employed [87–91]. Published veterinary surgical research is limited in this area but no significant benefit was demonstrated when triclosan-impregnated suture was used for closure of tibial plateau leveling stifle stabilization [92]. The choice of skin suture, intradermal suture, or skin staple placement in terms of inflammation or infection development at the surgery site is unclear, with no clear scientific agreement on the relative merits of any of these strategies [92–94].

6.11 Identification of Intraoperative Complications

The development of intraoperative complications is not uncommon in stifle surgery and is influenced by the inherent difficulty of the surgical technique employed, the surgeon's knowledge and experience in performing the chosen technique, and the individual challenges inherent in the broad range of patient size and differences in anatomy. In small, overweight, and heavily muscled breeds, the dissection of the lateral aspect of the stifle can be challenging. Meticulous attention to anatomical detail and surgical landmarks is essential in avoiding excessive tissue dissection trauma. Difficulties are encountered with dissection medial to the biceps femoris fascia and the fascia at the caudo-distal aspect of the stifle adjacent to, and distal to, the lateral fabella. In this site inadvertent damage to local blood vessels with resultant hemorrhage can obscure important fabellar and femoral anchor site anatomy and result in incorrect ECS placement. The common peroneal nerve is also found running over the gastrocnemius muscle head in this location and entrapment of the nerve course during ECS placement is possible when a circumfabellar LFTS suture is used.

The intraoperative techniques used to ensure ECS implants acutely eliminate or significantly reduce cranio-caudal stifle instability and excessive internal tibial rotation vary according to personal preference, the ECS procedure variant used, the ECS material employed, and the use of a suture tensioner with or without a tensiometer. There is no universally accepted technique at the current time and there are no scientific data that support one technique as being the most successful. Individual surgeons who hand-tighten ECS use their judgment and experience to determine the tension prior to either knotting or placing suture crimps. Use of a tensiometer to set overall suture tension to a predetermined measurable level increases objectivity when assessing operative suture tension. When used in two-strand suture constructs, the tensioner with tensiometer allows tension on the overall construct to be set and maintained with one suture strand while the nontensioned suture strand is secured to itself by knot or crimp. There is no evidence that the suture tension chosen at surgery is maintained post surgery once joint motion resumes and a post-operative loss of suture tension, and therefore joint stability, is possible [95].

It is important when attempting to restore the normal anatomical relationship between the femur and the tibia that prior to final securing of the implant, any inherent creep (increase in length) in the suture material and loss of established suture tension due to soft tissue compression be minimized by preplacement loading and tensioning of suture material, by flexing and extending the stifle multiple times after initial suture placement and retensioning of the ECS construct after this process. The stifle joint angle at final tensioning and securement should be in slight extension and not flexion [50].

6.11.1 Decision Making with Identification of Intraoperative Complications

The development of intraoperative complications forces the surgeon to pause and consider their options. It is very important that a conscious consideration of the challenge that has arisen be assessed in terms of what is required to remedy it versus the degree of impact the complication will have on patient outcome. The balance of these two factors dictates the surgeon's course of action. The extended surgical time in combination with the continued patient's surgical trauma must be considered before a significant alteration in the patient's procedure is undertaken. It is also important that the surgeon feels strongly that they can significantly improve on the patient's current operative status before changing the procedure's protocol and revising steps in the procedure.

6.11.2 Revision Strategies for Intraoperative Complications

When performing intraoperative revisions, there are three potential options for the surgical team:

- repeat original technique sequence
- augmentation of currently placed implants
- technique replacement.

With ECS stabilization, the most common intraoperative complication is failure to achieve acceptable intraoperative stabilization. In this case, the surgeon can typically commence with replacing or retensioning and fastening the stabilization sutures. If a LFTS technique has been used, this may mean replacing the suture and placing it in a more anatomically secure location at the fabellar site with a second attempt to improve the tensioning and suture securing process. The caveat to this strategy is that if this does not improve the perceived stifle instability, the technique should be replaced with another option, as this may indicate that LFTS is not an appropriate therapy for this patient. The replacement technique may be a FCBT technique or a deviation to a dynamic stabilization technique utilizing a secured osteotomy. If a FCBT technique has been employed initially, a second femoral bone tunnel can be contemplated. The lack of available bone surface area in the correct femoral condylar tunnel origin site in most patients is difficult, so extreme care must be taken to avoid a tunnel-induced fracture.

The individual challenge for the surgeon is that they should be able to comfortably perform multiple surgical options for stifle stabilization, otherwise they may not be able to appropriately rescue a stifle stabilization failure at the time of the index procedure. If failure to achieve resolution of the underlying stifle instability occurs with operative revision, the patient's ineffective implants should be removed, the surgical site should be lavaged and closed carefully, the patient recovered from anesthesia safely, and an in-depth and honest discussion initiated with the patient owners. The owners should be informed of the challenges faced and current inability to overcome them. It is essential the patient's ongoing stifle instability be prioritized when amending the treatment plan. Offering referral at this stage, if not comfortable with more advanced techniques, is a required step to allow the patient to receive appropriate care and the surgical issue encountered to be resolved if possible. Attempting to explain away the operative failure, not having an open and honest discourse with the owners, and failing to prioritize the patient's safe and effective care are unacceptable and unethical.

6.12 Evaluation and Identification of Immediate Post-operative Complications

In the first 2 weeks after ECS surgery, the development of complications is termed *immediate*. The most common issues during this stage include excessive patient pain, failure of the patient to commence limb use, and the development of a SSI.

6.12.1 Excessive Patient Discomfort

Patients who present in the first 2 weeks with excessive surgical site and limb pain should be carefully evaluated and the cause determined. The three most common underlying causes are excessive inflammatory activity, development of a SSI, and the presence of neuropathic hypersensitivity. To differentiate between these, a thorough and methodical examination of the patient's limb and surgery site is necessary. Deciding between sterile inflammation and early infection can be challenging. There is some limited evidence that persistent elevations in the measurable blood values for C-reactive protein (CRP) and serum amyloid A (SAA) may indicate post-operative infection in knee surgery patients from day 6 post surgery [96]. The presence of local fluid accumulation at the surgical site, pain, lameness, an exudative discharge from the surgical incision or an adjacent skin sinus are major warning signs for infection. More in-depth information on identification of SSIs can be found in Chapter 3. An excessive inflammatory response can occur in the absence of infection and is characterized by surgery site swelling, edema, heat, and pain.

Treatment strategies for infection-induced and inflammation-induced excessive post-operative pain are different and delineation between the two is essential for correct treatment plans. Delineation of sterile versus septic inflammation is confirmed with positive bacterial culture of the incisional discharge although this process can give a false-negative result if concurrent antibiotic administration is present. It is also recommended that the presence of concurrent septic arthritis be investigated utilizing arthrocentesis and joint fluid analysis (Figure 6.3).

Pre- and postsurgery neuropathic pain syndromes (NPSs) are poorly recognized in canine patients in comparison to human patients. Neuropathic pain has been documented and explored in the canine patient [97–99] and has many similarities with the same condition in people. Neuropathic pain is common before and after human knee surgery and is present in up to 20% of human patients post surgery [100]. Canine patients who have excessive surgery site and limb pain post surgery, particularly without evidence of significant inflammation or infection, should be examined for the presence of allodynia and hyperalgesia on palpation of the sciatic nerve tract as it descends the caudolateral thigh. It is not uncommon that human patients are pre- and post-medicated with a

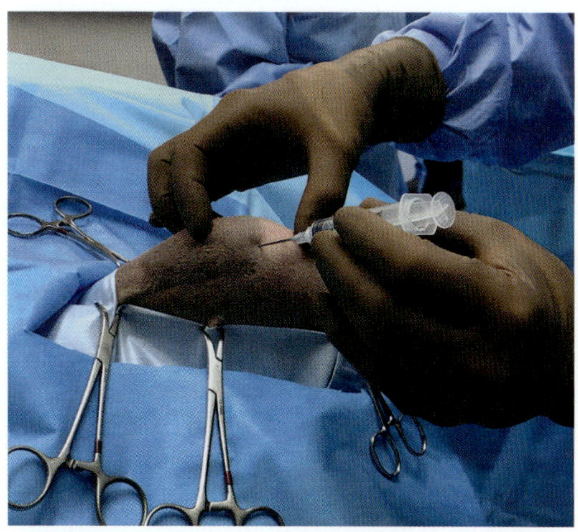

Figure 6.3 Arthrocentesis of a right stifle joint to detect the presence of septic arthritis post ECS surgery.

gabapentinoids to decrease the advent of neuropathic syndrome and decrease opioid administration post surgery [101–103]. Although there is limited scientific evidence to support the same strategy in canine patients, anecdotally there may be a benefit to a similar strategy and treatment of canine postsurgical neuropathic pain should be guided by our current understanding of available medications and patient responses [97–99].

The potential for entrapment of the common peroneal nerve at the time of surgery should also be considered if severe caudo-lateral stifle pain is elicited, and if this is a possibility, removal of the LFTS may be necessary.

6.12.2 Failure to Commence Limb Use

Predicting when patients will begin to use their surgical limb following ECS stabilization surgery is difficult and varies between patients, procedures, and performing surgeons. Time to weight bearing in individual patients will vary depending on the chronicity of pain present and our effectiveness in ameliorating its effect. Adequate pain control is important to encourage early limb use.

There may also be a behavioral component to nonweight-bearing behavior due to chronic disuse and pain syndromes. A behavioral cause for lack of limb use may be suspected if the limb is comfortable during examination, including range of motion and palpation of the stifle. The owner should be trained in methodology to encourage limb use, such as weight-shifting exercises. In addition, formal rehabilitation therapy is encouraged; more information can be found in Chapter 15.

The presence of persistent clinical meniscal pathology, termed *latent* meniscal damage or tear, that was not identified or dealt with appropriately at the time of surgery can also be a culprit in early post-operative inability or unwillingness to use the surgical limb [104–106]. The diagnosis of latent meniscal pathology is challenging, as diagnostic tests for this complication are either advanced procedures requiring specialist assistance or invasive (arthrotomy or arthroscopy). Additional information on diagnosing and managing meniscal damage can be found in Chapter 18.

6.12.3 Infection

Examining the surgical site carefully and attempting to determine if a superficial or deep SSI is present is important; this determination may require sedated or anesthetized wound examination. Delineating the SSI present in a postsurgical patient into a superficial versus deep SSI will be helpful in determining the best treatment plan to resolve the relevant infection.

Superficial infections are defined as above the muscular fascia layer and are localized for the most part to the dermal and subcutaneous tissue sites. Limited debridement, copious site flushing, and prolonged use of sensitive and effective antibacterials will resolve the majority of superficial SSIs without the need to reopen the deeper layers and potentially explant biofilm-contaminated implants. In deep SSI infections, the contaminated zone is at the implant location and may involve the underlying bone surface. A real risk of osteomyelitis is present and treatment strategies have to be aggressive, will involve more surgical procedures in most cases, and explantation of the implant with its biofilm will likely be necessary. Obtaining deep cultures, including submission of contaminated explanted implants, may be necessary to accurately identify the bacterial population present and what antibacterials will be effective against them (Figure 6.4). Repeat irrigation and debridement of significantly infected tissue and the use of long-term antibiotic therapy for 6–8 weeks are not unusual.

The decision to explant and culture ECS implants is a difficult one and must be carefully considered and discussed with clients in detail. The removal of implants in the early stages of infection should be reserved for patients which do not respond to parenteral antibiotics and local treatment of the surgery site and intraarticular space. Clients must be aware that early explantation of ECS implants will destabilize the stifle joint and likely introduce the need for further stabilization surgery following complete resolution of surgical infection. Timing of the second stabilization procedure and choice of what procedure to perform are crucial to patient success and the maintenance of a positive, beneficial client relationship. Failure to discuss the options in detail and possibly refer to a second surgeon who is more skilled and

(a) (b)

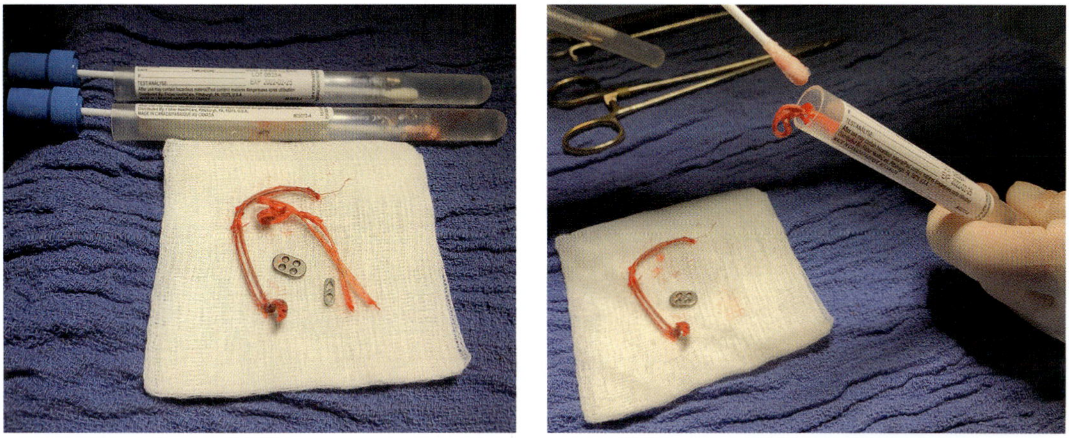

Figure 6.4 (a) Explanted multifilament polyblend polyethylene implant with corresponding tie and toggle securing buttons. (b) Implant placement into bacterial culturettes for culture and sensitivity testing.

experienced in a stifle stabilization procedure than the initial surgeon is a failure of the primary surgeon to act in an ethical and caring fashion and should be avoided in all cases.

A perception also exists in the veterinary surgical arena that multifilament ECS implants have a higher complication rate in terms of infection risk and ongoing damage to patient implant bone tunnels [6]. There is no definitive scientific evidence currently available in the canine or human literature that suggests that infection rates are higher with a multifilament versus monofilament implant or suture [106]. The choice of a nylon monofilament in a LFTS versus multifilament polyethylene sutures in an ECS construct should not be based on post-operative infection rate but rather on biomechanical comparison [59, 60] and individual surgeon' ability to overcome the technical challenges of placement.

It is also imperative to determine in a suspected SSI if there is a concurrent septic arthritis. Performance of joint arthrocentesis (Figure 6.3) with cytological examination of fluid smears along with comprehensive joint fluid analysis is indicated. The presence of degenerative neutrophils and visible bacteria indicates active joint infection. Culturing the joint fluid is recommended but obtaining a positive culture is challenging in many cases. The result of a false-negative culture from a joint fluid sample should be anticipated in approximately 50% of septic arthritis cases [107, 108]. In order to improve sensitivity of culture, some laboratories recommend storing joint fluid in blood culture media during transit. Alternatively, the submission of a sample of synovium may be required to obtain a positive culture result. Ideally, samples for culture would be collected prior to initiating (or after a break from) antibiotic therapy in order to isolate causative pathogens.

Once a sample has been collected for culture, broad-spectrum bactericidal antibiotics should be commenced while awaiting culture results. In the presence of suspected joint infection, it may be beneficial to perform joint lavage immediately post arthrocentesis. The placement of ingress and egress catheters or large-bore needles into separate stifle joint compartments and allowing 500–1000 mL of pressurized sterile isotonic fluid to irrigate the intraarticular space may be helpful in decreasing the intraarticular bacterial load (Figure 6.5). It is also possible that the joint is inflamed but not infected; blood and joint fluid laboratory analysis can also be used to help differentiate infectious from noninfectious joint inflammation [109].

6.13 Evaluation and Identification of Delayed, Midterm Post-operative Complications

Extracapsular suture complications that occur in the midterm range of 2 weeks to 6 months post surgery are termed *delayed* post-operative

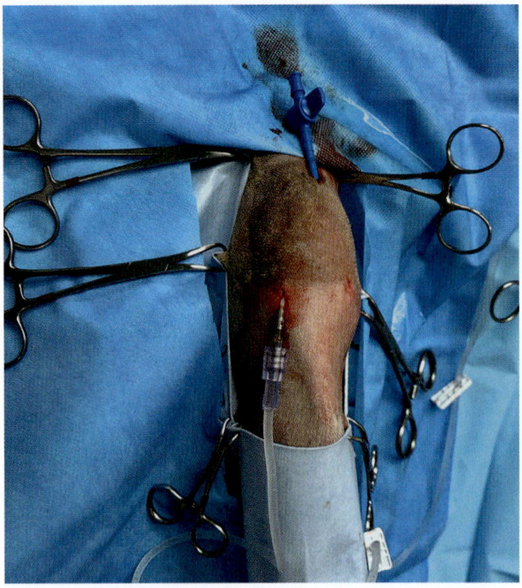

Figure 6.5 Therapeutic right stifle joint lavage in suspected septic arthritis post ECS stabilization. Saline delivery into lateral joint space with egress cannula medially in proximal joint space.

complications. The complications previously discussed in the immediate stage may persist or develop in this next time period. Persistent excessive patient discomfort can be caused by persistent inflammatory status of the intraarticular and/or extraarticular tissues. Concurrent infection is also an issue in some patients and it too may be inside the joint or in the extracapsular tissues. Persistent synovitis should be distinguished from septic arthritis by arthrocentesis and submission of synovial fluid for laboratory analysis. Examination of synovial fluid cytology along with documentation of cell types, cell characteristics such as degree of degeneration or toxicity, and relative cell counts will assist the surgeon in delineating between inflammatory synovitis and septic arthritis. The presence of fluid accumulation or a draining sinus at the surgical incision or adjacent to the surgical location may indicate SSI and collection of fluid accumulated at the surgery site with laboratory analysis and sinus tract culturing should be considered.

Aggressive treatment of intra- and extraarticular infection is crucial to preservation of the patient's stifle joint structures, including the cartilage beds and remaining normal intraarticular structures. As previously discussed, it is important to categorize the SSI present as superficial or deep and tailor treatment accordingly (see Chapter 3 for more information). If infection control is possible with accurate bacterial isolation, commencement of sensitive antibiotics and joint lavage or debridement as indicated, it may not be necessary to remove implants. However, the option to remove implants should be considered carefully. In most cases, the removal of ECS implants (Figure 6.4a) after 10–12 weeks will decrease joint stability but may not destabilize the affected stifle to a degree where further stabilization surgery is indicated. Patients in this category are assessed on a case-by-case basis and appropriate monitoring of both clinical improvements in lameness and joint function is instituted. Antibiotic therapy should be continued for 4–6 weeks. Following the cessation of antibiotics, the site must be monitored carefully for recurrence of clinical signs.

The presence of recurrence will require a change in treatment plan and explantation at that stage with implant culture is recommended. A decision to perform further joint stabilization should be postponed until complete recovery from infection is reached. Any doubt about whether this has occurred should prompt an extension in the observation period. Unfortunately, patients will often demonstrate significant lameness during this period and continued confinement and monitoring of the patient's progress by clients is crucial to long-term success. Excessive patient activity at this time on a grossly unstable joint will lead to joint damage and will compromise the results of further attempts to provide functional joint stability.

Neuropathic hypersensitivity can develop readily or persist into the delayed complication time period and may require extended treatment if persistent. Ongoing reassessment of sciatic nerve tract allodynia and hyperalgesia will allow clinicians to monitor for a lameness-inducing nerve pain syndrome and allow fine-tuning of medication treatment and physical rehabilitation efforts.

One of the critical reassessments that occur in the midterm recovery stage between 2 weeks and 6 months post surgery is the degree of stifle stability that the ECS procedure has provided to the patient. Careful, concise, and accurate assessment of cranio-caudal, medio-lateral, and rotational stifle stability is necessary during this period to determine change from the immediate post-operative period. Categorizing stifle stability in terms of mild, moderate, or severe instability for each of cranio-caudal, medio-lateral, and rotational stifle stability will allow an assessment of initial severity and progression of instability during subsequent exams during the midterm complication phase and beyond. Identifying loss of operative stability, that the patient's stifle is no longer functionally stable, is vital to the continued patient management plan. Some loss of operative stability with ECS procedures during this period is common among all the variants of the ECS procedure and may lead to permanent clinical dysfunction with lameness, compromise of athletic function, and progressive development of osteoarthritis.

It is well accepted that re-establishment of normal, native stability is likely not routinely possible with the ECS procedure. What is not well established is what degree of stability is needed for patients to be able to exercise normally and not have continued impairment to their function. The role of compensatory fibrosis of the periarticular tissues is thought to be the long-term stabilization mechanism and it is the fibrotic reaction in the joint capsule and adjacent connective tissue that supplements the ECS procedure and eventually replaces the role of the suture implant. How quickly this fibrosis develops, how well it preserves the stability achieved with the original implant placement, and how persistent its effect are vary between patients and are influenced by many factors.

In most cases, mild instability in any plane is well tolerated clinically and severe instability is not. The effect of moderate post-operative instability on the patient's stifle and limb function will depend heavily on the individual patient, and determination of the need for further surgical intervention will be an individual patient-based decision by the clinician managing the case.

If it is determined that the patient is not able to satisfactorily recover with the post-operative result present, the issue of follow-up surgery will need to be openly and honestly discussed with the client. Repeating the same ECS technique, replacing the primary ECS technique with another ECS technique or replacing the ECS technique with a different type of stabilization surgery are potential options. Assessing the relative merits of each option is challenging, requires knowledge and experience of other stabilization techniques and should be carefully and completely discussed with the client. Clients must be sufficiently educated about the options, have a good baseline of understanding to contribute to the decision making, and the ethical and medico-legal requirements of the profession must be adequately met. Referral of stabilization failures to specialist surgeons with broad-based, extensive stifle surgery experience must also be clearly discussed with clients and documented clearly in the patient's medical record to avoid professional challenge by veterinary supervisory boards. It is important that individual surgeons document their complications in sufficient detail and their discussions with clients are recorded in the medical record.

Follow-up revision procedures due to index procedure failure are challenging, have an increased rate of complications, and can also fail. Clients must understand this well and be able to guide their pet's care appropriately. Most revision procedures should not be attempted until the primary surgery site is well recovered, infection, if present, has been completely resolved, and the patient has demonstrated no significant surgical site issues for an appropriate time period. Rushing into a second procedure without sufficient pause is not appropriate and may worsen the current situation permanently.

A significant cause of postsurgical lameness and stifle joint discomfort following ECS is the development of a *subsequent* meniscal tear [105]. A subsequent meniscal tear is defined as meniscal damage sustained following the initial surgery (as opposed to a *latent* tear, which was missed at the initial surgery). Reaching a diagnosis of meniscal pathology can be challenging and significant research has been performed to clarify the relative accuracy of different diagnostic methods. The presence of a meniscal "click" or "catch" on stifle examination is strongly predictive of meniscal tear presence. However, the absence of a palpable meniscal click/catch is not a strong indicator for a normal meniscus [110–113].

Musculoskeletal ultrasound examination [114–116], computed tomography (CT) arthrography [117, 118], and low- [119, 120] and high-field magnetic resonance imaging (MRI) [121–124] have all been investigated for their accuracy in diagnosing canine meniscal pathology before surgery. Results vary between modalities and investigators but as a general rule, high-frequency ultrasound in the hands of an experienced operator and high-field MRI both had good accuracy. Expense and lack of availability (including expertise in stifle imaging) likely limit many surgeons from utilizing these modalities and many patients undergo joint exploration when analgesia treatment trials fail, and SSI is ruled out. The use of arthrotomy versus arthroscopy in detecting meniscal pathology has been evaluated and arthroscopic assessment with concurrent probing of the menisci is the most accurate technique [125, 126]. The availability of experienced arthroscopic stifle surgeons varies geographically but the improved visualization and increased accuracy of both diagnosis and treatment make this technique preferable to arthrotomy and referral to an arthroscopic surgeon should also be considered and offered to clients if readily available.

The development of patellar instability and luxation post stifle stabilization is not uncommon and is multifactorial in etiology. When present, it can be a significant cause of postsurgical lameness and patient discomfort. If persistent over time, cartilage damage to the articular surface of the patella and the medial or lateral trochlear ridges, depending on the direction of the patellar luxation, occurs. In patients who have predisposing abnormal femoral and tibial anatomy, the malalignment of the quadriceps axis influences patellar tracking and can result in patellofemoral malfunction. In patients whose patellar instability is not recognized prior to ECS surgery or who have a surgical complication post ECS surgery that destabilizes the patellofemoral relationship, the grade of instability and clinical severity are assessed for consideration of further surgery. The type, technical aspects, and relative success rates of combined tibiofemoral and patellofemoral stabilization surgery are beyond the scope of this chapter but need to be well understood and intelligently reviewed to determine the most appropriate course of action for the affected patient [127]. Failure to perform this review will predispose the patient to further issues and a possible treatment failure.

In patients who have undergone ECS surgery and in which a previously stable patellofemoral joint has become unstable, there are several possibilities. The most common cause of medial patellofemoral instability is breakdown of a lateral arthrotomy repair when the arthrotomy incision was advanced proximally to a level that the lateral patellofemoral band was transected and the subsequent surgical repair of that band failed. Similarly, lateral patellar luxation can occur if a medial arthrotomy destabilizes the medial patellofemoral band and the repair fails. In these cases, surgical reconstruction of the medial (or lateral) patellofemoral band often resolves the issue. Medial patellar luxation can also occur in cases where ECS failed to achieve good rotational stability post surgery. The tendency toward lack of rotational stability may be exacerbated in patients with distal femoral varus, distal femoral internal torsion or internal tibial torsion. Control of excessive internal tibial rotation is used in some patients with medial patellar luxation to decrease dynamic internal tibial rotation and improve patellar stability. Fortunately, regardless of the ECS technique used, rotational instability is improved in most patients post ECS surgery, although the degree with which it approaches normal rotational stability in individual patients varies [12, 13].

6.14 Evaluation and Identification of Long-Term Post-operative Complications

The persistence or development of ECS complications in the time period after 6 months post-operatively is designated *long term*. These complications are commonly reported by owners and not detected routinely by veterinary staff, as most patients are not examined routinely in this time period. It is important that owners are educated about possible complication issues in this period and are asked to proactively contact the surgeon's practice if they are concerned about the patient's status or recovery progress.

As previously discussed, post-operative stifle joint instability can persist or develop post-operatively and patients may demonstrate discomfort, lameness, and decreased function. Clinical examination is necessary to determine the degree of instability present. For the ECS procedure, a moderate or severe loss of cranio-caudal or rotational stability from the immediate or delayed post-operative periods is cause for concern. If unresponsive to reinstated exercise restriction for 4–6 weeks and/or a professional formal rehabilitation program, consideration should be given to another procedure to attempt to rectify the stifle instability. The choice of procedure type should be made carefully with full disclosure to clients of possible issues, including inability to restore stability, persistent lameness, and a possible increased risk of SSI that exists with subsequent surgery.

The development of late-onset SSI is not uncommon in the ECS surgical patient population and the presence of pain, lameness, swelling, and draining skin tracts at or adjacent to the surgical incision indicates its existence. The relative proportion of superficial versus deep SSI in the surgical patient 3 months or more post surgery appears to favor deep infection below the underlying fascial layer. These infections are often associated with implant biofilm and may also include bone involvement.

Radiographs of the surgical site are important in the early assessment of infection depth. Reactive periosteal new bone and lysis of adjacent cortical bone are strong indicators of osteomyelitis presence. Bacterial sampling for culture and susceptibility testing should be carefully performed and represents deep tissue contamination and not skin surface flora. Careful preparation of discharging sinus sites with clipping and antibacterial solutions prior to placement of the culture swab deep into the sinus tract may yield more accurate results. If deep infection is suspected, it is likely that explantation of the ECS implant will be necessary and clients should be prepared for that eventuality early and completely in the case discussion process.

Treating the infection initially with susceptible antibiotics and monitoring clinical response is appropriate but in the presence of joint sepsis, bony involvement or poor early response to antibiotic therapy, surgical explantation and infected tissue irrigation and debridement is appropriate. Antibiotic therapy should be continued for 3–6 weeks post surgery with routine revisits for assessment of infection resolution. If osteomyelitis is present, careful selection of effective antibiotics that penetrate bone is necessary. Failure to select appropriate antibacterial agents can lead to chronic, persistent bone infection that may be very difficult to resolve.

Following surgical implant removal, the patient should be allowed to recover completely from the infection process prior to reassessment of joint stability. In this later stage of overall recovery, it is common that the stifle will retain its pre-explantation stability with formed fibrous tissue at the implant location and generally in the joint capsule, providing acceptable joint stability in many patients. In others, instability may require a second procedure, but the timing and choice of the procedure type must be carefully weighed against the possibility of residual bacterial presence and persistent subclinical infection.

As previously discussed in the delayed complication section, subsequent meniscal tears are not an uncommon ECS postsurgical cause of patient lameness, stifle pain, and poor function. Rates vary in the surgical literature but most studies report a 5–10% long-term occurrence in ECS patients [105, 128, 129]. Reported cases include patients who develop clinical signs that are significant enough for re-presentation for veterinary examination. They do not include patients that have developed nonclinical tears and it is thought the actual subsequent tear rate may be significantly higher. Treatment of clinical subsequent tears may include conservative management with rest and reduced exercise for several months or surgical re-examination of the menisci and removal of damaged, unstable meniscal tissue. The presence of meniscal pathology should be carefully considered in patients which have acutely decompensated in their surgical limb use at some point post surgery. Failure to address significant tears that impinge upon femoral condylar and tibial plateau articular cartilage may result in significant damage to articular cartilage of these structures and exacerbate the degree of osteoarthritis present in the stifle joint.

A significant and well-documented issue with all stifle stabilization surgeries is the progression of osteoarthritis and chronic fibrosing joint capsule synovitis. Regardless of the technique utilized to stabilize the stifle, an appreciable progression of radiographic osteoarthritis in ECS patients is seen when patients have follow-up imaging studies [27, 28]. The clinical role of this progressive degeneration in the stifle structures is difficult to separate from residual instability, as they are most likely linked. Treatment of osteoarthritis is based on multimodal therapy and includes patient conditioning and weight loss, judicious use of nutraceuticals and prescription medications, and, more recently, biologic therapy. Patient response varies and is difficult to predict, an in-depth discussion with clients with sequential examinations to determine efficacy of treatment plans is recommended.

6.15 Conclusion

Overall, the rate of significant operative and post-operative complications in performance of ECS stabilization of the canine stifle in clinically affected dogs is routinely 5–8%. The occurrence and recognition of complications are very important in maintaining the success of the stabilization procedure for the individual surgical patient. Complication rates vary between surgeons and it is important for individual surgeons to carefully document their minor and major complications. Informing the patient's owners of your overall complication rate, your complication rate for the main complication classification categories and what will be the general sequence of events that occurs if a minor or major complication develops is ethical and professional and should be performed for every owner of every stifle instability patient that is offered stabilization surgery. A dedicated, long-term effort by the surgical team to recognize surgical complications as they arise, inform owners completely about their occurrence, and develop a complication treatment plan is necessary.

Every effort should be made to reduce complication rates and avoid their occurrence. Constant reassessment of surgical protocols, documentation of changes in protocol, and ongoing education of the surgical team are crucial in controlling complication rates. Establishment and maintenance of surgical protocol checklists to avoid breaches in surgical protocol are essential to long-term surgical unit success. Complication rates can be controlled and individual patients with complications can be resolved with attention to detail, ethical decision making, excellent patient follow-up, and a dedicated effort by all members of the practice team to follow well-established and successful surgical protocols.

Contributors

Sincere gratitiude and grateful recognition of effort made is extended to Selena Tinga, DVM, PhD, DACVS-SA for assistance in Chapter editing and content suggestions.

References

1. Smith, B. (2000). Extracapsular stabilisation. *Aust. Vet. J.* 78 (6): 382–383.
2. Tonks, C.A., Lewis, D.D., and Pozzi, A. (2011). A review of extra-articular prosthetic stabilization of the cranial cruciate ligament-deficient stifle. *Vet. Comp. Orthop. Traumatol.* 24 (3): 167–177.
3. Comerford, E., Forster, K., Gorton, K., and Maddox, T. (2013). Management of cranial cruciate ligament rupture in small dogs: a questionnaire study. *Vet. Comp. Orthop. Traumatol.* 26 (6): 493–497.
4. Duerr, F.M., Martin, K.W., Rishniw, M. et al. (2014). Treatment of canine cranial cruciate ligament disease. A survey of ACVS Diplomates and primary care veterinarians. *Vet. Comp. Orthop. Traumatol.* 27 (6): 478–483.
5. Bergh, M.S., Sullivan, C., Ferrell, C.L. et al. (2014). Systematic review of surgical treatments for cranial cruciate ligament disease in dogs. *J. Am. Anim. Hosp. Assoc.* 50 (5): 315–321.
6. von Pfeil, D.J.F., Kowaleski, M.P., Glassman, M., and Dejardin, L.M. (2018). Results of a survey of Veterinary Orthopedic Society members on the preferred method for treating cranial cruciate ligament rupture in dogs weighing more than 15 kilograms (33 pounds). *J. Am. Vet. Med. Assoc.* 253 (5): 586–597.
7. D'Amico, L.L., Lanz, O.I., Aulakh, K.S. et al. (2013). The effects of a novel lateral extracapsular suture system on the kinematics of the cranial cruciate deficient canine stifle. *Vet. Comp. Orthop. Traumatol.* 26 (4): 271–279.
8. Rey, J., Fischer, M.S., and Böttcher, P. (2014). Sagittal joint instability in the cranial cruciate ligament insufficient canine stifle. Caudal slippage of the femur and not cranial tibial subluxation. *Tierarztl. Prax. Ausg. K Kleintiere Heimtiere* 42 (3): 151–156.

9. Headrick, J.F., Zhang, S., Millard, R.P. et al. (2014). Use of an inverse dynamics method to compare the three-dimensional motion of the pelvic limb among clinically normal dogs and dogs with cranial cruciate ligament-deficient stifle joints following tibial plateau leveling osteotomy or lateral fabellar-tibial suture stabilization. *Am. J. Vet. Res.* 75 (6): 554–564.
10. Biskup, J.J., Griffon, D.J., Socie, M. et al. (2014). Ability of the Tightrope® and percutaneous lateral fabellar suture techniques to control cranial tibial translation. *Vet. Surg.* 43 (8): 959–965.
11. Tinga, S., Kim, S.E., Banks, S.A. et al. (2018). Femorotibial kinematics in dogs with cranial cruciate ligament insufficiency: a three-dimensional in-vivo fluoroscopic analysis during walking. *BMC Vet. Res.* 14 (1): 85.
12. Tinga, S. (2018). In-vivo femorotibial kinematics in dogs with cranial cruciate ligament insufficiency before and after surgical stabilization. PhD dissertation. University of Florida, Gainesville, FL, USA.
13. Tinga, S., Kim, S.E., Banks, S.A. et al. (2020). Femorotibial kinematics in dogs treated with lateral fabellotibial suture stabilization for complete cranial cruciate ligament rupture: an in-vivo fluoroscopic analysis during walking in nine dogs weighing more than 15kg (33 lbs). *J. Am. Vet. Med. Assoc.* 49: 187–199.
14. Laugier, M., Tremblay, J., Petit, Y. et al. (2019). Three-dimensional kinematic evaluation of Tightrope CCL in a canine in vitro cranial cruciate deficient stifle model. *Can. J. Vet. Res.* 83 (4): 317–321.
15. Quinn, M.M., Keuler, N.S., Lu, Y. et al. (2007). Evaluation of agreement between numerical rating scales, visual analogue scoring scales, and force plate gait analysis in dogs. *Vet. Surg.* 36 (4): 360–367.
16. Tivers, M.S., Commerford, E.J., and Owen, M.R. (2009). Does a fabella-tibial suture alter the outcome for dogs with cranial cruciate ligament insufficiency undergoing arthrotomy and caudal pole medial meniscectomy? *Vet. Comp. Orthop. Traumatol.* 22 (4): 283–288.
17. Snow, L.A., White, R., Gustafson, S. et al. (2010). ex vivo comparison of three surgical techniques to stabilize canine cranial cruciate ligament deficient stifles. *Vet. Surg.* 39 (2): 195–207.
18. Cook, J.L., Luther, J.K., Beetem, J. et al. (2010). Clinical comparison of a novel extracapsular stabilization procedure and tibial plateau leveling osteotomy for treatment of cranial cruciate ligament deficiency in dogs. *Vet. Surg.* 39 (3): 315–323.
19. Conzemius, M.G., Evans, R.B., Besancon, M.F. et al. (2005). Effect of surgical technique on limb function after surgery for rupture of the cranial cruciate ligament in dogs. *J. Am. Vet. Med. Assoc.* 226 (2): 232–236.
20. Gordon-Evans, W.J., Griffon, D.J., Bubb, C. et al. (2013). Comparison of lateral fabellar suture and tibial plateau leveling osteotomy techniques for treatment of dogs with cranial cruciate ligament disease. *J. Am. Vet. Med. Assoc.* 243 (5): 675–680.
21. Nelson, S.A., Krotscheck, U., Rawlinson, J. et al. (2013). Long-term functional outcome of tibial plateau leveling osteotomy versus extracapsular repair in a heterogeneous population of dogs. *Vet. Surg.* 42 (1): 38–50.
22. Mölsä, S.H., Hyytiäinen, H.K., Hielm-Björkman, A.K., and Laitinen-Vapaavuori, O.M. (2014). Long-term functional outcome after surgical repair of cranial cruciate ligament disease in dogs. *BMC Vet. Res.* 10: 266.
23. Berger, B., Knebel, J., Steigmeier-Raith, S. et al. (2015). Long-term outcome after surgical treatment of cranial cruciate ligament rupture in small breed dogs. Comparison of tibial plateau leveling osteotomy and extra-articular stifle stabilization. *Tierarztl. Prax. Ausg. K Kleintiere Heimtiere* 43 (6): 373–380.
24. Krotscheck, U., Nelson, S.A., Todhunter, R.J. et al. (2016). Long term functional outcome of tibial tuberosity advancement vs. tibial plateau leveling osteotomy and extracapsular repair in a heterogeneous population of dogs. *Vet. Surg.* 45 (2): 261–268.
25. Lussier, B., Gagnon, A., Moreau, M. et al. (2018). Peak vertical force in a stabilized canine cranial cruciate deficient stifle model: a one-year follow-up. *Can. J. Vet. Res.* 82 (2): 159–161.
26. Au, K.K., Gordon-Evans, W.J., Dunning, D. et al. (2010). Comparison of short- and long-term function and radiographic osteoarthrosis in dogs after post-operative physical rehabilitation and tibial plateau leveling osteotomy or lateral fabellar suture stabilization. *Vet. Surg.* 39 (2): 173–180.
27. Lazar, T.P., Berry, C.R., deHaan, J.J. et al. (2005). Long-term radiographiccomparison of tibial plateau leveling osteotomy versus extracapsular stabilization for cranial cruciate ligament rupture in the dog. *Vet. Surg.* 34 (2): 133–141.
28. Gilbert, S., Langenbach, A., Marcellin-Little, D.J. et al. (2019). Stifle joint osteoarthritis at the time of diagnosis of cranial cruciate ligament injury is higher in boxers and in dogs weighing more than 35 kilograms. *Vet. Radiol. Ultrasound* 60 (3): 280–288.
29. Havig, M.E., Dyce, J., Kowaleski, M.P. et al. (2007). Relationship of tibial plateau slope to limb function in dogs treated with a lateral suture technique for stabilization of cranial cruciate ligament deficient stifles. *Vet. Surg.* 36 (3): 245–251.
30. DeAngelis, M. and Lau, R.E. (1970). A lateral retinacular imbrication technique for the surgical correction of anterior cruciate ligament rupture in the dog. *J. Am. Vet. Med. Assoc.* 157 (1): 79–84.
31. Flo, G.L. (1975). Modification of the lateral retinacular imbrication technique for stabilizating cruciate ligament injuries. *J. Am. Anim. Hosp. Assoc.* 11: 570–573.
32. Olmstead, M.L. (1993). The use of orthopedic wire as a lateral suture for stifle stabilization. *Vet. Clin. North Am. Small Anim. Pract.* 23 (4): 735–753.

33. Störk, C.K., Gibson, N.R., Owen, M.R. et al. (2001). Radiographic features of a lateral extracapsular wire suture in the canine cranial cruciate deficient stifle. *J. Small Anim. Pract.* 42 (10): 487–490.
34. Choate, C.J., Lewis, D.D., Conrad, B.P. et al. (2013). Assessment of the craniocaudal stability of four extracapsular stabilization techniques during two cyclic loading protocols: a cadaver study. *Vet. Surg.* 42 (7): 853–859.
35. Biskup, J.J. and Griffon, D.J. (2014). Technical difficulties during the training phase for Tightrope® and percutaneous lateral fabellar suture techniques for cranial cruciate ligament repair. *Vet. Surg.* 43 (3): 347–354.
36. Sidhwa, F. and Itani, K.M. (2015). Skin preparation before surgery: options and evidence. *Surg. Infect* 16 (1): 14–23.
37. Letzelter, J., Hill, J.B., and Hacquebord, J. (2019). An overview of skin antiseptics used in orthopaedic surgery procedures. *J. Am. Acad. Orthop. Surg.* 27 (16): 599–606.
38. Chen, S., Chen, J.W., Guo, B., and Xu, C.C. (2020). Preoperative antisepsis with chlorhexidine versus povidone-iodine for the prevention of surgical site infection: a systematic review and meta-analysis. *World J. Surg.* 44: 1412–1424.
39. Kieser, D.C., Wyatt, M.C., Beswick, A. et al. (2018). Does the type of surgical drape (disposable versus non-disposable) affect the risk of subsequent surgical site infection? *J. Orthop.* 15 (2): 566–570.
40. Kramer, A., Assadian, O., and Lademann, J. (2010). Prevention of post-operative wound infections by covering the surgical field with iodine-impregnated incision drape (Ioban 2). *GMS Krankenhhyg. Interdiszip.* 5 (2): doc08.
41. Webster, J. and Alghamdi, A. (2013). Use of plastic adhesive drapes during surgery for preventing surgical site infection. *Cochrane Database Syst. Rev.* (1): CD006353.
42. Bejko, J., Tarzia, V., Carrozzini, M. et al. (2015). Comparison of efficacy and cost of iodine impregnated drape vs. standard drape in cardiac surgery: study in 5100 patients. *J. Cardiovasc. Transl. Res.* 8 (7): 431–437.
43. Liu, Z., Dumville, J.C., Norman, G. et al. (2018). Intraoperative interventions for preventing surgical site infection: an overview of Cochrane reviews. *Cochrane Database Syst. Rev.* 2: CD012653.
44. Karapınar, K. and Kocatürk, C.İ. (2019). The effectiveness of sterile wound drapes in the prevention of surgical site infection in thoracic surgery. *Biomed Res. Int.* 2019: 1438793.
45. Patrick, S., McDowell, A., Lee, A. et al. (2017). Antisepsis of the skin before spinal surgery with povidone iodine-alcohol followed by chlorhexidine gluconate-alcohol *versus* povidone iodine-alcohol applied twice for the prevention of contamination of the wound by bacteria: a randomised controlled trial. *Bone Joint J.* 99-B (10): 1354–1365.
46. Stine, S.L., Odum, S.M., and Mertens, W.D. (2018). Protocol changes to reduce implant-associated infection rate after tibial plateau leveling osteotomy: 703 dogs, 811 TPLO (2006-2014). *Vet. Surg.* 47 (4): 481–489.
47. Roe, S.C., Kue, J., and Gemma, J. (2008). Isometry of potential suture attachment sites for the cranial cruciate ligament deficient canine stifle. *Vet. Comp. Orthop. Traumatol.* 21 (3): 215–220.
48. Kunkel, K.A., Basinger, R.R., Suber, J.T., and Gerard, P.D. (2009). Evaluation of a transcondylar toggle system for stabilization of the cranial cruciate deficient stifle in small dogs and cats. *Vet. Surg.* 38 (8): 975–982.
49. Hulse, D., Hyman, W., Beale, B. et al. (2010). Determination of isometric points for placement of a lateral suture in treatment of the cranial cruciate ligament deficient stifle. *Vet. Comp. Orthop. Traumatol.* 23 (3): 163–167.
50. Fischer, C., Cherres, M., Grevel, V. et al. (2010). Effects of attachment sites and joint angle at the time of lateral suture fixation on tension in the suture for stabilization of the cranial cruciate ligament deficient stifle in dogs. *Vet. Surg.* 39 (3): 334–342.
51. Reichert, E.E., Kunkel, K.A., Suber, J.T. et al. (2013). Radiographic localization and isometry of the origin and insertion of the canine cranial cruciate ligament. *Vet. Surg.* 42 (7): 860–866.
52. Aulakh, K.S., Harper, T.A., Lanz, O.I. et al. (2013). Effect of tibial insertion site for lateral suture stabilization on the kinematics of the cranial cruciate ligament deficient-stifle during early, middle and late stance: an in vitro study. *Vet. Comp. Orthop. Traumatol.* 26 (3): 208–217.
53. Roe, S.C. (2013). The challenge of isometry for extracapsular devices. *Vet. Comp. Orthop. Traumatol.* 26 (4): VII.
54. Cinti, F., Signorelli, C., Lopomo, N. et al. (2015). Two different approaches for novel extracapsular cranial cruciate ligament reconstruction: an in vitro kinematics study. *J. Small. Anim. Pract.* 56 (6): 398–406.
55. Witte, P.G. (2015). Tibial anatomy in normal small breed dogs including anisometry of various extracapsular stabilizing suture attachment sites. *Vet. Comp. Orthop. Traumatol.* 28 (5): 331–338.
56. Lewis, D.D., Milthorpe, B.K., and Bellenger, C.R. (1997). Mechanical comparison of materials used for extra-capsular stabilisation of the stifle joint in dogs. *Aust. Vet. J.* 75 (12): 890–896.
57. Sicard, G.K., Hayashi, K., and Manley, P.A. (2002). Evaluation of 5 types of fishing material, 2 sterilization methods, and a crimp-clamp system for extra-articular stabilization of the canine stifle joint. *Vet. Surg.* 31 (1): 78–84.
58. Wallace, A.M., Cutting, E.D., Sutcliffe, M.P., and Langley-Hobbs, S.J. (2008). A biomechanical comparison of six different double loop configurations for use in the lateral fabella suture technique. *Vet. Comp. Orthop. Traumatol.* 21 (5): 391–399.

59. Burgess, R., Elder, S., McLaughlin, R., and Constable, P. (2010). in vitro biomechanical evaluation and comparison of FiberWire, FiberTape, OrthoFiber, and nylon leader line for potential use during extraarticular stabilization of canine cruciate deficient stifles. *Vet. Surg.* 39 (2): 208–215.
60. Rose, N.D., Goerke, D., Evans, R.B., and Conzemius, M.G. (2012). Mechanical testing of orthopedic suture material used for extra-articular stabilization of canine cruciate ligament-deficient stifles. *Vet. Surg.* 41 (2): 266–272.
61. Leishman, D.J. and Chudik, S.C. (2019). Suture tape with broad full-width core versus traditional round suture with round core: a mechanical comparison. *Arthroscopy* 35 (8): 2461–2466.
62. Lodato, D., Wardlaw, J., and Rowe, D. (2013). Retrospective study comparing two materials commonly used in the LFS technique for CCLR. *J. Am. Anim. Hosp. Assoc.* 49 (2): 108–114.
63. Gnandt, R.J., Smith, J.L., Nguyen-Ta, K. et al. (2016). High-tensile strength tape versus high-tensile strength suture: a biomechanical study. *Arthroscopy* 32 (2): 356–363.
64. Dunn, A.L., Buffa, E.A., Marchevsky, A.M. et al. (2012). Inter- and intra-operator variability associated with extracapsular suture tensioning: an ex vivo study. *Vet. Comp. Orthop. Traumatol.* 25 (6): 472–477.
65. Burton, A.F., Horstman, C., and Mason, D.R. (2015). Tensions generated in a lateral fabellotibial suture model. Comparison of methods of application of tension, fixation of tension and suture material. *Vet. Comp. Orthop. Traumatol.* 28 (6): 391–400.
66. Tonks, C.A., Pozzi, A., Ling, H.Y., and Lewis, D.D. (2010). The effects of extra-articular suture tension on contact mechanics of the lateral compartment of cadaveric stifles treated with the TightRope CCL or lateral suture technique. *Vet. Surg.* 39 (3): 343–349.
67. Jiang, J., Mat Jais, I.S., Yam, A.K. et al. (2017). A biomechanical comparison of different knots tied on fibrewire suture. *J. Hand Surg. Asian Pac. Vol.* 22 (1): 65–69.
68. Meyer, D.C., Bachmann, E., Lädermann, A. et al. (2018). The best knot and suture configurations for high-strength suture material. An in vitro biomechanical study. *Orthop. Traumatol. Surg. Res.* 104 (8): 1277–1282.
69. Anderson, C.C. 3rd, Tomlinson, J.L., Daly, W.R. et al. (1998). Biomechanical evaluation of a crimp clamp system for loop fixation of monofilament nylon leader material used for stabilization of the canine stifle joint. *Vet. Surg.* 27 (6): 533–539.
70. Moores, A.P., Beck, A.L., Jespers, K.J. et al. (2006). Mechanical evaluation of two crimp clamp systems for extracapsular stabilization of the cranial cruciate ligament-deficient canine stifle. *Vet. Surg.* 35 (5): 470–475.
71. Vianna, M.L. and Roe, S.C. (2006). Mechanical comparison of two knots and two crimp systems for securing nylon line used for extra-articular stabilization of the canine stifle. *Vet. Surg.* 35 (6): 567–572.
72. Maritato, K.C., Barnhart, M.D., Kazanovicz, A.J., and Naber, S.J. (2012). in vitro mechanical evaluation and comparison of two crimping devices for securing monofilament nylon and multifilament polyethylene for use in extracapsular stabilization of the canine stifle. *Vet. Comp. Orthop. Traumatol.* 25 (6): 466–471.
73. Aisa, J., Calvo, I., Buckley, C.T., and Kirby, B.M. (2015). Mechanical comparison of loop and crimp configurations for extracapsular stabilization of the cranial cruciate ligament-deficient stifle. *Vet. Surg.* 44 (1): 50–58.
74. Guénégo, L., Zahra, A., Madelénat, A. et al. (2007). Cranial cruciate ligament rupture in large and giant dogs. A retrospective evaluation of a modified lateral extracapsular stabilization. *Vet. Comp. Orthop. Traumatol.* 20 (1): 43–50.
75. Hulse, D., Saunders, B., Beale, B., and Kowaleski, M. (2011). Extra-articular stabilization of the cranial cruciate deficient stifle with anchor systems. *Tierarztl. Prax. Ausg. K Kleintiere Heimtiere* 39 (5): 363–367.
76. Raske, M. and Hulse, D. (2013). SwiveLock bone anchor stabilization of the cranial cruciate ligament deficient stifle in dogs: clinical outcome. *Open J. Vet. Med.* 3: 297–301.
77. Edmiston, C.E. Jr., McBain, A.J., Roberts, C., and Leaper, D. (2015). Clinical and microbiological aspects of biofilm-associated surgical site infections. *Adv. Exp. Med. Biol.* 830: 47–67.
78. Edmiston, C.E. Jr. and Leaper, D.J. (2016). Intra-operative surgical irrigation of the surgical incision: what does the future hold-saline, antibiotic agents, or antiseptic agents? *Surg. Infect.* 17 (6): 656–664.
79. van Meurs, S.J., Gawlitta, D., Heemstra, K.A. et al. (2014). Selection of an optimal antiseptic solution for intraoperative irrigation: an in vitro study. *J. Bone Joint Surg. Am.* 96 (4): 285–291.
80. Edmiston, C.E. Jr., Spencer, M., and Leaper, D. (2018). Antiseptic irrigation as an effective interventional strategy for reducing the risk of surgical site infections. *Surg. Infect. (Larchmt)* 19 (8): 774–780.
81. Edmiston, C.E. Jr., Bruden, B., Rucinski, M.C. et al. (2013). Reducing the risk of surgical site infections: does chlorhexidine gluconate provide a risk reduction benefit? *Am. J. Infect. Control* 41 (5 Suppl): S49–S55.
82. Schmidt, K., Estes, C., McLaren, A., and Spangehl, M.J. (2018). Chlorhexidine antiseptic irrigation eradicates *Staphylococcus epidermidis* from biofilm: an in vitro study. *Clin. Orthop. Relat. Res.* 476 (3): 648–653.

83. Arslan, N.C., Degirmenci, A.K., Ozdenkaya, Y., and Terzi, C. (2020). Wound irrigation with chlorhexidine gluconate reduces surgical site infection in pilonidal disease: single-blind prospective study. *Surg. Infect.* 21 (2): 143–149.
84. Ward, W.G. Sr., Cooper, J.M., Lippert, D. et al. (2014). Glove and gown effects on intraoperative bacterial contamination. *Ann. Surg.* 259 (3): 591–597.
85. Mischke, C., Verbeek, J.H., Saarto, A. et al. (2014). Gloves, extra gloves or special types of gloves for preventing percutaneous exposure injuries in healthcare personnel. *Cochrane Database Syst. Rev.* 3: CD009573.
86. Kim, K., Zhu, M., Munro, J.T., and Young, S.W. (2019). Glove change to reduce the risk of surgical site infection or prosthetic joint infection in arthroplasty surgeries: a systematic review. *ANZ J. Surg.* 89 (9): 1009–1015.
87. Chang, W.K., Srinivasa, S., Morton, R., and Hill, A.G. (2012). Triclosan-impregnated sutures to decrease surgical site infections: systematic review and meta-analysis of randomized trials. *Ann. Surg.* 255 (5): 854–859.
88. Wang, Z.X., Jiang, C.P., Cao, Y., and Ding, Y.T. (2013). Systematic review and meta-analysis of triclosan-coated sutures for the prevention of surgical-site infection. *Br. J. Surg.* 100 (4): 465–473.
89. Edmiston, C.E. Jr., Daoud, F.C., and Leaper, D. (2013). Is there an evidence-based argument for embracing an antimicrobial (triclosan)-coated suture technology to reduce the risk for surgical-site infections? A meta-analysis. *Surgery* 154 (1): 89–100.
90. de Jonge, S.W., Atema, J.J., Solomkin, J.S., and Boermeester, M.A. (2017). Meta-analysis and trial sequential analysis of triclosan-coated sutures for the prevention of surgical-site infection. *Br. J. Surg.* 104 (2): e118–e133.
91. Ahmed, I., Boulton, A.J., Rizvi, S. et al. (2019). The use of triclosan-coated sutures to prevent surgical site infections: a systematic review and meta-analysis of the literature. *BMJ Open* 9 (9): e029727.
92. Etter, S.W., Ragetly, G.R., Bennett, R.A., and Schaeffer, D.J. (2013). Effect of using triclosan-impregnated suture for incisional closure on surgical site infection and inflammation following tibial plateau leveling osteotomy in dogs. *J. Am. Vet. Med. Assoc.* 242 (3): 355–358.
93. Frey, T.N., Hoelzler, M.G., Scavelli, T.D. et al. (2010). Risk factors for surgical site infection-inflammation in dogs undergoing surgery for rupture of the cranial cruciate ligament: 902 cases (2005–2006). *J. Am. Vet. Med. Assoc.* 236 (1): 88–94.
94. Atwood, C., Maxwell, M., Butler, R., and Wills, R. (2015). Effects of incision closure method on infection prevalence following tibial plateau leveling osteotomy in dogs. *Can. Vet. J.* 56 (4): 375–381.
95. Böttcher, P., Fischer, C., Werner, H. et al. (2010). Stifle stability after lateral suture stabilisation using Ethibond Excel®: early destabilisation following cyclic passive joint motion (in German). *Tierarztl. Prax. Ausg. K Kleintiere Heimtiere* 38 (2): 61–69.
96. Löfqvist, K., Kjelgaard-Hansen, M., and Nielsen, M.B.M. (2018). Usefulness of C-reactive protein and serum amyloid A in early detection of post-operative infectious complications to tibial plateau leveling osteotomy in dogs. *Acta Vet. Scand.* 60 (1): 30.
97. Grubb, T. (2010). Chronic neuropathic pain in veterinary patients. *Top. Compan. Anim. Med.* 25 (1): 45–52.
98. Sanchis-Mora, S., Pelligand, L., Volk, H.A., and Abeyesinghe, S.M. (2015). Diagnosis and treatment of canine neuropathic pain. *Vet. Rec.* 177 (18): 470.
99. Moore, S.A. (2016). Managing neuropathic pain in dogs. *Front. Vet. Sci.* 3: 12.
100. Vergne-Salle, P. (2016). Management of neuropathic pain after knee surgery. *Joint Bone Spine* 83 (6): 657–663.
101. Zhai, L., Song, Z., and Liu, K. (2016). The effect of gabapentin on acute post-operative pain in patients undergoing total knee arthroplasty: a meta-analysis. *Medicine* 95 (20): e3673.
102. Fitzsimmons, M., Carr, E., Woodhouse, L., and Bostick, G.P. (2018). Development and persistence of suspected neuropathic pain after total knee arthroplasty in individuals with osteoarthritis. *PM R* 10 (9): 903–909.
103. Attal, N. (2019). Pharmacological treatments of neuropathic pain: the latest recommendations. *Rev. Neurol.* 175 (1–2): 46–50.
104. Plesman, R., Gilbert, P., and Campbell, J. (2013). Detection of meniscal tears by arthroscopyand arthrotomy in dogs with cranial cruciate ligament rupture: a retrospective, cohort study. *Vet. Comp. Orthop. Traumatol.* 26 (1): 42–46.
105. Ritzo, M.E., Ritzo, B.A., Siddens, A.D. et al. (2014). Incidence and type of meniscal injury and associated long-term clinical outcomes in dogs treated surgically for cranial cruciate ligament disease. *Vet. Surg.* 43 (8): 952–958.
106. Rappa, N.S. and Radasch, R.M. (2016). Post-operative complications associated with the Arthrex Canine Cranial Cruciate Ligament Repair Anchor System in small- to medium-sized dogs: a retrospective analysis (2009–2012). *Can. Vet. J.* 57 (8): 847–852.
107. Scharf, V.F., Lewis, S.T., Wellehan, J.F. et al. (2015). Retrospective evaluation of the efficacy of isolating bacteria from synovial fluid in dogs with suspected septic arthritis. *Aust. Vet. J.* 93 (6): 200–203.
108. Mielke, B., Comerford, E., English, K., and Meeson, R. (2018). Spontaneous septic arthritis

of canine elbows: twenty-one cases. *Vet. Comp. Orthop. Traumatol.* 31 (6): 488–493.

109. Hillström, A., Bylin, J., Hagman, R. et al. (2016). Measurement of serum C-reactive protein concentration for discriminating between suppurative arthritis and osteoarthritis in dogs. *BMC Vet. Res.* 12 (1): 240.
110. Tuuli, M.G., Stout, M.J., Martin, S. et al. (2016). Comparison of suture materials for subcuticular skin closure at cesarean delivery. *Am. J. Obstet. Gynecol.* 215 (4): 490.
111. Case, J.B., Hulse, D., Kerwin, S.C., and Peycke, L.E. (2008). Meniscal injury following initial cranial cruciate ligament stabilization surgery in 26 dogs (29 stifles). *Vet. Comp. Orthop. Traumatol.* 21 (4): 365–367.
112. Neal, B.A., Ting, D., Bonczynski, J.J., and Yasuda, K. (2015). Evaluation of meniscal click for detecting meniscal tears in stifles with cranial cruciate ligament disease. *Vet. Surg.* 44 (2): 191–194.
113. Gleason, H.E., Hudson, C.C., and Cerroni, B. (2020). Meniscal click in cranial cruciate deficient stifles as a predictor of specific meniscal pathology. *Vet. Surg.* 49 (1): 155–159.
114. Mahn, M.M., Cook, J.L., Cook, C.R., and Balke, M.T. (2005). Arthroscopic verification of ultrasonographic diagnosis of meniscal pathology in dogs. *Vet. Surg.* 34 (4): 318–323.
115. Arnault, F., Cauvin, E., Viguier, E. et al. (2009). Diagnostic value of ultrasonography to assess stifle lesions in dogs after cranial cruciate ligament rupture: 13 cases. *Vet. Comp. Orthop. Traumatol.* 22 (6): 479–485.
116. Franklin, S.P., Cook, J.L., Cook, C.R. et al. (2017). Comparison of ultrasonography and magnetic resonance imaging to arthroscopy for diagnosing medial meniscal lesions in dogs with cranial cruciate ligament deficiency. *J. Am. Vet. Med. Assoc.* 251 (1): 71–79.
117. Samii, V.F., Dyce, J., Pozzi, A. et al. (2009). Computed tomographic arthrography of the stifle for detection of cranial and caudal cruciate ligament and meniscal tears in dogs. *Vet. Radiol. Ultrasound* 50 (2): 144–150.
118. Tivers, M.S., Mahoney, P.N., Baines, E.A., and Corr, S.A. (2009). Diagnostic accuracy of positive contrast computed tomography arthrography for the detection of injuries to the medial meniscus in dogs with naturally occurring cranial cruciate ligament insufficiency. *J. Small Anim. Pract.* 50 (7): 324–332.
119. Böttcher, P., Brühschwein, A., Winkels, P. et al. (2010). Value of low-field magnetic resonance imaging in diagnosing meniscal tears in the canine stifle: a prospective study evaluating sensitivity and specificity in naturally occurring cranial cruciate ligament deficiency with arthroscopy as the gold standard. *Vet. Surg.* 39 (3): 296–305.
120. Böttcher, P., Armbrust, L., Blond, L. et al. (2012). Effects of observer on the diagnostic accuracy of low-field MRI for detecting canine meniscal tears. *Vet. Radiol. Ultrasound* 53 (6): 628–635.
121. Blond, L., Thrall, D.E., Roe, S.C. et al. (2008). Diagnostic accuracy of magnetic resonance imaging for meniscal tears in dogs affected with naturally occurring cranial cruciate ligament rupture. *Vet. Radiol. Ultrasound* 49 (5): 425–431.
122. Galindo-Zamora, V., Dziallas, P., Ludwig, D.C. et al. (2013). Diagnostic accuracy of a short-duration 3 Tesla magnetic resonance protocol for diagnosing stifle joint lesions in dogs with non-traumatic cranial cruciate ligament rupture. *BMC Vet. Res.* 9: 40.
123. Olive, J., d'Anjou, M.A., Cabassu, J. et al. (2014). Fast presurgical magnetic resonance imaging of meniscal tears and concurrent subchondral bone marrow lesions. Study of dogs with naturally occurring cranial cruciate ligament rupture. *Vet. Comp. Orthop. Traumatol.* 27 (1): 1–7.
124. Taylor-Brown, F., Lamb, C.R., Tivers, M.S., and Li, A. (2014). Magnetic resonance imaging for detection of late meniscal tears in dogs following tibial tuberosity advancement for treatment of cranial cruciate ligament injury. *Vet. Comp. Orthop. Traumatol.* 27 (2): 141–146.
125. Pozzi, A., Hildreth, B.E. 3rd, and Rajala-Schultz, P.J. (2008). Comparison of arthroscopy and arthrotomy for diagnosis of medial meniscal pathology: an ex vivo study. *Vet. Surg.* 37 (8): 749–755.
126. Plesman, R., Gilbert, P., and Campbell, J. (2013). Detection of meniscal tears by arthroscopy and arthrotomy in dogs with cranial cruciate ligament rupture: a retrospective, cohort study. *Vet. Comp. Orthop. Traumatol.* 26 (1): 42–46.
127. Fauron, A.H., Bruce, M., James, D.R. et al. (2017). Surgical stabilization of concomitant canine medial patellar luxation and cranial cruciate ligament disease. Effect of fixation method on post-operative complication rate and clinical outcome. *Vet. Comp. Orthop. Traumatol.* 30 (3): 209–218.
128. Christopher, S.A., Beetem, J., and Cook, J.L. (2013). Comparison of long-term outcomes associated with three surgical techniques for treatment of cranial cruciate ligament disease in dogs. *Vet. Surg.* 42 (3): 329–334.
129. Dycus, D.L., Wardlaw, J.L., Rowe, D., and Elder, S. (2013). In-vitro comparison of 3 knotting techniques for lateral fabellotibial suture stabilization. *Can. Vet. J.* 54 (4): 353–358.

7 Complications Associated with Extracapsular Stabilization Using Monofilament Material

R. Randy Basinger

7.1 Introduction

The definition of lateral extracapsular suture (LES) for the purposes of this chapter will be an extracapsular suture of nylon leader line (NLL) coursing from the lateral surface of the femur to the proximal cranial tibia. The suture is anchored proximally by encircling the lateral fabella or to a bone anchor in the caudolateral femoral condyle distal to the lateral fabella. It is anchored distally to bone tunnel(s) or a bone anchor in the proximal cranial tibia.

7.2 History of Lateral Extracapsular Suture

The LES is a common technique for repair of the cranial cruciate ligament (CCL)-deficient stifle that was developed in the 1970s [1, 2] and has been performed on tens of thousands of patients over the years. It is probably still the most common surgical procedure performed for treatment of this condition given that general practitioners as well as specialists perform the procedure. Over time, innovations have been made to the original procedure to make it technically easier and more reproducible. Different suture types and means to attach the suture to the femur and tibia, and methods to tension and secure the suture have been introduced [3–6].

Over the last 30 years, multiple studies have been published about outcomes, complications, comparison of different suture types, fastening methods, anchor types, isometric placement points, and comparison of outcomes to other techniques. No single surgical technique has consistently proven superior. In a number of studies, LES compares favorably to other current techniques [7, 8] and only recently was tibial plateau leveling osteotomy (TPLO) shown to be superior to LES in a controlled study [9].

When the American College of Veterinary Surgeon Diplomates and general practice veterinarians were surveyed in 1999, the majority of dogs under 9.1 kg were still treated by LES [10]. In the same study, LES was still commonly performed in large dogs although more osteotomy procedures were done compared to small dogs. Despite all the options available for CCL disease repair today, LES is still a commonly performed repair technique. This is especially true with general practice veterinarians due to the relative simplicity of the procedure, the low cost of instrumentation and

Complications in Canine Cranial Cruciate Ligament Surgery, First Edition. Edited by Ron Ben-Amotz and David L. Dycus.

implants to perform the procedure, and the decreased cost to the client compared to osteotomy techniques. Because of the antirotational effect of LES, it is also a useful procedure when there is a coexistent medial patellar luxation (MPL), with or without CCL disease, or when excessive internal rotation is still present after an osteotomy procedure. Finally, the monofilament nature of NLL makes infection risk lower than multifilament suture types due to lower bacterial adherence compared to multifilament sutures [11, 12].

Lateral extracapsular suture is likely to remain a viable surgical treatment option, especially for general practice veterinarians, smaller dogs, and when excessive internal rotation of the tibia or MPL exists.

This chapter will cover patient selection considerations for LES along with preoperative planning tips to minimize complications. In addition, intraoperative technical considerations, complications, identification, and revision strategies will be discussed as well as identification and management of postoperative complications. Tips to avoid intraoperative and postoperative complications will be presented.

7.3 Patient Selection Considerations for Lateral Extracapsular Suture

Historically, LES was performed on all types of veterinary patients largely due to a lack of other treatment options. While many patients did very well, others did not, and critical evaluation over the last 50 years began to shed some light on factors that influenced the outcome of the procedure. Refinements in surgical technique, implants, and equipment occurred which helped with some of the technical and implant complications covered later, but some patients consistently did not due as well as others. How one defines "complication" of a specific procedure also determines whether some outcomes are complications or not.

When multiple procedures exist for the same condition, this author feels it may be fair to consider it a complication if the selected procedure does not consistently meet the expected level of return to function of the other procedures that treat the same condition. Multiple studies compared outcome difference between LES and TPLO or other surgery techniques, with variable conclusions but generally showing LES to be an effective treatment for CCL disease, often showing it to have outcomes no different from or better than other procedures currently in use [13–19]. It is important that the client be aware of the expected outcome for a given procedure compared to other options based on clinical studies, and our own subjective assessment of the other variables of the patient's and owner's situation and expectations that influence outcome but are not included in published studies.

This author's approach is generally to recommend TPLO for almost all dogs if finances permit, based on its more consistent ability to return dogs closer to normal function and minimize subsequent osteoarthritis (OA) development [13] compared to LES. However, I do emphasize that LES is certainly a very good procedure and likely to improve comfort and function in patients for clients unwilling to pursue osteotomy procedures. If the patient is small or has concurrent MPL or excessive internal rotation, LES is more frequently recommended. I would not generally recommend bilateral simultaneous LES repair in dogs with bilateral CCL disease due to slower return to weight bearing and concerns of stabilization failure.

It is generally accepted that body weight is a major factor determining expected level of function of dogs with LES, with those weighing more than about 25–30 kg being more likely to have TPLO over LES [10]. Body weight is also a factor in the likelihood of developing complications. In a study of 305 dogs, those heavier than 33.7 kg were more likely to develop complications with LES, defined as an undesirable outcome associated with the surgical procedure or occurring after the surgery that was confirmed via physical examination of the dog at the hospital [20].

In this same study, younger dogs were also reported to be more likely to develop complications. It was theorized that their greater activity level or difficulty in postoperative restraint could be the cause of their increased risk of complications. Overall, 17.4% of patients developed a complication in this study, and 7.2% required an additional surgery [20]. Other studies have reported overall complication rates between 9% and 25% [6].

The progression of OA is greater with LES than TPLO [13]. Due to our current lack of good salvage procedures for end-stage stifle OA, managing CCL disease to minimize OA development is critical. This includes proper timing of surgical treatment before OA is established, maintaining meniscal integrity, choosing procedures for CCL disease repair most likely to minimize OA development, and being conscientious about follow-up and weight management.

Dogs with high tibial plateau angles (TPAs) seem more likely to develop problems with repair breakdown, despite one study showing no difference [21]. Measurement of TPA should be part of the minimum database before a specific procedure for CCL disease repair is recommended. More on measuring the TPA can be found in Chapter 10. Many surgeons have performed LES on a small dog who we felt should have done well with a lateral suture repair only to have the suture(s) break in the first 2 weeks postoperatively (PO). When evaluation of TPA became commonplace and we looked at these patients, we found many of them had excessive TPA angles (>34°) and were likely to overpower any LES repair (Figure 7.1).

Postoperative physical rehabilitation has been shown to improve outcomes for patients with CCL disease repaired with LES [22]. In a survey with 376 respondents, 71% of veterinarians recommended postoperative rehabilitation and were more than twice as likely to recommend rehabilitation for LES than osteotomy techniques [23]. The client must be aware of this, and if postoperative rehabilitation cannot be done for some reason, it may affect the LES outcome and prompt consideration of another treatment. While a full rehabilitation protocol is beyond the scope of this book, additional information on rehabilitation can be found in Chapter 15.

7.4 Preoperative Planning Tips to Minimize Complications

- Obtain a thorough history of the patients' current lifestyle and expectations for lifestyle after surgery.
- In young dogs, consider the increased risk of complications with LES and higher risk of OA development long term given the expected length of life after surgery.
- In large dogs, recommend an osteotomy technique over LES as likely to give the best outcome.
- Evaluate the TPA and consider a repair technique other than LES if the TPA is high (>26°) or excessive (>34°) (Figure 7.1a).
- Determine the pet owner's ability to undertake formal rehabilitation postoperatively for their pet.

7.5 Intraoperative Technical Considerations, Complications, and Revision Strategies

Lateral extracapsular suture repair techniques have been described previously [1, 2, 6–8]. One modification that the author finds very useful is to avoid the morbidity of a full lateral arthrotomy and instead perform two limited approaches to separately accomplish the two goals of the procedure.

The skin incision for the procedure can be either medial or lateral. A medial "mini-arthrotomy" is done to evaluate, probe, and excise any damaged meniscal tissue and release the medial meniscus if desired. This incision is closed with several interrupted sutures and the skin incision is reflected laterally. Alternatively, this step can be done via arthroscopy.

For placement of the LES, the caudolateral femoral condyle and fabella are approached by a linear incision directed from the proximal cranial tibia directly toward the fabella, exposing the path that the LES will take and avoiding excessive dissection and a large arthrotomy. If needed, the incision can be carried caudoproximal past the fabella to gain good exposure, though the surgeon will have to split some of the fibers of the biceps muscle at its insertion on the lateral fascia of the joint. This approach provides greater exposure for atraumatic circumfabellar suture placement or easy access to the F2 isometric point on the femoral condyle for bone anchor placement. Good exposure and accurate needle passage around the fabella can also minimize the chance of iatrogenic peroneal nerve damage, which has been reported as a possible complication to LES [20].

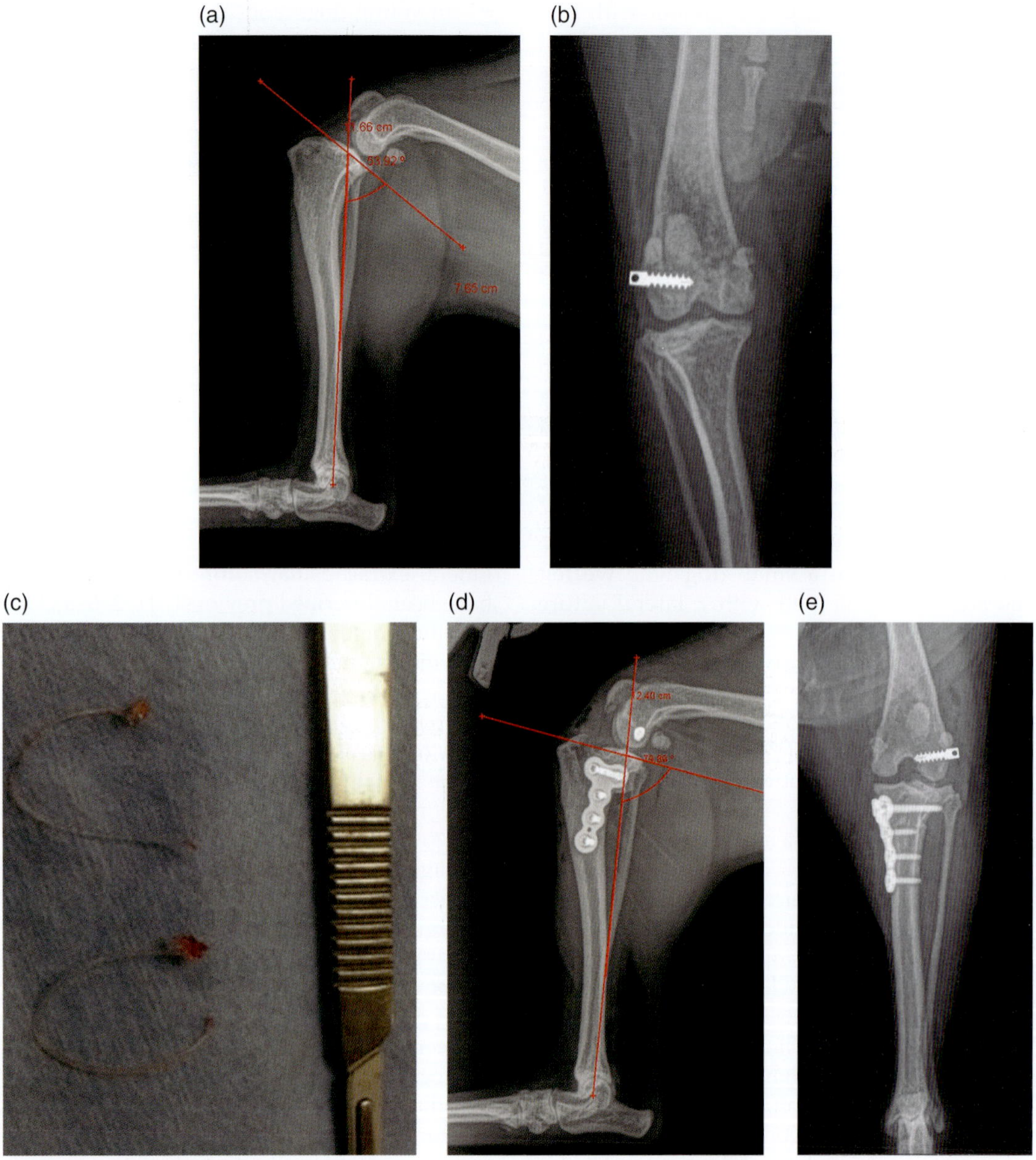

Figure 7.1 (a) Preoperative lateral radiograph of a 4.3 kg Yorkie with TPA = 36°. (b) Postoperative caudal cranial radiograph documenting bone anchor placement. (c) Two-week postoperative, acutely lame – 2 × 9 kg NLL breakage at knot. (d) Postoperative lateral view of revision with TPLO. (e) Postoperative caudal-cranial view of revision with TPLO.

Regardless of the surgical technique used, the goal of the procedure is to evaluate and treat any meniscal injuries, and then place the LES so that it will minimize cranial translation of the tibia in relation to the femur while periarticular fibrosis imparts long-term stability to the joint.

Diagnosis and management of meniscal injuries is covered in Chapter 18. A significant complication of any CCL disease repair surgery would be to miss a meniscal injury requiring treatment. More specific to LES repair with NLL than other techniques is deciding whether or not to release the medial meniscus. Given that NLL will stretch, and most repairs will have some cranial tibial subluxation return over time, the risk of subsequent or postliminary meniscal tears is probably higher with this technique. The meniscal release procedure was advised to decrease the risk of postliminary meniscal injury. It is effective in decreasing the risk of subsequent meniscal tears with TPLO [24] and LES [20]. However, the released medial meniscus is less able to limit cranial tibial subluxation which further challenges the LES repair. Releasing the medial meniscus also concentrates femorotibial contact stress in the caudal portion of the medial compartment, resulting in decreased contact area and increased peak pressure, predisposing to OA development [25].

While there is considerable controversy regarding medial meniscal release, it is fair to say that there is further stress on the LES repair and an increased risk of OA development when meniscal release is performed, and an increased risk of postliminary meniscal tears when the meniscus is not released. An older dog or one in which the possibility of a second surgery to treat a postliminary meniscal tear is not an option might be the most reasonable patient for which to consider meniscal release in conjunction with LES.

After the fabella and proximal tibia have been exposed for placement of the LES, the surgeon must decide whether the fabella or a bone anchor will be used as the proximal anchor point. When the fabella is chosen as the proximal LES attachment point, care must be taken to avoid disruption of the attachment of the fabella to the caudal aspect of the femur. This is especially true in small patients for which LES is commonly chosen. In a study of dogs <7 kg, the mean lateral fabellar diameter was only 2.9 mm, and one dog had an absence of a lateral fabella [26]. Occasionally, bipartite fabella are noted as well. In an effort to minimize the chance of LES failure due to disruption of the attachments of the fabella to the femur, this author uses a bone anchor (Figure 7.1b) instead of the fabella in instances where the fabella is absent, bipartite, or in patients less than 7 kg where fabellar diameter is quite small. Intraoperative disruption of these attachments can be identified by noting that the fabella displaces laterally or distolaterally when a "testing" load is applied to the circumfabellar NLL by exerting manual force distocranially before securing it, or if displacement of the fabella is seen while checking for drawer after placement, tensioning, and securing of the NLL. If this occurs, another method of femoral suture fixation should be used such as a bone anchor (Figure 7.1b) or transcondylar toggle, or a different technique besides LES should be considered.

Disruption of the fabellar–femoral attachment can be minimized by using a swaged-on needle with the NLL and obtaining good exposure to place the circumfabellar suture atraumatically. Picking the smallest needle size that will encircle the fabella is important to minimize soft tissue interposition when placing the suture. Using a needle that is too large can result in entrapping soft tissues, which will lead to subsequent loosening or entrapment of unwanted tissue such as the peroneal nerve. The use of bulky, eyed needles should be avoided. NLL is superior to other nylon lines such as fishing line because it has a higher load to failure, greater stiffness, and recovers tension better [11, 27]. Sterilization by steam or ethylene oxide has minimal effects on the mechanical properties of NLL [11, 28]. Currently, NLL is available with a swaged-on needle in 18, 23, 27, 36, and 45 kg sizes. For smaller patients where 9 or 14 kg NLL would be chosen, a tensioning device and crimping system and 9 and 14 kg NLL on swaged-on needles are now available (Everost Orthopedics, Steris Animal Health, Birmingham, AL).

When a bone anchor is chosen as the femoral LES attachment, the surgeon must select an appropriate anchor design that will durably hold in the cancellous bone of the caudal femoral condyle and withstand the high cyclic loading it will experience (Figure 7.2a,b). An eyelet style anchor (Figure 7.2b) is generally used with NLL [29]. Alternatively, a transcondylar toggle anchor has also been described to anchor the NLL in the distal femur [26]. The size of the hole in the toggle or eyelet of the anchor determines the maximum size of the NLL that can be used with that anchor style. The abrasion characteristics of each eyelet design are determined by the geometry and polishing of the eyelet [29]. Using anchor orientation that allows for the NLL to have the greatest radius of curvature through the eyelet over a beveled

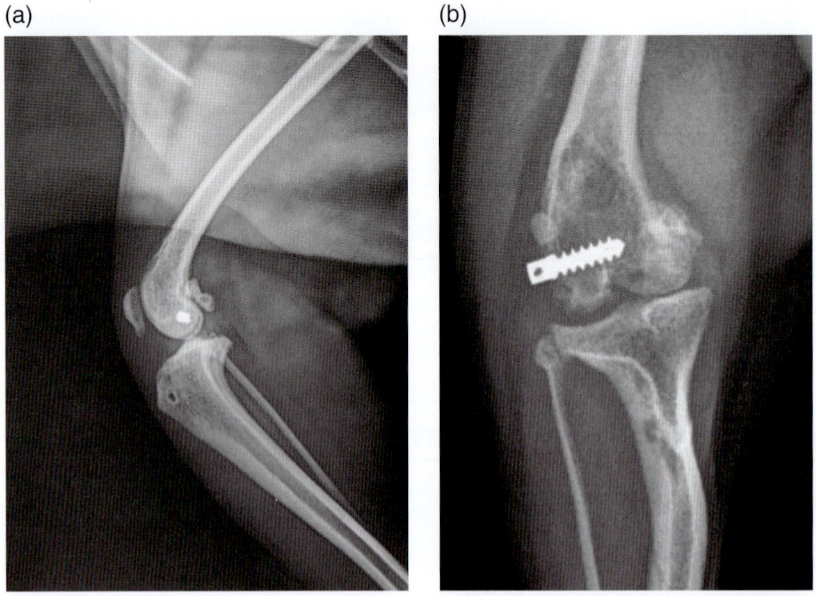

Figure 7.2 Bone anchor 3 years post placement in a 4.9 kg patient. (a) Lateral view. (b) Caudal-cranial view.

surface would seem prudent to minimize the chance of NLL breakage from eyelet abrasion. Unfortunately, no studies are currently available to compare all the commercially available veterinary bone anchors' strength for this use in canine cancellous bone, though some have been tested mechanically in cancellous bone substitute [29].

Bone anchors have the advantage of giving the surgeon precise control for placement at the point of greatest isometry, and an alternative suture placement if the fabella is absent. The most isometric point for a femoral bone anchor is F2 (Figure 7.3) which is located at the distal pole of the lateral fabella just cranial to the caudal cortex of the condyle [30–32]. A tip for locating F2 on caudal aspect of the femoral condyle is to "walk" a 22 G needle caudally along the condyle just distal to the fabella until it drops off caudally and temporarily leave the needle in place. The bone anchor is placed one "needle hub" width cranial to that.

A disadvantage of bone anchors is that they can fail due to the soft nature of the cancellous bone where they are placed and the high loads they experience (Figure 7.4a,b). Until comparison studies are done, it seems prudent to use the longest possible eyelet anchor with a cancellous thread profile.

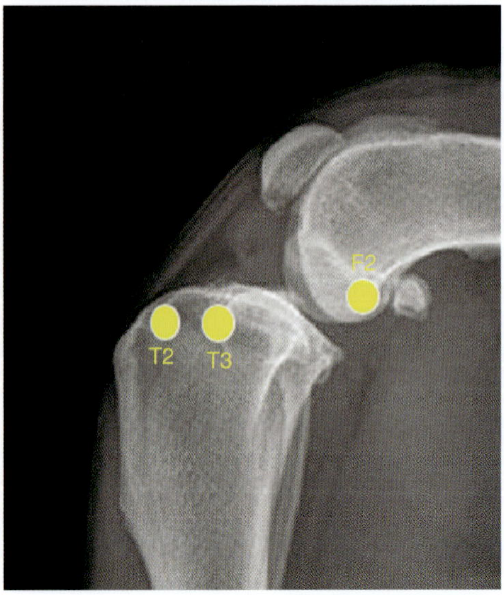

Figure 7.3 Isometric points on femur and tibia.

The tibial attachment point of the LES is typically one or two bone tunnels in the proximal cranial tibia. If two bone tunnels are used, they must be placed far enough apart to prevent the NLL pulling through the bone. A bone anchor can be used in this location as well. The most isometric points on the tibia are T2 and T3 [30–32], just cranial and caudal to the extensor

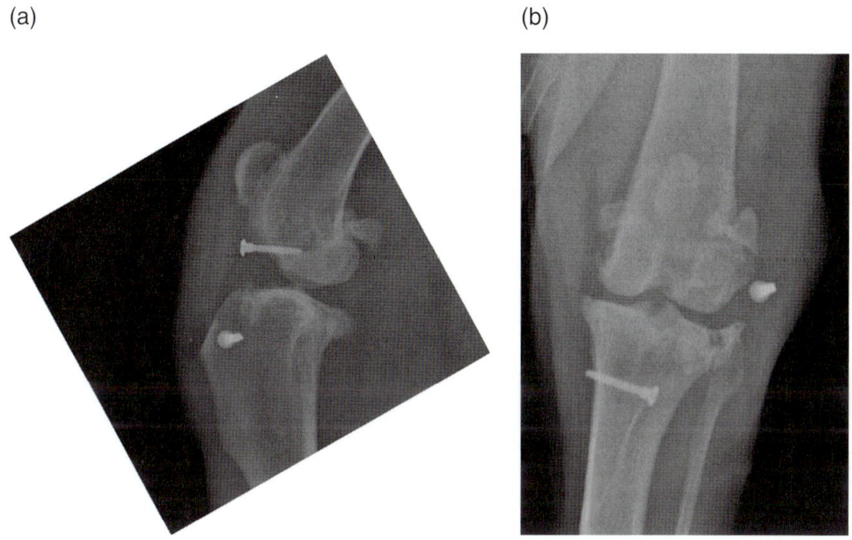

Figure 7.4 Femoral bone anchor failure. (a) Lateral view. (b) Caudal-cranial view.

groove (Figure 7.3). When a single bone tunnel is used, the NLL passes through the tibial bone tunnel and then courses caudally toward the lateral fabella just caudal to the patella tendon. When a fabellotibial suture is placed with one bone tunnel, this elongated rectangle shape placement encloses the F2 and T2 and T3 isometric points, suggesting that this placement is fairly isometric (Figure 7.5). When two bone tunnels are used, the axis of this rectangle is shifted distally, and may be less isometric.

Once the NLL is placed, it must be tensioned and secured. Tensioning can be done manually or with a mechanical tensioning device. The use of a device is recommended as it allows precise tensioning to eliminate drawer in multiple stifle flexion angles without limiting range of motion (ROM) and evaluation of suture tightness throughout the ROM (isometry) before securing the NLL. When tensioned manually, it is not possible to evaluate that tension's effect on stability, nor its isometry prior to securing the NLL, hence requiring removal and replacement of the NLL if it is not satisfactory.

Securing the suture is best accomplished with a crimp. When mechanically tested, the 27 and 36 kg NLL had less elongation, greater stiffness and initial loop tension, and higher load to failure than knotting [4, 5, 33, 34]. Also, a crimp has a much lower profile than the 5–6 throws required to securely knot NLL, which will reduce

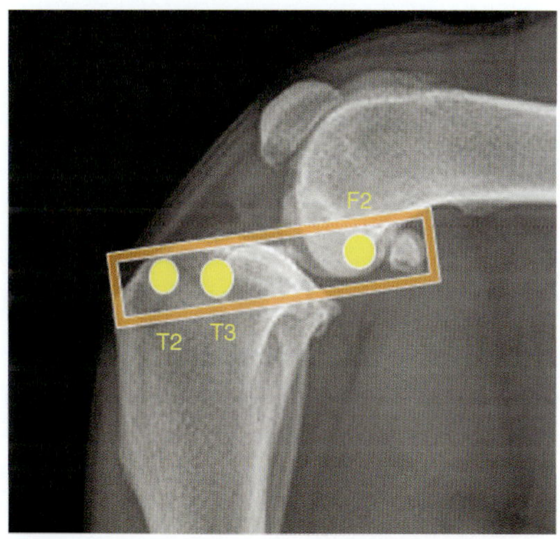

Figure 7.5 Path of LES enclosing femoral and tibial isometric points.

local tissue irritation and the potential for persistent swelling or sinus over the knot on the lateral stifle. Care must be taken with oval crimp tubes to crimp them properly (Figure 7.6a,b). If the crimping is not done correctly it may fail prematurely. Improperly crimped NLL should be removed, replaced, and crimped properly.

There is no universally accepted recommendation for appropriate size of NLL based on patient size. It is generally accepted that one should aim for at least equaling the patient's body weight in

(a)

(b)

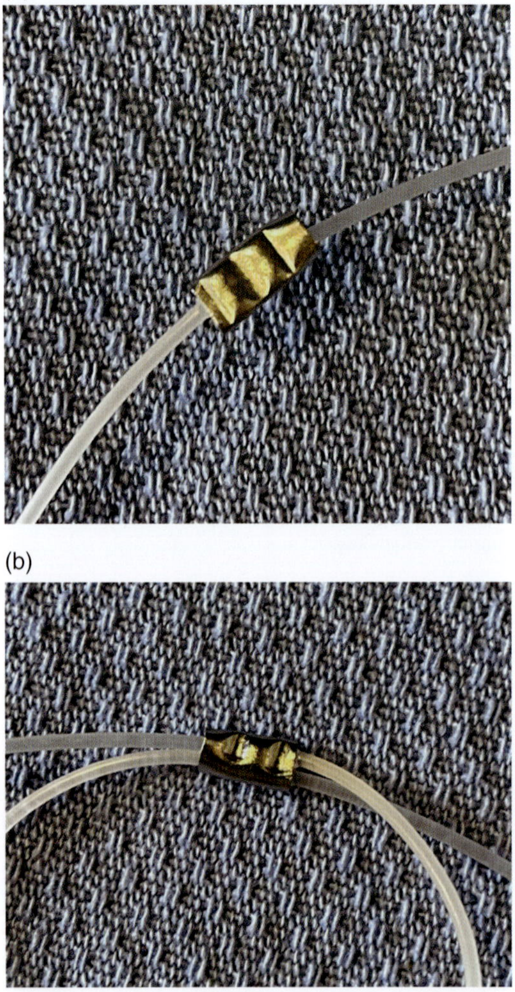

Figure 7.6 (a) Properly crimped oval crimp tube. (b) Improperly crimped oval crimp tube. Source: Photos courtesy of Dr David L. Dycus.

NLL strength and doubling the patient's weight is often done [8]. Placement of one larger versus two smaller sutures is based on the size of the fabella relative to the needle on the NLL to minimize fabellar attachment disruption, and when the patient's weight requires more than one strand to equal 1–2 times NLL strength.

After placement, tensioning, and securing of the NLL, critical assessment of the mechanics and isometry of the repair should be undertaken before closure. Cranial drawer testing should be negative throughout stifle ROM. If some residual drawer remains, the surgeon should evaluate and revise the repair as follows.

- If only 1–2 mm of drawer exists, it may be acceptable, but the surgeon should recognize that with LES with NLL, this is likely to increase over time.
- If more than 1–2 mm of cranial drawer exists or the drawer exists in multiple stifle angles, the NLL should be replaced with more tension prior to securing it.
- If the NLL is tight in some positions of stifle flexion but loose in others, the suture has not been placed isometrically.

Because the stifle is not a simple hinge joint but rather has a sliding and rotational component in addition to the rolling component, there is not a set of points on the femur and tibia that are truly isometric [8]. However, marked differences in the tightness of the NLL with different joint angles should prompt the surgeon to reevaluate the femoral and tibial anchor points. Is the circumfabellar suture properly placed snug to the fabella? If not, it should be replaced. If a bone anchor is used, is it in the F2 position, which can be evaluated by confirming it just distal to the fabella and caudally placed on the femoral condyle? If the anchor is not at F2, it should be replaced. Improper tibial bone tunnel or anchor positioning is common and typically too far distal. Evaluation and repositioning of the bone tunnel or anchor should be done if it is incorrect. If the placement point was at the T3 position and intraoperatively verified to be there but the NLL is not uniformly tight throughout stifle flexion and extension, then placing it at T2 and reevaluating NLL tension is suggested. If the placement point was at the T2 position and intraoperatively verified to be there but the NLL is not uniformly tight throughout stifle flexion and extension, then placing it at T3 and reevaluating NLL tension is suggested.

With tensioning devices, it is possible to get the suture so tight that it will limit stifle ROM. Typically, this is noted as a limitation to extension or even locking in flexion. Tension should be released until normal ROM is present but there is negligible drawer. If the NLL has already been secured, it should be removed and replaced. If the balance between maintenance of ROM and elimination of drawer cannot be achieved, evaluating the NLL attachment points for isometry and replacement at more isometric points are required. If this cannot be achieved, conversion to another procedure for CCL stabilization should be done.

7.6 Tips to Prevent Intraoperative Complications

- Obtain good exposure of the meniscus and probe carefully to avoid missing meniscal pathology (detailed information can be found in Chapter 18).
- Consider medial meniscal release in an older patient or in those where revision surgery is not an option if a postliminary meniscal tear occurs.
- Obtain good exposure of the fabella and place a circumfabellar suture precisely using a swaged-on needle of appropriate size.
- Use a needle to locate the caudal edge of the femoral condyle distal to the fabella for F2 bone tunnel or bone anchor placement.
- Expose the bone of the proximal cranial tibia to the tubercle of Gerty to accurately determine the T2 or T3 locations for bone tunnel or anchor placement.
- Use a tensioner to allow critical evaluation of the NLL's ability to counter drawer and maintain ROM prior to securing it.
- Use crimps instead of knotting to best maintain desired NLL tension.
- Use crimps instead of knotting to minimize the complication of swelling or sinus formation over the NLL.
- Be sure oval crimp tubes are positioned in the crimper properly before crimping.
- Critically palpate for drawer throughout stifle range of motion and evaluate for uniform suture tension and normal range of motion prior to closure.

7.7 Identification and Management of Postoperative Complications

Incision issues were reported with 8.8% of 363 LES cases [20] and are managed similarly to incisions elsewhere. Because of the underlying implants (NLL, crimps, anchors), prompt recognition and aggressive treatment of incisional issues are indicated. If a bandage is used in the postoperative period, it is another potential source of complications. Bandage-related complications are handled similar to issues with bandages used for other purposes. For routine LES repair, the author covers the incision with a strip of Telfa™ pad held in place with Tegaderm™ or Primapore™ for the initial 24–48 hours. No additional bandaging is done.

Lateral extracapsular suture fixation failure is a serious postoperative complication of this procedure. The frequency of this complication is unknown but in one large study, only one intraoperative failure of fixation was identified [20]. Fixation failure can occur slowly or acutely and from several causes. The common feature of fixation failure is the return of drawer and poor function due to instability.

Obtaining a thorough history is helpful in elucidating the cause of the failure. Did the patient never do well or did they have a setback in limb use that has persisted? Has there been swelling or sinus formation over the lateral suture site? Is there any audible click? Is there discomfort when palpating for drawer or over the NLL path? Physical examination should focus on determining if and how much drawer has returned and in what stifle positions. Evaluating for any catch, click, or pop during ROM can incriminate the menisci as possible causes of the setback.

Radiographs should be taken to evaluate for effusion, OA progression, the position of the lateral fabella and crimp or bone anchor, and the position of the tibia in relationship to the femur (e.g., cranial displacement). Displacement of the fabella laterally or distally will indicate loosening or failure of that anchor point. Crimp position and bone anchors should be similar to postoperative radiographic positioning. If the crimp is not radiographically aligned with the course the NLL took at the time of initial surgery, it suggests breakage of the NLL, displacement off the fabella or slippage through the crimp (Figure 7.7). New or excessive effusion can support the suspicion of a meniscal tear, especially if the stifle is relatively stable. Aspiration of any swelling over the LES implant and arthrocentesis can be useful to rule out infection.

When cranial drawer has returned, it is important to interpret this finding along with the history and clinical function of the patient. Most dogs with LES will develop some return of drawer over the first 6–8 weeks when they are being rechecked as part of their routine postoperative follow-up. Suture creep and

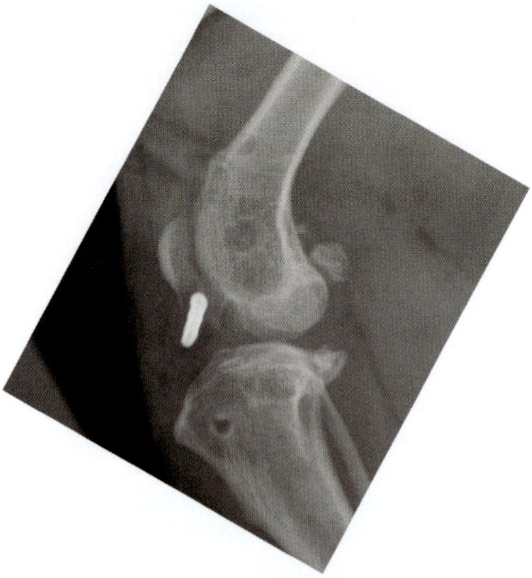

Figure 7.7 LES failure with crimp displacement.

stretch are going to occur with NLL more than some other materials, but cranial drawer return due to this alone should be in the 2–3 mm range. If knotting is used instead of crimps, there can be some elongation at the knot. The NLL can also loosen as it "seats" into the straightest alignment between its two anchor point as it pressure necroses through interposed soft tissues. Finally, the fabellofemoral attachment to the femur can loosen or fail. If the patient is doing clinically well, some degree of drawer is tolerated as normal for LES. If significant drawer has returned along with unacceptable clinical function, surgical revision is indicated. The type of failure will determine what type of revision strategy is appropriate.

Suture breakage is a common cause of LES failure. Typically, this occurs at the level of the knot or crimp. When the suture has broken, the surgeon should determine whether the NLL was of appropriate strength for that patient and consider replacing it with a stronger NLL or adding a second suture. Alternatively, a suture of a type other than NLL that is stronger could be considered. Finally, if the preoperative assessment for this patient did not include TPA measurement, it should be measured prior to repeating the LES. If the TPA is high or excessive, another type of repair should be recommended. This author would revise the repair with TPLO (Figure 7.1d,e). If the NLL is intact but has pulled off the lateral fabella or the fabella is displaced from the femur, a bone anchor can be used in the distal femur at F2 (Figure 7.2). If a bone anchor was used and has pulled out or loosened, replacement with a new anchor or switching to a bone tunnel or the lateral fabella as the femoral anchor point is done.

Swelling over the LES path on the lateral condyle of the femur may occur postoperatively and can be marked. In the author's experience, it is more likely to occur when NLL is knotted rather than crimped. The author also feels that the incidence of sterile swelling over the knot or crimp is less when the knot or crimp is placed on the distal arm of circumfabellar sutures due to the ability to obtain more substantial soft tissue closure of the biceps and lateral fascia over the knot or crimp. When an acute swelling occurs along with a setback in limb use, it can indicate failure of the LES construct which is typically NLL breakage. Persistent swelling with a stable stifle and good function is usually ignored and often improves some over time. If the swelling is warm, uncomfortable or begins to drain, infection is suspected. Aseptic aspiration for cytology and culture is indicated. Sterile persistent swelling over the NLL path is managed by implant removal and palpation for maintenance of adequate stability. If the stifle is not stable, LES can be repeated or another technique employed to stabilize the stifle.

Implant-associated infection (IAI) can occur in the immediate postoperative period or even months later. In one study, the incidence was 3.9% [20] which is similar to infection rates for other clean surgeries in veterinary medicine. The monofilament nature of NLL is less likely to become infected than other multifilament or braided nonabsorbable sutures due to low bacterial adherence [11, 12]. With IAI, there is typically swelling, discomfort or a draining tract over the NLL path and decreased limb use. If the IAI occurs as a late complication and there has been at least 6–8 weeks for pericapsular fibrosis to occur, removal of the NLL, crimps, and bone anchors is indicated. The explanted material is cultured, and 3–4 weeks of appropriate antibiotic therapy is instituted. If the stifle is not stable and function remains unsatisfactory with elimination of infection, the surgical site and joint should be aspirated for repeat culture. When the culture is negative, the stifle can be stabilized by repeating LES or another repair technique. The author would not support placement of a nonabsorbable braided or multifilament suture into a site that has been previously infected. If the culture remains positive, another round of antibiotics is started and the process is repeated. If the IAI occurs in the early postoperative period of 6–8 weeks before pericapsular fibrosis could occur, the joint and surgery site are cultured and antibiotics are started. If the infection resolves clinically, the antibiotics can be continued for 6–8 weeks until pericapsular fibrosis has occurred and then the implants can be removed. The stifle is assessed for stability and followed as previously discussed.

If a missed or postliminary meniscal tear is suspected, the stifle should be explored via arthroscopy or arthrotomy for meniscal evaluation and treatment. Magnetic resonance imaging or ultrasonography may be used to noninvasively document meniscal tears prior to surgical exploration.

7.8 Tips to Prevent Postoperative Complications

- Send all patients home with good instructions for home care.
- Use a sterile incisional covering for the first 24–48 hours to prevent early contamination of the surgical incision.
- Insist on continuous use of an Elizabethan collar until suture removal.
- Use crimps instead of knots to secure the NLL to maximize NLL fixation security and minimize persistent swelling or sinus formation over bulky stiff knots.
- Consider the use of meniscal release to decrease the incidence of postliminary meniscal tears.

7.9 Conclusion

Overall, LES is a safe and effective treatment for CCL disease. Attention to the details of preoperative planning, surgical execution, and follow-up will minimize the incidence of complications. Prompt identification and treatment of any complications will minimize their impact on the patient's outcome.

References

1. DeAngelis, M. and Lau, R.E. (1970). A lateral retinacular imbrication technique for the surgical correction of anterior cruciate ligament rupture in the dog. *J. Am. Vet. Med. Assoc.* 57: 79.
2. Flo, G.L. (1975). Modification of the lateral retinacular imbrication technique for stabilizing cruciate ligament injuries. *J. Am. Anim. Hosp. Assoc.* 11: 570.
3. Wallace, A.M., Cutting, E.D., Sutcliffe, M.P. et al. (2008). A biomechanical comparison of six different double loop configurations for use in the lateral fabella suture technique. *Vet. Comp. Orthop. Traumatol.* 21: 39.
4. Sicard, G.K., Hayashi, K., and Manley, P.A. (2002). Evaluation of 5 types of fishing material, 2 sterilisation methods, and a crimp-clamp system for extra-articular stabilization of the canine stifle joint. *Vet. Surg.* 31: 78.
5. Anderson, C.C., Tomlinson, J.L., Daly, W.R. et al. (1998). Biomechanical evaluation of a crimp clamp system for loop fixation of monofilament nylon leader material used for stabilization of the canine stifle joint. *Vet. Surg.* 27: 533.
6. Cook, J.L., Luther, J.K., Beetem, J. et al. (2010). Clinical comparison of a novel extracapsular stabilization procedure and tibial plateau leveling osteotomy for treatment of cranial cruciate ligament deficiency in dogs. *Vet. Surg.* 39: 315.
7. Cook, J.L. (2010). Extracapsular stabilization. In: *Advances in Veterinary Surgery: The Canine Cruciate* (ed. P. Muir). Oxford: Wiley Blackwell.
8. Kowaleski, M.P., Boudieau, R.J., and Pozzi, A. (2012). Stifle joint. In: *Veterinary Surgery: Small Animal* (eds. K.M. Tobias and S.A. Johnston). St Louis, MO: Elsevier.
9. Gordon-Evans, W.J., Griffon, D.J., and Bub, C. (2013). Comparison of lateral fabellar suture and tibial plateau leveling osteotomy techniques for dogs with cranial cruciate ligament disease. *J. Am. Vet. Med. Assoc.* 243: 675.
10. Duerr, F.M., Martin, K.W., Rishniw, M. et al. (2014). Treatment of canine cruciate disease – a survey of ACVS Diplomates and primary care veterinarians. *Vet. Comp. Orthop. Traumatol.* 27 (06): 478.
11. Caporn, T.M. and Roe, S.C. (1996). Biomechanical evaluation of the suitability of monofilament nylon fishing and leader line for extra-articular stabilization of the canine cruciate deficient stifle. *Vet. Comp. Orthop. Traumatol.* 9: 126.
12. Korvick, D.L., Johnson, A.L., and Schaeffer, D.J. (1994). Surgeons' preference in treating cranial cruciate ligament ruptures in dogs. *J. Am. Vet. Med. Assoc.* 205: 1318.
13. Lazar, T.P., Berry, C.R., deHaan, J.J. et al. (2005). Long-term radiographic comparison of tibial plateau leveling osteotomy versus extracapsular

stabilization for cranial cruciate ligament rupture in the dog. *Vet. Surg.* 34: 133.
14. Moore, K.W. and Read, R.A. (1995). Cranial cruciate ligament rupture in the dog: a retrospective study comparing surgical techniques. *Aust. Vet. J.* 72: 281.
15. Gambardella, P.C., Wallace, L.J., and Cassidy, F. (1985). Lateral suture technique for management of anterior cruciate ligament rupture in dogs: a retrospective study. *J. Am. Anim. Hosp. Assoc.* 31: 289.
16. Chauvet, A.E., Johnson, A.L., Pijanowski, G.J. et al. (1996). Evaluation of fibular head transposition, lateral fabellar suture, and conservative treatment of cranial cruciate ligament rupture in large dogs: a retrospective study. *J. Am. Anim. Hosp. Assoc.* 32: 247.
17. Budsberg, S.C., Verstraete, M.C., Soutas-Little, R.W. et al. (1988). Force plate analyses before and after stabilization of canine stifles for cruciate injury. *Am. J. Vet. Res.* 46: 1522.
18. Conzemius, M.G., Evans, R.B., Besancon, M.F. et al. (2005). Effect of surgical technique on limb function after surgery for rupture of the cranial cruciate ligament in dogs. *J. Am. Vet. Med. Assoc.* 226: 232.
19. Au, K.K., Gordon-Evans, W.J., Dunning, D. et al. (2010). Comparison of short- and long-term function and radiographic osteoarthrosis in dogs after postoperative physical rehabilitation and tibial plateau levelling osteotomy or lateral fabellar suture stabilization. *Vet. Surg.* 39: 173.
20. Casale, S.A. and McCarthy, R.J. (2009). Complications associated with lateral fabellotibial suture surgery for cranial cruciate ligament injury in dogs: 363 cases (1997–2005). *J. Am. Vet. Med. Assoc.* 234: 229.
21. Havig, M.E., Dyce, J., Kowaleski, M.P. et al. (2007). Relationship of tibial plateau slope to limb function in dogs treated with a lateral suture technique for stabilization of cranial cruciate deficient stifles. *Vet. Surg.* 36: 245.
22. Marsolais, G.S., Dvorak, G., and Conzemius, M.G. (2002). Effects of postoperative rehabilitation on limb function after cranial cruciate ligament repair in dogs. *J. Am. Vet. Med. Assoc.* 220: 1325.
23. Eiermann, J., Kirby-Shaw, K., Evans, R.B. et al. (2020). Recommendations for rehabilitation after surgical treatment of cranial cruciate ligament disease in dogs: a 2017 survey of veterinary practitioners. *Vet. Surg.* 49: 80.
24. Thieman, K.M., Tomlinson, J.L., Fox, D.B. et al. (2006). Effect of meniscal release on rate of subsequent meniscal tears and owner-assessed outcome in dogs with cruciate disease treated with tibial plateau leveling osteotomy. *Vet. Surg.* 35: 705.
25. Pozzi, A., Kim, S., and Lewis, D. (2010). Effect of transection of the caudal menisco-tibial ligament on femorotibial contact mechanics. *Vet. Surg.* 39: 489.
26. Kunkel, K.A.R., Basinger, R.R. et al. (2009). Evaluation of a transcondylar toggle system for stabilization of the cranial cruciate ligament stifle in dogs and cats. *Vet. Surg.* 38: 975.
27. Nwadike, B.S. and Roe, S.C. (1998). Mechanical comparison of suture material and knot type used for fabello-tibial sutures. *Vet. Comp. Orthop. Traumatol.* 11: 47.
28. Lewis, D.D., Milthorpe, B.K., and Bellenger, C.R. (1997). Mechanical comparison of materials used for extracapsular stabilisation of the stifle joint in dogs. *Aust. Vet. J.* 75: 890.
29. Kunkel, K.A.R., Rusly, R., Basinger, R.R. et al. (2013). In vitro acute load to failure and eyelet abrasion testing of a novel veterinary screw-type mini-anchor design. *Vet. Surg.* 42: 217.
30. Hulse, D.A. (1995). The stifle joint. In: *Small Animal Orthopedics* (ed. M.L. Olmstead), 395. St Louis, MO: Mosby.
31. Roe, S.C., Kue, J., and Gemma, J. (2008). Isometry of potential suture attachment sites for the cranial cruciate ligament deficient canine stifle. *Vet. Comp. Orthop. Traumatol.* 21: 215.
32. Reichert, E.E., Kunkel, K.A.R., Suber, J.T. et al. (2013). Radiographic location and isometry of the origin and insertion of the canine cranial cruciate ligament. *Vet. Surg.* 42: 860.
33. Banwell, M.N., Kerwin, S.C., Hosgood, G. et al. (2005). In vitro evaluation of the 18 and 36 kg Securos cranial cruciate ligament repair system. *Vet. Surg.* 34: 283.
34. Peycke, L.E., Kerwin, S.C., Hosgood, G. et al. (2002). Mechanical comparison of six loop fixation methods with monofilament nylon leader line. *Vet. Comp. Orthop. Traumatol.* 15: 210.

8 Complications Associated with Extracapsular Stabilization using Multifilament Material

Matt Corse and Ian G. Holsworth

8.1 Introduction

Surgeons must understand the goals and vulnerabilities of each procedure they perform to maximize the probability of a successful outcome. Orthopedic surgery is a process that requires deliberate preoperative planning, intraoperative execution, and postoperative management to consistently produce the intended outcome. Surgeons must have a comprehensive understanding of common errors and pitfalls of a given procedure to avoid, manage, and correct complications. This chapter provides specific preoperative, intraoperative, and postoperative guides for the surgeon to help direct successful navigation through the process of performing extracapsular stabilization using synthetic multifilament material to manage canine cranial cruciate ligament (CCL) rupture in the dog.

8.1.1 Preoperative Goals of Extracapsular Stabilization

- Predict the probability of success of the procedure in the individual patient.

8.1.2 Intraoperative Goals of Extracapsular Stabilization

- Evaluate and manage the meniscus.
- Produce a mechanically sound knee.
- Minimize risk of infection.

8.1.3 Postoperative Goals of Extracapsular Stabilization

- Maintain a mechanically sound knee.
- Avoid infection.
- Restore the patient to normal activity in a predictable manner.

8.2 Preoperative Planning

8.2.1 Introduction

It is a responsibility of the surgeon to determine whether a patient is appropriate for the procedure they plan to perform. Some patient characteristics may clearly identify them as inappropriate for a procedure, but more frequently patients have features with less conclusive risk profiles that the

Complications in Canine Cranial Cruciate Ligament Surgery, First Edition. Edited by Ron Ben-Amotz and David L. Dycus.

surgeon must consider carefully to help them decide whether or not to proceed. For this reason, it oversimplistic to provide a list of disqualifiers for a given procedure. Instead, the surgeon must consider how specific patient factors may impact operative and postoperative objectives and vulnerabilities of the procedure they wish to perform.

When performing extracapsular stifle stabilization procedures using multifilament material, a successful outcome requires a well-executed surgery, bone tunnel maturation and periarticular fibrosis formation in the recovery period, and the avoidance of bacterial colonization of implants. The surgeon's preoperative objective should be to determine whether these intraoperative and postoperative goals can be achieved with a high degree of certainty. To do so, surgeons should consider four questions during preoperative patient assessment.

1. Can I easily perform the procedure in this patient?
2. Does the patient have features that will stress the repair?
3. Does the patient have predisposing risk factors for infection?
4. Will this patient and this client be compliant postoperatively?

Failing to satisfactorily ask these questions or misjudgment in answering them during the preoperative period will result in deleterious consequences either at surgery or during the recovery period.

8.2.1.1 *Can I Easily Perform the Procedure in This Patient?*

Regardless of surgeon experience, the technical ease of extracapsular stifle stabilization varies with patient size, body conformation, and body condition score. Size of implants relative to the patient, ideal bone tunnel angles, and ease of dissection to identify isometric points should be considered preoperatively.

- Very small patients: implants and bone tunnels may be too large to be accurately placed in an isometric position. Some bone anchors are too large for smaller patients. The surgeon needs to have a comprehensive knowledge of the implant options in their toolbox, and size tolerances specific to each implant.
- Small patients with chondrodystrophoid (aka "hockey-stick") distal femoral morphology: in small patients with 90° caudal femoral metaphyseal deviation, it may not be possible to create a 30–45° tunnel from the femoral isometric point (Figure 8.1). Selecting a flatter trajectory of the bone tunnel or anchor socket that is more perpendicular to the joint line can result in:
  - implants or bone tunnels unintentionally being directed into the joint
  - increased implant stresses risking implant failure
  - increased abrasion on bone tunnels and socket exit sites predisposing to bone tunnel widening.
- Dogs with dense body weight and small bone morphology: muscular dogs with relatively small bone morphology (like English Bulldogs) make identification of

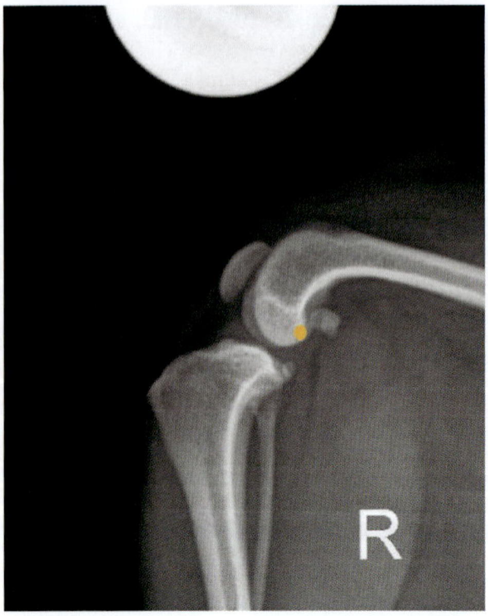

Figure 8.1 90° "hockey stick" morphology of the distal femur of a toy-breed dog. A 25 mm radiopaque calibration ball provides a size reference. The orange dot represents the optimal initiation point for the femoral bone tunnel. This distal femoral morphology combined with small patient size lead to the creation of a bone tunnel angled 30–45° away from the joint.

isometric points and optimal directing of bone tunnels challenging.

- Morbidly obese patients: morbidly obese dogs can challenge the technical ease of identifying optimal isometric points.

8.2.1.2 Does the Patient Have Physical Features That Will Stress the Repair?

In dogs, the answer to this question is always yes, but some patients will have characteristics that may stress the repair more than others. Biomechanical factors should be considered when planning stifle surgery in the dog. As described by Slocum, the magnitude of cranial tibial thrust is enhanced by tibial plateau slope and the weight of the dog and is counteracted by passive restraint from the CCL and active restraint from the biceps femoris muscle and hamstring muscle group [1]. When extracapsular stifle stabilization is performed to manage CCL rupture, the suture implants function in part to passively restrain cranial tibial thrust. Evaluating these opposing biomechanical factors for each potential surgical candidate should influence surgeon decision making.

- Long-legged dogs: because stifle extension produces a less favorable lever arm for the caudal thigh muscles to resist cranial tibial thrust, tall, long-legged dogs with a straighter stifle conformation may expose extracapsular stabilization implants to relatively higher loads as compared to shorter, squat dogs that generate more effective active muscle restraint to tibial thrust.
- Dogs with dense body weight and small bone morphology: dogs like English Bulldogs that have heavy body weight relative to their smaller skeletal frame may require larger implants than their bone size can accommodate.
- Morbidly obese patients: increased patient body weight enhances the magnitude of cranial tibial thrust, exposing extracapsular implants to higher loads.
- Dogs with steep tibial plateau angles: tibial plateau angle (TPA) is not the sole determinant of load on the joint, but it is a metric that should be considered prior to every stifle surgery [2]. Taken in relation to other patient features (for example, considering the mechanics of a tall, long-legged dog with long joint levers versus a shorter, squat dog with shorter joint levers), patients with steep TPAs may be better suited for corrective osteotomy procedures than extracapsular stabilization. Although there is no red line TPA directing whether one type of stifle surgical repair would be indicated over another, these authors recommend looking closely at all contributing patient factors, particularly when TPA exceeds 30°.

8.2.1.3 Does the Patient Have Predisposing Risk Factors for Infection?

Surgical site infections (SSIs) that are deep, implant associated and involve multifilament implant material are often major complications that can have catastrophic results. Bacterial colonization of surgical implants can occur during surgery, by local extension of superficial incisional infections postoperatively, or by hematogenous colonization in the postoperative period. Because of the devastating consequences of implant-associated SSI, the surgeon must have comprehensive processes in the preoperative, intraoperative, and postoperative periods to minimize patient risk of implant colonization.

In the preoperative period, the surgeon is responsible for screening each patient for infection risk factors that may disqualify them from the procedure. Chapter 2 provides in-depth information on ways to minimize SSIs. The surgeon must review patient medical records, perform a thorough physical exam (including evaluation of skin for any current pyoderma), and conduct a thorough client interview to assess their willingness and capacity for postoperative compliance. It is recommended to perform a complete blood work in order to rule out any systemic diseases that might preclude performance of the surgical procedure.

- Patients with active or recurrent infections: pyoderma and recurrent urinary tract infection are two common forms of recurrent infection observed in dogs. Dogs with recurrent pyoderma that have had medical treatment may have an increased skin flora of antibiotic-resistant bacteria

that can increase the risk of a postoperative incisional infection. In addition, recurrent pyoderma can predispose to infection from hematogenous implant colonization at any point later in life. Similar risk for hematogenous infection can result from recurrent urinary tract infections. In patients with active pyoderma or urinary tract infection, the authors would recommend delaying extracapsular stifle stabilization until the infection is treated. Patients with recurrent pyoderma or recurrent urinary infections that are well controlled with medication or diet should remain on their treatment. In patients with recurrent skin, urinary tract, or other sources of infection, the surgeon must weigh relative risk and potential consequence of a surgical infection to determine whether to proceed with the procedure.
- Immunocompromised patients: although studies have not documented an increased risk of postoperative infection in patients immunosuppressed from endocrine disease (Cushing disease, diabetes mellitus) or with conditions treated with immunosuppressive drugs, the authors recommend evaluating these patients cautiously when considering extracapsular stifle stabilization surgery using multifilament material.

8.2.1.4 Will This Patient and Client Be Compliant Postoperatively?

- Noncompliant clients unwilling to prevent licking: patient self-trauma to their incision (i.e., licking) is an avoidable but common cause of poor postoperative incisional healing in dogs. Clients must commit to strict use of an Elizabethan collar or other lick-preventing device in the postoperative period while their pet's incision is healing. The surgeon must clearly and persuasively educate about the significant and often costly consequences that can occur from a patient licking their incision. The surgeon must also assess a client's willingness for compliance, as patients owned by clients unwilling to commit to this responsibility may be disqualified from the procedure.
- Noncompliant clients unwilling to activity restrict their pet: long-term mechanical integrity of the stifle repaired with extracapsular stabilization techniques depends on both bone tunnel maturation and periarticular fibrosis formation in the postoperative period. The bone tunnel maturation process requires 6–8 weeks of deliberate activity restriction to avoid damage to the wall of the bone tunnels during the vulnerable postoperative period. Periarticular fibrosis formation requires a similar time frame to sufficiently protect the synthetic suture implants from both cyclical fatigue and acute compromise from premature overactivity. Because of the importance of these processes, the surgeon must communicate about the postoperative plan with the client with persuasive and uncompromising clarity before proceeding with surgery. Surgeon failure to preoperatively identify and exclude clients who are unwilling to adhere to postoperative activity restriction may result in a deleterious outcome.
- Noncompliant patients that cannot be activity restricted: extremely rambunctious dogs and dogs with severe separation anxiety are at higher risk of premature limb overuse. Sedation should be used liberally in these patients to help them through the recovery process. For these patients, it is highly advisable to perform a preoperative trial of the sedation and activity confinement protocol. This will help determine whether the protocol will be sufficient to control the patient postoperatively and assist in deeming them an acceptable candidate for the procedure.

8.2.2 Preoperative Planning Summary

Ultimately, every patient requires careful assessment in the preoperative period to help the surgeon decide if the patient is an appropriate candidate for an extracapsular stifle stabilization using multifilament material [2]. Only by weighing the technical requirements of the surgery, the spectrum of patient features that influence surgery and recovery, the factors that could compromise repair, and the client commitment to the process can the surgeon reasonably predict the likelihood of a successful outcome.

8.3 Intraoperative Procedure

8.3.1 Intraoperative Objectives of Extracapsular Stifle Stabilization with Multifilament Material

1. Evaluate and manage meniscus.
2. Identify optimal isometric points.
3. Create appropriate bone tunnels and/or anchor sites.
4. Apply appropriate tension to implants.
5. Evaluate and manage implant and tissue creep.
6. Maintain meticulous aseptic technique throughout the procedure.

As with all surgical techniques to manage CCL rupture, careful meniscal evaluation and treatment is a critical component of any extracapsular stabilization surgery. Failure to recognize meniscal tears and treat them when present may result in poor recovery and ultimately failed outcome. Surgeons who are insufficiently trained in meniscal evaluation and treatment should not perform stifle surgery. More information on meniscal treatment decisions can be found in Chapter 18.

Additional intraoperative focus must be aimed at identifying optimal isometric points, creating appropriate bone tunnels and/or anchor sites, applying appropriate tension to implants, and maintaining meticulous aseptic technique throughout the procedure. Failure to execute any of these goals will lead to a predictable detrimental outcome.

8.3.2 Intraoperative Mechanical Objectives

The goal of extracapsular stifle stabilization is to restore mechanics as closely as possible to normal [3–6].

1. Tarsal range of motion should be unimpeded throughout flexion and extension without restriction or conflict.
2. Stifle range of motion should be unimpeded throughout flexion and extension without palpable areas of restriction or conflict.
3. Cranial drawer and cranial tibial thrust should be 3 mm or less.
4. The tibia should not be fixed in external rotation, and the surgeon should be able to internally rotate the stifle 10–20° after tensioning suture implants.

Failure to achieve these goals can indicate a technical error in isometry, an error in implant/bone anchor placement, or errant implant tensioning. Intraoperative assessment of limb mechanics must be performed by the surgeon during each procedure to validate that mechanical goals have been achieved, and if problems are identified the surgeon must determine the correction required.

8.3.2.1 Identifying and Correcting Intraoperative Mechanical Errors

8.3.2.1.1 Impaired Tarsal Range of Motion:
Following extracapsular stifle stabilization with multifilament implants, stifle and tarsal range of motion should be unimpeded. Restricted tarsal range of motion following implant placement requires close inspection of the tibial bone tunnel and tibial implant path, as this typically indicates entrapment of the long digital extensor tendon (LDE) (Figure 8.2). Whether the origin of the tibial bone tunnel is at Gerdy's sister (i.e., the tibial bony prominence demarcating the caudal border of the extensor groove) or within the proximal aspect of the extensor groove, the LDE should be reflected cranially to avoid entrapment. If Gerdy's sister is used for the origin of the tibial bone tunnel, it is possible to improperly direct the tunnel cranially in a manner that breaks directly into the extensor groove which could allow the implant to cross over the LDE, entrapping it. LDE entrapment necessitates replacement of the implant with the LDE properly retracted cranially or redrilling a more caudally directed tibial bone tunnel.

8.3.2.1.2 Stifle Conflict Palpable During Range of Motion:
Following implant placement, restriction or conflict palpable at any point through stifle range of motion requires close inspection of isometric points. When femoral and tibial anchor points are isometric, the distance between these points and the resulting suture tension should remain constant throughout full

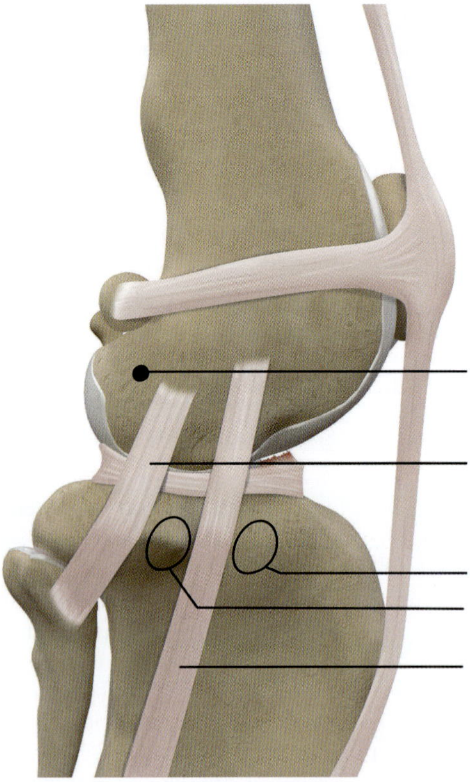

Figure 8.2 Lateral stifle anatomy relevant to localization of implantation sites of femoral and tibial bone tunnels/socket.

stifle range of motion [7–15]. This creates smooth unrestricted stifle motion. Suture tension in nonisometrically placed suture implants will tighten or loosen through different zones of the range of motion, creating stifle conflict. Poor isometry can result in bone tunnel widening, implant failure, stifle joint mechanical compromise, and ultimately a poor functional outcome for the patient. When stifle conflict is identified, the surgeon must determine the cause of the isometric error and make the necessary correction.

Evaluating Isometric Error

For the femur, the most common isometric error is starting the femoral bone tunnel/anchor point too far cranially. This creates an insufficient caudoproximal to craniodistal suture implant trajectory across the stifle joint, resulting in a poor mechanical and isometric outcome. Sufficient lateral femoral condyle exposure to allow accurate assessment of the femoral bone tunnel/bone anchor site relative to the distal femorofabellar joint space must be performed at every surgery. Sufficient lateral femoral exposure requires visualization of the transition of the nonarticular and articular cartilage of the femoral condyle just distal to the femorofabellar joint.

To achieve this exposure, the biceps fascia is incised and retracted caudally. Grasping the lateral fabella with thumb forceps, the distal aspect of the femorofabellar joint is tented and sharply incised with a stab incision with a #15 blade to expose the joint space. Once the femorofabellar joint space is identified, distal joint capsule dissection is extended by remaining just caudal and parallel to the lateral collateral ligament. The femoral bone tunnel should be made in the lateral condyle just distal to the femorofabellar joint at the transition between nonarticular and articular portions. Because there is a tendency to create the femoral tunnel too far cranial, the authors recommend trending the tunnel placement more towards the articular portion of the transition. The femoral tunnel should be angled towards the medial femur at the level of the proximal aspect of the trochlear groove.

For the tibia, the most common errors are starting the tibial bone tunnel either too far caudal or too far distal. This also results in insufficient caudoproximal to craniodistal suture implant trajectory across the stifle joint and a detrimental isometric consequence. Sufficient identification of the LDE tendon, lateral meniscus, and Gerdy's sister must be performed at every surgery to guarantee an appropriate isometric tibial bone tunnel site (Figure 8.2).

Evaluation of Isometry Using the Suture Tensioner

When performing extracapsular stifle stabilization with multifilament material like the TightRope® (Figure 8.3) or Knotted SwiveLock® (Figure 8.4), using a suture tensioner with tensiometer (Figure 8.5) can provide the surgeon with an objective tool to assess for suture tension changes throughout stifle range of motion. The stifle should be maintained in slight extension when tensioning the suture [10]. Once the desired suture tension is applied to the suture implants using the suture tensioner, the knee can be flexed and extended with the suture tensioner still in place. With optimal isometric suture placement, the tensiometer reading should remain static throughout stifle range of motion, without fluctuating up or down. If the tensiometer reading deviates greater than 3–4 lb/ft, isometric points should be critically reassessed and corrected before proceeding.

8.3.2.1.3 Excessive Cranial Drawer or Cranial Tibial Thrust:

Following extracapsular implant placement and tensioning, the knee should be stable with less than 3 mm of cranial drawer present. An excess of 3 mm of cranial drawer indicates:

- a problem in isometry
- insufficient stifle tensioning
- tensioning the implants while the stifle was positioned in excessive cranial drawer
- failing to address implant or tissue creep
- the presence of soft tissue between toggle/suture buttons and the bone.

Isometric Error

If excessive cranial drawer is present after implant placement, the surgeon should start with careful inspection of tibial and femur isometric points as previously described (see Chapter 6 for more information on isometric points). If an errant isometric point or tunnel is identified, a new site should be drilled and

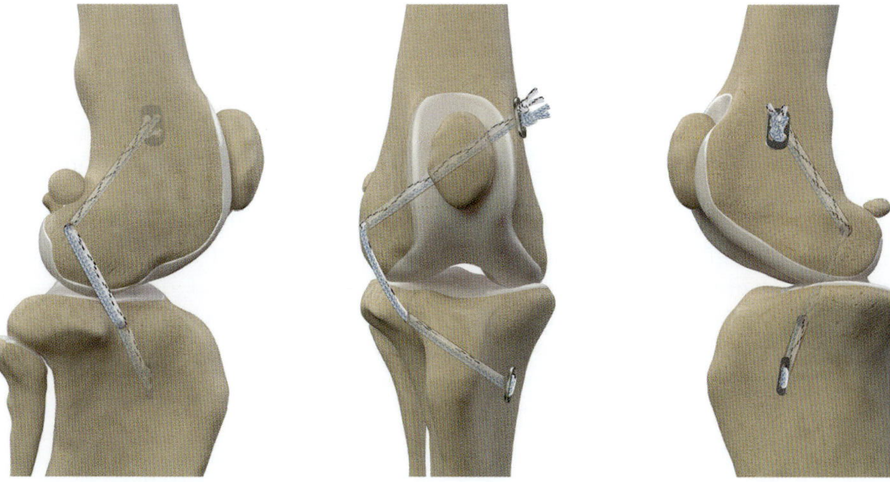

Figure 8.3 TightRope implant placed on the lateral aspect of the stifle in correct TightRope® ECS technique with two strands of 2 mm FiberTape® tensioned appropriately and secured by multi-throw square knot over a four-hole tie-button on the medial femur.

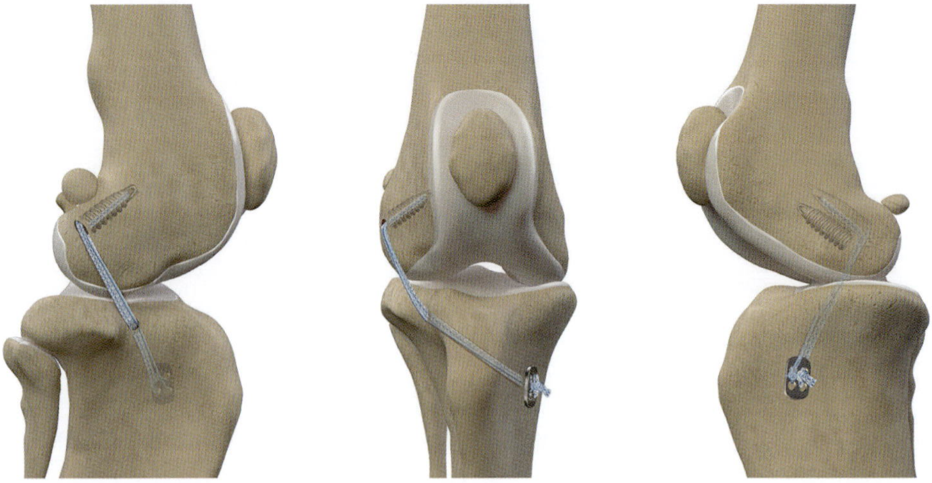

Figure 8.4 SwiveLock® implant placed on the lateral aspect of the stifle in correct Knotted SwiveLock® ECS technique with two strands of 2 mm FiberTape anchored at the femoral socket and tensioned appropriately and secured by multi-throw square knot over a four-hole tie-button on the medial tibia.

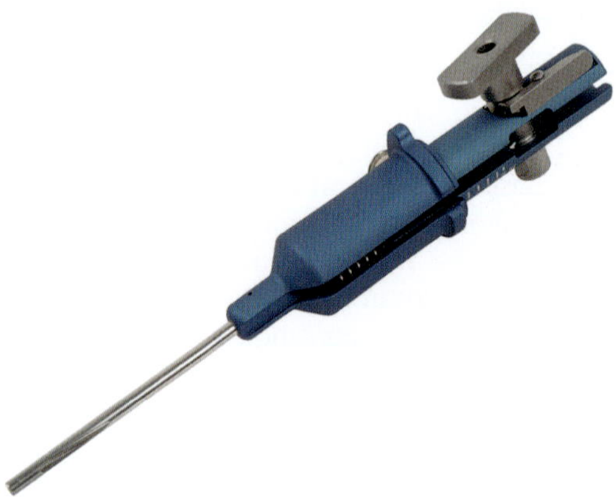

Figure 8.5 Tensioner with tensiometer suture tensioning device (Arthrex® AR-1529).

implants replaced if possible. If proper isometric points and bone tunnels are confirmed and cranial drawer persists, the surgeon must evaluate whether they insufficiently tensioned the implants, tensioned implants while the stifle was positioned in cranial drawer, failed to sufficiently address implant or tissue creep prior to securing the implants, or interposed soft tissue between suture toggles/buttons and bone.

Insufficient Tensioning

Use of a tensioner with tensiometer allows incremental tension application, assessment of knee mechanics achieved, and adjustment. In addition, when using the suture tensioner, the surgeon may cycle the knee once tension is applied to assess and manage implant or soft tissue creep (see section on creep, below).

Tensioning with the Stifle in Excessive Drawer

For dogs with an extremely unstable stifle and a large amount of cranial drawer, it is possible to tension implants with the tibia unintentionally positioned in a cranially subluxated position (i.e., tensioned while in cranial drawer). In this circumstance, after suture implants are tensioned, the tibia can easily displace caudally into a reduced position, functionally alleviating all tension on the implants. If excessive cranial drawer is present after tensioning implants, the surgeon should start by making sure that the stifle was reduced when sutures were tensioned. If it is determined that the tibia was in cranial drawer when implants were tensioned, an assistant should hold the tibia in a reduced position while implants are tensioned.

Implant and Tissue Creep

Soft tissue and/or implant creep can lead to excessive cranial drawer after implant placement [16–22]. Once implants are placed, tightened, and secured, the surgeon should be able to cycle the stifle 20–30 times through the range of motion (flexion/extension, internal/external rotation, cranial/caudal displacement) without alteration in stifle stability. If cycling the stifle leads to the development of cranial drawer, creep should be suspected.

Managing Creep Using the Suture Tensioner

Using a suture tensioner with tensiometer gives the surgeon a tool to assess and manage creep. Once the desired suture tension is applied to the suture implants using the suture tensioner, the stifle can be cycled 20–30 times through the range of motion with the suture tensioner still in place. If creep has been eliminated, the tensiometer reading should not drop after cycling and there should be less than 3 mm of cranial drawer present on stifle palpation. If cycling results in a loss of suture tension and excessive cranial drawer, the implants should be retensioned to the desired level, the stifle should be re-cycled, and stifle stability should be reassessed. This process should be repeated until creep is eliminated and the stifle remains stable after cycling. If this process does not eliminate cranial drawer, the surgeon should evaluate for other causes of excessive cranial drawer including poor isometry, tensioning the implants with the stifle positioned in cranial drawer, or the presence of soft tissue between toggle/suture buttons and the bone.

Rescuing a Knotless SwiveLock Stabilization

A limitation of the Knotless SwiveLock® (Figure 8.6) is that creep is difficult to adjust for prior to securing the implants. If excessive drawer is identified intraoperatively following a Knotless SwiveLock® stabilization (due to either insufficient tensioning or insufficient elimination of creep), the Knotless SwiveLock® can be converted to a Knotted SwiveLock® implant without use of additional implants (Figure 8.4).

At the conclusion of a Knotless SwiveLock®, if the stifle is determined to be stable after cycling the joint and assessing mechanics, the long remaining strands of FiberTape® extending from the SwiveLock® are cut flush with the bone anchor and the stabilization is complete. If residual instability remains at the conclusion of a Knotless SwiveLock®, the long strands of FiberTape® extending from the bone anchor are not cut and instead are passed back through the tibial bone tunnel from lateral to medial. On the medial tibia, the implant strands are fed through the suture button, tensioned, cycled, and, when creep is eliminated, tied, completing the conversion of the Knotless SwiveLock® to a Knotted SwiveLock® (Figure 8.7). Use of a tensioner

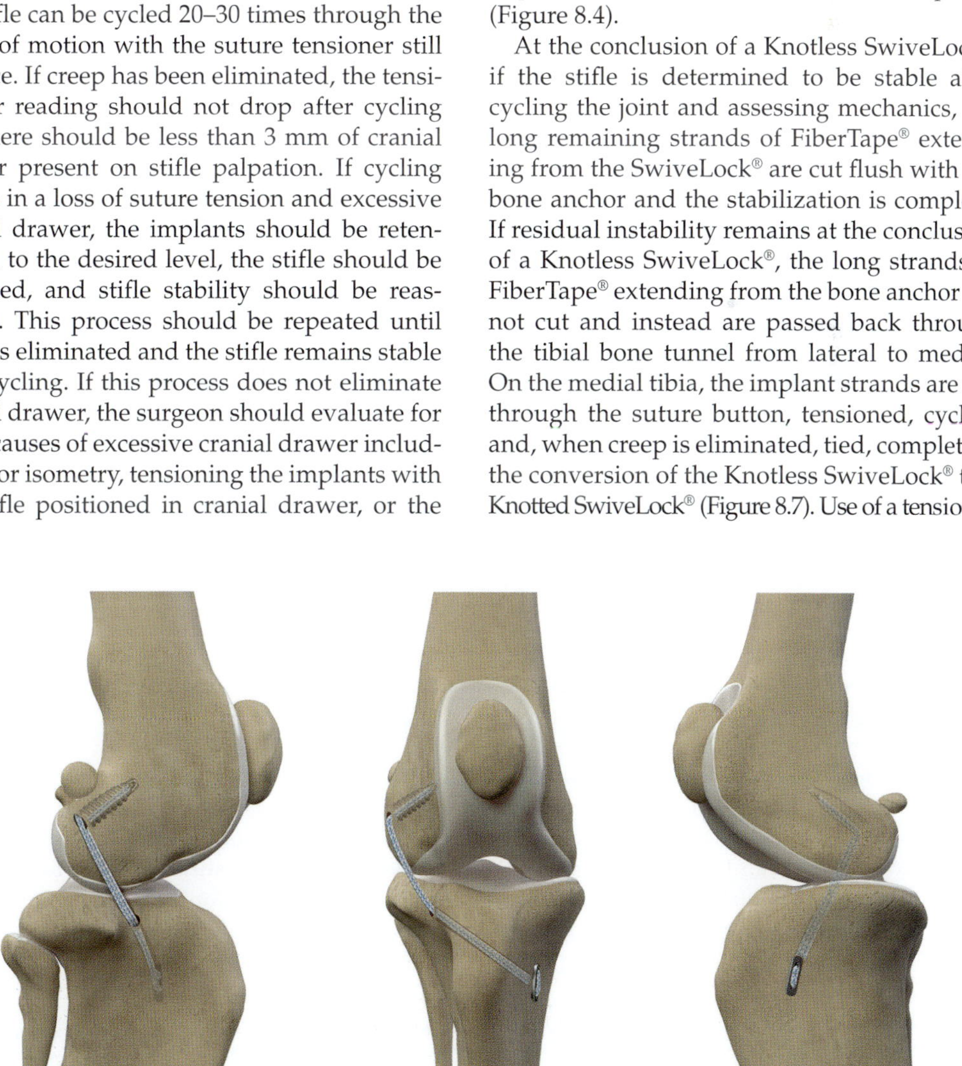

Figure 8.6 SwiveLock® implant placed on the lateral aspect of the stifle in correct Knotless SwiveLock® ECS technique with one strand of 2 mm FiberTape® anchored at the femoral socket with a two-hole toggle button on the medial tibia.

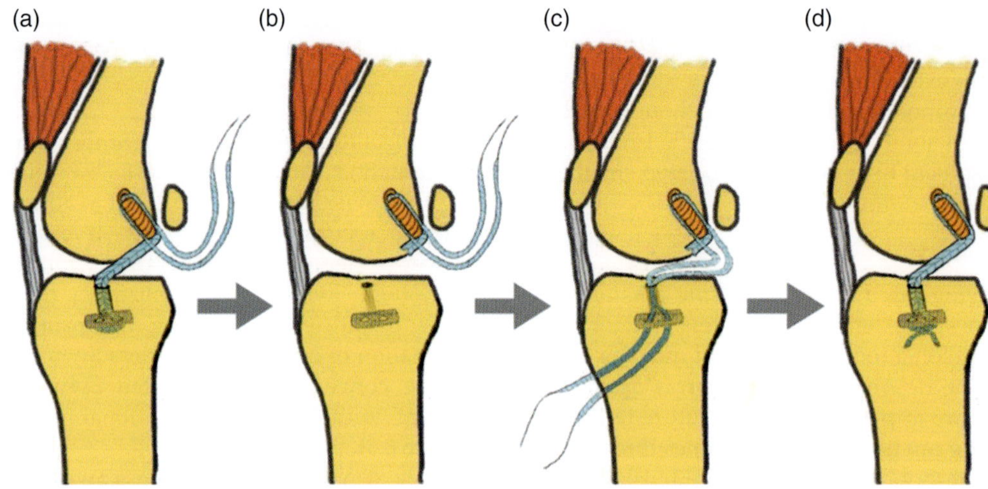

Figure 8.7 Rescuing a Knotless SwiveLock® by converting to a Knotted SwiveLock®. At the conclusion of a Knotless SwiveLock®, if the knee is determined to be unstable, the long strands of FiberTape® extending from the bone anchor are not cut (a). The loose suture crossing the joint is cut at the level of the bone anchor and removed from the toggle button (b). The long strands of FiberTape® are passed back through the tibial bone tunnel from lateral to medial (c). On the medial tibia, the implant strands are fed through the suture button, tensioned, cycled, and when creep is eliminated, tied, completing the conversion of the Knotless SwiveLock® to a Knotted SwiveLock® (d). Source: Artwork courtesy of Matt Corse.

with tensiometer when performing a Knotted SwiveLock® allows incremental tension application and management of creep as previously described.

Presence of Soft Tissue Between Toggle/Suture Buttons and the Bone

Stifle stabilization using the TightRope® technique was initially described using minimal or closed approaches for bone tunnel creation and placement of toggle buttons. Although this is possible, careful surgical dissection allows safe and efficient access to isometric points and toggle button sites to allow precise implant placement. When performing extracapsular repair using toggle buttons or bone buttons, the surgeon should always gain direct visual access to each site to ensure that no soft tissue is interposed between buttons and bone (Figure 8.8).

8.3.2.1.4 Tibia Fixed in External Rotation

A secondary function of the CCL is preventing excessive internal tibial rotation. Although extracapsular stifle stabilization is effective at eliminating excessive internal tibial rotation, 10–20° of internal rotation should be maintained. When the tibia is fixed in external rotation, it not only restricts normal stifle mechanics but also serves as an intraoperative indicator that the lateral joint compartment may be getting overcompressed from implant overtension. Because implant overtensioning may cause lateral joint compartment collapse, bone tunnel abrasion, implant failure, and patient discomfort, the surgeon should reduce tension on the implants if the tibia is fixed in external rotation.

8.3.2.2 Meticulous Aseptic Technique

It is vital to maintain meticulous aseptic technique throughout stifle surgery to minimize risk of implant colonization [23–26]. Use of perioperative antibiotics, gentle soft tissue handling, and minimizing anesthetic and surgical time are essential aseptic principles that must be implemented when performing stifle surgery. Additional precautions to reduce implant colonization risk when performing extracapsular stifle stabilization surgery with multifilament materials include the following:

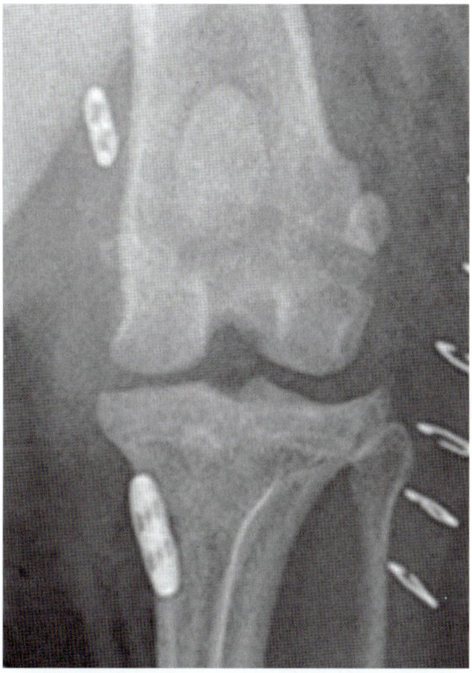

Figure 8.8 Postsurgical caudo-cranial radiographic image of a TightRope® construct with the toggle button proximally and the tie button distally. Note that the femoral toggle button is elevated from the bone, indicating soft tissue interposition. This implant should be immediately replaced with the toggle button directly contacting the femur.

- Avoiding direct contact with patient skin throughout the procedure by using adhesive plastic material (i.e., Ioban™ dressing) or sew-in drapes. Synthetic implant material should not contact patient skin prior to implantation.
- Do not remove the multifilament implant from the package until tunnels and anchor sites are completely prepared already for implantation.
- Apply a new pair of sterile surgical gloves immediately before handling multifilament suture material implants.

Surgeons unprepared or unwilling to practice meticulous aseptic technique should not perform stifle surgery.

8.3.3 Intraoperative Summary

At the conclusion of extracapsular stifle stabilization with multifilament implants, the surgeon must be satisfied that all intraoperative objectives were met to give the patient the highest probability for a successful outcome. The surgeon must be keenly aware of all intraoperative objectives and willing to make intraoperative adjustments when necessary. Poor surgical execution or failure to produce the desired mechanical goals will lead to a predictable detrimental outcome.

8.4 Postoperative Considerations

- Maintain a mechanically sound stifle.
- Detect and manage infection.
- Restore patient to normal activity in a predictable manner.

A comprehensive postoperative plan for managing extracapsular stifle stabilization patients should be focused on maintaining a mechanically sound stifle and restoring the patient to a normal activity level in a predictable manner. To realize these goals, the surgeon must understand changing healing objectives and vulnerabilities at different phases of the postoperative period. In addition, the surgeon must establish firm expectations for limb function after surgery and have strategies ready if expectations are not met or if complications occur.

8.4.1 Maintain a Mechanically Sound Stifle

Maintaining a mechanically sound stifle after extracapsular bone-to-bone stifle stabilization surgery requires periarticular fibrosis formation and bone tunnel maturation to occur. Failure of either of these processes can lead to mechanical destabilization of the joint, pain, and limb dysfunction. Because there is a critical need for bone tunnel maturation and periarticular fibrosis formation to maintain stifle stability, the design of a postoperative plan should largely center around these processes.

8.4.1.1 Periarticular Fibrosis Formation

Due to normal biomechanical forces generated in the canine stifle with weight bearing, multifilament extracapsular stabilizing implants are exposed to cyclical loads throughout the recovery process [27]. An explosive, high-energy force exceeding the ultimate strength of the implant can result in acute destructive implant failure. Lower-energy chronic, repetitive activities, on the other hand, cause cyclical fatigue that weaken implants over time.

Periarticular fibrosis formation refers to the development of fibrous tissue around the joint and extracapsular suture implants that augment joint stability created by the extracapsular repair. Postoperative extracapsular patients allowed overactivity prior to sufficient periarticular fibrosis formation risk weakening and breakage of the implant and disruption of mechanical stability of their postoperative stifle. Because of the time required for sufficient periarticular fibrosis to occur, the authors recommend 6–8 weeks of short-duration, low-intensity activity followed by 4 weeks of low-intensity, increasing-duration activity followed by 4 weeks of increasing-intensity, increasing-duration activity. Surgeons can vary specifics of this structure but must keep in mind that maintaining a mechanically sound stifle after extracapsular stabilization requires a sufficient amount of structurally supportive periarticular fibrosis formation to occur.

8.4.1.2 Bone Tunnel Maturation

During extracapsular stifle stabilization, bone tunnels are created in relatively soft metaphyseal bone of the distal femur and proximal tibia. Because materials of most multifilament suture implants passing through the bone tunnels are typically stiff, joint motion in the recovery period can allow the suture material to cut into the adjacent soft metaphyseal bone. When this occurs, bone tunnel widening occurs (Figure 8.9) which compromises the mechanical integrity of the fixation and can result in joint instability. To prevent this, bone tunnel maturation must occur. Bone tunnel maturation refers to osseous remodeling and hardening of the inner wall of the bone tunnels that occur over time after surgery. Maturation of the bone tunnels increases resistance to bone tunnel widening and ultimately enables patients to return to increased activity.

Bone tunnel maturation is contingent on technical execution by the surgeon producing a mechanical sound stifle at surgery, avoiding infection, and giving the patient a sufficient period of deliberate controlled activity following surgery.

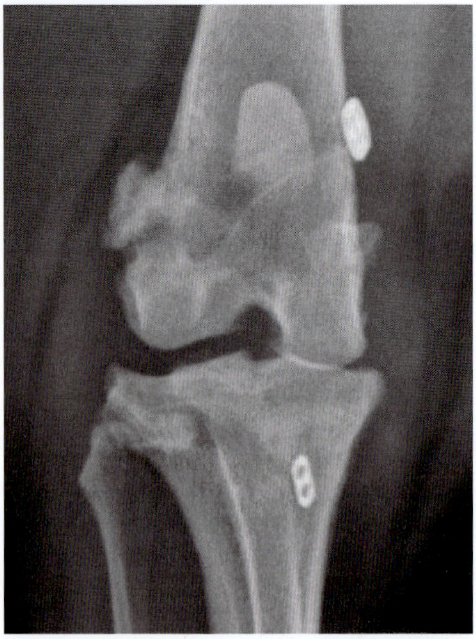

Figure 8.9 Bone tunnel widening most prominently observed on the lateral aspect of the femoral tunnel. The smooth tapering appearance of the widened tunnel is most consistent with a mechanical source. Differentials in this dog would include overtightened implants, nonisometrically placed bone tunnels, and limb overuse.

8.4.1.2.1 What is Necessary for Bone Tunnel Maturation to Occur?

Bone tunnel maturation requires a time period after surgery where the implant-to-bone tunnel relationship is not excessively stressed. The implant-to-bone tunnel relationship can become overwhelmed and compromised from suboptimal mechanics created at surgery, postoperative infection, or premature overuse of the joint.

8.4.1.2.2 Surgical Considerations for Bone Tunnel Maturation

Origins of Bone Tunnels at Optimal Locations to Maximize Joint Isometry

When femoral and tibial anchor points are isometric, suture tension will remain relatively constant throughout stifle range of motion.

Nonisometrically placed suture implants will tighten or loosen through different zones of the range of motion, creating stifle conflict which can result in suture cutting into metaphyseal bone and causing bone tunnel widening.

Bone Tunnel Angulation

Bone tunnels should be angled 30–45° away from the joint. Angling the tunnel away from the joint allows a smooth transition as the suture exits the bone tunnel. Bone tunnels closer to parallel to the adjacent joint surface predispose to suture material cutting into the bone where the suture exits the tunnel, causing bone tunnel widening (Figure 8.10).

Bone Tunnel Size and Implant Type

Selection of implants and their associated bone tunnel diameter must be made relative to patient size. Implants can be too large for very small patients. Oversized implants can prevent accurate isometric tunnel placement, predisposing to bone tunnel widening. Implant selection should follow established weight-based guides.

Flat suture implants are superior to round suture implants. Round suture material has a higher risk than flat suture implants to saw into too soft metaphyseal bone [20]. The surgeon must be knowledgeable about implant options available for the procedure.

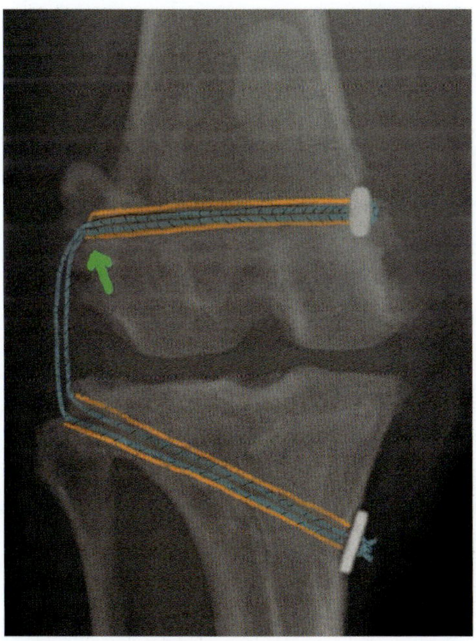

Figure 8.10 Note that the angle of the femoral bone tunnel is parallel to the joint. This tunnel angle increases the risk of suture cutting into the bone at the lateral exit point of the femoral tunnel (green arrow). This can cause the bone tunnel to widen, shortening the path the suture has to travel and resulting in loosening of the stifle.

8.4.2 Infection

Infection associated with implants can cause osteolysis around bone tunnels, resulting in significant bone tunnel widening. Because severe bone tunnel widening will result in a catastrophic disruption of repair stability, early detection and treatment of implant-associated infections are critical. Detection and management of infection are addressed later in this chapter.

8.4.3 Postoperative Activity Restrictions

Until bone tunnel maturation has occurred, bone tunnels are vulnerable to widening from either a single episode of high-intensity burst activity or excessive repetitive cyclical loading. For this reason, the surgeon, rehabilitation team, and client should not aim to restore patients to normal activity duration or intensity until bone tunnel maturation has occurred. Although different postoperative activity plans can be considered, to optimize the environment for bone tunnel maturation and periarticular fibrosis to occur, the authors recommend 6–8 weeks of short-duration, low-intensity activity followed by 4 weeks of low-intensity, increasing-duration activity followed by 4 weeks of increasing-intensity, increasing-duration activity. Surgeons can vary specifics of this structure but must keep in mind that maintaining a mechanically sound stifle after extracapsular stabilization requires a sufficient amount of structurally supportive periarticular fibrosis formation to occur.

8.4.4 Postoperative Benchmarks of Expectation

When performing stifle surgery, the surgeon should establish benchmarks of expectation at specific postoperative time points in the recovery period. This allows the surgeon to survey the quality of recovery and to signal when complications are occurring. Although numerous metrics can be used to assess quality of recovery, subjective assessment of limb use should be a primary metric evaluated by the surgeon.

8.4.4.1 Limb Use Expectation: 2 Weeks Postoperative

The time point after stifle surgery when patients transition from nonweight bearing to weight bearing varies from patient to patient. The surgeon should expect that some patients will start using their operated leg on the day of surgery while others will not start using it until several weeks postoperatively. This variation is reasonable and expected given the range of factors that can influence immediate postoperative pain and how it subsides after surgery.

The surgeon should expect all patients to be at least weakly weight bearing by 2 weeks postoperative, subjectively bearing at least 25–35% normal weight at a slow walk. Although many patients will exceed this minimal expectation at the 2-week follow-up exam, weak but consistent weight bearing should be the low bar of expectation tolerated by the surgeon for this stage of recovery. If a patient fails to meet this minimal expectation at the 2-week postoperative time point, the surgeon must assess the patient for medical reasons to explain the underperformance. Differentials for poor limb use at the 2-week follow-up include:

- pain
- infection
- mechanical abnormality.

Unacceptable limb usage at the 2-week follow-up signals that something is wrong and that action should be taken. The surgeon's evaluation should include a conversation with the client to update the patient's history, performing a detailed orthopedic exam, and additional diagnostics.

8.4.4.1.1 History Considerations

What Analgesics is the Client Administering?

Insufficient pain management may result in poor limb use after surgery [28–30]. The surgeon must examine which medications the client has been administering, including dose, frequency, and last date each drug was administered. Surgeons should not assume that because a medication was prescribed, it was actually administered. Optimally, a multimodal analgesic plan was prescribed following surgery and that plan was executed by the client. If insufficient analgesia was administered, renewing an analgesic plan can contribute to returning the patient to an expected course of recovery.

Was the Patient Using the Leg at Any Point of the Recovery?

If a patient has never used their leg following surgery, differentials include insufficient postoperative analgesia, presence of a latent meniscal tear from inadequate meniscal examination and management at surgery [31–33], infection, or a mechanical problem with the repair (i.e., residual instability, implant overtightening, or areas of conflict through the range of motion from poor implant isometry). If a patient had been using their leg well and then stopped, differentials include a nondestructive limb overuse event for that stage of recovery (i.e., a joint sprain that will recover in a short time period), a subsequent meniscal tear, SSI, or a mechanical problem with the repair (loose or broken implants, bone tunnel widening). Understanding the chronology of limb disuse after surgery will help the surgeon navigate these differentials.

How Has the Patient Been Confined and How Much Activity Has the Patient Been Getting?

Poor limb use can result from premature limb overuse (i.e., too much activity) or insufficient opportunity to use and rehabilitate the leg (i.e., too rigid confinement). To make this determination, the surgeon must enquire about how the patient is being activity limited (crate, pen, small room, or free access to house), whether a leash is used during all activities, and whether there have been breaches in security where overuse could have occurred. Whether participating in a home rehabilitation plan or a regimented physical rehabilitation program, the surgeon needs to understand the types and volume of activity the patient has been exposed to.

Recognizing if the patient has been exposed to too much activity or too little limb use opportunity can help the surgeon determine how activity adjustments may contribute to an underachieving patient's return to expected recovery performance.

Has an E-collar or Other Device Been Used?
Incisional irritation and subsequent infection from licking can significantly impede a patient's recovery. If licking has occurred, to prevent ongoing incisional self-trauma it must be determined whether an anti-lick device is being used, if there are times the device is not being used, or whether the patient can traumatize the incision while using the device.

8.4.4.1.2 Physical Examination and Orthopedic Examination

Evaluate the Entire Limb
Although it seems like a reasonable assumption that the limb disuse is stemming from the operated knee, always examine the entire limb to make sure that there are no extenuating problems elsewhere to account for the disuse. This would be unexpected, but always check to be certain.

Evaluate for Evidence of Infection
Three types of SSI must be considered in patients failing to meet the limb use benchmark of expectation 2 weeks after stifle surgery.

- Superficial incisional SSI: the incision should be inspected for redness, discharge, or gapping. The incision and surrounding skin should be examined for erythema and thickening which could indicate whether licking or other patient self-trauma has occurred.
- Deep implant-associated SSI: examine the limb for evidence of pain, redness, or swelling. Apply direct palpation over suture implants and anchor sites to assess for sensitivity over implants.
- Joint infection: septic arthritis has to be a differential for any patient failing to meet expectations for limb use during recovery, particularly when other causes of the unacceptable limb use are not identified. There is a false assumption that a septic knee will always result in fever, lethargy, excessive joint swelling, pain on direct palpation of the knee, lymph node enlargement, or elevated white blood cells. Although one or several of these symptoms can occur, a joint infection can be present in the absence of all these conditions. Collection of joint fluid by arthrocentesis and performing joint fluid analysis including cytology is the only conclusive diagnostic to rule in or rule out a septic joint.

Limb Mechanics Assessment
- Excessive cranial drawer: less than 3 mm of cranial drawer should be present following extracapsular stifle stabilization procedures. Poor limb use associated with excessive cranial drawer can result from joint instability, predisposition of the patient to subsequent meniscal tears, and/or sensitivity to loose implants irritating periarticular soft tissues.
- Suture implant conflict: palpable conflict between the extracapsular suture implants and adjacent soft tissue structures occurs with nonisometric implant positioning. Suture implant conflict can cause pain from periarticular soft tissue impingement, soft tissue abrasion, or by causing mechanical restriction through some phases of the range of motion.
- Restricted stifle mechanics (fixed external tibial rotation): overtightening extracapsular suture implants at surgery can mechanically restrain the stifle in external rotation and cause excessive compression to the lateral stifle joint compartment. Overtightened suture implants can impede patient recovery by causing mechanical dysfunction to the joint, joint pain from compression of the lateral joint compartment, and potential metaphyseal bone pain from suture implants cutting into bone tunnels (i.e., bone tunnel widening).
- Restricted tarsal mechanics: entrapment of the LDE tendon at surgery will restrict tarsal flexion, altering postoperative mechanics and compromising recovery.

8.4.4.1.3 Additional Diagnostics

Follow-Up Radiographs

Orthogonal view stifle radiographs should be taken in patients that fail to meet expectation at any time point. Bone toggle/tie-button positioning, amount of stifle effusion, and bone tunnel size and character should all be evaluated when interpreting follow-up stifle radiographs. Bone toggle/tie-button positioning as compared to the immediate postoperative study can indicate if the suture implants have loosened or broken.

- Quantifying the amount of radiographic stifle effusion can suggest that an inflammatory process is occurring in the joint, but cannot discern whether it is normal for the given stage of recovery, the result of osteoarthritis in the joint, the result of limb overuse, the result of poor limb mechanics, the result of a meniscal tear, or the result of septic arthritis.
- Bone tunnel size and character should be evaluated as the presence of bone tunnel widening is often an indication of significant surgical site issue. Because most causes of bone tunnel widening require time to occur, it is rare to observe meaningful bone tunnel widening at a 2-week follow-up exam.
- Interpreted in the context of history, physical exam, and other diagnostic findings, stifle radiographs can provide useful insights in narrowing down the differentials for poor limb use after surgery. Stifle radiographs should be taken in all patients failing to meet postsurgical benchmarks of expectation.

Arthrocentesis

Joint sepsis is an important differential for any patient failing to meet limb use expectations following stifle surgery. Stifle arthrocentesis should be considered in all underperforming patients. Arthrocentesis is the conclusive diagnostic to investigate a possible septic joint, and frustratingly, poor limb use may be the only prevailing symptom of septic arthritis.

The gross appearance and consistency of the joint fluid should be closely inspected when joint fluid has been collected. Normal joint fluid should be clear and should have a viscous consistency. Joint fluid that appears turbid or cloudy, or has a watery consistency should be presumed to be infected (Figure 8.11) [34].

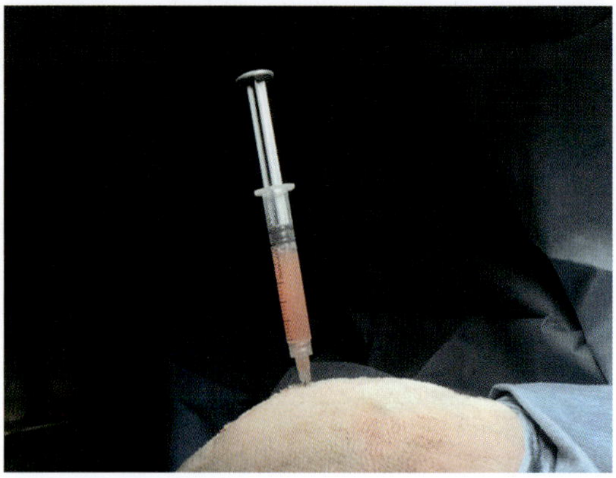

Figure 8.11 A joint tap should be performed in all patients failing to meet the surgeon's benchmark of expectation in the postoperative period. Turbid, cloudy fluid with watery consistency warrants joint fluid culture, flushing the joint using ingress and egress needles, and antibiotic therapy.

Basic cytological examination of joint fluid is a simple procedure even for the least cytologically inclined surgeon. Normal joint fluid should contain small lymphocytes and mononuclear cells, typically in low numbers. Osteoarthritic joint fluid should also contain small lymphocytes and mononuclear cells. For both normal and osteoarthritic joints, there should be less than 10% neutrophils present. The presence of abundant neutrophils with a concurrent degenerative neutrophil presence in the postoperative knee patient supports the presumptive diagnosis of septic arthritis and should prompt bacterial culture and sensitivity testing, joint irrigation, and the initiation of empirical antibiotic therapy.

Joint Irrigation

Joint irrigation with lactated Ringer's solution (LRS) or isotonic saline using ingress and egress needles is an important component of septic arthritis management in the postoperative patient. Clinical benefit is gained from flushing cytotoxins and inflammatory mediators from the septic joint, and antibiotic treatment alone may be insufficient in treating septic joint patients without starting with joint irrigation. Although LRS may be preferable to 0.9% sodium chloride because it is considered to be more physiological, either isotonic solution would be considered appropriate for joint irrigation in the septic joint. Needle size will vary depending on patient size, and pressure bags, mechanical pumps, or arthroscopic pumps can be used for ingress. Fluid volume used to flush will vary based on patient size (usually 500–1000 mL), and ingress flush fluids are continued until egress fluids are consistently clear.

Empirical Antibiotic Therapy

When joint fluid appearance is consistent with infection, empirical antibiotics should be initiated. In stable patients that are limping but otherwise doing well, a first-line empirical oral antibiotic should be initiated while culture results are pending. In sick or systemically unstable patients, hospitalization for intravenous broad-spectrum antibiotics and supportive care may be necessary.

Deciding whether to extend the empirical antibiotic course or change to another antibiotic medication should be based on the clinical response to initial treatment and bacterial culture results. Duration of the antibiotic treatment course should be based on stage of healing from surgery, safety of antibiotic being used, and patient tolerance of antibiotic being used. When a joint is found to be septic following extracapsular bone-to-bone stifle stabilization surgery, the surgeon should presume that implant colonization has occurred. Because infection has a highly deleterious effect on bone tunnel maturation, antibiotics should ideally be continued without interruption until bone tunnel maturation has occurred. In addition, when implant colonization has occurred, recurrence of infection is very likely at some point after discontinuation of antibiotics. For this reason, antibiotics should also ideally be continued until sufficient periarticular fibrosis formation has occurred in the event that implants need to be explanted. A 4–8-week course of antibiotics should be considered when septic arthritis is identified during the recovery period from extracapsular stifle stabilization surgery.

In summary, the minimal benchmark of expectation at the 2-week follow-up exam following extracapsular bone-to-bone stifle stabilization surgery is that every patient should be weak but weight bearing. If a patient fails to meet this expectation, a thorough history should be taken, a physical and orthopedic examination should be performed, follow-up radiographs should be taken, and the joint should be tapped. The goal of this process is to identify the source of poor limb use and implement a targeted treatment regimen to help get the patient back on course.

8.4.4.2 Six Weeks Postoperative Follow-Up

Six weeks following extracapsular stifle stabilization surgery is generally considered a sufficient timeframe for bone tunnel maturation and periarticular fibrosis formation to occur to safely allow an increase in duration of activity. Because there is no way to objectively quantify the amount of periarticular fibrosis or bone tunnel maturation that has occurred, and because premature limb overuse prior to sufficient bone tunnel maturation and the development of periarticular fibrosis can lead to bone tunnel widening, implant failure, destabilization of the stifle, and a subsequent poor outcome, the authors would suggest that 6 weeks means not sooner than 6 weeks and more accurately would be represented by a week 6 to week 8 timeframe.

8.4.4.2.1 Limb Use Expectation: Six Weeks Postoperative

At 6 weeks postoperative, patients should have substantially improved limb use compared to the 2-week follow-up exam, bearing approximately 70–90% normal weight. Subjectively, weight bearing at 6 weeks postoperative should be fair but not normal. Because most rehabilitation plans for extracapsular bone-to-bone stabilization with synthetic implants require 6 weeks of low-duration, low-intensity activity to provide an environment for bone tunnel maturation and periarticular fibrosis formation to occur, it is expected that most patients will not be back to normal by 6 weeks postoperatively. Effectively communicating with clients this fair but not normal limb function expectation at 6 weeks postoperative will help reduce anxieties and temper impatience that often occur during a restricted postoperative activity period.

Notably, some clients inaccurately believe that it is acceptable to increase their pet's activity prior to the 6-week postoperative mark because they are subjectively happy with how well their pet is doing. It is vital to preemptively communicate that time is the trigger for increasing volume and intensity of activity, not how well the limb is being used. Without sufficient bone tunnel maturation and periarticular fibrosis formation, premature limb overuse puts patients that were doing well at risk of a failed mechanical outcome.

8.4.4.2.2 Poor Limb Use: Six Weeks Postoperative

As previously stated, the authors would suggest that the 6 weeks postoperative exam be performed not sooner than 6 weeks, and more accurately within the week 6 to week 8 time interval. Differentials for poor limb use at 6 weeks post surgery include surgery site pain, neuropathic pain, osteoarthritis pain, infection, meniscal tear, implant-associated discomfort, and mechanical abnormalities. The patient assessment process should again include a thorough history, physical and orthopedic exam, and additional diagnostics.

8.4.4.2.2.1 History

History for the patient that is not meeting expectation at the 6-week follow-up exam should center around the patient's trend of limb use, activity level, and medications.

- Trend of limb use: understanding whether the patient never trended in a favorable clinical direction after surgery or if they had been doing well before acutely deteriorating can help prioritize differentials.
- Activity level: the surgeon should investigate how the patient has been activity limited, types and volume of activity the patient has had access to, and whether there was any correlation between lameness onset with activity.
- Medications: understanding whether the quality of limb use responds significantly to pain medications can help narrow the differential list. Note that when a client reports that medications seem to make their dog feel better but they do not use their leg more effectively, this should be considered an insignificant or poor response to pain medication in the postoperative stifle patient. Limb use is the primary metric of interest.

8.4.4.2.2.2 Physical and Orthopedic Examination

A physical and orthopedic exam should be performed on patients underperforming at the 6-week postsurgical time point to evaluate for mechanical abnormalities and/or pain associated with stifle palpation or implant locations. Stifle radiographs, stifle ultrasound imaging or joint exploration to reexamine the meniscus, joint fluid analysis and culture, implant explantation and culture and joint restabilization are considerations for patients that are clinically doing poorly 6–8 weeks after surgery.

- Excessive cranial drawer: excessive cranial drawer can cause persistent lameness from joint instability and can predispose to a postoperative or subsequent meniscal tear. Loose implants in stifles with excessive cranial drawer can abrade soft tissues, causing implant-associated pain. Stifle radiographs, stifle exploration to reexamine the meniscus, joint fluid analysis and culture, implant explantation and culture and joint restabilization are considerations for these patients.
- Implant-associated pain: implant-associated pain typically occurs if there is deep SSI and infection at the implant site or if implants are loose. Stifle radiographs and culture of the implants should be performed in patients with implant-associated pain.
- Restricted stifle mechanics: overtightened extracapsular suture implants can result in joint pain from compression of the lateral compartment of the stifle and/or metaphyseal bone pain from suture implants cutting into bone tunnels (i.e., bone tunnel widening). Follow-up stifle radiographs should be taken, and the surgeon should consider either removing the implants or attempting physical rehabilitation and removing implants at a later time if the patient responds poorly to physical rehabilitation. More information on complications associated with physical rehabilitation can be found in Chapter 15.

8.4.4.2.2.3 Additional Diagnostics

Stifle Radiographs

Stifle radiographs should be taken in all underperforming postoperative knee patients at 6–8 weeks post surgery to assess for toggle/button positioning, joint effusion, and bone tunnel width and character.

- Bone toggle/button positioning compared to the immediate postoperative study can indicate if the suture implants have loosened or broken.
- Stifle effusion suggests that an inflammatory process is occurring in the joint, but cannot discern whether it is normal for the given stage of recovery or the result of osteoarthritis in the joint, limb overuse, poor limb mechanics, a meniscal tear, or infection.
- Bone tunnel widening can result from premature limb overuse, nonisometrically placed implants, bone tunnels angled too parallel to the joint, overtightened implants, and infection. Widened tunnels with smooth bone tunnel margins stem from limb mechanical causes, and typically require dialing back activity volume and/or intensity (Figure 8.9). Tunnel widening with irregular margins often indicates infection, and requires culture and appropriate antibiotic therapy. Dogs with gross enlargement of bone tunnels due to infection should have implants removed immediately, as their usefulness to stifle stability cannot be restored and their presence will serve as an ongoing source of irritation and infection (Figure 8.12).

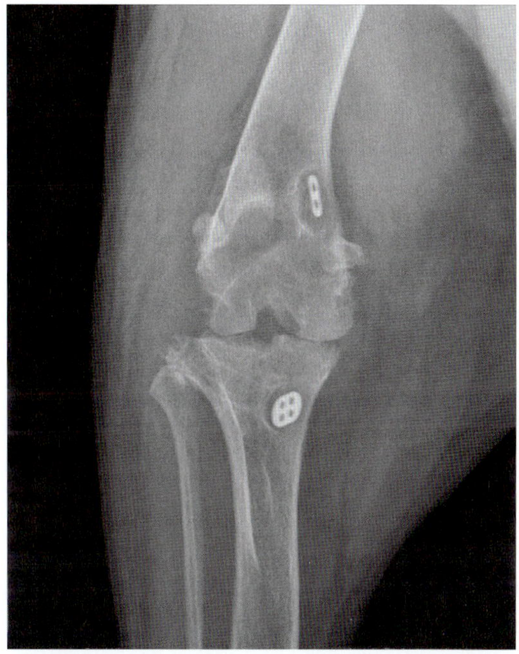

Figure 8.12 Bone tunnel widening caused by infection. Note the severe bone tunnel widening with irregular margins. Note the radiolucency surrounding the metallic buttons which can indicate significant implant loosening. Medical treatment will not salvage this repair, and implant removal is an essential component of infection management for this patient.

Arthrocentesis

A joint tap of the stifle should be considered in all patients doing poorly at 6–8 weeks after knee surgery. Development of a joint infection can occur at any time after knee surgery [35], and treatment should include culture of the joint fluid, flushing the joint with ingress/egress needles, and systematic antibiotics. If a septic joint is identified, the surgeon should assume that implant colonization has occurred. If this proves to be true, recurrence of infection will occur at some point after discontinuation of antibiotics. For this reason, when an infection is identified at this stage of recovery, it is ideal to continue antibiotics until lameness resolves and the patient is allowed to complete 4–8 weeks of successful rehabilitation without increased risk of setback from infection recurrence.

If lameness persists during antibiotic administration and infection treatment is not deemed successful, then early explantation should be considered. If infection recurs after discontinuation of this longer course of antibiotics, the infection should be re-treated and implants should be explanted.

8.4.4.2.3 Managing Implant-Associated Pain

Implant removal is necessary if it is the source of mechanical irritation or when bacterial colonization has occurred. Because long-term maintenance of stifle stability depends on periarticular fibrosis, removing implants does not necessarily cause meaningful increases in instability. If a condition exists that necessitates implant removal, they should be removed. Revision or an alternative method of stifle stabilization only is necessary if ongoing lameness from the residual instability occurs.

8.4.4.2.4 Managing Restricted Stifle Range of Motion

In patients with lameness from restricted stifle motion from overtightened suture implants, a graded physical rehabilitation plan should be implemented to try to restore stifle range of motion. Because overtightened implants carry the risk of causing bone tunnel widening, the surgeon should monitor the patient's recovery process with serial radiographs on an alternate-week basis to help guide the physical rehabilitation therapist on whether efforts are appropriate or need to be scaled back. If physical rehabilitation fails to restore limb function to an acceptable level or progressive bone tunnel widening is observed, implants should be removed. Revision or pursuing an alternate mode of stifle repair (stifle osteotomy technique) should be considered if lameness persists after implant removal.

8.4.4.2.5 Managing Excessive Stifle Instability

The presence of excessive cranial drawer can cause lameness in three potential ways: the loose implants can cause periarticular soft tissue pain, the instability can predispose to a postliminary meniscal tear, or the residual instability in the knee can be the source of pain.

- Physical rehabilitation: in an underperforming postoperative patient with excessive cranial drawer, it is reasonable to initiate a course of pain medications and attempt physical rehabilitation. If these efforts do not produce sufficient resolution of lameness, the extracapsular suture implants should be removed and the joint should be examined surgically for the potential presence of a meniscal tear.
- Removing loose implants: the presence of loose extracapsular implants can cause pain and lameness by irritating periarticular soft tissues. Although it may feel like a failure to remove implants, if they are no longer an asset to the stability of the stifle, they should be removed. Because loose implants can be a significant source of discomfort and lameness, removing loose implants has the potential to restore comfort and function to the patient.
- Joint exploration: because the residually unstable stifle is at risk for developing a subsequent meniscal tear, joint exploration for meniscal inspection and management will be a critical step to restore limb function.
- Joint restabilization: by managing the meniscus (if a meniscal tear is present) and removing the loose implants, the surgeon has eliminated two important sources of lameness associated excessive residual instability. If lameness persists, then the surgeon must conclude that the instability itself is the source of the lameness, and revision of the extracapsular repair or pursuing an alternative mode of stifle stabilization (a corrective osteotomy technique) must be considered.
- Debriefing residual instability: when a postoperative patient has residual instability, the surgeon must debrief to determine the likely cause of the unstable stifle. The surgeon must consider whether technical factors like patient conformation, patient size, or implant choices challenged the surgery. The surgeon must review whether patient features like excessive TPA, excessive body weight, dense body weight to bone size, or poor compliance stressed the integrity of the repair. Did infection occur and could it have been prevented or treated more effectively? Was the postoperative plan appropriate to create an environment for periarticular fibrosis formation and bone tunnel maturation? Taking time to contemplate and reflect on our patients with complications is vital to help determine if the patient would be appropriate for revision or better suited for an alternative type of stifle stabilization (like a corrective osteotomy technique) and guide decision making on the management of future similar patients.

8.4.4.2.6 Acute Onset of Lameness in the Recovery Period

With increased activity, postoperative stifle patients may develop acute episodes of lameness at any point in their life. Mechanical abnormalities can occur and should be identifiable based on physical examination. In the stable postoperative stifle, acute lameness of this nature can occur from either a joint sprain or a subsequent meniscal tear [32].

Differentiating a Joint Sprain from a Subsequent Meniscal Tear

A joint sprain is an acute flare-up of pain, inflammation, and lameness that occurs when a postoperative patient has minor stifle joint trauma or overuses their limb without compromising the integrity of the repair. A sprain can happen at any phase of recovery, but generally is less likely to occur later in the recovery period after patients have fully rehabilitated their knee. Lameness stemming from a sprain will improve with time, rest, and antiinflammatory medications.

Similar to a sprain, a subsequent meniscal tear causes an acute onset of pain, inflammation, and lameness, and can occur at any time during the recovery period. Whereas a patient with a stifle sprain will return to their presprain status with rest, time, and antiinflammatory therapy, a patient with a significant meniscal tear will not.

When a patient becomes acutely lame during the postoperative period and the stifle palpates as mechanically sound and effusion is present radiographically, it is reasonable to initiate a course of antiinflammatory pain medications and a period of rest. If the lameness resolves and does not recur, it was a sprain. If the lameness does not improve or recurs when activity is reinitiated, a meniscal tear should be more strongly suspected and joint exploration should be considered [31, 36].

8.4.4.3 Limb Use Expectation: 14 Weeks Postoperative

The benchmark of expectation at 14 weeks postoperative from an extracapsular stifle stabilization is return to 90+% of normal function.

By producing a mechanically sound knee, providing an environment for bone tunnel maturation and periarticular fibrosis formation, avoiding/managing infection, and gradually restoring patient activity, the expectation at 14 weeks postoperative from an extracapsular stifle stabilization procedure is a return to full function. When a patient fails to meet this expectation, there is an underlying reason that warrants consideration. Strategies to evaluate and manage patients that fail to meet the 14-week postoperative benchmark are similar to earlier time points, and the surgeon must determine whether a mechanical abnormality, meniscal injury, or other source of pain is at play. Outcomes less than full function, even when deemed to be acceptable, should still be considered a compromise of the expected objective.

8.5 Conclusion

Surgery is a process that requires a comprehensive understanding of every step, from the preoperative examination through the final follow-up. Approaching extracapsular stifle stabilization in an organized manner enables the surgeon to disqualify patients that are poor candidates, maximize execution of intraoperative mechanical objectives, create an environment for healing and return to function to occur, and manage complications when they occur. As surgeons, we have a responsibility to our patients and clients to avoid problems when we can, recognize complications if they occur, and utilize our resources and resourcefulness to correct complications when we are able.

References

1. Vezzoni, A. (2004). TPLO by Slocum: a successful approach in the treatment of cranial cruciate injuries. *World Small Animal Veterinary Association World Congress Proceedings*. www.vin.com/apputil/content/defaultadv1.aspx?meta=Generic&pId=11181&id=3852273.
2. Havig, M.E., Dyce, J., Kowaleski, M.P. et al. (2007). Relationship of tibial plateau slope to limb function in dogs treated with a lateral suture technique for stabilization of cranial cruciate ligament deficient stifles. *Vet. Surg*. 36 (3): 245–251.

3. Biskup, J.J. and Griffon, D.J. (2014). Technical difficulties during the training phase for Tightrope® and percutaneous lateral fabellar suture techniques for cranial cruciate ligament repair. *Vet. Surg.* 43 (3): 347–354.
4. Tinga, S. (2018). In-vivo femorotibial kinematics in dogs with cranial cruciate ligament insufficiency before and after surgical stabilization. PhD dissertation. University of Florida, Gainesville, FL, USA.
5. Tinga, S., Kim, S.E., Banks, S.A. et al. (2020). Femorotibial kinematics in dogs treated with lateral fabellotibial suture stabilization for complete cranial cruciate ligament rupture: an in-vivo fluoroscopic analysis during walking in nine dogs weighing more than 15kg (33 lbs). *J. Am. Vet. Med. Ass.* 49: 187–199.
6. Laugier, M., Tremblay, J., Petit, Y. et al. (2019). Three-dimensional kinematic evaluation of Tightrope CCL in a canine in vitro cranial cruciate deficient stifle model. *Can. J. Vet. Res.* 83 (4): 317–321.
7. Roe, S.C., Kue, J., and Gemma, J. (2008). Isometry of potential suture attachment sites for the cranial cruciate ligament deficient canine stifle. *Vet. Comp. Orthop. Traumatol.* 21 (3): 215–220.
8. Kunkel, K.A., Basinger, R.R., Suber, J.T., and Gerard, P.D. (2009). Evaluation of a transcondylar toggle system for stabilization of the cranial cruciate deficient stifle in small dogs and cats. *Vet. Surg.* 38 (8): 975–982.
9. Hulse, D., Hyman, W., Beale, B. et al. (2010). Determination of isometric points for placement of a lateral suture in treatment of the cranial cruciate ligament deficient stifle. *Vet. Comp. Orthop. Traumatol.* 23 (3): 163–167.
10. Fischer, C., Cherres, M., Grevel, V. et al. (2010). Effects of attachment sites and joint angle at the time of lateral suture fixation on tension in the suture for stabilization of the cranial cruciate ligament deficient stifle in dogs. *Vet. Surg.* 39 (3): 334–342.
11. Reichert, E.E., Kunkel, K.A., Suber, J.T. et al. (2013). Radiographic localization and isometry of the origin and insertion of the canine cranial cruciate ligament. *Vet. Surg.* 42 (7): 860–866.
12. Aulakh, K.S., Harper, T.A., Lanz, O.I. et al. (2013). Effect of tibial insertion site for lateral suture stabilization on the kinematics of the cranial cruciate ligament deficient-stifle during early, middle and late stance: an in vitro study. *Vet. Comp. Orthop. Traumatol.* 26 (3): 208–217.
13. Roe, S.C. (2013). The challenge of isometry for extracapsular devices. *Vet. Comp. Orthop. Traumatol.* 26 (4): VII.
14. Cinti, F., Signorelli, C., Lopomo, N. et al. (2015). Two different approaches for novel extracapsular cranial cruciate ligament reconstruction: an in vitro kinematics study. *J. Small Anim. Pract.* 56 (6): 398–406.
15. Witte, P.G. (2015). Tibial anatomy in normal small breed dogs including anisometry of various extracapsular stabilizing suture attachment sites. *Vet. Comp. Orthop. Traumatol.* 28 (5): 331–338.
16. Böttcher, P., Fischer, C., Werner, H. et al. (2010). Stifle stability after lateral suture stabilisation using Ethibond Excel®: early destabilization following cyclic passive joint motion (in German). *Tierarztl. Prax. Ausg. K. Kleintiere. Heimtiere.* 38 (2): 61–69.
17. Lewis, D.D., Milthorpe, B.K., and Bellenger, C.R. (1997). Mechanical comparison of materials used for extra-capsular stabilisation of the stifle joint in dogs. *Aust. Vet. J.* 75 (12): 890–896.
18. Burgess, R., Elder, S., McLaughlin, R., and Constable, P. (2010). In vitro biomechanical evaluation and comparison of FiberWire, FiberTape, OrthoFiber, and nylon leader line for potential use during extraarticular stabilization of canine cruciate deficient stifles. *Vet. Surg.* 39 (2): 208–215.
19. Rose, N.D., Goerke, D., Evans, R.B., and Conzemius, M.G. (2012). Mechanical testing of orthopedic suture material used for extra-articular stabilization of canine cruciate ligament-deficient stifles. *Vet. Surg.* 41 (2): 266–272.
20. Leishman, D.J. and Chudik, S.C. (2019). Suture tape with broad full-width core versus traditional round suture with round core: a mechanical comparison. *Arthroscopy* 35 (8): 2461–2466.
21. Lodato, D., Wardlaw, J., and Rowe, D. (2013). Retrospective study comparing two materials commonly used in the LFS technique for CCLR. *J. Am. Anim. Hosp. Assoc.* 49 (2): 108–114.
22. Gnandt, R.J., Smith, J.L., Nguyen-Ta, K. et al. (2016). High-tensile strength tape versus high-tensile strength suture: a biomechanical study. *Arthroscopy* 32 (2): 356–363.
23. Edmiston, C.E. Jr., McBain, A.J., Roberts, C., and Leaper, D. (2015). Clinical and microbiological aspects of biofilm-associated surgical site infections. *Adv. Exp. Med. Biol.* 830: 47–67.
24. Ward, W.G. Sr., Cooper, J.M., Lippert, D. et al. (2014). Glove and gown effects on intraoperative bacterial contamination. *Ann. Surg.* 259 (3): 591–597.
25. Mischke, C., Verbeek, J.H., Saarto, A. et al. (2014). Gloves, extra gloves or special types of gloves for preventing percutaneous exposure injuries in healthcare personnel. *Cochrane Database Syst. Rev.* 3: CD009573.
26. Kim, K., Zhu, M., Munro, J.T., and Young, S.W. (2019). Glove change to reduce the risk of surgical site infection or prosthetic joint infection in arthroplasty surgeries: a systematic review. *ANZ J. Surg.* 89 (9): 1009–1015.
27. Choate, C.J., Lewis, D.D., Conrad, B.P. et al. (2013). Assessment of the craniocaudal stability of four extracapsular stabilization techniques during two cyclic loading protocols: a cadaver study. *Vet. Surg.* 42 (7): 853–859.

28. Grubb, T. (2010). Chronic neuropathic pain in veterinary patients. *Top. Companion Anim. Med.* 25 (1): 45–52.
29. Sanchis-Mora, S., Pelligand, L., Volk, H.A., and Abeyesinghe, S.M. (2015). Diagnosis and treatment of canine neuropathic pain. *Vet. Rec.* 177 (18): 470.
30. Moore, S.A. (2016). Managing neuropathic pain in dogs. *Front Vet. Sci.* 3: 12.
31. Plesman, R., Gilbert, P., and Campbell, J. (2013). Detection of meniscal tears by arthroscopy and arthrotomy in dogs with cranial cruciate ligament rupture: a retrospective,cohort study. *Vet. Comp. Orthop. Traumatol.* 26 (1): 42–46.
32. Ritzo, M.E., Ritzo, B.A., Siddens, A.D. et al. (2014). Incidence and type of meniscal injury and associated long-term clinical outcomes in dogs treated surgically for cranial cruciate ligament disease. *Vet. Surg.* 43 (8): 952–958.
33. Rappa, N.S. and Radasch, R.M. (2016). Postoperative complications associated with the arthrex canine cranial cruciate ligament repair anchor system in small- to medium-sized dogs: a retrospective analysis (2009–2012). *Can. Vet. J.* 57 (8): 847–852.
34. Scharf, V.F., Lewis, S.T., Wellehan, J.F. et al. (2015). Retrospective evaluation of the efficacy of isolating bacteria from synovial fluid in dogs with suspected septic arthritis. *Aust. Vet. J.* 93 (6): 200–203.
35. Mielke, B., Comerford, E., English, K., and Meeson, R. (2018). Spontaneous septic arthritis of canine elbows: twenty-one cases. *Vet. Comp. Orthop. Traumatol.* 31 (6): 488–493.
36. Pozzi, A., Hildreth, B.E. 3rd, and Rajala-Schultz, P.J. (2008). Comparison of arthroscopy and arthrotomy for diagnosis of medial meniscal pathology: an ex vivo study. *Vet. Surg.* 37 (8): 749–755.

Section IV

Osteotomy Repair Techniques

9 Complications Associated with Cranial Closing Wedge Osteotomy

Bill Oxley

9.1 Introduction

Cranial closing wedge osteotomy (CCWO) was the first dynamic stabilization technique described for the treatment of cruciate disease by Barclay Slocum and Theresa Devine in 1984 [1]. The same authors described radial tibial plateau leveling osteotomy (TPLO) in 1993 [2], and subsequent studies of the originally reported techniques revealed radial TPLO to be associated with lower overall complication and reoperation rates [3–6]. However, more recently, key alterations to the original technique (including the use of locking TPLO plates and modified wedge geometry) have resulted in similar major complication rates of approximately 5–8% for both procedures [7]. Many surgeons prefer CCWO to TPLO in small dogs due to the larger size of the proximal osteotomy segment, although the procedure can be used in dogs of any size, and those with excessive tibial plateau angles (TPAs), without technical modification or adjunctive procedures [8, 9]. Additionally, CCWO can be easily adapted to concurrently manage medial patellar luxation and proximal tibial deformities.

This chapter will describe CCWO preoperative planning and surgical technique, highlighting potential pitfalls that can lead to preventable complications. The recognition and management of postoperative complications will then be reviewed.

9.2 Preoperative Planning

The importance of accurate and thorough preoperative planning cannot be overemphasized in the context of avoidance of not only intraoperative but also many postoperative complications. Good planning not only reduces the risk of surgical errors but facilitates less tangible benefits such as minimized tissue handling and reduced surgical time which are equally important in the reduction of complication rates.

Preoperative planning starts with appropriately positioned mediolateral and craniocaudal radiographs including the stifle, tibia, and talocrural joint. Criteria for optimal positioning are identical to those described in Chapter 10 for radial TPLO. The ability to accurately measure distances on the radiograph is essential and thus the use of a magnification marker and/or digital calibration is mandatory.

Complications in Canine Cranial Cruciate Ligament Surgery, First Edition. Edited by Ron Ben-Amotz and David L. Dycus.

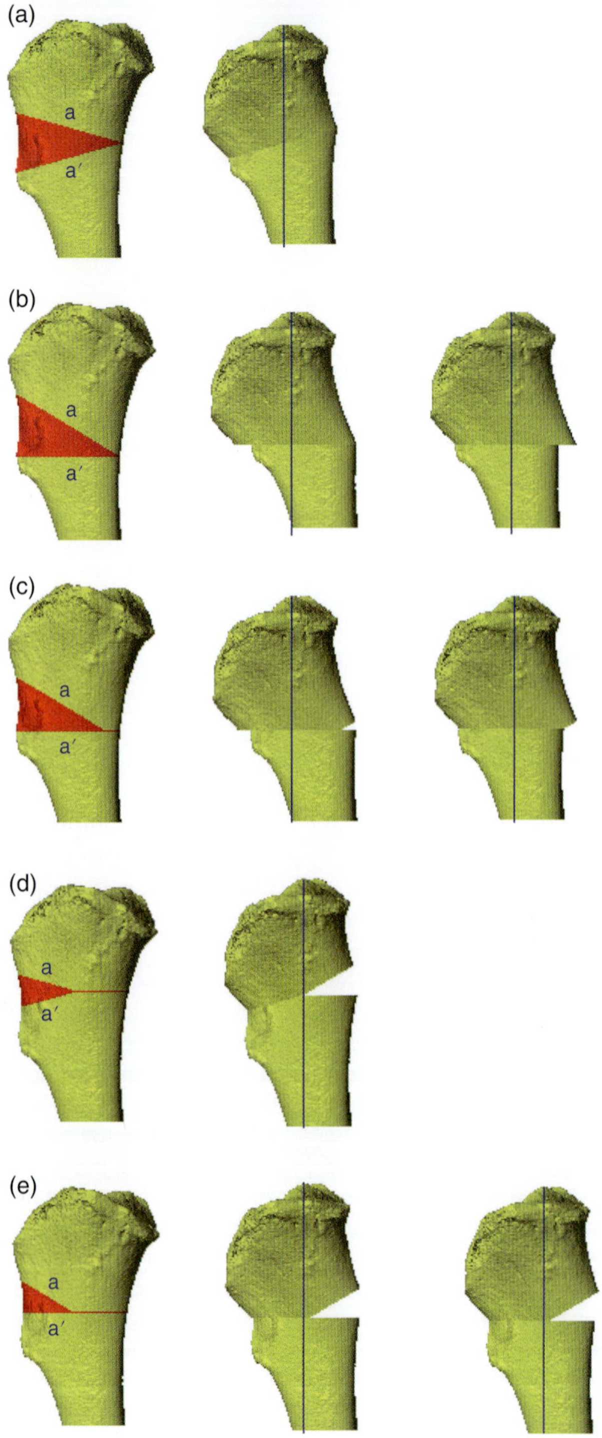

Figure 9.1 Various CCWO wedge geometries. In all cases, the wedge angle is 30°. (a) Closing symmetrical (isosceles) wedge [7]. Note that the proximal (a) and distal (a′) osteotomies are the same length and meet at the caudal cortex. (b) Closing asymmetrical wedge [1, 10]. Note that a ≠ a′, and that the osteotomies meet at the caudal cortex. Since the wedge is asymmetrical, the osteotomy surfaces differ in length and either the cranial or caudal cortices may be aligned. Aligning the cranial cortices shifts the long axis as indicated by the vertical blue line. Note the similar axis shift between the isosceles wedge and the asymmetrical, cranial cortical aligned geometries. (c) Neutral/closing asymmetrical wedge [8, 11, 12]. Note that a = a′ but that the osteotomies meet cranial to the caudal cortex, but more caudal than the midpoint between the cortices. Again, since the wedge is asymmetrical, either the cranial or caudal cortices may be aligned. As with the original asymmetrical wedge, cranial cortical alignment with a caudal overhang is preferred to reduce long axis shift. (d) Neutral symmetrical (isosceles) wedge. Note that a = a′ and the osteotomies meet at the midpoint between the cortices. (e) Neutral asymmetrical wedge. Note that a ≠ a′ and the osteotomies meet at the midpoint between the cortices. Since the difference in length between a and a′ is small, the difference in long axis shift between the cranial and caudal cortical alignment options is also small.

Various different CCWO osteotomy geometries have been described (Figure 9.1) [1, 7, 8, 10–12]. The original technique employed a closing asymmetrical wedge with its base perpendicular to the long axis of the tibia [1, 10]. Since the wedge is asymmetrical, the osteotomy surfaces differ in length, and either the cranial or caudal cortices are aligned, causing an "overhang" at the opposite cortex (Figure 9.1b). Alignment of the cranial cortices minimizes tibial long axis shift. Reported modifications include a closing symmetrical (isosceles triangle) wedge [7], and several neutral/closing asymmetrical wedge variations [8, 11, 12]. While each of these variations has specific potential advantages, none has been shown to be definitively superior in terms of indication (normal and excessive TPA), biomechanics, complication rates or functional outcome. All CCWO variations will cause relative distalization of the patella in the trochlea, although this is rarely of clinical significance. It is important to note that the degree of patella baja induced is proportional to the overall angular correction rather than the cranial wedge length as has been suggested, and is thus the same for closing, neutral, and indeed opening wedges. Given the relative similarity of the various modified techniques, it is improbable that any one technique will prove to be definitively superior, and the choice will likely remain one of surgeon preference.

A further variation on the original CCWO technique is to concurrently perform radial TPLO [13]. This technique has been recommended in cases with excessive TPA (>34°) since it permits plateau leveling without the very large proximal segment rotation necessary during radial TPLO or the large distalization of the patella during CCWO. However, the technique is technically challenging and associated with a high complication rate. More recently, CCWO as a stand-alone alone technique has been reported with a much lower overall complication rate [8]. Although patella baja was not assessed in that study, no specific complications associated with patella position were reported and long-term functional outcomes were very good. CCWO is therefore recommended in cases with excessive TPA; both the symmetrical isosceles and asymmetrical neutral variations can be used without additional technique modifications.

9.2.1 Isosceles Modified Cranial Closing Wedge Osteotomy (mCCWO) Planning

The author is most familiar with the isosceles closing wedge technique which will be described here, but the general principles of planning and execution will apply equally to other variations.

The osteotomy is templated by drawing an isosceles triangle-shaped wedge as proximally as possible on the tibia while preserving sufficient bone stock for plate fixation and remaining an adequate distance distal to the tibial tuberosity. In dogs weighing more than 20 kg, a 10 mm distance is recommended, but in smaller dogs a minimum of 5 mm is acceptable (Figure 9.2). To achieve a tibial plateau angle of 5°, for starting TPAs of 20° or less the planned wedge angle should be the TPA −5°. To compensate for greater tibial long axis shift associated with larger starting TPAs, the planned wedge angle should be increased by 1° for each increase of 5° (Table 9.1). For example, a 31° wedge angle is recommended for a 33° starting TPA.

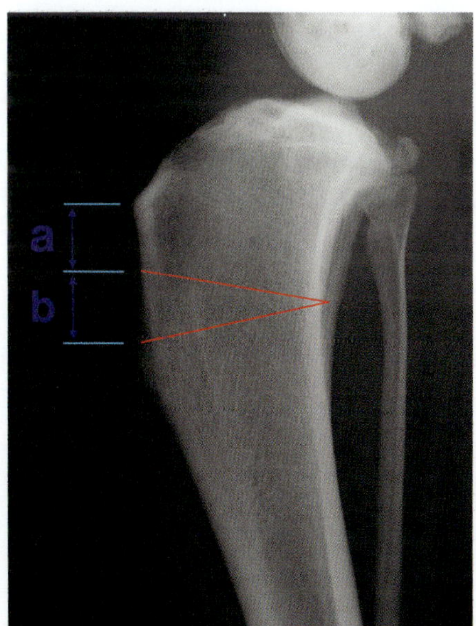

Figure 9.2 Preoperative planning. An isosceles triangle wedge is templated with its proximal point on the cranial cortex located 5 mm distal to the proximal point of the tibial tuberosity in dogs weighing <20 kg, and 10 mm distal to that point in heavier dogs (distance 'a'). Distance 'b' is then measured along the cranial cortex between the proximal and distal osteotomy lines.

Table 9.1 Planned wedge angles based on preoperative tibial plateau angle (TPA).

TPA	Wedge angle
≤20°	TPA – 5°
21–25°	TPA – 4°
26–30°	TPA – 3°
31–35°	TPA – 2°
36–40°	TPA – 1°

The sequence is continued for higher TPAs.

Templating is performed to ensure that the proximal segment is large enough to accommodate the proximal portion of an appropriately sized plate; if necessary, the wedge can be replanned a few millimeters distally. In dogs weighing more than 50 kg, placement of a second, cranial plate should be considered. The increase in overall strength afforded by orthogonal plating is well established [14]; however, for stabilization of a CCWO osteotomy, a cranial plate is particularly well positioned to oppose "rock-back" of the proximal osteotomy segment. As a secondary implant, even in very big dogs, a relatively small plate can be used (typically 2.4 mm). While placement of a single proximal locking screw may suffice, two screws are recommended; this will require distalization of the osteotomy by approximately 3–4 mm.

If desired, the caudal point of the wedge where the equal length osteotomy lines intersect can be planned to be 1–2 mm cranial to the caudal cortex (Figure 9.3). Although not essential, if this caudal bridge of bone is preserved during the osteotomies, it will deform and act as a hinge as the ostectomy is closed, reducing the risk of torsional malalignment, enabling inspection of osteotomy plane parallelity before reduction, and facilitating maintenance of segment alignment for plating.

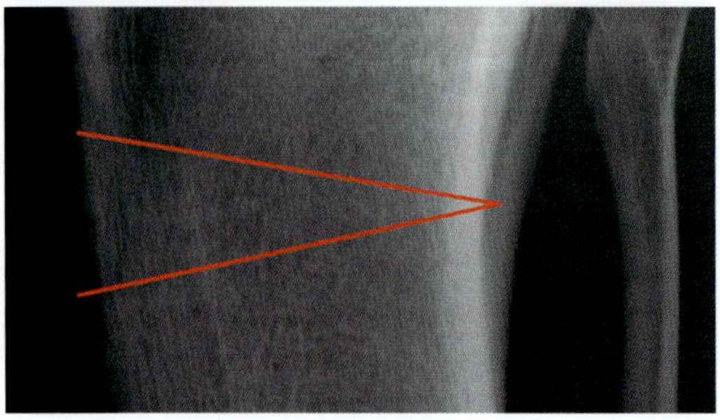

Figure 9.3 The proximal and distal osteotomies meet at a point 1–2 mm cranial to the caudal cortex.

Two distance measurements along the cranial tibial cortex are made and recorded for intraoperative reference. The first measurement is the distance between the proximal extent of the tibial tuberosity and the proximal osteotomy line, and the second is the length of the base of the isosceles triangle (Figure 9.2).

9.3 Intraoperative Complications

The majority of potential complications that may occur during the surgical procedure are ultimately avoidable. Key principles include thorough preoperative planning, knowledge of the relevant anatomy, and careful attention to an appropriate surgical sequence which safely accomplishes the goals of surgery while minimizing tissue injury and surgical time.

9.3.1 The Surgical Approach

The surgical approach for CCWO is almost identical to that previously described for TPLO. If mini arthrotomy for meniscal inspection is to be performed, the medial incision is started at the level of the distal pole of the patella; if not, it is commenced slightly proximal to the tibial tuberosity. The distal extent of the incision is determined by the required exposure for placement of the planned plate. It is rarely necessary to expose the medial saphenous artery and vein which are typically just distal to the incision.

An incision is made in the crural fascia a few millimeters caudal to the cranial border of the medial tibia. This incision is therefore caudal to the patella tendon insertion which should be clearly visible. Working from cranial to caudal, the fibrous pes ancerinus (the combined insertion of the sartorius, gracilis, and semitendinosus muscles) is elevated from the bone, taking care to preserve the medial collateral ligament which inserts at the caudal border of the cortex (Figure 9.4a). At this point, the entire pes ancerinus can be reflected caudally; this may be facilitated by a limited proximal extension of the fascial incision along the cranial border of the sartorius muscle.

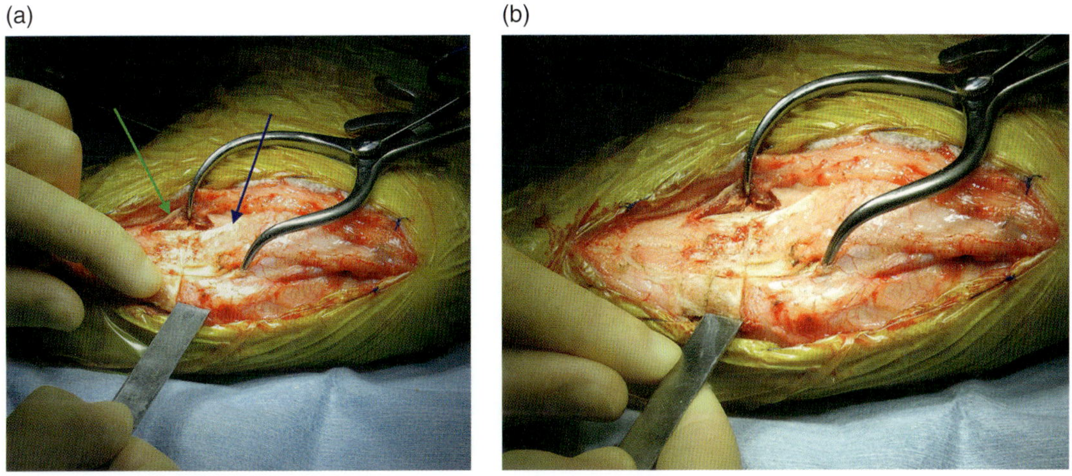

Figure 9.4 (a) The position of the proximal osteotomy on the cranial cortex is identified by measuring the preplanned distance distally from the point of insertion of the patellar tendon. In the image, a TPLO rotation gauge of the appropriate length is shown, but a ruler or calipers could be used. Note the change in color indicating the insertion of the patellar tendon at the proximal corner of the gauge. The bone is marked using any suitable method. The blue arrow indicates the medial collateral ligament; note the typical location of the proximal osteotomy a few millimeters distal to this. The green arrow indicates the position of the popliteal muscle elevation; note the limited proximal–distal extent. (b) The position of the distal osteotomy is measured from the proximal osteotomy position. Note that the proximal osteotomy position has been scored with the oscillating saw blade, and the gauge placed so as to include the kerf width. In this image, the distal position has been marked using diathermy.

Opinions differ as to the necessity during radial TPLO of partial popliteal muscle elevation for swab placement for protection of the cranial tibial artery, but this step is strongly recommended during CCWO. This is due to the caudolateral angulation of the oscillating saw blade which is helpful to complete the caudal corticotomy. A periosteal elevator should be introduced between the cortex and the muscle at the level of the planned apex of the wedge (typically a few millimeters distal to the base of the collateral ligament insertion) (Figure 9.4a). The aponeurotic attachment to the bone is often quite fibrous and particular attention is warranted to ensure correct placement of the elevator to prevent unnecessary injury to the muscle or indeed the artery itself. The tip of the elevator is advanced caudally in contact with the cortex until it is felt to pass over the caudal border of the bone, often meeting some slight resistance halfway. The elevator is then moved proximally and distally a short distance, creating a space for insertion of a moist swab. This available space is small and need only be gently packed; a whole standard swab is generally far too large, and the excess is folded caudally or cut off.

9.3.2 Ostectomy Position

Correct positioning of the wedge ostectomy is a key step as an incorrect location could increase the risk of tibial tuberosity or other proximal segment fracture and could also hamper plate application. The planned positions of both osteotomies are identified with reference to the insertion point of the patellar tendon. This point is identified by the generally well-demarcated transition line between the white striated appearance of the tendon and the cortical bone distally (Figure 9.4a). The planned distance distally from this point to the exit point of the proximal osteotomy is measured and the cortex marked (Figure 9.4a). This is easier if the tightly adherent fascia is elevated for a length a few millimeters more than the wedge base.

The further distance distally to the exit point of the distal osteotomy is then measured and marked (Figure 9.4b). In very small patients, the doubled width of the kerf of the saw blade can represent a significant proportion of the length of the base of the wedge (Figure 9.5). This can lead to removal of a larger wedge than planned and thus an excessively low final TPA. To avoid this, care is taken that the blade is positioned distal to the proximal measured cortical mark and vice versa. Next, the equal length "legs" of the wedge are measured from their origins on the cranial cortex to intersect either at the caudal cortex or 1–2 mm cranial to this if planned. The intersection point can be found using a wedge osteotomy gauge (commercially available isosceles triangle gauges of various angles), an orthopedic ruler, or with experience by eye. The osteotomy positions are marked on the cortex, and if wished can be scored with the oscillating saw blade (Figure 9.6a).

Finally, a 0.8 or 1 mm wire is preplaced through 1.1 or 1.5 mm holes drilled a few millimeters proximal and distal to the cranial osteotomy positions (Figure 9.6b). This requires

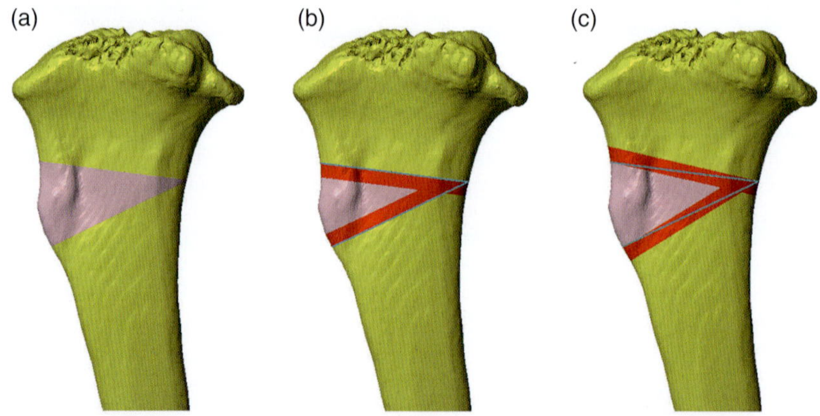

Figure 9.5 **(a)** A 32° wedge is planned in a small dog. The length of the base of the wedge (along the cranial cortex) is 5 mm. **(b)** A 1 mm thick oscillating saw blade is used to make the osteotomies. When the blade is started *within* the planned 5 mm wedge base, the kerf of the cut (indicated in red) does not increase the size of the wedge from that planned (light blue). **(c)** When the blade is started *outside* the planned wedge base, but aimed to a common exit point caudally, the kerf of the cut increases the length of the wedge base to 7 mm, and the wedge angle to 43°.

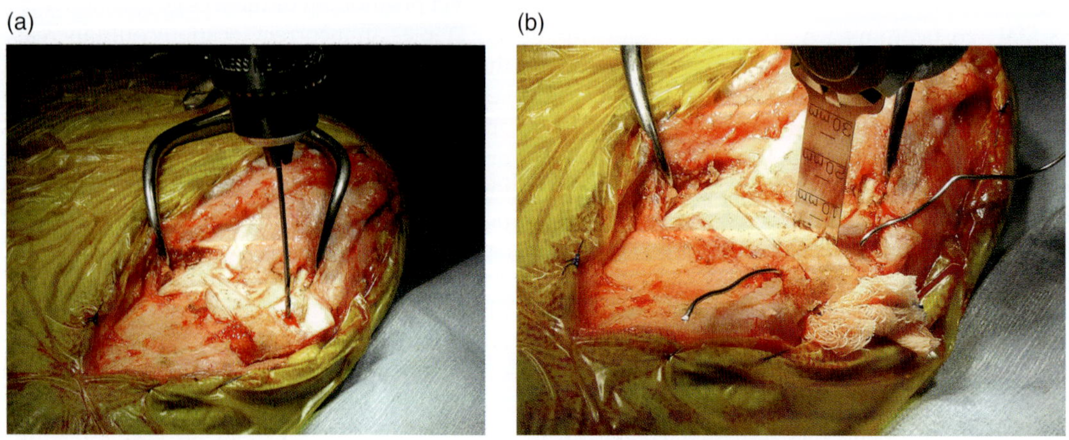

Figure 9.6 **(a)** The osteotomy positions have been scored with the oscillating saw blade. A small corner of fascia has been elevated to give access for the drill bit to create a 1.5 mm diameter hole for the reduction wire loop. **(b)** A simple wire loop has been preplaced. The cranial tibial muscle has been elevated at the level of the wedge and a swab placed to protect it from the saw blade.

limited elevation of the cranial tibial muscle, which if wished can be easily extended beneath the wedge and a moistened swab placed to protect the muscle from the exiting saw blade.

9.3.3 The Osteotomies

Attention to several key steps will minimize the risk of complications as the two osteotomies are made. Of particular importance is ensuring that the oscillating saw blade is maintained perpendicular to the cortex during both osteotomies. Any difference in the proximal/distal tilt of the blade (i.e., its angle in the dorsal plane) between the osteotomies will result in varus or valgus deformity when the ostectomy is reduced. Before the first osteotomy is started, the tibia should be positioned such that the medial cortex is horizontal to the surgical table. Swabs can be placed to maintain this orientation, and if available an assistant can hold the crus distally to maintain alignment. A vertical saw orientation, in other words perpendicular to the cortex, is the easiest for a surgeon to judge and maintain, and as long as the tibial orientation does not change materially between the two osteotomies then the osteotomy surfaces should be parallel in the dorsal plane. If there is any concern, a spare saw blade can be inserted into the first osteotomy and its orientation used as a guide for the optimal angle of the second osteotomy.

Particular care should be taken that the portion of the caudolateral cortex representing the apex of the wedge is removed (Figure 9.7). While the cortex at this point is relatively thick, the wedge is narrow and tapering and therefore vulnerable to breaking. If this occurs, a small fragment remains behind in a position that is not visible without specific visualization. Such a fragment will impede optimal reduction of the osteotomy surfaces, resulting in a varus deformity. The wedge should be inspected after removal for the presence of the caudolateral apex as shown in Figure 9.7. If this is absent, the corresponding area at the base of the ostectomy should be visualized and any residual cortex removed.

If a caudal cortical hinge is to be maintained, a slightly oblique caudolateral oscillating saw blade orientation can facilitate completion of

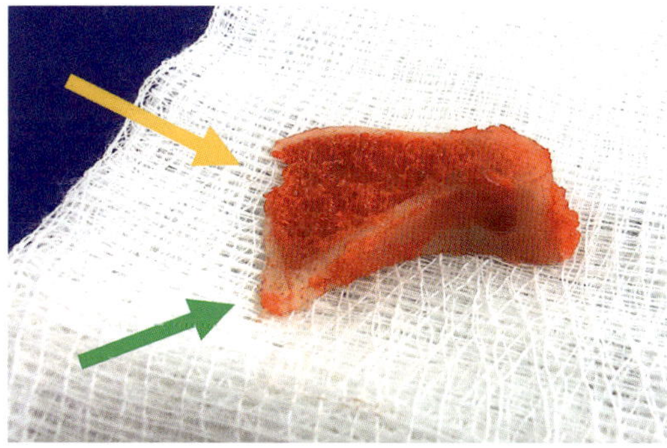

Figure 9.7 The optimal appearance of a CCWO wedge. Note the presence of the caudolateral cortex representing the apex of the wedge (green arrow). The cortex is absent from the wedge caudomedially (orange arrow) as this has been maintained as a "hinge" for osteotomy closure.

the osteotomy of the more lateral portion of the angled caudal cortex. This has the potential to bring the saw blade into closer contact with the cranial tibial artery than a purely laterally directed TPLO or oscillating saw orientation and is the reason that swab packing in that position is recommended. If this precaution is taken, iatrogenic arterial laceration is rare but should this occur, packing with a hemostatic agent may be effective. If this fails, the artery will require ligation. Sufficient surgical access can be gained by distraction of the osteotomy segments. Firm external pressure applied to the caudal aspect of the stifle by an assistant will usually significantly reduce or stop ongoing hemorrhage such that the artery can be identified and ligated.

If a caudal hinge has been maintained, the parallelity of the two osteotomy surfaces can be visually assessed following removal of the wedge. Alternatively, the wedge itself can be similarly assessed, whether or not a hinge is present. If necessary, a small amount of bone can be removed from one of the osteotomy surfaces to make it parallel to the other. It is important to note that it is the parallelity of the osteotomies, rather than their exact angle in relation to the dorsal plane, that determines whether malalignment results after reduction. For example, a slight proximomedial to distolateral osteotomy plane angle will not induce deformity or affect reduction as long as this angle is the same for both osteotomies. The use of a new oscillating saw blade for each surgery,

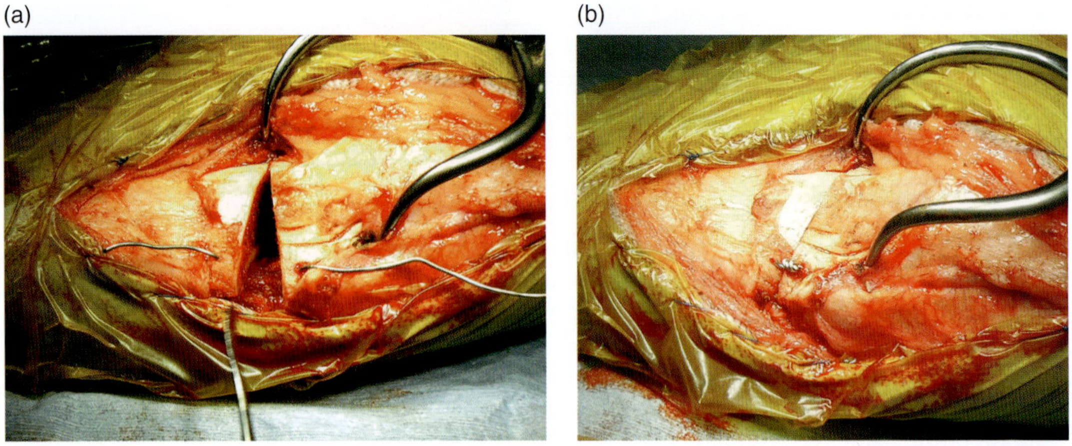

Figure 9.8 **(a)** The wedge and packing swabs have been removed. Note the intact caudomedial cortical hinge. **(b)** The wire has been twisted resulting in closure and maintained reduction of the osteotomy ready for plate application.

and lavage during the osteotomies, are recommended to reduce the risk of thermal necrosis which may delay bone healing and increase the risks of implant failure and infection [15].

Following completion of the osteotomies, any swabs placed to protect soft tissues are removed. This is an easily forgotten step but of critical importance as a retained swab will inevitably lead to formation of a gossypiboma. Establishing a set routine is helpful, and the use of tagged swabs can be considered in addition to the routine swab count before closure. Using swabs with radiopaque markers will reveal a retained swab at postoperative radiography, allowing immediate return to surgery for retrieval.

The final step before plating is reduction of the osteotomy. If an interfragmentary wire has been preplaced, this is twisted to form a simple loop which will progressively close the osteotomy gap as it is tightened, and then maintain reduction for plating (Figure 9.8). As an alternative reduction method, modified pointed reduction forceps can be used. It is very difficult to maintain reduction using a temporary stabilizing pin and this technique is not recommended.

In contrast to radial TPLO where tibiofibular joint ankylosis or a robust fibula can prevent planned rotation [16], difficulties with CCWO osteotomy reduction are very rare even when such features are present or with very large wedges when TPA is excessive.

A number of ancillary devices have been described to facilitate osteotomy creation and reduction. A variable-angle, slotted osteotomy guide has been shown to increase the accuracy of the resected wedge compared to a freehand technique [17] and could be used when performing either symmetrical or asymmetrical closing wedges. Use of a TPLO jig to facilitate optimal reduction has also been described [9] and could be considered at the surgeon's discretion.

9.3.4 Limb Alignment and Osteotomy Gaps

Following reduction, assessments of both limb alignment and for the presence of an osteotomy gap are made. It is vital to remember that limb malalignment and osteotomy gaps can occur together or independently of one another. For example, if the two osteotomies are nonparallel in the dorsal plane, they can still be perfectly reduced without a gap, but a deformity will result.

Several scenarios are possible:

1. Nonparallel osteotomies/perfect reduction.
   - No osteotomy gap.
   - Frontal plane deformity will result.
2. Nonparallel osteotomies/imperfect reduction.
   - Osteotomy gap.
   - Frontal plane deformity may be exacerbated or reduced by the imperfect reduction (Figure 9.9).
3. Parallel osteotomies/perfect reduction.
   - Optimal outcome (Figure 9.10).

(a) (b)

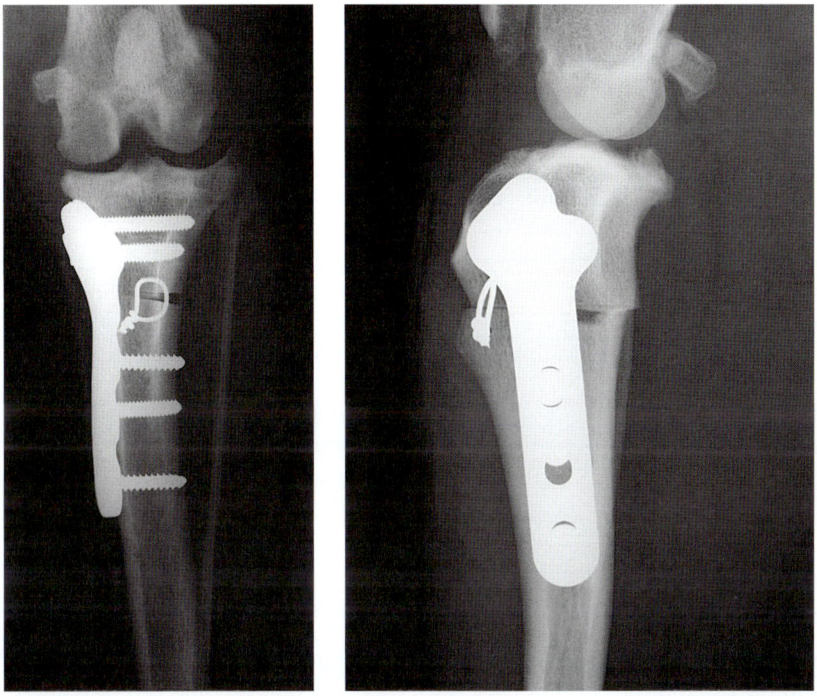

Figure 9.9 Postoperative (a) craniocaudal and (b) mediolateral projections showing nonparallel osteotomy planes. Had reduction been perfect, a valgus deformity would have been induced. In fact, the imperfect reduction with a lateral osteotomy gap was compensatory and limb alignment was normal.

(a) (b)

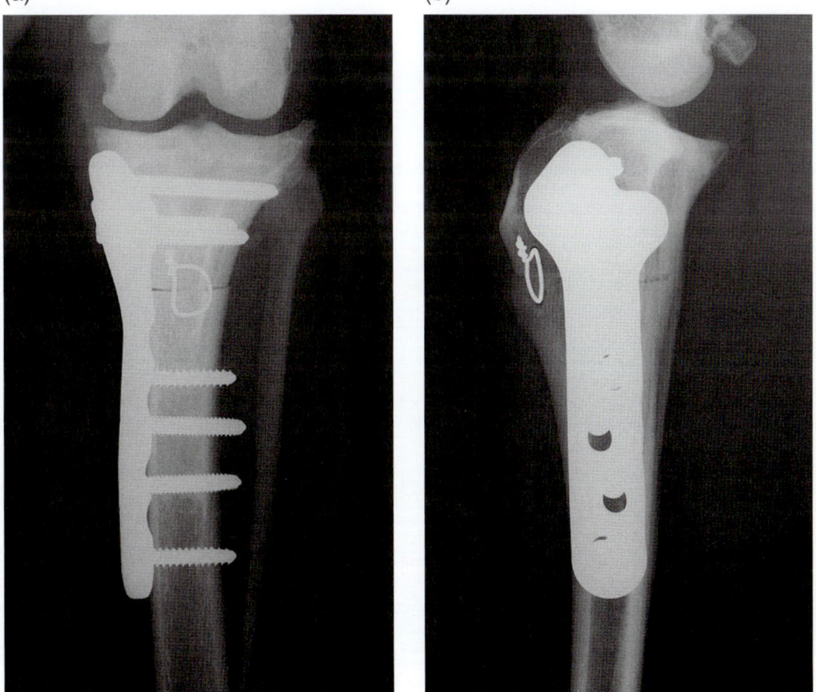

Figure 9.10 Postoperative (a) craniocaudal and (b) mediolateral projections showing optimally reduced parallel osteotomy planes. Limb alignment is normal in all planes and there are no osteotomy gaps. Note the intact caudomedial cortical hinge.

4. Parallel osteotomies/imperfect reduction.
   - Osteotomy gap.
   - Frontal plane deformity will result.
   - An example of this scenario is failure to remove the caudolateral corner of the wedge. This will prevent full lateral reduction, but the readily visible medial cortex will reduce perfectly. However, varus deformity will result.
5. Torsional malreduction.
   - May occur in combination with any of the above.

Following osteotomy reduction, the tibia should be checked for both alignment (frontal plane and torsional) and the presence of osteotomy gaps. An advantage of the use of the interfragmentary wire for reduction is that it permits the surgeon to observe the relative orientations of the medial cortices of the proximal and distal segments as the wedge progressively closes. If the orientations do not vary, an induced deformity is improbable. With experience, the expected relative cortical orientations become familiar, although a mild varus deformity can be deceptively difficult to appreciate. If in any doubt, tibial alignment should be assessed from a cranial as well as a medial perspective, and torsional alignment checked by ensuring the planes of movement of both the stifle and tarsus are sagittal. Should frontal plane deformity with no osteotomy gap be noted, it will be necessary to trim a small amount from the appropriate cortex until correct frontal plane alignment results after reduction.

Osteotomy gaps resulting from inconsistent saw orientation are generally small (1–2mm) and only partially affect reduction (Figure 9.11a,b). These are not generally of concern and typically heal uneventfully (Figure 9.11c,d). If a larger gap (>2mm) is present, the cause should be established, and limb alignment checked. If alignment is poor then the appropriate steps are taken to rectify the situation; however, if alignment is good the surgeon must decide whether to revise the osteotomy and/or reduction or to accept the presence of a gap. As with any osteosynthesis, a *cis*-cortical gap is less deleterious than a gap affecting the *trans*-cortex, although this effect is mitigated by the presence of an intact fibula. However, if in any doubt, placement of a second cranially located plate should be considered. At least one and sometimes two locking screws can be placed between the tuberosity and the osteotomy.

Figure 9.9 shows a moderate *trans*-cortical gap resulting from imperfect reduction of nonparallel osteotomies; had reduction been perfect, a valgus deformity would have been induced. Given the normal limb alignment, it is possible that intraoperatively the surgeon was unaware of this gap; however, if it had been

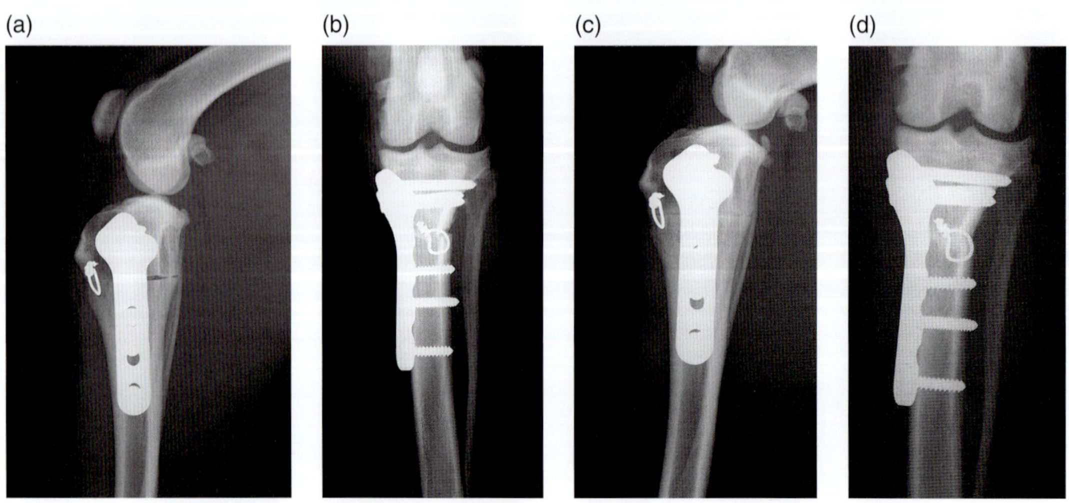

Figure 9.11 **(a,b)** Postoperative projections reveal a small lateral osteotomy gap resulting from inconsistent saw orientation during the osteotomies. **(c,d)** Clinical recovery was uneventful and follow-up radiographs after 8 weeks show unaltered segment orientation and advanced osteotomy healing.

noted, alternative options would have included revision of the distal osteotomy or application of a second plate. Inspection of the lateral osteotomy is possible from a cranial direction following limited elevation of the cranial tibial muscle; this is not routinely recommended but should be performed if reduction is not routine or if limb alignment is abnormal.

9.3.5 Plate Application

Use of a locking plate will increase the resistance of the osteosynthesis to cyclic loading [10], and its use is recommended. The anatomical shape of a TPLO plate is well suited for CCWO stabilization, and additional features such as the distal angulation of the proximal screw are also helpful. The size of the proximal CCWO segment is greater than that resulting from a radial TPLO. This permits the plate to be applied further from the joint, rendering the occurrence of intraarticular screws very rare.

Following reduction of the osteotomy and verification of appropriate tibial alignment, the plate templated during preoperative planning is applied to the cortex with an appropriate gap between the most distal screw in the proximal part of the plate and the osteotomy (Figure 9.12). If preoperative templating has been performed accurately, there will be ample space between the proximal screw and the joint, but if in doubt, especially in small dogs, a needle can be used to identify the joint margin. Ideally, plate positioning is slightly cranially biased (to more optimally resist rock-back) while remaining a safe distance caudal to the tibial tuberosity.

In some cases, a layer of firm fibrotic tissue is present adjacent to the medial metaphyseal cortex ("medial buttress"). The surface of this layer is sometimes more sharply medially angled than the precontour of the TPLO plate, and the natural response is to contour the plate further to conform to the surface. However, this action would direct the proximal screw toward the joint. Instead, resection of the fibrotic tissue beneath the plate is recommended (the optimally positioned plate can be used as a stencil to mark the area to be removed) (Figure 9.12a). Due to the slightly more distal plate position compared to radial TPLO, it is rare that additional contouring of this type is necessary

(a)

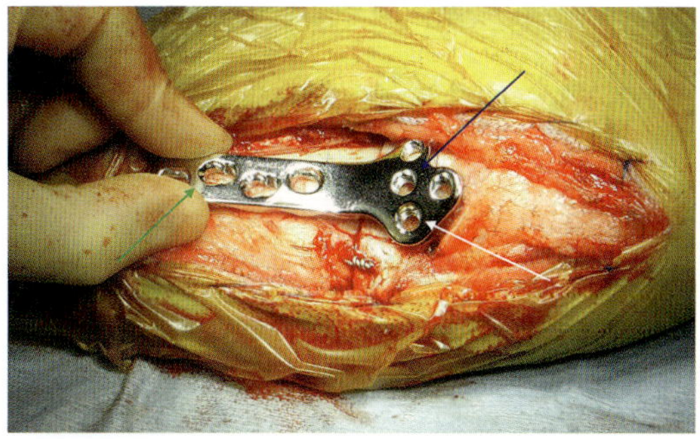

(b)

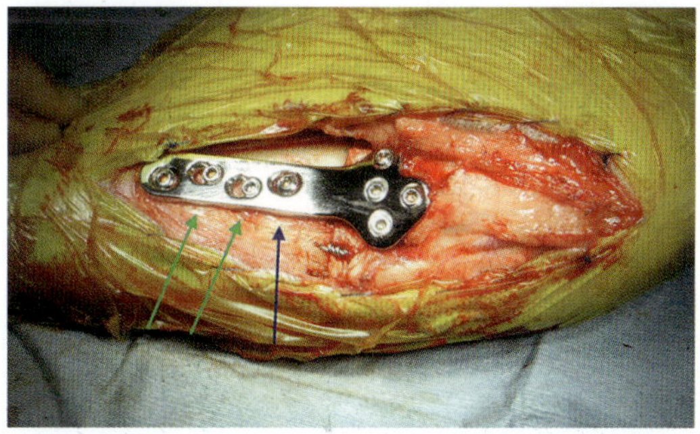

Figure 9.12 (a) A broad 3.5 mm locking TPLO plate is offered up to the cortex. In the proximal part of the plate, note the relative positions of the distal (blue arrow) and cranial (white arrow) screws to the osteotomy and tibial tuberosity respectively. The underlying medial buttress has been resected beneath the outline of the plate. Note also the slight lateral contour of the plate at the level of the distal plate hole between the surgeon's finger and thumb (green arrow). Care is taken that the distal end of the plate is positioned centrally between the cranial and caudal cortices. (b) The plate following screw placement. Note the position of the proximal cortical screw in the plate hole indicating compression (blue arrow), and the presence of two locking screws distally (green arrows).

during CCWO. However, for the same reason, a slight lateral contour at the level of the distal plate hole is optimal in nearly all cases.

Application of compression across the osteotomy is recommended. However, achieving perfect contouring of the proximal half of the plate to metaphyseal cortex is very difficult, and tightening of a cortical screw in that position could therefore cause displacement of the osteotomy segments. To minimize this risk, contouring of the distal half of the plate to the more cylindrical diaphysis is optimized, while proximally the plate is contoured to be close to but not necessarily in perfect contact with the cortex. If proximal locking screws are then first placed, followed by a compression screw distally, unwanted segment displacement will be minimal. If wished, the plate can be held in position by first placing a lightly tightened distal cortical screw in a loaded position; after proximal locking screws are placed, this screw can be fully tightened. This strategy also allows the distal part of the plate to be centered on the midline of the diaphysis before its position is fixed. Placement of at least one locking screw in the distal half of the plate is recommended to optimize resistance of the osteosynthesis to cyclic loading. Figure 9.12a shows an optimally positioned broad 3.5 mm locking TPLO plate.

Concurrent treatment of medial patellar luxation with CCWO is possible via tibial tuberosity transposition after plating. This requires careful preoperative planning of the position of the tibial tuberosity osteotomy to ensure the cranial segment is of sufficient size while leaving space for the plate more caudally (Figure 9.13). This can be challenging when the metaphysis is narrow. In such situations, some distalization of the osteotomy to permit three proximal screws in a straight plate can be considered, as can the addition of a cranial locking plate which can stabilize the main caudal segment but also in some cases the transposed tuberosity.

9.3.6 Wound Closure

The importance of good wound closure technique in the avoidance of complications is easily overlooked. Failure to close dead space can lead to persistent wound discharge or seroma formation, which in turn will predispose to infection. Failure of deep suture layers, especially the pes ancerinus/crural fascia repair, will create potentially dramatic dead-space volumes and is likely to adversely affect ultimate mechanical function.

The pes ancerinus should be sutured to the crural fascia at its cut edge on the cranial border of the tibia using a slowly dissolvable material such as polydioxanone. In some dogs, the fascia is thin and tightly adhered to the tibial cortex, offering poor suture purchase, in which case the suture is placed into fascia more laterally over the border of the cranial tibial muscle.

The subcuticular fat layer is carefully closed in one or two layers, ensuring no dead space remains, followed by the skin. A sterile adhesive dressing should be applied before sterility

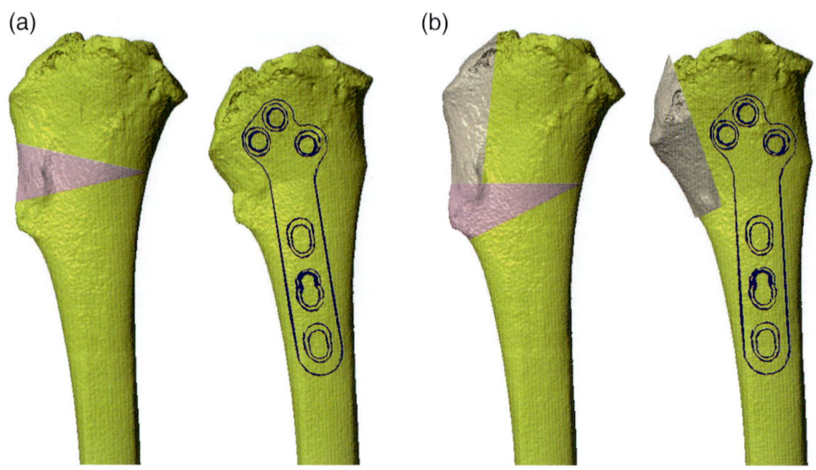

Figure 9.13 **(a)** Routine symmetrical wedge planning. The wedge is planned 10 mm distal to the tibial tuberosity. Plate positioning is slightly cranially biased on the proximal segment to more optimally resist rock-back. **(b)** Planning modifications for concurrent tibial crest transposition. The position of the wedge is moved slightly distally and, due to the taper of the bone at the base of the crest, its angle relative to the long axis of the tibia is adjusted to maintain the isosceles geometry. A further osteotomy of the tibial crest is planned to ensure that the cranial segment is of sufficient size while leaving space for the plate caudally. The tibial crest is stabilized routinely using pins and tension band wire, or in some cases a cranially applied plate can be used.

is broken, and maintained for 48 hours. It is the author's preference not to apply additional dressings, although if wished a padded bandage may be applied for 12–48 hours.

9.4 Postoperative Complications

At the time of discharge, clients should be advised verbally and in writing of signs suggestive of the occurrence of a complication, and the importance of prompt reporting and, if necessary, re-presentation of the dog discussed.

In general, early complications (within the first 2 weeks) are more likely to be less severe and include minor wound problems (e.g., self-trauma and suture loosening) and seroma. More severe complications have a peak incidence at approximately 3–4 weeks following surgery, although at any point a history of suddenly increased lameness should prompt reassessment.

9.4.1 Acute Nonspecific Arthritis

Acute nonspecific arthritis is a presumptive diagnosis of exclusion made when investigations of recurrent lameness fail to yield a diagnosis, and when lameness subsequently improves over a period of a week or so. This most commonly occurs at 2–4 weeks following surgery, often secondary to sudden increases in permitted exercise as owners perceive lameness to be improving.

Unfortunately, the degree of lameness in such cases can be quite marked and cannot always be reliably differentiated from a more severe complication on the basis of clinical assessment alone. A period of reduced exercise may be attempted but given the potential differential diagnoses such as infection where prompt intervention is optimal, many owners will opt for early investigation. Typically, synoviocentesis and radiography are recommended, with arthroscopy considered for meniscal assessment if lameness fails to improve.

9.4.2 Late Meniscal Injury

The rate of clinically significant late meniscal injury following CCWO is not precisely known but is probably around 5% [7]. These cases can present at any time following surgery, and with variable signs ranging from acute marked recurrent lameness to a slight intermittent limp or suboptimal return to function. Diagnosis is by initial exclusion of other complications followed typically by arthroscopy or arthrotomy. The prognosis is very good following debridement of the torn portion of the meniscus. Further discussion regarding the meniscus can be found in Chapter 18.

9.4.3 Infection

Surgical site infections involve the joint itself, the bone, or both, and occur at a rate of approximately 5% [7]. Some such infections resolve with extended oral antibiotic therapy, but a proportion require surgical intervention. Surgical site infections are discussed in detail in Chapters 2 and 3.

9.4.4 Fractures

Fractures of the tibia, fibula, and patella are rare following CCWO. The large proximal osteotomy segment without isolation of the tibial tuberosity probably explains the low rate of tuberosity fractures compared to radial TPLO. Despite this, care should be taken not to position the cranial plate screw immediately adjacent to the tuberosity as this could provide a stress riser promoting fracture.

The cause of the very low rate of fibular fracture is unknown but may be related to the differing effects of radial TPLO and CCWO on the tibial anatomical axis. If the tibia is assumed to have a sagittal plane center of rotation of angulation (CORA) located somewhere in the metaphysis, the dome osteotomy of a radial TPLO centered over the intercondylar eminence will cause a caudal shift in the anatomical axis of the proximal segment compared to the distal segment, potentially inducing a shear force and greater loading in the fibula. By contrast, the CCWO osteotomy position is approximated to the CORA and axis translation does not occur (Figure 9.14).

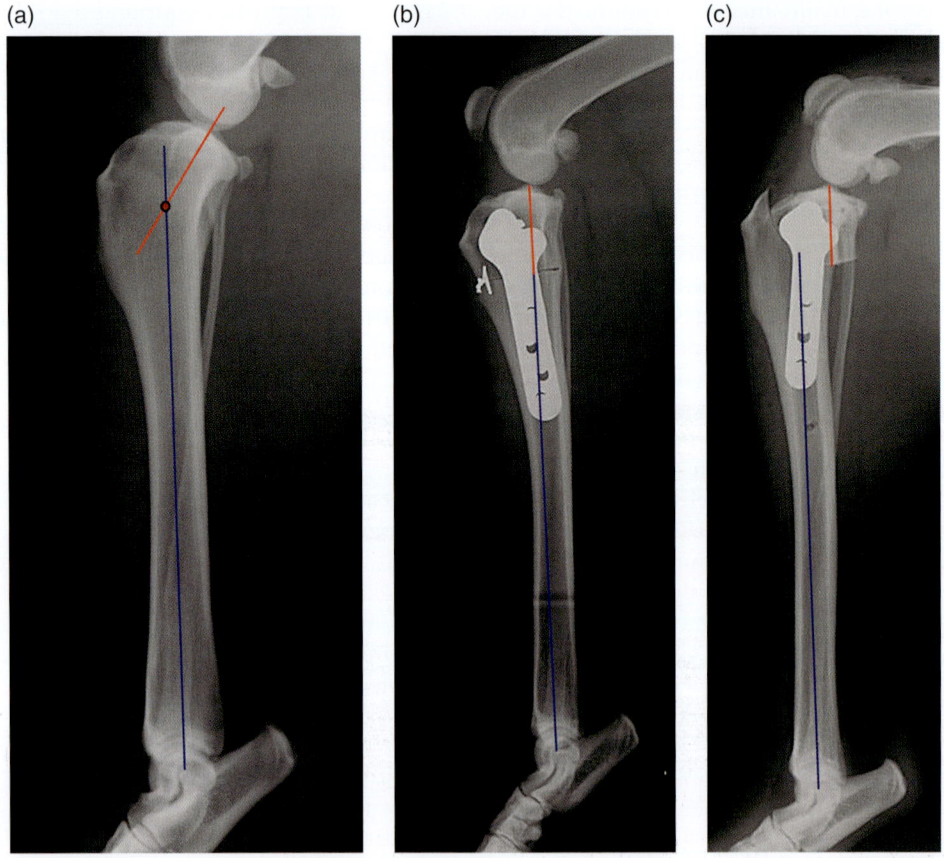

Figure 9.14 (a) In the context of tibial plateau leveling, sagittal plane anatomical axes suggest a proximal metaphyseal CORA location. (b) When CCWO is performed, the angulation correction axis (ACA) and osteotomy position are close to the CORA and the proximal and distal anatomical axes align. (c) When radial TPLO is performed, the ACA is located over the intercondylar eminence and is therefore distant to the CORA. The proximal and distal anatomical axes become coplanar but with caudal translation of the proximal segment. The proximal fibula must displace caudally with the proximal tibial segment; note the more caudal fibular position compared to the CCWO projection. This necessitates rotation at the proximal tibiofibular joint, may induce a shear force within the fibula, and may expose the fibula to greater loading, all factors which may increase the risk of fracture.

9.4.5 Implant Failure

The most common manifestation of implant failure following CCWO is "rock-back" of the proximal segment. This refers to loss of reduction of the osteotomy due to caudal tilting of the proximal osteotomy segment (Figure 9.15a). Any indication of loss of reduction of the osteotomy suggests fixation failure and will necessitate surgical revision; delaying intervention in the hope that healing will progress, even if the patient is partially weight bearing, is usually futile.

Revision should comprise implant removal, restoration of appropriate reduction of the osteotomy, and placement of a new medial plate (Figure 9.15b). Typically, some degree of debridement of callus is necessary, although further osteotomies are rarely needed. Bone graft may be applied at the surgeon's discretion. Placement of a second plate cranially or craniomedially may also be considered.

Occasionally, radiographs will reveal reduced radiopacity at the osteotomy site but without loss of reduction (Figure 9.16). This may occur for several reasons including thermal necrosis or a high strain environment in a very small osteotomy gap but may also be an indication of early implant failure and instability. This situation is typically characterized as delayed union, and these cases may progress to union but should be monitored closely and revised promptly should loss of reduction occur.

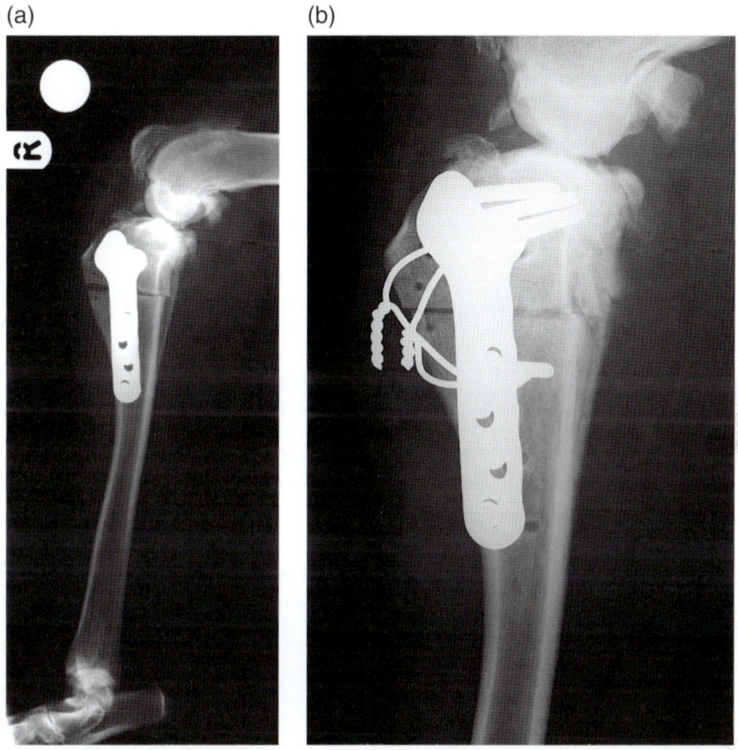

Figure 9.15 (a) "Rock-back" following CCWO describes loss of reduction of the osteotomy with caudal tilting of the proximal segment. (b) The original implant has been removed, the osteotomy reduced, and a new plate applied more proximally, avoiding the original screw holes. Application of a second plate should have been considered.

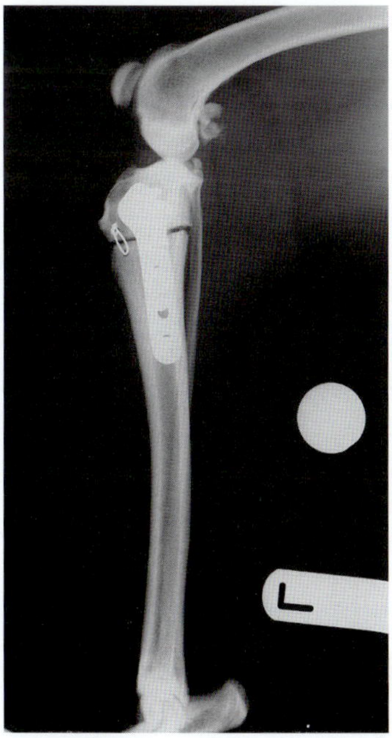

Figure 9.16 Reduced radiopacity at the osteotomy site without loss of reduction.

9.4.6 Patellar Instability/Luxation

Medial or lateral patellar instability is a rare but serious complication of CCWO, with no cases in the 173 dogs for which outcomes of modified CCWO have been reported [7–9, 12]. The two most common causes are alteration in the line of action of the quadriceps mechanism (usually due to torsional malreduction of the osteotomy) or persistent internal tibial rotation, although in some cases no obvious predisposing factor can be identified.

Optimal treatment will depend on the cause, and whether associated additional problems are present such as pivot shift in the case of persistent tibial rotation, or clinically significant gait abnormality if torsional deformity has been induced. In these scenarios, placement of a lateral retinacular suture, or osteotomy revision, may be considered, although in the majority of cases tibial tuberosity transposition is performed. Since the osteotomy passes through the tibial crest, tibial crest transposition must be delayed until radiographic healing is confirmed, typically at least 8 weeks after surgery. Due to the risk of fracture at the original osteotomy site, plate removal is not recommended for at least 6 months (ideally a year); if the plate will impede the tibial crest osteotomy, it should be replaced by a new plate applied more caudally.

9.4.7 Pivot Shift

Pivot shift seems to be rare following CCWO, with four cases reported in a single paper [9], giving a cumulative incidence of 2.3% [7–9, 12]. Pivot shift probably occurs for the same reason postulated for radial TPLO – failure of the technique to address the rotational component of the instability resulting from cranial cruciate ligament deficiency. Conservative management may be appropriate [9] or if necessary, placement of a lateral retinacular suture could be considered.

References

1. Slocum, B. and Devine, T. (1984). Cranial tibial wedge osteotomy: a technique for eliminating cranial tibial thrust in cranial cruciate ligament repair. *J. Am. Vet. Med. Assoc.* 184 (5): 564–569.
2. Slocum, B. and Slocum, T.D. (1993). Tibial plateau leveling osteotomy for repair of cranial cruciate ligament rupture in the canine. *Vet. Clin. North Am. Small Anim. Pract.* 23 (4): 777–795.
3. Fitzpatrick, N. and Solano, M.A. (2010). Predictive variables for complications after TPLO with stifle inspection by arthrotomy in 1000 consecutive dogs. *Vet. Surg.* 39 (4): 460–474.
4. Gatineau, M., Dupuis, J., Plante, J., and Moreau, M. (2011). Retrospective study of 476 tibial plateau levelling osteotomy procedures. Rate of subsequent 'pivot shift', meniscal tear and other complications. *Vet. Comp. Orthop. Traumatol.* 24 (5): 333–341.
5. Corr, S.A. and Brown, C. (2007). A comparison of outcomes following tibial plateau levelling osteotomy and cranial tibial wedge osteotomy procedures. *Vet. Comp. Orthop. Traumatol.* 20 (4): 312–319.
6. Kuan, S., Smith, B., and Black, A. (2009). Tibial wedge ostectomy: complications of 300 surgical procedures. *Aust. Vet. J.* 87 (11): 438–444.
7. Oxley, B., Gemmill, T.J., Renwick, A.R. et al. (2013). Comparison of complication rates and clinical outcome between tibial plateau leveling osteotomy and a modified cranial closing wedge osteotomy for treatment of cranial cruciate ligament disease in dogs. *Vet. Surg.* 42 (6): 739–750.
8. Frederick, S.W. and Cross, A.R. (2017). Modified cranial closing wedge osteotomy for treatment of cranial cruciate ligament insufficiency in dogs with excessive tibial plateau angles: technique and complications in 19 cases. *Vet. Surg.* 46 (3): 403–411.
9. Campbell, K.A., Payne, J.T., Doornink, M.T., and Haggerty, J. (2016). Outcome of tibial closing wedge osteotomy in 55 cranial cruciate ligament-deficient stifles of small dogs (<15 kg). *Vet. Surg.* 45 (8): 1056–1062.
10. Apelt, D., Pozzi, A., Marcellin-Little, D.J., and Kowaleski, M.P. (2010). Effect of cranial tibial closing wedge angle on tibial subluxation: an ex vivo study. *Vet. Surg.* 39 (4): 454–459.
11. Wallace, A.M., Addison, E.S., Smith, B.A. et al. (2011). Modification of the cranial closing wedge ostectomy technique for the treatment of canine cruciate disease. Description and comparison with standard technique. *Vet. Comp. Orthop. Traumatol.* 24 (6): 457–462.
12. Christ, J.P., Anderson, J.R., and Youk, A.O. (2018). Modified cranial closing wedge ostectomy in 25 dogs. *Vet. Surg.* 47 (5): 683–691.
13. Talaat, M.B., Kowaleski, M.P., and Boudrieau, R.J. (2006). Combination tibial plateau leveling osteotomy and cranial closing wedge osteotomy of the tibia for the treatment of cranial cruciate ligament-deficient stifles with excessive tibial plateau angle. *Vet. Surg.* 35 (8): 729–739.
14. Schmierer, P.A., Smolders, L.A., Zderic, I. et al. (2019). Biomechanical properties of plate constructs for feline ilial fracture gap stabilization. *Vet. Surg.* 48 (1): 88–95.
15. Gallagher, A.D. and Mertens, W.D. (2012). Implant removal rate from infection after tibial plateau leveling osteotomy in dogs. *Vet. Surg.* 41: 705–711.
16. Zuckerman, J.S., Dyce, J., Arruda, A.G. et al. (2018). Fibular osteotomy to facilitate proximal tibial rotation during tibial plateau leveling osteotomy. *Vet. Surg.* 47 (7): 923–931.
17. Shamir, S.K., Wolynski, J.G., Duncan, C.G. et al. (2019). ex vivo evaluation of a novel surgical guide on the accuracy of closing wedge osteotomies. *Vet. Surg.* 48 (8): 1429–1436.

10 Complications Associated with Tibial Plateau Leveling Osteotomy

Ron Ben-Amotz and Joshua S. Zuckerman

10.1 Introduction

Cranial cruciate ligament (CCL) rupture is the most common cause of pelvic limb lameness in dogs. Although numerous surgical techniques have been described to address this condition, the tibial plateau leveling osteotomy (TPLO) remains one of the most commonly performed among both board-certified and non board-certified surgeons [1–3]. TPLO was first described by Slocum in 1983 as a modification of the cranial closing wedge osteotomy (CCWO), and the theory behind the procedure has since been further evaluated in numerous cadaveric studies [4–6]. These studies tried to justify and confirm the theory that use of a radial osteotomy to level the plateau (to an angle of approximately 6.5°) neutralizes cranial tibial thrust, thus restoring stifle stability in the stance phase [7–9]. More recent studies, however, have found that about 30% of postoperative TPLOs continue to exhibit some degree of cranial tibial subluxation during the stance phase [10, 11].

10.2 Literature Review of Complications

Over the last four decades, many studies have reported the clinical outcome of patients following TPLO, with reported complication rates ranging from 9.7% to 39% [12–17].

Incisional complications, tibial tuberosity fractures, and implant failure were the most commonly reported complications after TPLO surgery [14, 16]. Swelling, bruising, and seroma formation may occur in the short or intermediate time period after surgery. Although these may not typically be considered major complications, they carry the potential for significant patient morbidity such as pain and lameness. Meticulous soft tissue handling and dead-space closure (Halsted's principles) will reduce their occurrence. Tibial diaphyseal fractures, avulsion fractures of the tibial tuberosity, patellar fracture, fibular fracture, and patella luxation are categorized as bony related complications [18–21]. Other reported complications are categorized as implant related, including intraarticular placement of a jig pin, K-wire, or screw that can cause damage to the articular cartilage. Implants may also fail (bend, break, loosen) which can result in significant loss of limb function [12, 13]. Therefore, their immediate identification and prompt treatment are of utmost importance. Careful surgical planning, accurate execution of the surgical procedure, and increased surgeon experience will reduce the incidence of complications.

Complications in Canine Cranial Cruciate Ligament Surgery, First Edition. Edited by Ron Ben-Amotz and David L. Dycus.

10.3 Complications Specific to Tibial Plateau Leveling Osteotomy: Tips to Minimize Complications

The purpose of this chapter is to provide a comprehensive review of the reported complications and to provide the reader with a stepwise approach to prevention, early recognition, and treatment of these complications. The complications discussed will be divided into the timeframes in which they are most likely to occur: the preoperative, intraoperative, and both immediate (<14 days) and delayed (>14 days) postoperative periods.

10.3.1 Preoperative: Radiographic Positioning

High-quality, well-positioned mediolateral and craniocaudal radiographs are necessary for thorough surgical planning [22]. These films should include the distal third of the femur, the stifle joint, and the tarsus to ensure appropriate positioning. To facilitate accurate positioning and mitigate the potential for motion artifacts, we strongly recommend that films are obtained with the patient under heavy sedation or a short general anesthetic protocol. We also strongly recommend use of a calibration marker placed adjacent to the tibia to ensure the accuracy of digital measurements [23].

To position the limb for the mediolateral (sagittal) radiograph, the tibia should be parallel to the beam/cassette, with both the stifle and tarsus flexed to 90° angles. During positioning, it is imperative to ensure that neither the femur nor tibia is rotated. In order to minimize projection artifact, the beam should be centered over the stifle joint. Provided there is no deformity present, both the tibial and femoral condyles should appear perfectly superimposed (Figure 10.1a). An appropriately positioned mediolateral radiograph allows not only for accurate measurement of the tibial plateau angle (TPA), but also for assessment of distal femoral deformities (both varus/valgus and rotational). It should also be used to determine an approximation of the appropriate radial saw blade to be used and for determining the location of the anticipated osteotomy. When digital radiography is used, additional software applications may be used to quantify the magnitude of the required tibial plateau rotation, and to determine whether this rotation will exceed the accepted "safe point" (the insertion point of the patellar tendon). Often, these software applications include templates of various TPLO plates, allowing the surgeon to preemptively determine the most appropriate implant size and the approximate location of the implant relative to the planned osteotomy (Figure 10.1b).

When the limb is positioned for a radiograph in the craniocaudal (frontal) plane, the stifle joint should be extended and the tibia should again be held parallel to the beam/cassette with care taken to avoid internal or external rotation. In a well-positioned film, the proximal aspect of the calcaneus should be observed bisecting the medial cortex of the distal tibia and the fabellae should be centered over the lateral and medial femoral condyles. Radiographs in this plane allow for identification and quantification of any angular or rotational deformities that may be present, as well as for identification of the location of the fibular head relative to the proximal tibia, which may be used as an intraoperative reference point to aid in screw placement and avoidance of articular penetration (Figure 10.1c).

10.3.2 Intraoperative

Overall, many of the reported intraoperative complications are the result of technical error. The authors believe that with surgeon experience, careful preoperative planning, and careful attention to procedural execution, many of these complications can be mitigated.

10.3.2.1 Surgical Approach (Recognition and Avoidance of Important Anatomical Structures)

As is the case with any surgical procedure, the potential for soft tissue complications (bruising, hematoma, seroma formation) may be minimized by careful attention to Halsted's principles, with particular attention given to gentle tissue handling.

During the initial approach, the saphenous neuromuscular bundle should be identified and

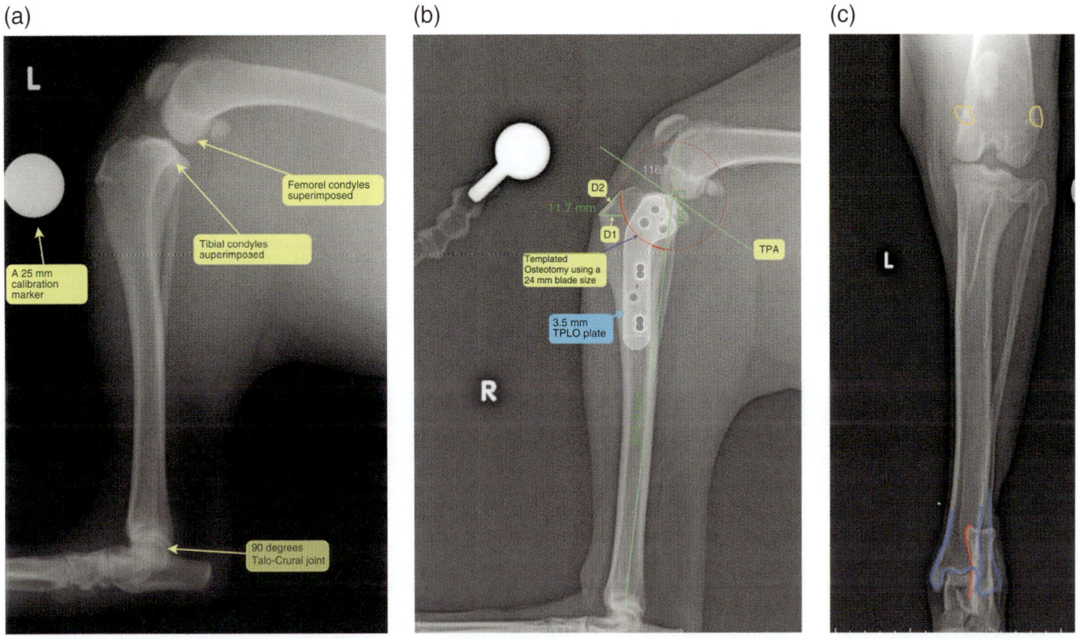

Figure 10.1 (a) Appropriate limb positioning for a radiograph in the mediolateral (sagittal) plane. The stifle joint and the tarsocrural joint are flexed to a 90° angle and the tibia is positioned parallel to the cassette. Both the tibial and femoral condyles (medial and lateral) are superimposed. In dogs with femoral or tibial angular or torsional deformities, this usually cannot be accomplished. In this image, a ball marker has been used for calibration purposes. (b) The mediolateral projection is used for accurate measuring of the tibial plateau angle (TPA), determination of the appropriate saw blade size, plate size, and for the determination of the D1/D2 reference lines. Source: vPOP-pro, VetSOS Education Ltd, veterinary preoperative orthopedic planning software. (c) Limb positioning for a radiograph in the craniocaudal (frontal) plane. The proximal and medial aspects of the calcaneus should be observed bisecting the distal tibial cortices and the fabellae should be centered over the lateral and medial femoral condyles.

preserved (Figure 10.2). This is especially important when TPLO is performed in small patients, in which case this structure may be found in a more superficial position and closer to the intended incision than anticipated. As the approach to the tibia continues, one must be meticulous in elevation of the aponeurosis attachments of the caudal part of the sartorius, semitendinosus, and gracilis muscles (Figure 10.2b,c) which will allow for robust soft tissue closure and therefore implant coverage, ultimately aiding in the reduction of soft tissue complications in the immediate postoperative period. During elevation of the muscle, it is imperative to identify the medial collateral ligament that lies deep to it at the caudomedial aspect of the proximal tibia. In some dogs, this structure may be obscured by a thin layer of fascia/fat that can be carefully removed with a gauze sponge in a gentle rubbing motion (Figure 10.2d).

Next, the popliteus muscle should be partially elevated from the caudal aspect of the proximal tibia using a large periosteal elevator. In order to minimize muscle trauma and bleeding, the author (RBA) recommends elevating the muscle along with its associated fascia (Figure 10.2e). Care must be taken to ensure the periosteal elevator maintains contact with the caudal cortex of the tibia during elevation, as deviation into the caudal or lateral soft tissue may result in significant hemorrhage (discussed later).

10.3.2.2 Osteotomy Planning

Calibrated preoperative radiographs are necessary to accurately determine the required plate size and for determining the appropriate location of the osteotomy [24]. Templated radiographs allow the surgeon to define D1, D2, and

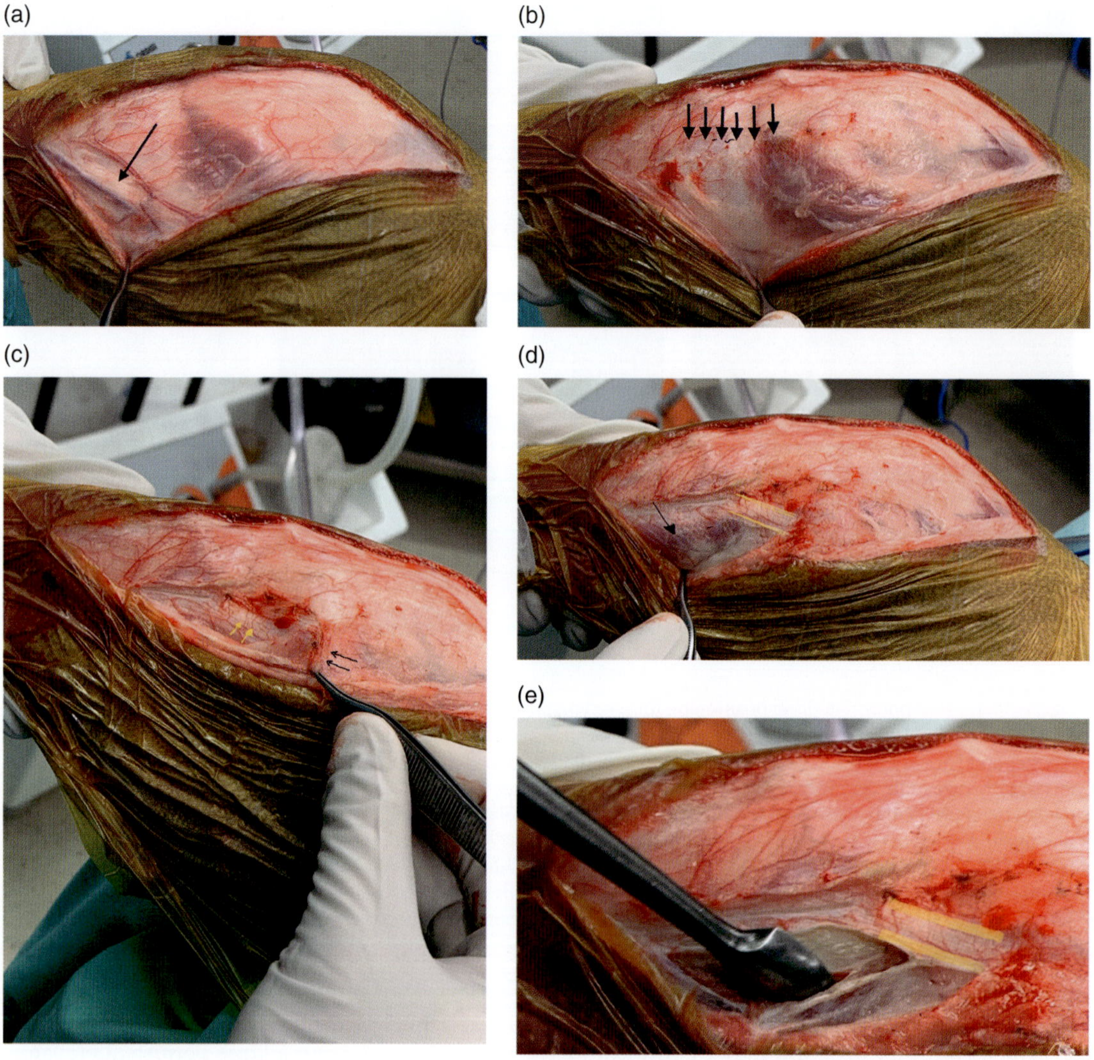

Figure 10.2 (a) The saphenous neurovascular bundle (black arrow). (b) Identification of the aponeurosis of the semitendinosus, gracilis, and caudal part of the sartorius muscles. The black arrows indicate the location of the aponeurosis incision. The incision should commence distal to the aponeurosis attachment directly over the tibial diaphysis and continue proximally while remaining as close to the bone as possible to prevent muscle laceration. (c) Elevation of the muscular aponeurosis attachment to the proximal medial tibia. The black arrows indicate caudal reflection of the aponeurosis. Yellow arrows: medial collateral ligament. (d) Note the location of the medial collateral ligament (outlined in yellow) and the popliteus muscle (black arrow, cranial to the forceps). (e) Popliteus muscle elevation using a periosteal elevator. Note that the fascia is elevated along with the muscle. The medial collateral ligament is bordered by yellow lines.

the size of the blade required to achieve the planned osteotomy based on these measurements [25–27]. Due to the somewhat variable morphology of the proximal tibia in dogs, it is important to confirm the accuracy of the preplanned measurements intraoperatively before performing the cut, ensuring the planned osteotomy line will not only intersect D1 and D2 but will also result in a cut that exits the caudal cortex of the tibia at a 90° angle.

In order to identify the point of origin of D1, the insertion point of the patellar tendon on the proximal tibia (Sharpey's fibers) must be carefully identified. In order to identify D2, an incision is made caudal to the medial edge of the patellar tendon just proximal to its attachment

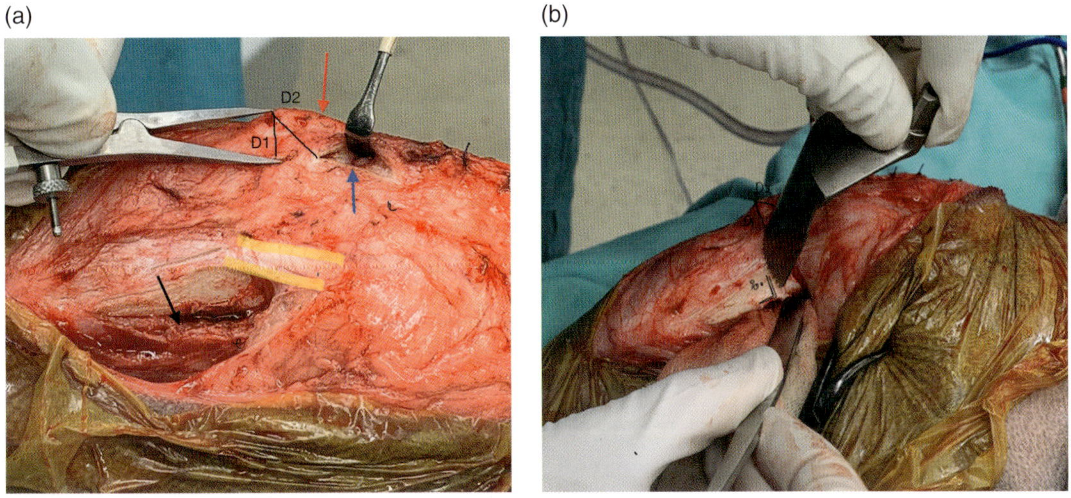

Figure 10.3 (a) To mark D1, the caliper is placed with one arm at the insertion point of the patellar tendon (Sharpey's fibers) and opened to the premeasured D1 value on the preoperative radiographs. For D2, the infrapatellar bursa (blue arrow) is opened, taking care to protect the patellar tendon (red arrow) by cranial retraction with a Senn–Miller retractor. The caliper arm is then extended to mark D2. The medial collateral ligament and the popliteus muscle are marked with yellow lines and a black arrow respectively. (b) Once D1 and D2 are marked, the appropriate size TPLO blade is selected. Care is taken to identify its exit point at a 90° angle to the caudomedial tibial cortex. In this image, a gauze sponge has been carefully packed between the elevated popliteus muscle and the caudal tibial cortex in order to decrease the risk of iatrogenic trauma to the cranial tibial artery (the distal continuation of the popliteal artery) during the osteotomy.

on the tibia, exposing the infrapatellar bursa (this also allows further cranial retraction of the patellar tendon, therefore decreasing the risk of iatrogenic trauma as the osteotomy is performed. The D2 point is then marked (Figure 10.3a). The blade may then be positioned so that it intersects both D1 and D2, allowing the surgeon to visualize the planned osteotomy. The blade should exit the caudal cortex at 90° (Figure 10.3b).

10.3.2.3 Thermal Necrosis

Thermal necrosis may result in delayed healing and bone necrosis, and increases the risk of infection [27]. It is imperative to use copious lavage during any portion of the procedure in which significant heat may be generated at the bone–metal interface, including the osteotomy procedure, application of both the rotational and antirotational pins, and as screw holes are drilled.

10.3.2.4 Hemorrhage (Laceration of the Cranial Tibial Artery)

Hemorrhage resulting from iatrogenic trauma to the cranial tibial artery has been reported (Figure 10.4) [28–30]. Despite some disagreement

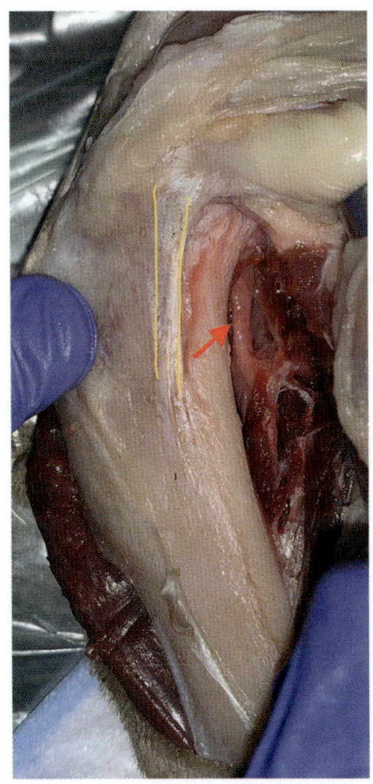

Figure 10.4 In this cadaveric image, one can identify the popliteal artery located at the caudolateral border of the tibia (red arrow) at the level of the stifle joint. The cranial tibial artery is located at the caudolateral border of the tibia distal to the joint. Yellow lines mark the medial collateral ligament.

among surgeons, the risk of arterial laceration is likely decreased by placing a radiopaque gauze sponge between the tibia and the elevated cranial tibial muscle laterally and the elevated popliteus muscle caudally [31, 32]. After the osteotomy has been completed, the sponges must be removed and the sites copiously lavaged with sterile saline to reduce retention of microscopic cotton particulate debris in the surgical site [12].

If mild hemorrhage is identified once the sponge has been removed, packing the site with an epinephrine-impregnated sponge or use of another hemostatic agent such as Gelfoam® should result in cessation of the bleeding. More significant hemorrhage may require the use of hemoclips or suture. Identification of the lacerated artery may require further elevation and/or caudal retraction of the popliteus muscle combined with distraction of the osteotomy site. If this is ineffective, a lateral approach to the proximal tibia may be necessary to facilitate identification and control of hemorrhage at its source.

10.3.2.5 Patellar Tendon Laceration

In order to minimize this catastrophic complication, the author (RBA) uses blade and implant templates on preoperative radiographs (Figure 10.1b) to ensure the appropriate blade size is selected. If specialized templating software is not available, one can draw a circle (found in the menu of most commonly used digital radiography programs) at the site of the planned osteotomy on the mediolateral radiograph. The radius of the circle should correspond with available blade sizes, and the circle should be centered on the intercondylar eminences of the proximal tibia. Once placed, the proximal "exit point" of the circle should be identified and used to confirm it does not intersect with the patellar tendon (Figure 10.1b). In surgery, the proximal exit point of the osteotomy (D2) is identified following elevation of the infrapatellar bursa (Figure 10.3a). It is imperative to use a Senn retractor to retract the tendon cranially (away from the blade) as the cut is performed (Figure 10.3a). The surgical assistant should immediately make the surgeon aware of any "metal on metal" sounds or vibration of the Senn as this may indicate that the blade is at risk of coming into contact with the patellar tendon.

10.3.2.6 Rotational and Antirotational Pin Placement

A 3.2 mm (1/8 inch) pin (or smaller for small-breed dogs) should be placed just caudal and proximal to the osteotomy in the proximal tibial segment. To further identify the appropriate placement site, a small depression in the bone just proximal to the osteotomy is palpated. The orientation of pin placement is from proximal and cranial to distal and caudal at an approximately 30–40° oblique angle (Figure 10.5a).

A 1.6 mm (0.062 inch) Kirshner wire (or smaller for small-breed dogs) is placed adjacent to the patellar tendon attachment line (Sharpey's fibers) in the midpoint of the tibial crest in the frontal plane (Figure 10.5b). This will reduce the incidence of postoperative fracture of the tibial tuberosity [18]. All soft tissues are protected with a drill guide while the pin is advanced. The pin should be directed toward the caudal cortex proximal to the osteotomy line and distal to the joint surface. Placement of a 25 G needle into the distal aspect of the stifle joint is an effective and minimally invasive method for outlining the border of the joint (Figure 10.5c). Care should be taken to avoid completely advancing the needle into the joint in order to minimize the risk for iatrogenic meniscal damage.

Once the plate is placed (with at least four cortices engaged in each bone segment), the K-wire can be removed. It is important to evaluate the integrity of the pin once removed in order to assess for any implant breakage. If this occurs, further caudal retraction of the popliteus muscle will allow inspection to determine if the remnant of the pin is present exiting the caudal tibia. If present, it may be removed with a large needle driver and manual traction. If the tip cannot be found, it is likely that it is completely embedded within the bone and its retrieval is not critical. It is imperative to use copious lavage during placement of both the rotational and antirotational pins.

10.3.2.7 Broken Drill Bits

Careful angulation of drill bits is necessary to avoid interference with other screws and the antirotational pin. This can be mitigated when locking plates are used, as the screw plate angle is predetermined. If a broken bit or pin is

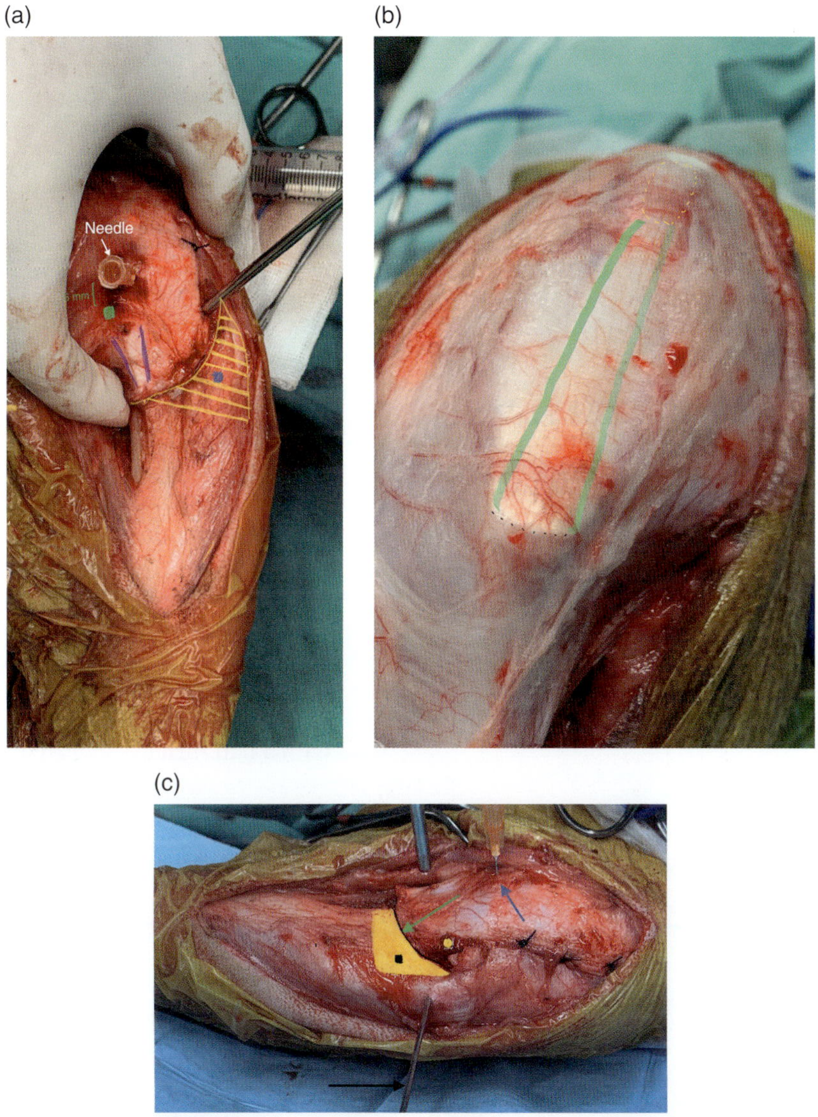

Figure 10.5 (a) Identification of the insertion point for rotational pin placement. The rotational pin is placed at a 30–40° angle in the proximal tibial segment directed from cranio-proximal to caudo-distal. The pin should slightly penetrate the caudal cortex of the proximal tibial segment. The exit point may be identified with an index finger, taking care to avoid laceration of the glove during pin placement. For joint identification, a 25 G needle is "walked" proximally along the cranial border of the medial collateral until it is felt "dropping" into the joint. Care is taken to avoid introducing the entire needle into the joint as this can result in iatrogenic meniscal laceration. The green box represents the location of the entry point of the proximal jig pin. The jig pin is placed 5 mm distal to the articular surface (using the needle as a reference point) and caudal to the medial collateral ligament. The hatched yellow area represents a trapezoidal tibial crest. The light blue box represents the site for antirotational suture placement in case of identification of pivot shift. The medial collateral ligament is bordered by purple lines. (b) Identification of Sharpey's fibers (black dotted line). This should be identified as a transverse tissue line that delineates the transition from the patellar tendon (bordered in green lines) to bone at the insertion point. (c) The osteotomy line (green arrow, black line), needle placement for joint identification (blue arrow), Sharpey's fibers, and location of the holding pin (black arrow). Note the trapezoidal shape of the tibia below the osteotomy line (yellow color), bordered by the osteotomy, patellar tendon insertion, and the tibial crest. The black box indicates the antirotational suture placement site. The small yellow circle indicates a previously placed antirotational pin.

present within the bone, it is generally possible to bypass it with slight redirection of the drill or screw. In most cases, broken drill bits that are well seated within the bone will not result in patient morbidity, and therefore their retrieval is not necessary. However, a broken bit or pin that extends out of the bone carries the risk for soft tissue irritation that may result in morbidity, pain, and even further implant migration. Therefore, in these cases, we recommend that the offending implant be removed.

Further elevation of the cranial tibial muscle on the lateral tibial surface can assist in identification of the exposed drill bit. A hand chuck can then be used to firmly secure and remove the broken tip.

10.3.2.8 Complications of Implant Positioning

Inappropriate implant placement carries inherent risks. Common examples of inappropriate plate and screw application during TPLO include the following.

10.3.2.8.1 Inadequate Number of Cortices Engaged/Fissuring of the Trans Cortex During Screw Placement

Nonlocking screws that fail to penetrate the far (trans) cortex will result in less robust fixation both below and above the osteotomy line [33–35]. In order to achieve bicortical purchase, it is advised to add 2 mm of screw length to the measured depth of the drill hole when selecting the screw for placement.

Fissure or fracture of the trans cortex as screws engage the bone can result in delayed healing and, in rare cases, even implant failure (Figure 10.6). In one paper, the incidence of transcortical fractures was higher when self-tapping screws were used compared to non self-tapping screws placed after the drill hole was tapped manually. It was speculated that the flute of the tap used for non self-tapping screws is longer than the flute of a self-tapping screw [32]. When a self-tapping screw is used, before engaging the far (trans) cortex, it is advised to advance the screw in small movements (alternating a quarter turn counterclockwise with a half turn clockwise) until the screw

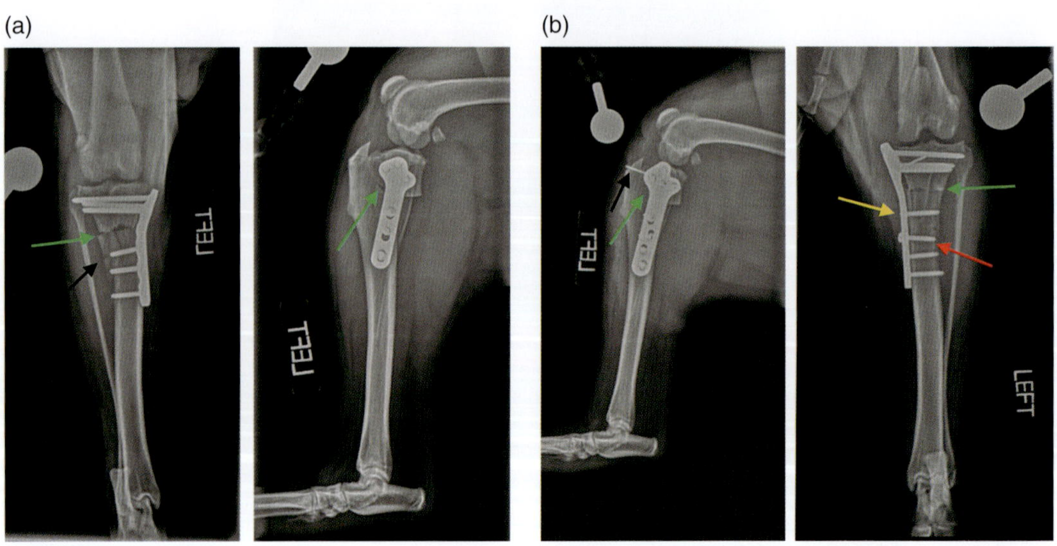

Figure 10.6 **(a)** Postoperative TPLO using a six-hole Synthes locking plate. The black arrow indicates a large medial and caudal cortical fragment noted once the screw was engaged into the trans cortex. The green arrow marks the loss of reduction at the osteotomy. **(b)** An 0.062 K-wire was placed adjacent to Sharpey's fibers and into the proximal tibial segment before the plate was removed to aid in reduction (black arrow). The plate was removed. The fragment was stabilized using point-to-point reduction forceps. A 3.5 broad locking Synthes plate was then applied. Notice that the first screw distal to the osteotomy was placed in lag fashion (yellow arrow), thus reducing the fragment into place. The second screw distal to the osteotomy is directed in a craniodistal direction to avoid the previously drilled screw hole (red arrow). The antirotational pin was left in place. The osteotomy gap has been reduced (green arrow). Source: All images courtesy of Dr. Brian Beale.

is seated in the far cortex. This technique will help minimize an abrupt "push" of the screw into the far cortex, therefore decreasing the risk of cortical fissuring or even fracturing.

If an audible crack is heard as the screw is engaged, the screw should be removed and a lateral approach to the tibia should be performed to aid in the identification of any potential fissures that have resulted. If a fissure is present, the plate should be removed and a cerclage wire applied (using standard cerclage wire application technique and principles). If the screw placement has resulted in a fracture and the fragment is of a large size, it is advised to repair the fragment with a screw placed in lag fashion (either through the plate (Figure 10.6b) or independent from the plate). Any other screws placed through the plate should then be directed away from the fracture site to avoid further displacement. If In most cases, if the fragment is small, simply redirecting the screw away from the fragment is sufficient.

10.3.2.8.2 Screws That Penetrate the Osteotomy Line Might Interfere with Osteotomy Healing

The effects of placement of a screw through a fracture have been reported. These include an increased risk of delayed and nonunion of the fracture site [36]. When there is any suspicion that a screw has been placed through the osteotomy line, the surgeon should remove the screw and redirect it. In cases where this is identified during postoperative radiographic evaluation, it is advised that the patient be returned to surgery and the offending screw redirected. In Figure 10.7a, double plating was used after a TPLO was performed (>70 kg dog). In the postoperative

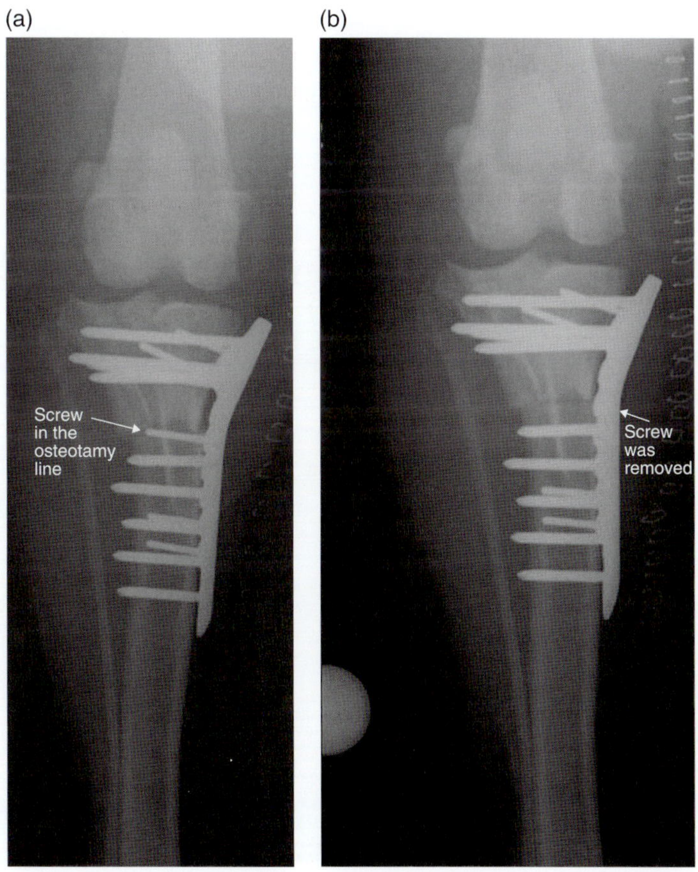

Figure 10.7 (a) Postoperative craniocaudal radiographs in which a screw is noted penetrating the osteotomy line (white arrow). (b) In order to minimize potential osteotomy healing complications, the screw was removed via a small incision directly over the screw head (white arrow).

radiographs, one screw was identified in the osteotomy line; therefore, it was removed as there were a sufficient number of screws to achieve biomechanical stability (Figure 10.7b).

10.3.2.8.3 Screws That Penetrate the Joint

Precontoured locking TPLO plates are designed with a slight angulation at the neck of the plate to account for the natural contour of the proximomedial tibia, theoretically allowing the surgeon to place the plate directly on the bone without requiring additional bending. [31]. These plates are designed to be placed proximally, just distal to the articular surface. The proximal head screw is angled away from the articular surface (Figure 10.8a). In some cases (for example, if a large medial buttress is present), the surgeon may elect to further contour the plate to improve contact at the distal bone–plate interface. This can result in redirection of the proximal screw hole (Figure 10.8b) such that the screw may penetrate the articular surface [33] (Figure 10.9a,b). In order to decrease the risk of this potential error, we recommend taking the following precautions even for plates that have not undergone additional contouring.

- The joint can be identified using a 25 gauge needle. The needle is "walked" from distal to proximal beginning at the midportion of the medial collateral ligament until the tip enters the joint. In order to minimize the risk of meniscal damage, the needle should not be fully advanced into the joint.
- Placing the index finger of the nondominant hand on the fibular head during drilling. Once the hole has been completed, the depth gauge is inserted to measure its length. The surgeon should be able to feel the tip of the depth gauge as it exits the far cortex and appreciate its location relative to the position of the fibular head. If access to the preoperative radiographs is available intraoperatively, the surgeon may then evaluate the calibrated craniocaudal film to appreciate the distance from the lateral joint surface to the fibular head. This will allow a subjective determination of the screw trajectory relative to the joint surface.
- Once the screw hole is drilled, the depth gauge may be used to "feel" the bone along the proximal aspect of the hole as it is advanced toward the far cortex. If the drill hole feels completely surrounded by solid bone, it is unlikely that it has penetrated into the joint.
- If the surgeon is concerned that placement of a locking screw in the proximal hole will result in penetration of the joint, a nonlocking screw may be substituted, therefore

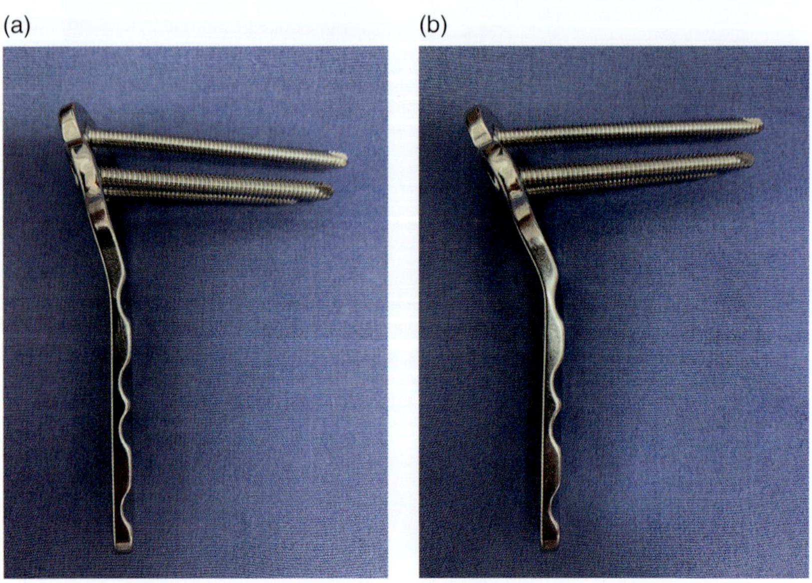

Figure 10.8 **(a)** Precontoured plate. Note the direction on the proximal three screws. **(b)** The same plate following additional contouring. Note the direction change of the proximal three screws.

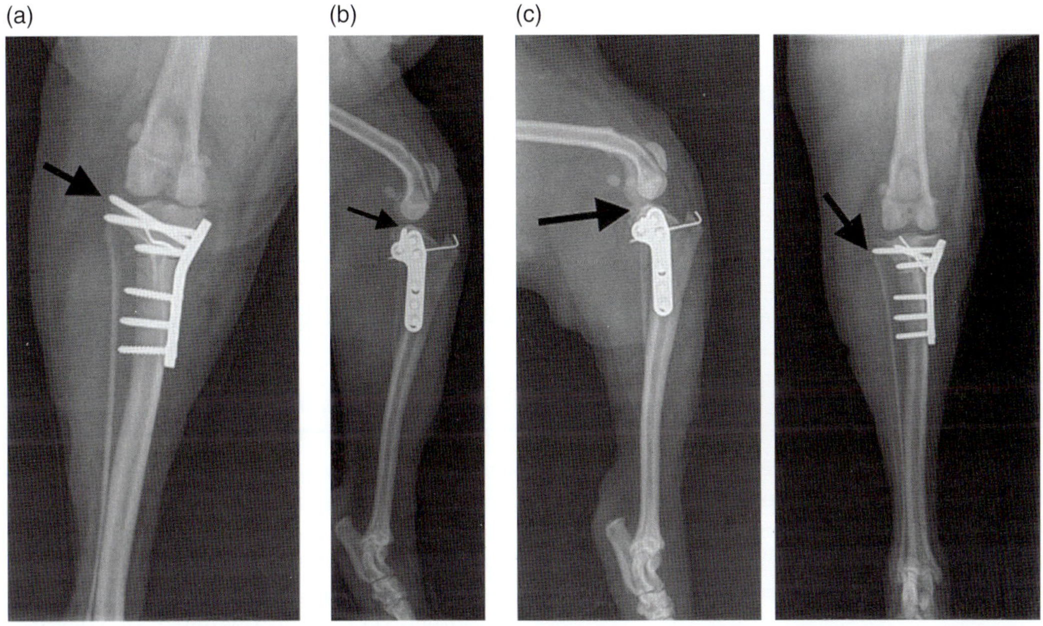

Figure 10.9 (a–c) Immediate postoperative TPLO using a 2.4 locking plate. Note the "nose" screw penetration into the articular surface (black arrow). The patient was returned to the operating room and a shorter (monocortical) screw was placed. Postoperative radiographs confirmed adequate screw positioning (black arrow). Source: All images courtesy of Dr. Rory Paton.

allowing the surgeon to direct the screw away from the joint. Care should be taken not to interfere with the other screws in the proximal segment when the proximal screw is drilled. Alternatively, the locking screw can be shortened using the preoperative craniocaudal radiographs for accurate screw length measurement.

- If there is a concern that a screw is penetrating the joint surface, the screw should be removed and a shorter (monocortical) screw should be placed instead (Figure 10.9c).

10.3.2.8.4 Jig Pin Placement into the Joint

In order to minimize the risk of articular penetration of the proximal jig pin, the steps listed below should be followed (Figure 10.5a, green box).

1. Identify the joint using a 25 gauge needle.
2. Identify the medial collateral ligament.
3. Place the proximal jig pin 5 mm distal to the articular surface (using the needle as a reference point) and caudal to the medial collateral ligament.
4. To assure perpendicular placement, reflect the ligament cranially (pin is held in oblique position first). The surgeon must place it parallel to the proximal tibial joint surface and perpendicular to the sagittal plane of the tibia.

10.3.2.9 The Osteotomy Gap

The osteotomy should be assessed to ensure the proximal and distal segments are adequately apposed after the rotation is achieved as well as once the plate is placed over the bone. If a gap is present after the antirotational pin is placed, a point-to-point bone-holding forceps can be used to reduce the gap. When this is done, it is very important to evaluate the osteotomy during forceps placement as the applied force may result in loss of rotation. If this is identified, we recommend removing the antirotational pin and repeating the rotation process.

When nonlocking screws are placed in the distal part of the plate, it is imperative to contour the plate so the distal portion of the plate sits in contact with the medial tibial cortex. Failure to do so will result in loss of reduction, osteotomy gap formation, and potentially change in angulation resulting in deformity as the screws are tightened. If a gap in the osteotomy is present once the screws are tightened, one should assess the gap dimensions. This can be done by gently placing a number 11 blade into the gap and feeling if the blade is stopped by an appropriately compressed gap at the far cortex. If a >2 mm gap is present across the osteotomy line (for example, there is no bone contact of the lateral cortex), the authors recommend grafting the osteotomy gap. The authors' preference is using an autogenous cancellous bone graft taken from the proximal humerus. If the donor site has not been prepared beforehand, a graft can be harvested from the distal femoral metaphysis using care not to damage important structures (such as the medial collateral ligament). Alternatively, an allogenic bone graft may be used.

10.3.2.10 Medial Patellar Luxation

It is imperative to evaluate overall limb alignment prior to performing surgery. In some cases in which an angular deformity is present but not corrected, medial patellar luxation may result [37]. Tibial torsion can be quantified clinically by visual inspection of the relative alignment of the hock and stifle joints, but for the most accurate determination, computed tomography is advised. It is also very important to evaluate for any angulation (varus) deformity of the distal femur. Discussion regarding surgical correction of a distal femoral varus deformity is beyond the scope of this chapter [38, 39].

Correction of mild deformities may be achieved by manipulation of the jig pin. In order to correct for a varus deformity, the distal jig arm is slid medially (away from the tibia) along the jig pin, and to correct for valgus the distal jig arm is shifted laterally (toward the tibia) along the pin. Modest torsional correction may be accomplished by bending the distal pin using handheld plate-bending pliers, applied in such way that the convexity of the bend is located cranially (to correct the internal tibial torsion). Regardless of the deformity being addressed, the position of the patella should be monitored throughout the process to ensure that the deformity has not been over- or under-corrected. These corrections will result in appropriate apposition of the osteotomy, and should maintain contact at the lateral cortex. Use of a bone graft at the resultant medial gap and use of a locking plate can optimize the outcome. If a nonlocking plate is used, meticulous contouring of the plate and optimization of the screw–bone interface are of paramount importance.

Trochlear block/wedge recession and soft tissue reconstruction (medial capsular release as well as lateral fascia imbrication) are straightforward ancillary procedures that may be performed without risk to the tibial osteotomy site. In cases of more severe patellar luxation, combination of tibial tuberosity transposition (TTT) as well as TPLO is achievable as long as meticulous technique and implants of adequate strength are used to create a robust enough construct to minimize the risk of postoperative tibial crest fixation failure [40, 41] (Figure 10.10). In a recent paper, modified TPLO for treatment of concurrent medial patellar luxation (MPL) was evaluated in 76 stifles. This technique utilized rotation as well as medial proximal tibial plateau translation. The outcome was reported to be good, with comparable complication rates to the traditional repairs for MPL [42].

10.3.2.11 Pivot Shift

In a recent study, it was found that in 15/16 dogs, the TPLO procedure was associated with persistently abnormal femorotibial kinematics during walking. Both caudal and cranial tibial subluxation were common after TPLO. The coupling of cranial tibial translation and internal tibial rotation that was found after a TPLO might provide evidence to suggest that consideration should be given to addressing both axial rotational and craniocaudal translational instability when treating CCL rupture [10].

In dogs, it is postulated that pivot shift occurs when internal tibial rotation is not adequately controlled, resulting in cranial subluxation of the tibial plateau in association with a sudden lateral change in direction of the stifle joint during weight bearing. The incidence of pivot shift after TPLO in dogs has been previously reported between 0.3% and 3.1% [43]. In order to fully evaluate for the presence of pivot shift, once the TPLO plate has been placed, the tibial compression test should be reassessed intraoperatively.

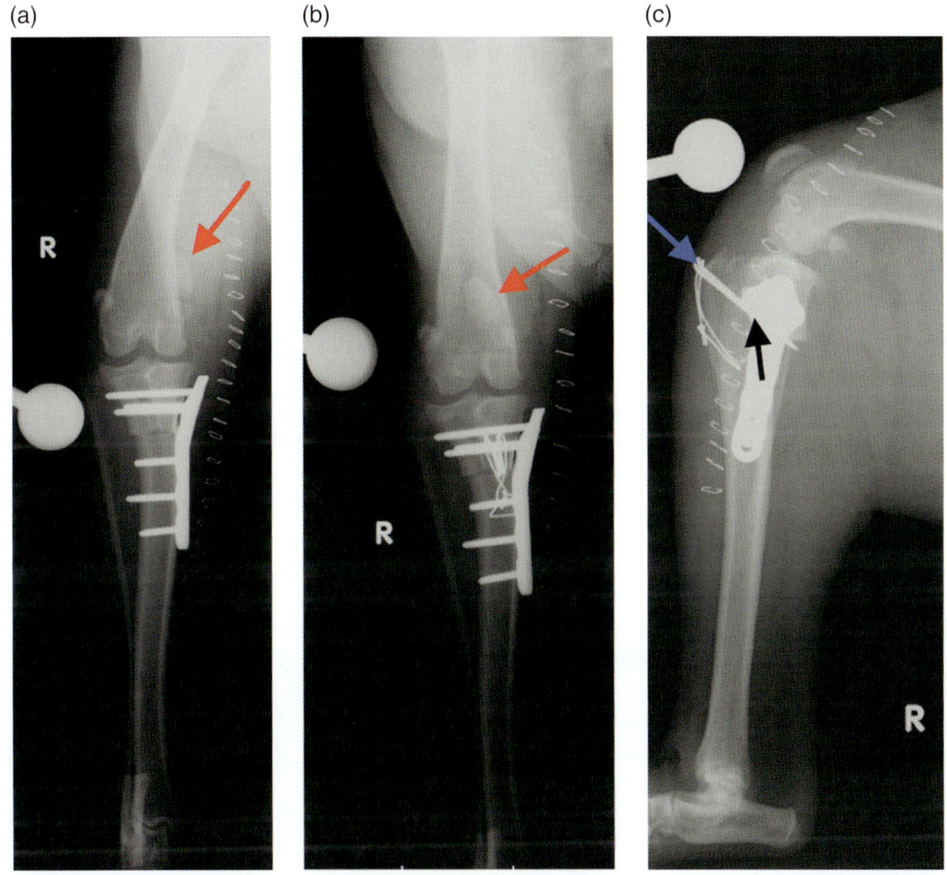

Figure 10.10 (a) Immediate postoperative craniocaudal radiographs showing a medially positioned patella (red arrow). The patella was palpated and noted to luxate each time the stifle was flexed (b) The dog was returned to the operating room and an osteotomy and tibial tuberosity transposition (TTT) were performed. Note the appropriate positioning of the patella within the trochlear groove (red arrow). (c) Lateral radiographs showing an appropriate sagittal crest osteotomy. Once the crest was lateralized, it was secured with two K-wires and a tension band wire (blue arrow). Note that in this case the K-wires are too close to the radial osteotomy (black arrow). Care should be taken to direct the K-wires distal to the osteotomy.

When excessive internal tibial rotation is observed and palpated as an abrupt craniolateral tibial subluxation from below the lateral femoral condyle, a lateral fabellotibial suture (LFTS) should be added [44]. Some companies now produce a modified TPLO plate that facilitates placement of an internal brace (suture) via a hole located in the implant (InternalBrace™, Arthrex Vet Systems). For cases that require LFTS placement with a traditional TPLO plate, the suture should pass through a hole drilled in the tibial crest cranial to the plate [43]. The suture should be tightened until internal tibial rotational instability is eliminated

10.3.2.12 Inability to Rotate to the Planned Rotation

Inadequate rotation of the proximal tibial segment during TPLO may result in failure to reduce cranial tibial thrust. In some cases, however, the surgeon may find that significant resistance is encountered as the proximal tibial segment is rotated, preventing the planned rotation from being achieved. Factors that contribute to rotational resistance have been documented and include bony fusion of the proximal tibiofibular joint (tibiofibular synostosis) and a fibular width that is 24% or greater of the tibial width at the level of the osteotomy [44]. The presence of synostosis may be appreciated on preoperative craniocaudal and occasionally mediolateral radiographs.

If rotational constraints are encountered during the procedure, it is not recommended to "force" the rotation, as this may place a greater strain on the fibula, potentially increasing the risk for postoperative fibular fracture, and thus unnecessary patient discomfort. Rather, a lateral approach by either a small separate incision or retraction of the existing incision has been described to gain access to the proximal fibula, allowing the surgeon to transect it with either a sagittal saw or bone-cutting forceps. During this approach, it is imperative that the peroneal nerve is identified and carefully retracted to protect it from iatrogenic trauma (Figure 10.11a). Transection of the fibula should allow for the planned rotation of the proximal tibial segment to be completed. Due to the loss of lateral support that occurs following transection of the fibula and the documented postoperative rotational loss ("rock-back") that occurs following TPLO with fibular fracture, bolstering the TPLO with a second plate and screw fixation is recommended to ensure adequate construct strength (Figure 10.11b,c) [45].

10.3.2.13 Malalignment

In addition to its potential use in correcting mild varus/valgus deformities, use of a jig may aid in ensuring appropriate fragment alignment during and following rotation of the proximal tibial segment [46, 47]. In addition, higher incidence of fibular penetration occurs when locking TPLO plates are used without the use of a jig [48]. Despite this, Bell and Ness reported that the use of a jig did not improve the precision of TPLO surgery [46]. When the jig is used, particular care must be taken during insertion of the jig pins, which should be placed perfectly perpendicular to the tibial diaphysis. Angulation of the proximal jig pin may result in inadvertent violation of the articular surface, increasing the risk for damage to intraarticular structures [49]. It is also imperative that the distal jig pin is inserted such that it only penetrates the cis cortex of the bone. If the jig pin penetrates both the cis and trans cortices of the tibia, an unfilled

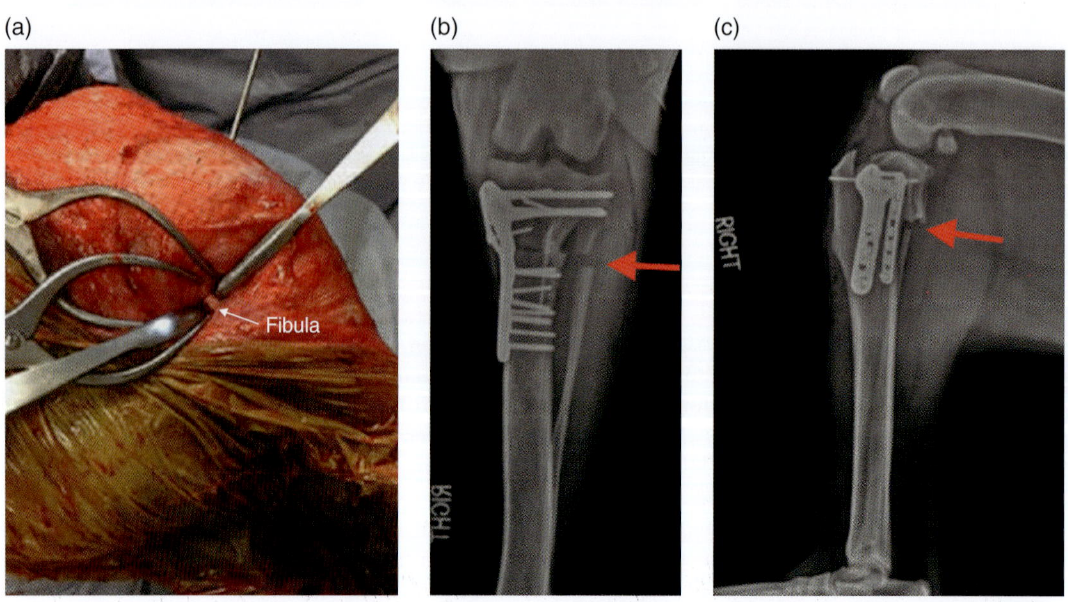

Figure 10.11 **(a)** The skin has been retracted laterally and the fibula is exposed (white arrow). The bone is isolated by two Hohmann retractors prior to transection in order to protect the peroneal nerve. **(b,c)** Postoperative radiographs showing TPLO with fibular osteotomy (red arrow). In order to minimize potential rotational loss (due to loss of lateral support), a second plate and screws were placed.

hole will be left in its place when the jig is removed. This creates a weak point in the bone that may increase the risk of postoperative fracture of the tibial diaphysis [50].

Once the jig has been correctly assembled, the surgeon may use the proximal jig pin as a reference point when performing the osteotomy. If the proximal pin has been inserted perpendicular to the bone, the saw should be angled such that the osteotomy will proceed along the same angle (90° to the diaphysis) as it is completed.

10.3.3 Postoperative Complications

10.3.3.1 Immediate Postoperative Complications (<14 days)

10.3.3.1.1 Identification of a Surgical Sponge at the Surgical Site

The use of a gauze sponge is recommended in order to protect the soft tissue envelope while the osteotomy is performed [30]. However, in order to prevent retention of microscopic particulate cotton debris, alternatives to cotton-gauze sponges have been recommended as protective devices. If a protective sponge is used, it is imperative to retrieve the sponge prior to proximal tibial rotation as it can prevent adequate rotation (Figure 10.12). If a gauze sponge is noted on the immediate postoperative radiographs (note: only a radiopaque gauze sponge will be readily apparent) it is imperative to return the patient to the operating room for retrieval [30].

10.3.3.1.2 Incisional Seroma/Infection

Postoperative application of a modified Robert-Jones bandage has been previously reported to be ineffective in reduction of postsurgical swelling [51]. The author (RBA), however, uses the application of the bandage to prevent contact between the incision and the hospital environment. Twenty-four hours after surgery, the bandage is removed and cold compresses are utilized to decrease swelling and pain.

Incisional seroma formation in the authors' experience occurs most commonly when there is a break in the surgical sutures of the fascia, or secondary to overactivity of the patient. For cases in which a seroma forms, the swollen region should be aseptically prepared for aspiration and fluid analysis. It is not required to fully drain the fluid, but enough must be obtained for cytological evaluation. If the findings are consistent with a seroma, we advise warm compression as well as reduction in excessive activities. In most cases, this resolves in 5–7 days.

For implant-associated surgical site infections, please refer to Chapter 3.

10.3.3.1.3 Screws in the Joint/Osteotomy

Screws that penetrate the joint or violate the osteotomy should be identified on the immediate postoperative radiographs. If noted, the patient should be returned to the operating room and the offending screws should be either redirected or replaced with a shorter screw (Figure 10.9).

10.3.3.1.4 Medial or Lateral Patellar Luxation

Patellar luxation has been reported as a potential complication following a TPLO procedure. This can be a direct result of the TPLO procedure (due to tibial torsion or angular deformity created during the procedure, osteotomy gap formation, or malalignment), preexisting subclinical tibial or femoral angulation, or simply due to lack of adequate orthopedic examination prior to the procedure (for example, MPL was present before the procedure).

Once the TPLO plate is positioned and secured, the tibial compression test should be performed and patellar tracking should be assessed. If the patella is palpated outside the trochlear groove during flexion and extension of the stifle, there should be concern regarding inappropriate patellar tracking (for example, medial and/or lateral luxation). It is the author's preference (RBA) to correct this by performing a sagittal tibial tuberosity osteotomy that commences at the cranioproximal aspect of the radial osteotomy and ends at the distal aspect of the tibial crest. Once the crest is transposed to the appropriate location (laterally for medial patellar luxation, medially for lateral patellar luxation), it should be secured to the tibial shaft with pins and a tension band fixation. Additional corrections (recession trochleoplasty, lateral fascia imbrication, medial capsular release) are performed if deemed necessary (Figure 10.10a,b).

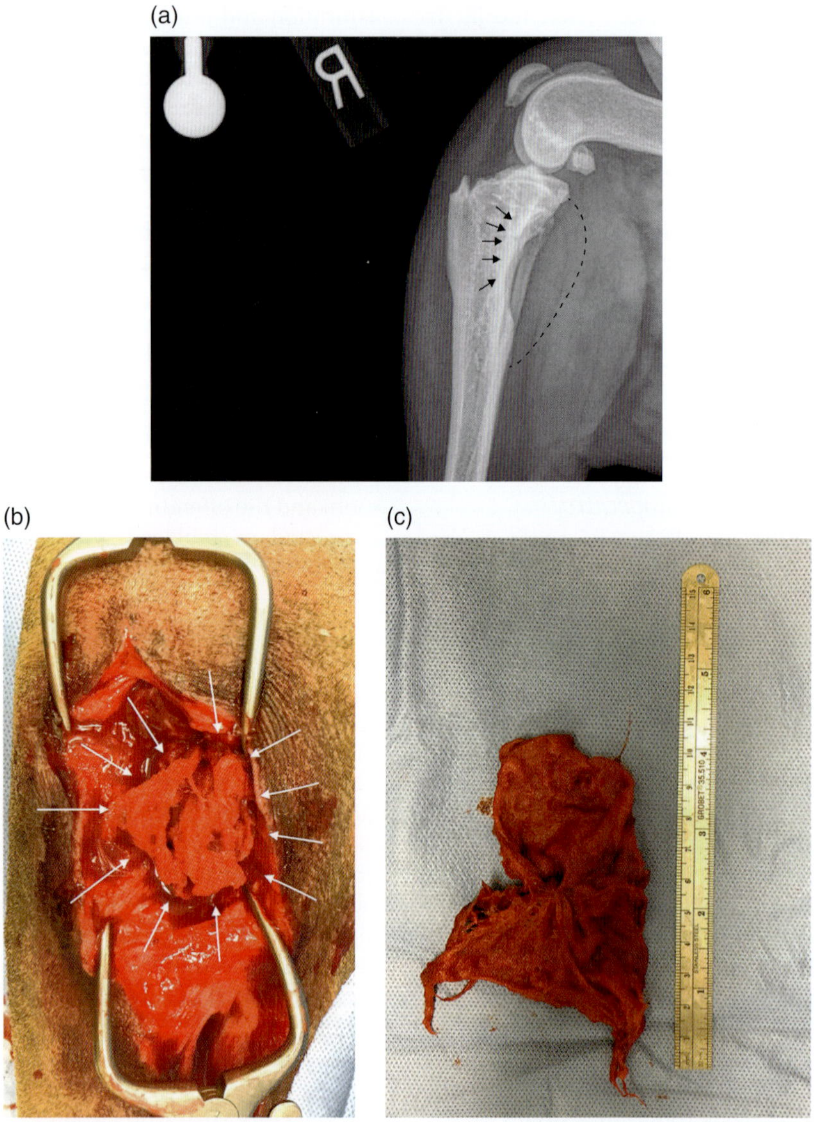

Figure 10.12 (a) Fourteen months post TPLO radiographs following a chronic draining tract along the medial aspect of the right tibia (the TPLO plate had previously been removed). Osteolysis with subchondral sclerosis (short arrows) along the caudal and proximal aspects of the tibia and a mass effect (outlined by black lines) in the adjacent soft tissue that displaces the popliteus and gastrocnemius muscles caudally. Additionally, irregular margins of the tibia at the proximal and distal aspect of this mass effect are suggestive of a periosteal reaction. (b) Intraoperative image of the dog in Figure 10.9a, showing the surgical sponge (outlined by white arrows). (c) The sponge appearance after removal. Source: All images courtesy of Dr. David L. Dycus.

10.3.4 Delayed Postoperative Complications (>14 days)

10.3.4.1 Fibular Fracture

The incidence of fibular fracture is reported to be 0.1–15% and it may occur either during or after the TPLO procedure [21]. The fibula, located caudal and lateral to the tibia, may add stability to the tibial plateau after a TPLO. The joint formed between the proximal fibula and tibia allows the plateau's rotation during a TPLO. In cases in which ankylosis of this joint has formed, increased resistance during rotation of the tibial plateau may occur. This resistance to rotation may increase the risk of fibular fracture as the tibia is rotated. Prophylactic fibular osteotomy or ostectomy has been advised in order to overcome fibular resistance to rotation (discussed in section 10.3.2.12). Unfilled holes drilled through the fibula have also been implicated in postoperative fibular fracture during both the immediate and late convalescent period [52]. If the proximal screw hole penetrates the fibula, it is advised that the entire depth of the hole (including its extent through the fibula) is measured and that a screw is placed that travels through both bones so that the hole is completely filled. Higher body weight, larger preoperative TPA, larger reduction in TPA, and performing a TPLO without the use of a jig have also been identified as risk factors for fibula fractures. In the authors' experience, postoperative fibular fracture results in a mild morbidity, but should not affect the overall surgical outcome.

Fibular fracture can also occur secondary to fixation failure. In these cases, they are managed conservatively while the other concomitant fractures (tibia) are surgically addressed.

10.3.4.2 Incisional and Implant-Related Infection

Please refer to Chapter 3 for information regarding the identification and treatment of surgical site infections.

10.3.4.3 Medial or Lateral Patellar Luxation

Patellar luxation has been reported as a potential complication following a TPLO procedure [37]. If persistent lameness following TPLO is noted, patellar tracking should be evaluated. If there is concern for medial and/or lateral patellar luxation at this stage (>14 days postoperatively), the authors suggest surgically addressing the condition once the tibial osteotomy has fully healed.

10.3.4.4 Latent or Postliminary Meniscal Tear

Please see Chapter 18 on addressing latent or postliminary meniscal tears.

10.3.5 Tibial Tuberosity Fracture

Fracture of the tibial tuberosity has been reported in 0.4–9% of dogs following TPLO and may occur at any time during the postoperative period [18]. An acute onset of lameness accompanied by pain and/or palpable soft tissue swelling in the region of the tibial tuberosity should raise suspicion for a fracture, though this complication is occasionally encountered as an incidental finding when recheck radiographs are obtained [53, 54]. If the fracture is acute and the tuberosity is displaced, surgery is indicated to reduce it and apply fixation in the form of pins and a tension band (Figure 10.13a,b). In certain cases, the fractured segment may be too small to offer adequate purchase for implant placement, in which case strict rest may suffice to allow for an acceptable return to function.

Although this is a complication that occurs in the postoperative period, decisions made during the initial procedure may help decrease overall risk. Appropriate blade size selection, attention to the planned D1 and D2 measurements, careful positioning of the saw blade ensuring that a wide tibial crest remains following completion of the osteotomy, as well as accurate positioning of the antirotational pin (at or above Sharpey's fibers) will decrease the risk of tuberosity fracture (Figure 10.13c). The recommended D1 width (tibial tuberosity width from the patellar insertion point to the osteotomy line) should be 10 mm or larger in medium- to large-breed dogs [18]. In smaller breeds, due to the size of the bone, such width is not achievable; therefore a "trapezoid shape" bone should be observable once the blade is positioned over the bone (Figure 10.5a, hatched yellow lines). It has also been shown that dogs that undergo simultaneous bilateral TPLO are at an increased risk for tibial tuberosity fracture, therefore staged surgeries are recommended to mitigate this risk. In one paper it was found that the incidence of tibial tuberosity fracture decreases when the antirotational pin is left in situ [18].

10.3.6 Patellar Fracture

Patellar fracture has been reported in 0.09–2% of dogs following a TPLO procedure [55]. These cases typically present with a history of acute

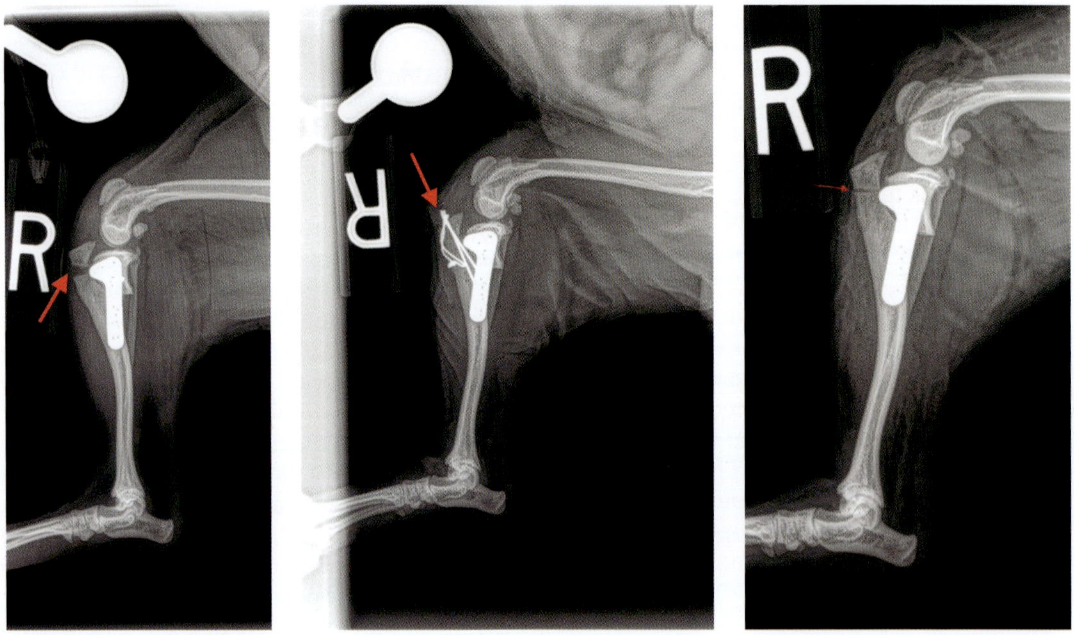

Figure 10.13 (a) Tibial tuberosity fracture in a small-breed dog 2 weeks following a TPLO procedure (red arrow). The dog became acutely lame with no known trauma. (b) The fracture was reduced and secured with two K-wires and tension band wire (red arrow). (c) Immediate postoperative TPLO radiographs. The red arrow points at the drilled track left after the antirotational pin was removed. Note the distal position in relation to the tibial tuberosity; this pin position can act as a stress riser and increase the incidence of tibial tuberosity fracture during the convalescent period. Source: All images courtesy of Dr. David L. Dycus.

recurrence of lameness following TPLO but may also be identified incidentally on recheck radiographs. It has been suggested that altered stifle biomechanics result in these stress fractures [56]. These fractures are typically avulsion fractures with a transverse to short oblique configuration at the apex of the patella (Figure 10.14). In most cases, they are accompanied by significant thickening of the patellar tendon. In the authors' experience, they can often be successfully managed conservatively with cage rest and administration of nonsteroidal antiinflammatory medications. Despite no evidence of fracture union, there is typically no evidence of persistent lameness.

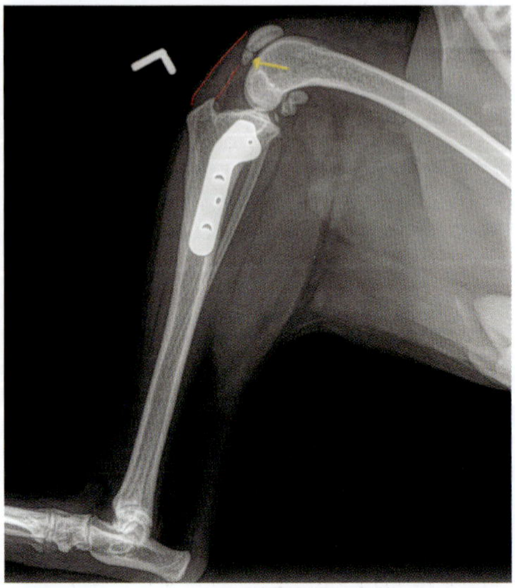

Figure 10.14 Apical patella fracture (yellow arrow) and patellar tendon thickening (outlined in red). Source: Image courtesy of Dr. David Lane.

10.3.7 Patellar Tendon Thickening

Patellar tendinopathy is an overuse condition. In dogs, this can be seen as thickening of the distal portion of the patellar tendon using imaging modalities such as radiography and ultrasound or by direct palpation of the tendon (Figure 10.15) [57, 58]. Carey et al. reported patellar tendon thickening grades as mild

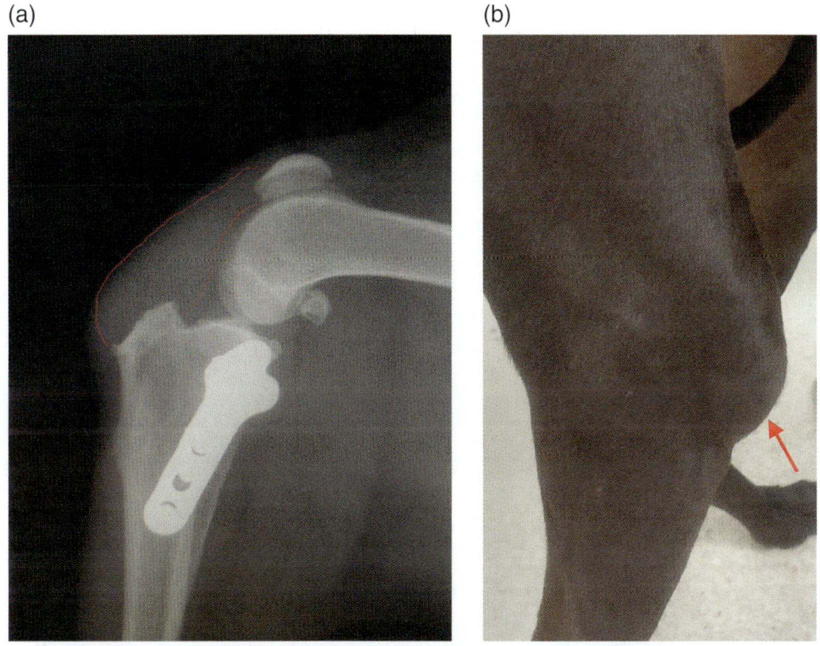

Figure 10.15 (a,b) Four months post TPLO procedure in a German Shorthaired Pointer. At this stage, the dog is not restricted. There is good limb function, normal muscle mass, and stable tibial thrust. The patellar tendon is both visibly and palpably thickened (red arrow). Radiographs of this dog confirmed the presence of severe patellar thickening (outlined in red). Source: Images courtesy of Dr. Ben Clarke.

(normal up to double thickness), moderate (6–11 mm) or severe (>12 mm or no identifiable borders) [56]. Clinical lameness secondary to patellar tendinopathy occurs infrequently relative to the frequency with which thickening of the patellar tendon is appreciated on radiographs. In humans, the condition can occasionally result in patellar tendon rupture or patellar fracture. In dogs that have undergone TPLO, patellar tendon thickening has been associated with a cranially located osteotomy position and postoperative tibial tuberosity fracture [59]. Radiographically apparent thickening of the patellar tendon and tendinopathy is seen in up to 80% of TPLO cases [56]. The mechanism is related to a decrease in the moment arm of the extensor mechanism which results in an increased force required for the patellar tendon to achieve the same torque [60].

Currently, there are no treatment guidelines for patellar tendinopathy in dogs post TPLO procedure. If the condition is present and believed to be the underlying cause of lameness, it should largely resolve with time or physiotherapy and administration of antiinflammatory medications. In addition, local treatment with platelet-rich plasma (PRP) or the use of extracorporeal shock wave therapy have been reported [60].

10.3.8 Loss of Reduction/Alignment (Rock-Back)/Catastrophic Tibial Fracture with Implant Failure

"Rock-back" following TPLO can indicate early implant loosening (Figure 10.16a,b). Early recognition is important as this can develop into a catastrophic implant failure with subsequent loss of stability at the osteotomy site. "Rock-back" can result in a significant increase in the TPA with valgus or varus angulation and secondary loss of stifle stability (Figure 10.16c). Such cases generally have a history of an acute onset of lameness during the healing period. Any worsening or acute lameness during the postoperative period should be taken seriously and warrants further investigation.

Any loss of reduction of the osteotomy indicates fixation failure and will necessitate

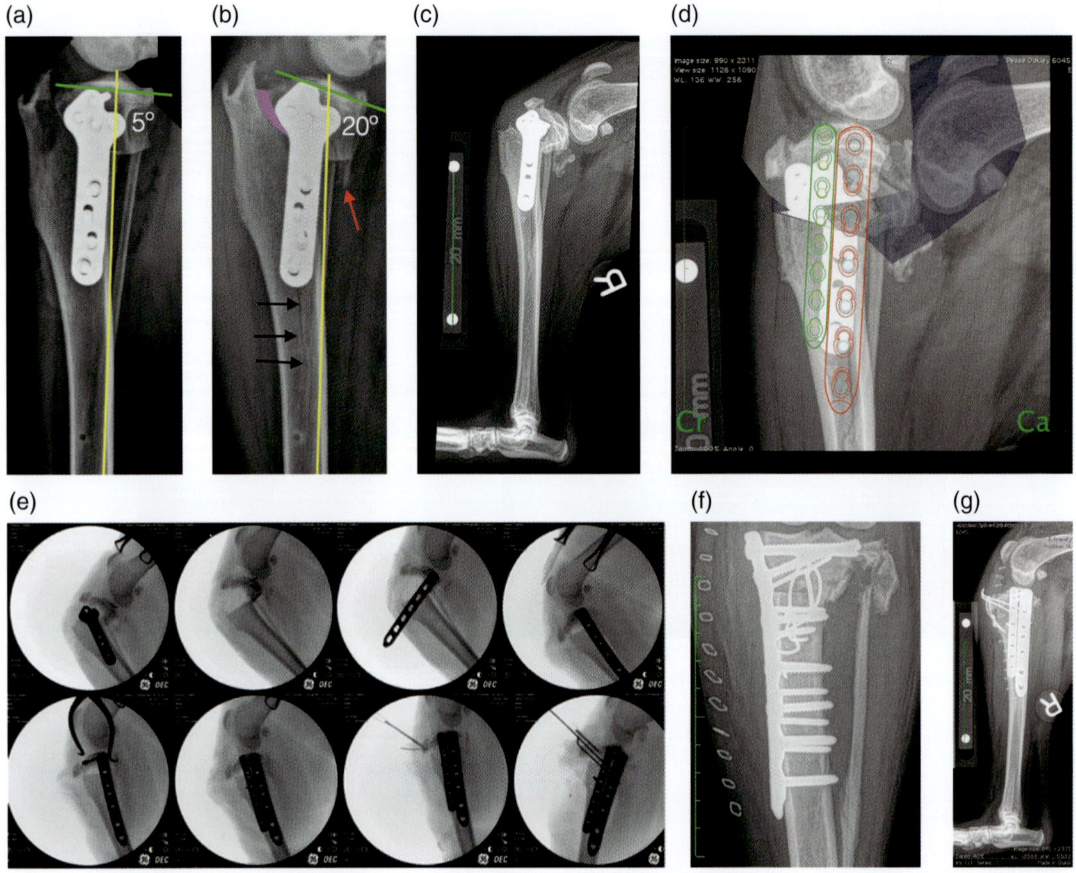

Figure 10.16 **(a,b)** Immediate postoperative TPLO radiographs indicating targeted TPA of 5°. An acute onset of lameness during the immediate post-operative period developed. The radiographs revealed a fibular fracture (red arrow, loss of lateral support) with subsequent change in the TPA (20°), which indicates "rock-back" (purple shading). Note the fissure propagation from the distal bone screw toward the distal jig pin hole (black arrows). In this case, prompt surgical revision is indicated (addition of a caudal plate, application of cerclage wires for the fissures). Source: Images (a)-(b) courtesy of Dr. Brian Beale. **(c)** Failed TPLO procedure resulting in caudal displacement (increased tibial plateau angle) as well as varus collapse of the proximal tibial segment with loss of implant support. **(d)** A software planning program was used to plan the reduction and realignment of the proximal tibial fragment. The bone has been templated with 3.5 and 2.7 mm locking plates. **(e)** Fluoroscopic images showing implant removal, reduction with a 3.5 mm LCP® plate, and augmentation with an adjacent cranially placed 2.7 mm LCP®. An identified tibial tuberosity fragment was reduced using pins and a tension band wire repair technique. **(f,g)** Postoperative lateral and craniocaudal radiographs of the fracture repaired in Figure 10.16e. The segmental proximal fibular fracture was not repaired. Source: Images (c)–(g) courtesy of Dr. Ross Lirtzman.

surgical revision. This should be performed at an early stage as a delay in the hope that osteotomy will progress to union is typically futile. Revision should consist of implant removal, restoration of appropriate reduction of the osteotomy, and placement of a new plate. If other fractures are recognized (such as tibial tuberosity fracture), they should be surgically addressed at the same time (Figure 10.16d–g).

Catastrophic implant failure with loss of reduction necessitates immediate recognition and surgical revision. Most failures are caused by technical error or inappropriate implant positioning. The authors suggest ensuring that adequate metaphyseal bone is used for screw purchase in the proximal tibial segment. Proximal and cranial plate tilting of the proximal aspect of the plate can result in inadequate screw–bone purchase (close to the osteotomy, intraarticular

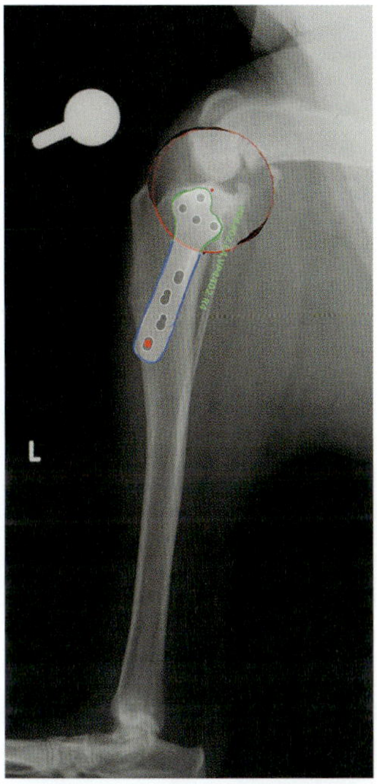

Figure 10.17 Mediolateral projection is used for accurate measuring of the tibial plateau angle (TPA) post TPLO with plate templating. Note the cranial position of the distal portion of the plate (blue) in order to compensate for metaphyseal bone purchase at the proximal tibial segment (green). This can result in a screw drill track close to the cranial cortex (red full circle). Source: vPOP-pro, VetSOS Education Ltd, veterinary preoperative orthopedic planning software.

penetration). In contrast, if the proximal part of the plate is tilted caudally to allow better screw–bone purchase, it can result in a cranial plate tilt at the distal bone segment, especially when the required rotation is large (Figure 10.17). When this occurs, the most distal screw will be positioned close to the cranial cortex, which may result in a diaphyseal tibial fracture (Figure 10.18). Newly designed plates utilize a caudal angulation of the proximal aspect of the plate that allows adequate metaphyseal bone purchase even with a relatively large rotation. In addition, this will mitigate the need for cranial tilting of the plate in the distal bone fragment (Figure 10.19).

In cases of implant failure (Figure 10.20a,b), the implants should be removed and the surgical site revised. The primary goal is to restore alignment with rigid stabilization even when control of the TPA is not achievable. Care should be taken to avoid previously

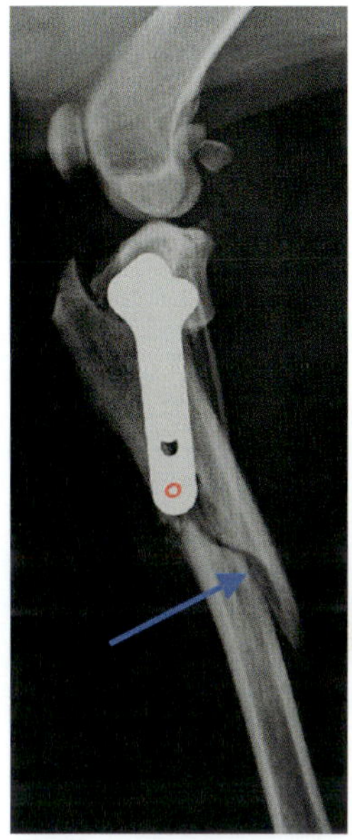

Figure 10.18 Two weeks postoperative TPLO patient that sustained a fall. A spiral fracture of the tibial diaphysis that propagated from the distal screw hole (red open circle) is present. Note the proximity of the distal screw to the cranial tibial cortex. Source: Image courtesy of Dr. Brian Beale.

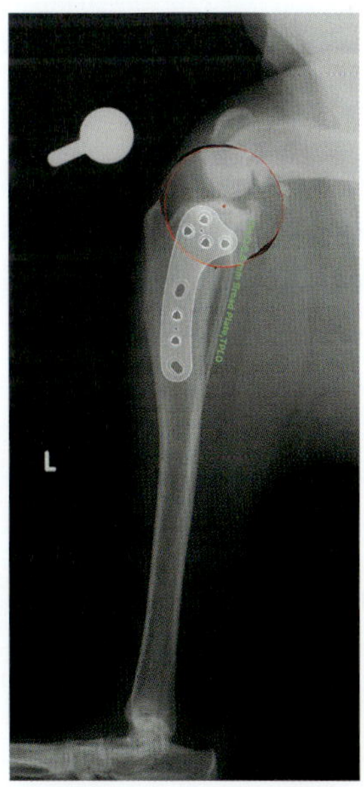

Figure 10.19 Mediolateral projection is used for accurate measuring of the tibial plateau angle (TPA) post TPLO with plate templating. A curved plate (Biomedrix) allows accurate screw placement in the proximal tibial metaphyseal bone and the distal bone segment, caudal to the cortical margin. Source: vPOP-pro, VetSOS Education Ltd, veterinary preoperative orthopedic planning software.

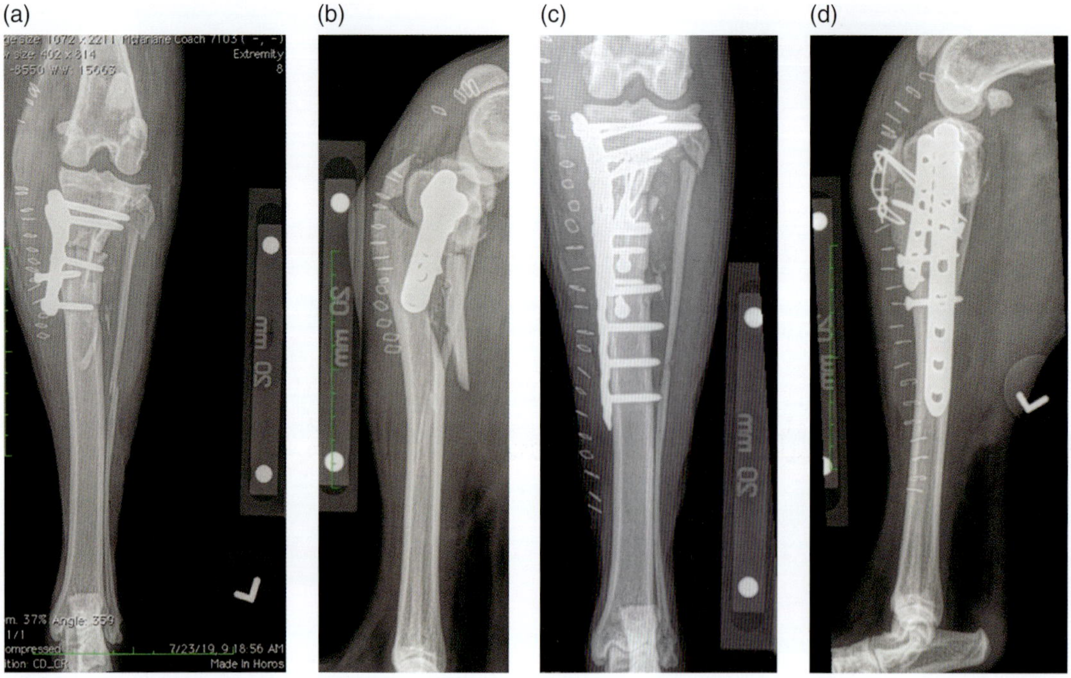

Figure 10.20 **(a,b)** Ten-day postoperative radiographs showing a catastrophic failure following a TPLO procedure. There is a tibial tuberosity fracture, fibular fracture, "rock-back" with valgus angulation and a butterfly fracture of the tibial diaphysis (caudally displaced). **(c,d)** Postoperative radiographs of the limb following revision surgery: The TPLO plate and broken screws were removed. The caudodistal fragment was secured using three screws in lag fashion (one screw was placed in a caudal to cranial direction and two screws were placed in the cranial to caudal direction). The proximal tibial segment was then secured to the distal fragment using two (3.5 and 2.7 mm) LCP® plates. The tibial tuberosity was reduced and secured to the tibia with two K-wires and a tension band wire. Source: All images courtesy of Dr. Ross Lirtzman.

drilled screw holes. If possible, the use of two plates is strongly advised to enhance the repair stability (side by side plating or orthogonally placed plates) (Figure 10.20c,d). In some cases, particular those with complex or nonreconstructible fractures a hybrid external skeletal fixator may also be considered. (Figure 10.21).

10.3.9 Implant-Associated Sarcoma

Although uncommon, implant-associated sarcoma has been described, and a specific association between TPLO and the development of proximal tibial osteosarcoma has been reported [61, 62]. Therefore, it is important for proximal tibial osteosarcoma to be included among the differential diagnoses for a new or worsening hindlimb lameness in dogs that previously underwent TPLO on the affected limb [60]. The treatment for implant-associated sarcoma is discussed elsewhere and is beyond the scope of this chapter.

10.3.10 Long Digital Extensor Tendon Luxation

Although rare, luxation of the long digital extensor (LDE) tendon as a complication secondary to TPLO has been reported in four dogs. The most likely hypothesis is that the luxation was caused by iatrogenic injury to the restraining ligament on its cranial or caudal attachment during surgery (soft tissue elevation). In cases of LDE luxation reported clinical signs were lameness, clicking sound on flexion and extension of the stifle joint, and/or localized pain and swelling over the craniolateral region of the proximal tibia. All reported cases were treated with surgical intervention (either

(a) (b)

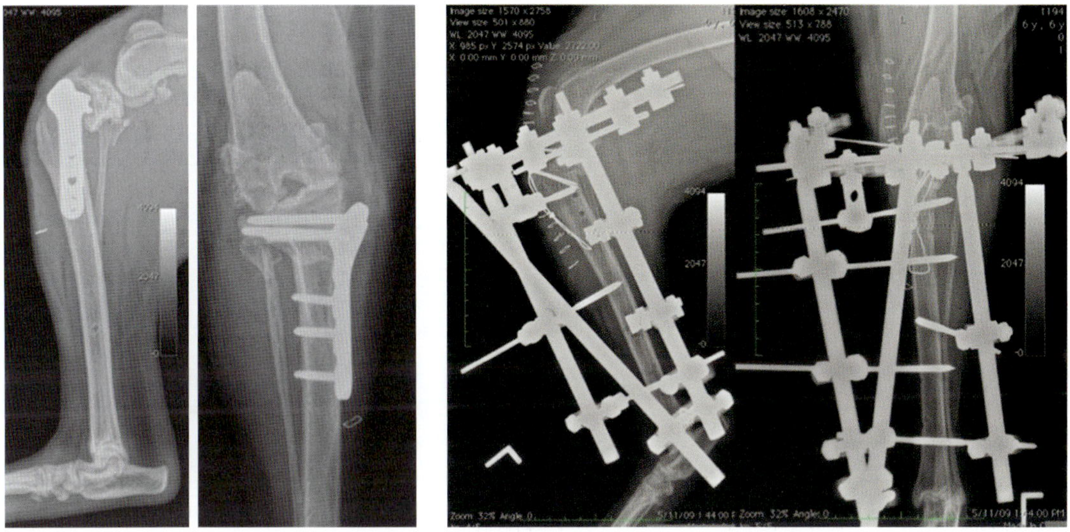

Figure 10.21 (a) Postoperative TPLO failure. There is marked caudal displacement of the proximal tibial segment, fibular fracture, and valgus deformity. (b) Postoperative radiographs show fracture repair of the case presented in Figure 10.21a. The fracture was reduced and stabilized using a hybrid external skeletal fixator (ring and linear external skeletal fixator). Source: Images courtesy of Dr. Ross Lirtzman.

tenodesis or release) with excellent clinical response [63].

10.4 Return to Function

Many biomechanical studies have evaluated the efficacy of the TPLO procedure on stifle stability. The TPLO procedure can improve sagittal plane femorotibial subluxation during weight bearing in dogs with naturally occurring CCL ruptures. However, in 30% of dogs, it was found that TPLO does not consistently resolve the cranial tibial subluxation during standing despite uniform improvement in limb function after surgery [10]. Heidorn et al. reported that the prognosis was good for competitive agility dogs undergoing TPLO and that none of the dogs that returned to competition sustained an injury of the affected limb during the follow-up period [64].

Many studies report objective measures of gait assessment following TPLO [65]. In order to achieve our functional goals, it has been suggested that early physiotherapy may achieve significantly greater thigh muscle circumference and stifle range of motion, reduce pain, and increase short-term use [66–69]. A detailed discussion of rehabilitation is beyond the scope of this chapter, and indeed this book. The complications associated with rehabilitation following TPLO are discussed in Chapter 15.

References

1. von Pfeil, D.J.F., Kowaleski, M.P., Glassman, M., and Dejardin, L.M. (2018). Results of a survey of Veterinary Orthopedic Society members on the preferred method for treating cranial cruciate ligament rupture in dogs weighing more than 15 kilograms (33 pounds). *J. Am. Vet. Med. Assoc.* 253 (5): 586–597.
2. Bergh, M.S., Sullivan, C., Ferrell, C.L. et al. (2014). Systematic review of surgical treatments for cranial cruciate ligament disease in dogs. *J. Am. Anim. Hosp. Assoc.* 50 (5): 315–321.
3. Kim, S.E., Pozzi, A., Kowaleski, M.P. et al. (2008). Tibial osteotomies for cranial cruciate ligament insufficiency in dogs. *Vet. Surg.* 37: 111–125.
4. Slocum, B. and Devine, T. (1984). Cranial tibial wedge osteotomy: a technique for eliminating cranial tibial thrust in cranial cruciate ligament repair. *J. Am. Vet. Med. Assoc.* 184: 564–569.

5. Slocum, B. and Slocum, T.D. (1993). Tibial plateau leveling osteotomy for repair of cranial cruciate ligament rupture in the canine. *Vet. Clin. North Am. Small Anim. Pract.* 23: 777–795.
6. Slocum, B. and Devine, T. (1983). Cranial tibial thrust: a primary force in the canine stifle. *J. Am. Vet. Med. Assoc.* 183: 456–459.
7. Kim, S.E., Pozzi, A., Banks, S.A. et al. (2009). Effect of tibial plateau leveling osteotomy on femorotibial contact mechanics and stifle kinematics. *Vet. Surg.* 38: 23–32.
8. Shahar, R. and Milgram, J. (2006). Biomechanics of tibial plateau leveling of the canine cruciate-deficient stifle joint: a theoretical model. *Vet. Surg.* 35: 144–149.
9. Reif, U., Hulse, D.A., and Hauptman, J.G. (2002). Effect of tibial plateau leveling on stability of the canine cranial cruciate-deficient stifle joint: an in vitro study. *Vet. Surg.* 31: 147–154.
10. Tinga, S., Kim, S.E., Banks, S.A. et al. (2018). Femorotibial kinematics in dogs with cranial cruciate ligament insufficiency: a three-dimensional in-vivo fluoroscopic analysis during walking. *BMC Vet. Res.* 14 (1): 85.
11. Zann, G.J., Kim, S.E., Pozzi, A., and Banks, S.A. (2020). The effect of tibial plateau leveling osteotomy on patellofemoral kinematics in dogs: an in vivo study. *Vet. Surg.* 49 (1): 207–221.
12. Garnett, S.D. and Daye, R.M. (2014). Short-term complications associated with TPLO in dogs using 2.0 and 2.7 mm plates. *J. Am. Anim. Hosp. Assoc.* 50 (6): 396–404.
13. Stauffer, K.D., Tuttle, T.A., Elkins, A.D. et al. (2006). Complications associated with 696 tibial plateau leveling osteotomies (2001–2003). *J. Am. Anim. Hosp. Assoc.* 42: 44–50.
14. Pacchiana, P.D., Morris, E., Gillings, S.L. et al. (2003). Surgical and postoperative complications associated with tibial plateau leveling osteotomy in dogs with cranial cruciate ligament rupture: 397 cases (1998–2001). *J. Am. Vet. Med. Assoc.* 222: 184–193.
15. Priddy, N.H. II, Tomlinson, J.L., Dodam, J.R. et al. (2003). Complications with and owner assessment of the outcome of tibial plateau leveling osteotomy for treatment of cranial cruciate ligament rupture in dogs: 193 cases (1997–2001). *J. Am. Vet. Med. Assoc.* 222: 1726–1173.
16. Coletti, T.J., Anderson, M., Gorse, M.J. et al. (2014). Complications associated with tibial plateau leveling osteotomy: a retrospective of 1519 procedures. *Can. Vet. J.* 55: 249–254.
17. Bergh, M.S. and Peirone, B. (2012). Complications of tibial plateau levelling osteotomy in dogs. *Vet. Comp. Orthop. Traumatol.* 25: 349–358.
18. Bergh, M.S., Rajala-Schultz, P., and Johnson, K.A. (2008). Risk factors for tibial tuberosity fracture after tibial plateau leveling osteotomy in dogs. *Vet. Surg.* 37: 374–382.
19. Tomlinson, J. (2005). Fractures of the patella. In: *AO Principles of Fracture Management in the dog and cat* (eds. A. Johnson, J. Houlton and R. Vannini), 305–308. New York: Thieme.
20. Jay, M.R., Mattoon, J.S., Gilbert, P.J. et al. (2019). Radiographic evaluation of patellar ligament length after tibial plateau leveling osteotomy in dogs. *Am. J. Vet. Res.* 80 (6): 607–612.
21. Taylor, J., Langenbach, A., and Marcellin-Little, D.J. (2011). Risk factors for fibular fracture after TPLO. *Vet. Surg.* 40 (6): 687–693.
22. Fettig, A.A., Rand, W.M., Sato, A.F. et al. (2003). Observer variability of tibial plateau slope measurement in 40 dogs with cranial cruciate ligament-deficient stifle joints. *Vet. Surg.* 32: 471–478.
23. Read, R.L., Duncan, C.G., Wallace, A.D. et al. (2012). Assessment of on-screen measurements, magnification, and calibration in digital radiography. *J. Am. Vet. Med. Assoc.* 241: 782.
24. Windolf, M., Leitner, M., Schwieger, K. et al. (2008). Accuracy of fragment positioning after TPLO and effect on biomechanical stability. *Vet. Surg.* 37 (4): 366–373.
25. Kowaleski, M.P., Apelt, D., Mattoon, J.S. et al. (2005). The effect of tibial plateau leveling osteotomy position on cranial tibial subluxation: an in vitro study. *Vet. Surg.* 34: 332–336.
26. Wheeler, J.L., Cross, A.R., and Gingrich, W. (2003). in vitro effects of osteotomy angle and osteotomy reduction on tibial angulation and rotation during the tibial plateau-leveling osteotomy procedure. *Vet. Surg.* 32: 371–377.
27. Gholampour, S., Shakouri, E., and Deh, H.H.H. (2018). Effect of drilling direction and depth on thermal necrosis during tibia drilling: an in vitro study. *Health Care* 26 (4): 687–697.
28. Moles, A. and Glyde, M. (2009). Anatomical investigation of the canine cranial tibial artery: a potential source of severe haemorrhage during proximal tibial osteotomies. *Vet. Comp. Orthop. Traumatol.* 22: 351–355.
29. Pozzi, A., Samii, V., and Horodyski, M.B. (2011). Evaluation of vascular trauma after tibial plateau levelling osteotomy with or without gauze protection. A cadaveric angiographic study. *Vet. Comp. Orthop. Traumatol.* 24: 266–271.
30. Clarke, S.P., Calvo, I., and Farrell, M. (2009). ex vivo evaulation of the effect of tibial plateau osteotomy on the proximal tibial soft tissue envelope with and without the use of protective gauze sponges. *Veg. Surg.* 38: 636–644.
31. Krotscheck, U., Thompson, M.S., Ryan, K.K., and Mohammed, H.O. (2012). Comparison of TPA, bone healing, and intra-articular screw placement using conventional nonlocked application of surgeon-contoured versus locked application of precontoured TPLO plates in dogs. *Vet. Surg.* 41 (8): 931–937.

32. Boekhout, C. and Cross, A. (2012). Incidence of transcortical tibial fractures with self-tapping and non-self-tapping screws in a canine TPLO model. *Vet. Surg.* 41 (7): 898–901.
33. Barnes, D.C., Trinterud, T., Owen, M.R., and Bush, M.A. (2016). Short-term outcome and complications of TPLO using anatomically contoured locking compression plates in small/medium-breed dogs with "excessive" tibial plateau angle. *J. Small Anim. Pract.* 57 (6): 305–310.
34. Chiu, K.W., Amsellem, P.M., Yu, J. et al. (2019). Influence of fixation systems on complications after tibial plateau leveling osteotomy in dogs greater than 45.4 kilograms (100 lb). *Vet. Surg.* 48 (4): 505–512.
35. Conkling, A.L., Fagin, B., and Daye, R.M. (2010). Comparison of tibial plateau angle changes after tibial plateau leveling osteotomy fixation with conventional or locking screw technology. *Vet. Surg.* 39: 475–481.
36. Gurusamy, K., Parker, M.J., and Rowlands, T.K. (2005). The complications of displaced intracapsular fracture of the hip: the effect of screw positioning and angulation on fracture healing. *J. Bone Joint Surg. Br.* 87 (5): 632.
37. Flesher, K., Beale, B.S., and Hudson, C.C. (2019). Technique and outcome of a modified tibial plateau levelling osteotomy for treatment of concurrent medial patellar luxation and cranial cruciate ligament rupture in 76 stifles. *Vet. Comp. Orthop. Traumatol.* 32 (1): 26–32.
38. Brower, B.E., Kowaleski, M.P., Peruski, A.M. et al. (2017). Distal femoral lateral closing wedge osteotomy as a component of comprehensive treatment of medial patellar luxation and distal femoral varus in dogs. *Vet. Comp. Traumatol.* 30 (1): 20–27.
39. Dudley, R.M., Kowaleski, M.P., Drost, W.T. et al. (2006). Radiographic and computed tomographic determination of femoral varus and torsion in the dog. *Vet. Radiol. Ultrasound* 47: 546–552.
40. Birks, R.R. and Kowaleski, M.P. (2018). Combined tibial plateau levelling osteotomy and tibial tuberosity transposition: an ex vivo mechanical study. *Vet. Comp. Orthop. Traumatol.* 31 (2): 124–130.
41. Leonard, K.C., Kowaleski, M.P., Saunders, W.B. et al. (2016). Combined tibial plateau levelling osteotomy and tibial tuberosity transposition for treatment of cranial cruciate ligament insufficiency with concomitant medial patellar luxation. *Vet. Comp. Tramato.* 29 (6): 536–540.
42. Flesher, K., Beale, B.S., and Hudson, C.C. (2019). Technique and outcome of a modified tibial plateau levelling osteotomy for treatment of concurrent medial patellar luxation and cranial cruciate ligament rupture in 76 stifles. *Vet. Comp. Orthop. Traumatol.* 32 (1): 26–32.
43. Schaible, M., Ben-Amotz, R., Caceres, A. et al. (2017). Combined tibial plateau levelling osteotomy and lateral fabellotibial suture for cranial cruciate ligament rupture with severe rotational instability in dogs. *J. Small Anim. Pract.* 58 (4): 219–226.
44. Gatineau, M. and Dupuis, J.P. (2011). Retrospective study of 476 tibial plateau levelling osteotomy procedures. Rate of subsequent "pivot shift", meniscal tear and other complications. *Vet. Comp. Orthop. Traumatol.* 24: 333–341.
45. Zuckerman, J.S., Dyce, J., Arruda, A.G. et al. (2018). Fibular osteotomy to facilitate proximal tibial rotation during tibial plateau leveling osteotomy. *Vet. Surg.* 47 (7): 923–931.
46. Bell, J.C. and Ness, M.G. (2007). Does use of a jig influence the precision of tibial plateau leveling osteotomy surgery? *Vet. Surg.* 36 (3): 228–233.
47. Mariano, A.D., Kowaleski, M.P., and Boudrieau, R.J. (2016). Novel TPLO alignment jig/saw guide reproduces freehand and ideal osteotomy positions. *PLoS One* 11 (8): e0161110.
48. Flynn, P., Duncan, C.G., Palmer, R.H., and Duerr, F.M. (2014). in vitro incidence of fibular penetration with and without the use of a jig during tibial plateau leveling osteotomy. *Vet. Surg.* 43 (4): 495–499.
49. Cavalcanti, J.V.J., Kim, S.E., and Colee, J. (2020). Intra-articular proximal jig pin placement during tibial plateau leveling osteotomy. *Open Vet. J.* 9 (4): 335–338.
50. Burton, N.J., Fitzpatrick, N., and Wallace, A.M. (2013). Evaluation of cut accuracy and cis cortical damage for tibial plateau leveling osteotomy performed with and without aid of a novel saw guide: an in vitro study. *Vet. Surg.* 42 (1): 28–37.
51. Unis, M.D., Roush, J.K., Blincki, K.L., and Baker, S.G. (2010). Effect of bandaging on post-operative swelling after tibial plateau leveling osteotomy. *Vet. Comp. Orthop. Traumatol.* 23 (4): 240–244.
52. Morgan, M.J. and Frazho, J.K. (2018). Comparison of TPLO tibial tuberosity fractures with and without an in situ rotational pin. *BMC. Res. Notes* 11 (1): 368.
53. Mehrkens, L.R., Hudson, C.C., and Cole, G.L. (2018). Factors associated with early tibial tuberosity fracture after tibial plateau leveling osteotomy. *Vet. Surg.* 47 (5): 634–639.
54. Rutherford, S., Bell, J.C., and Ness, M.G. (2012). Fracture of the patella after TPLO in 6 dogs. *Vet. Surg.* 41 (7): 869–875.
55. Hamilton, K., Tarlton, J., Parsons, K. et al. (2015). Effect of osteotomy position and tibial plateau rotation on the tensile force required for failure of the canine quadriceps mechanism. *Vet. Surg.* 44: 763–771.
56. Carey, K., Aiken, S.W., DiResta, G.R. et al. (2005). Radiographic and clinical changes of the patellar

tendon after tibial plateau leveling osteotomy 94 cases (2000–2003). *Vet. Comp. Orthop. Traumatol.* 18: 235–242.
57. Mattern, K.L., Berry, C.R., Peck, J.N. et al. (2006). Radiographic and ultrasonographic evaluation of the patellar ligament following tibial plateau leveling osteotomy. *Vet. Radiol. Ultrasound* 47: 185–191.
58. Kanno, N., Ochi, Y., Ichinohe, T. et al. (2019). Effect of the centre of rotation in tibial plateau levelling osteotomy on quadriceps tensile force: an ex vivo study in canine cadavers. *Vet. Comp. Orthop. Traumatol.* 32 (2): 117–125.
59. Dan, M.J., Crowley, J., Broe, D. et al. (2019). Patella tendinopathy zoobiquity – what can we learn from dogs? *Knee* 26 (1): 115–123.
60. Selmic, L.E., Ryan, S.D., Ruple, A. et al. (2018). Association of tibial plateau leveling osteotomy with proximal tibial osteosarcoma in dogs. *J. Am. Vet. Med. Assoc.* 253 (6): 752–756.
61. Straw, M.J. (2005). What is your diagnosis? Fracture/implant-associated osteosarcoma following TPLO procedures. *Small Anim. Pract.* 46 (9): 457–459.
62. Boudrieau, R.J., McCarthy, R.J., and Sisson, R.D. Jr. (2005). Sarcoma of the proximal portion of the tibia in a dog 5.5 years after tibial plateau leveling osteotomy. *J. Am. Vet. Med. Assoc.* 227: 1613–1617.
63. Sjöström L., H.P.J. (2007). Luxation of the long digital extensor tendon as a complication to tibial plateau leveling osteotomy. A presentation of four cases. *Vet. Comp. Orthop. Traumatol.* 3: 224–226.
64. Heidorn, S., Canapp, S., Zink, C. et al. (2018). Rate of return to agility competition for dogs with cranial cruciate ligament tears treated with tibial plateau leveling osteotomy. *J. Am. Vet. Med. Assoc.* 253: 1439–1444.
65. Amimoto, H., Koreeda, T., and W.N. (2019). Evaluation of recovery of limb function by use of force plate gait analysis after tibial plateau leveling osteotomy for management of dogs with unilateral cranial cruciate ligament rupture. *J. Vet. Res.* 80 (5): 461–468.
66. Drygas, K.A., McClure, S.R., Goring, R.L. et al. (2011). Effect of cold compression therapy on postoperative pain, swelling, range of motion, and lameness after tibial plateau leveling osteotomy in dogs. *J. Am. Vet. Med. Assoc.* 238: 1284–1291.
67. Renwick, S.M., Renwick, A.I., Brodbelt, D.C. et al. (2018). Influence of class IV laser therapy on the outcomes of tibial plateau leveling osteotomy in dogs. *Vet. Surg.* 47 (4): 507–515.
68. Barnes, K., Faludi, A., Takawira, C. et al. (2019). Extracorporeal shock wave therapy improves short-term limb use after canine tibial plateau leveling osteotomy. *Vet. Surg.* 48 (8): 1382–1390.
69. Gallagher, A., Cross, A.R., and Sepulveda, G. (2012). The effect of shock wave therapy on patellar ligament desmitis after tibial plateau leveling osteotomy. *Vet. Surg.* 41 (4): 482–485.

11 Complications Associated with CORA-Based Leveling Osteotomy

David L. Dycus and Don Hulse

11.1 Introduction

The center of rotation of angulation (CORA)-based leveling osteotomy (CBLO) is a recently described osteotomy procedure to stabilize the cranial cruciate ligament (CCL)-deficient stifle [1–3]. The concept of the CBLO is to modify the normal canine procurvatum to function with the normal recurvatum to eliminate cranial tibial thrust. The normal canine tibia has a proximal curvature (procurvatum) and as such a CORA exists. This means that the proximal anatomical longitudinal axis is not aligned with the distal longitudinal axis. It is the intersection of the proximal and distal anatomical lines (Figure 11.1) that defines the position of the CORA [3]. The angle formed at the intersection of the two lines will determine the magnitude of the CORA (Figure 11.2). As the angulation correction axis (ACA) is centered at the CORA, correction of the magnitude of the CORA will lead to the desired tibial plateau angle (TPA) and thus stabilization of cranial tibial subluxation through alignment of the proximal and distal longitudinal axes (Figure 11.3) [3].

Reported advantages of the CBLO include ample bone stock for fixation in both small/toy breeds and giant-breed dogs, compression of the osteotomy resulting in stable/early healing [4], improved alignment, no secondary translation, near normal articular cartilage appearance on second-look arthroscopy [5], facilitation of leveling in skeletally immature dogs with open proximal tibial physis [6], ease of procedure in dogs with an excessive TPA, facilitation of correction with concurrent patella luxation or patients with a compromised tibial crest, and allowing application of intraarticular auto/allografts.

11.2 Literature Review of Complications

With any new procedure, the scientific evidence is emerging in regard to the advantages as well as the disadvantages. Currently, several aspects of the CBLO are being investigated, such as looking at the ease of the CBLO in patients with an excessive TPA, utilization of tibial tuberosity transposition with the CBLO in patients with patella luxation, and determination of the biomechanical strength of various fixations for the CBLO. Therefore, while some complications and prevention of complications have been identified, others may emerge in the future. An

Complications in Canine Cranial Cruciate Ligament Surgery, First Edition. Edited by Ron Ben-Amotz and David L. Dycus.

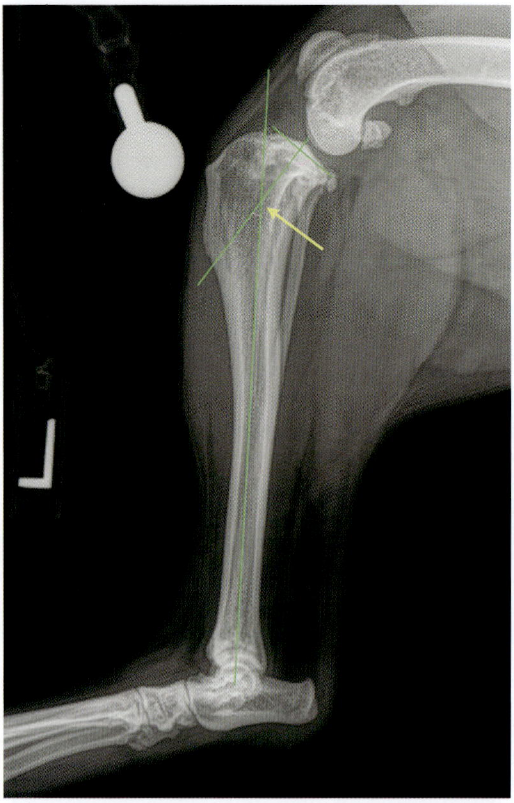

Figure 11.1 A lateral radiograph of the left stifle. Notice how the proximal anatomical longitudinal axis is not aligned with the distal longitudinal axis (green lines). The yellow arrow is the intersection of the proximal and distal longitudinal axis. This intersection is the location of the CORA.

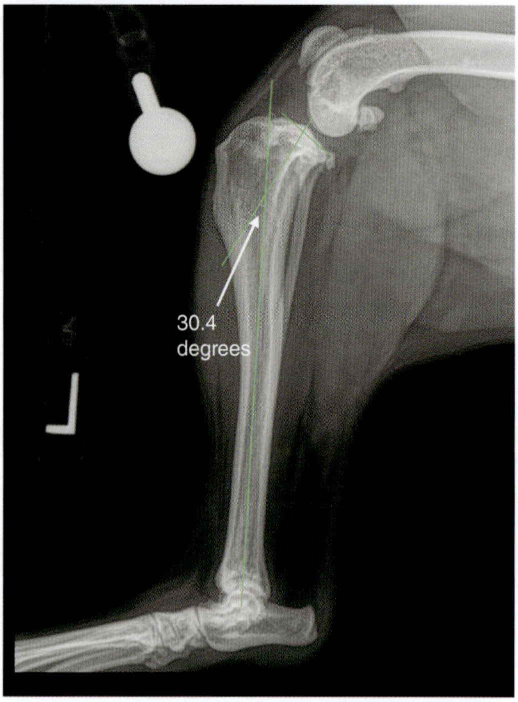

Figure 11.2 The same lateral radiograph as in Figure 11.1; the angle formed at the intersection of the proximal and distal longitudinal axis is the magnitude of the CORA (white arrow). In this example it is 30.4°.

owner evaluation of the CBLO revealed that 77% of the dogs had full function, 19% had acceptable function, and 4% had unacceptable function.

Complications were noted in 16% of the cases, and included incisional issues, late-onset meniscal tear, and implant-related complications [7]. The cases (3/11) that developed incisional issues were resolved with empirical antibiotic administration. In 8/11 cases that needed additional surgery, it was found that the majority (6/8) had late-onset meniscal tears. The two remaining cases (2/8) that required additional surgery had implant-related issues. In one of these cases the compression screw had become loose and was replaced without further incident. The other case was a juvenile dog that developed a tibial valgus secondary to screw malposition into the proximal tibial physis. The dog went on to undergo a tibial corrective surgery. All cases that required a second surgery returned to normal function [7].

11.3 Complications Specific to CORA-Based Leveling Osteotomy

Potential complications are suspected to be similar to other osteotomy procedures, including infection, patellar tendon thickening, postoperative meniscal tears, and pivot shift. These complications are covered elsewhere in this book and will not be discussed here. Complications identified to date specific to the CBLO include discomfort from utilizing a compression screw that is too long, impingement of the cranial distal tuberosity of the proximal segment with the cranial tibial cortex of the distal segment, opening of the cranial aspect of the osteotomy due to pull of the quadriceps, and induction of angulation and/or torsional proximal tibial changes.

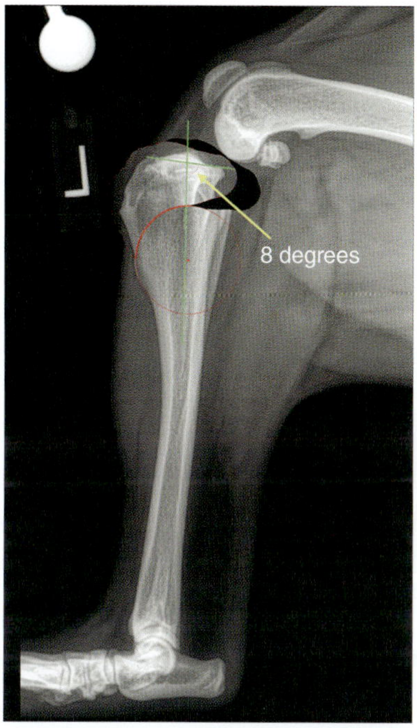

Figure 11.3 A lateral radiograph of the left stifle revealing preoperative planning of rotation of the proximal tibial segment to achieve the desired postoperative TPA (yellow arrow) and thus allowing alignment of the proximal and distal longitudinal axis. In this example the planned postoperative TPA is 8.0°.

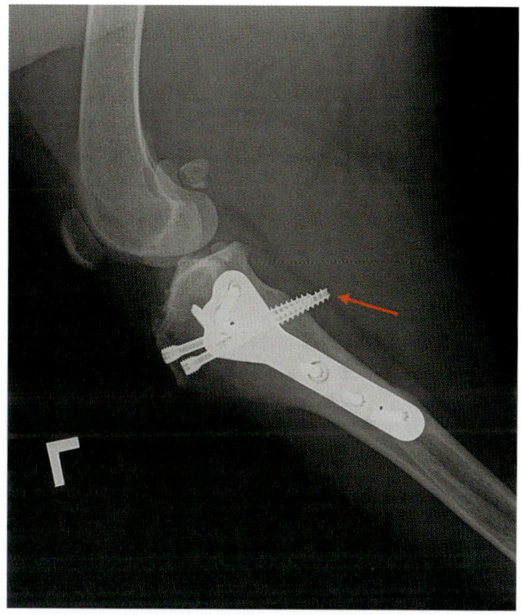

Figure 11.4 A lateral radiograph of the left stifle following complete osteotomy healing. Note the long headless compression screw (red arrow). The screw was impinging on the popliteal and gastrocnemius muscle, causing discomfort. Removal of the screw resulted in resolution of the discomfort.

Given the pull of the quadriceps, it is recommended to use adjunctive fixation across the osteotomy in conjunction with the CBLO plate. This is commonly achieved with a compression or lag screw. This adjunctive fixation is placed before the addition of the CBLO plate. The goal is for the screw to begin at or just proximal to the patellar tendon insertion, cross the osteotomy in a perpendicular fashion and exit the caudal tibial cortex. Failure of the screw to cross the osteotomy perpendicular could result in loss of compression.

Prior to placement of the compression screw, the length is measured using a standard depth gauge. It is important to remember that compression should occur across the osteotomy site so using a screw size that is equal to the depth gauge measurement will likely result in a screw that is 1–2 mm too long. If the popliteal muscle is elevated from the caudal tibial cortex then palpation or visualization of the screw can be seen. Once the screw has been placed and compression achieved, it should be noted how far caudally the screw penetrates the caudal tibial cortex. If a cannulated screw is used and noted to be too long, it should be cut flush with the caudal tibial cortex. If a noncannulated screw is used, then it can be backed out and a shorter one placed. Care should be taken not to damage the screw hole or allow movement of the osteotomy when replacing the compression screw. A compression screw that is too long (Figure 11.4) can irritate the gastrocnemius muscle, causing discomfort. Alternatively, if the screw is too long, it can cause pain while sitting due to the force of the screw into the gastrocnemius as the stifle if flexed.

If discomfort is noted following a CBLO due to a long screw, then it should be removed once osteotomy healing is complete. One author (DLD) evaluated a patient as a second opinion 1 year following a CBLO. This patient would randomly cry out in pain when walking and when sitting. The occurrence of this discomfort was noted immediately postoperatively. As a result, there was moderate to severe muscle atrophy of the operated limb due to chronic

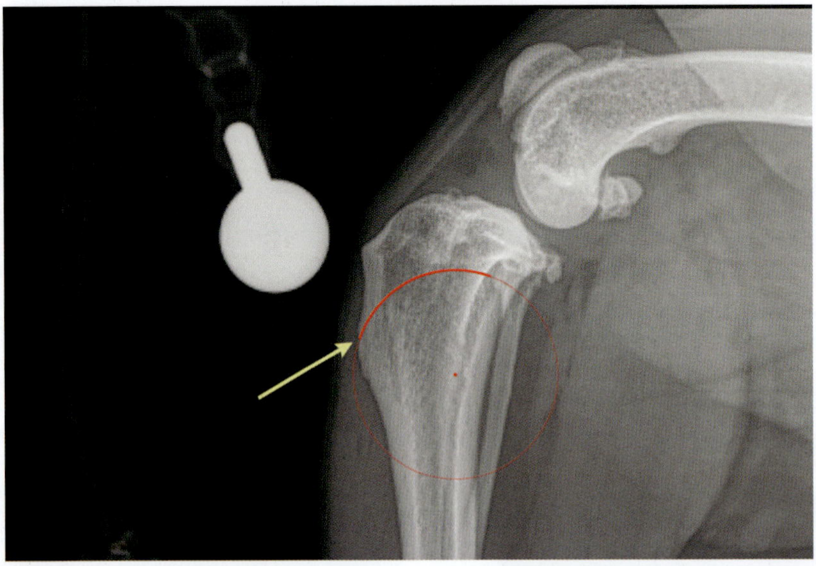

Figure 11.5 The goal of the cranial exit of the osteotomy is that it is tangent to the cranial tibial cortex (yellow arrow) while leaving as much of the tibial tuberosity as possible.

disuse. While stability of the stifle was noted, range of motion was reduced in flexion with a "hard-end feel" and pain. Radiographs of the patient revealed two headless compression screws that were too long (Figure 11.4). Removal of the screws led to complete resolution of the clinical signs and improved limb usage.

An osteotomy that is tangent to the cranial tibial cortex is recommended (Figure 11.5) while leaving as much of the tibial tuberosity as possible. During the cranial rotation, this can result in impingement of the cranial distal tuberosity of the proximal segment with the cranial tibial cortex of the distal segment. Planning of the osteotomy with the millimeters of rotation needed can help minimize this. This is particularly true in patients with a larger CORA magnitude and thus larger rotation. If impingement is noted during rotation or rotation cannot be completed, then the most cranio-distal aspect of the proximal segment can be removed to allow rotation. This can be accomplished with a small osteotome and mallet. Forcing rotation with impingement present can result in fissuring of the cranio-distal aspect of the proximal segment (Figure 11.6) or, worse, fracture of the tibial tuberosity or tibial diaphysis.

A major force acting on the osteotomy and thus leading to implant breakdown is the pull

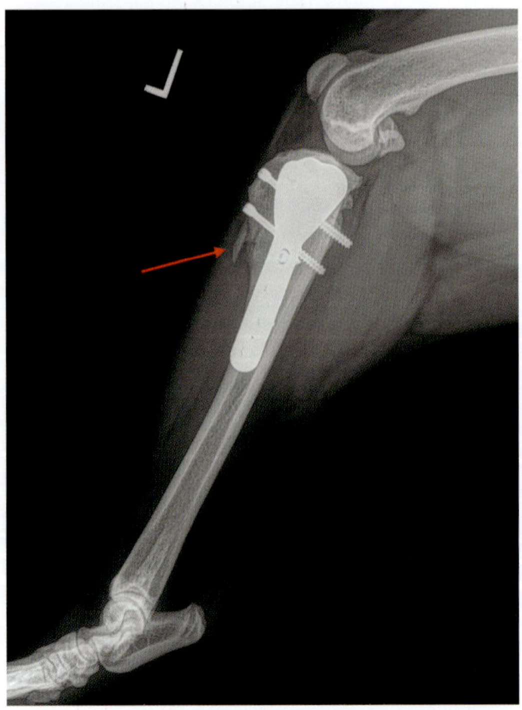

Figure 11.6 Impingement of the cranial cortex of the proximal fragment resulted in fissuring. No additional treatment was needed; however, attention to osteotomy placement intraoperatively is needed to avoid creating an osteotomy that is sloped and exiting the cranial cortex too far distally.

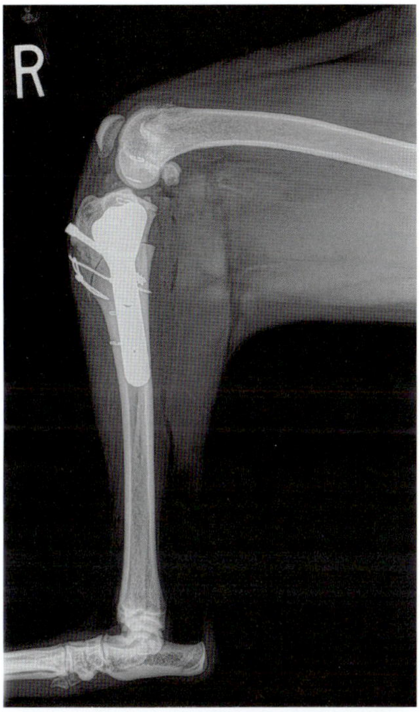

Figure 11.7 Immediate lateral postoperative radiograph following a right CBLO. The current recommendation for stability is placement of a CBLO plate, headless compression screw, and a tension band fixation.

of the quadriceps. Therefore, ample fixation of the CBLO is warranted. Unfortunately, the exact amount of force to be counteracted is not known. Current research is focusing on the biomechanics of various forms of fixation to determine what is the most stable. However, at the current time the recommendation for fixation is utilization of a compression/lag screw with a bone plate and screws and augmentation of a tension band fixation (Figure 11.7).

The failure caused by lack of adequate fixation is most commonly noted by widening of the cranial aspect of the osteotomy. This is most commonly noted by widening of the cranial aspect of the osteotomy (Figure 11.8). This could be an incidental finding or result in acute worsening of limb usage. If there is widening of the cranial aspect of the osteotomy, this will also lead to a loss of TPA and could render the stifle unstable. Revision surgery would be recommended if there is instability of the proximal segment. This is determined by taking a traditional lateral radiograph of the stifle and then a hyperflexed lateral radiograph of the stifle.

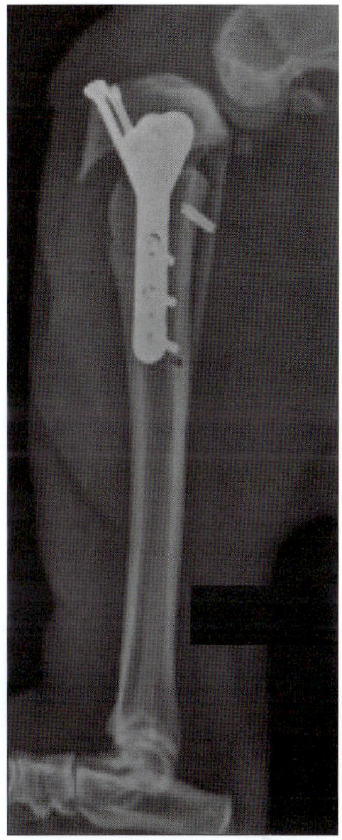

Figure 11.8 Ten-day postoperative lateral radiograph of a 170 lb dog following a CBLO. Notice the widening of the osteotomy leading to loss of reduction and an increase in the tibial plateau angle. In addition, there is evidence of a broken screw. This complication likely occurred due to inadequate stabilization.

Widening of the osteotomy on the hyperflexed view could indicate instability of the proximal segment. In addition, revision surgery may be recommended if there is loss of the TPA resulting in positive cranial tibial thrust or if there is severe acute worsening of limb usage. Ensuring robust fixation across the osteotomy with attention to counteraction of the pull of the quadriceps is needed to minimize widening of the osteotomy gap.

Rotation of the proximal segment cranially in relation to the distal segment is needed for the CBLO to be effective. Similar to a tibial plateau leveling osteotomy (TPLO), this results in a step at the osteotomy site. With a TPLO, there should be a medial step of the distal segment. This is due to the caudal rotation and the shape of the proximal tibia. With caudal rotation of the proximal segment, the cranio-proximal

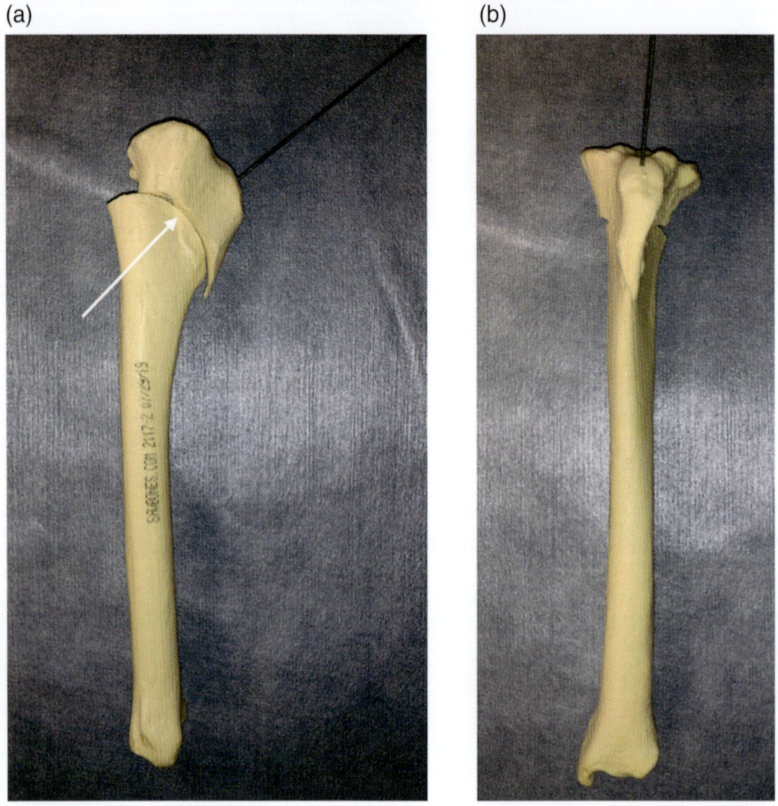

Figure 11.9 **(a)** Medial aspect of the tibia of a bone model demonstrating the lateral step of the distal segment (white arrow). **(b)** Frontal view of the tibia of a bone model revealing appropriate joint alignment of the proximal and distal tibial articular surfaces following rotation and ensuring the lateral step of the distal segment.

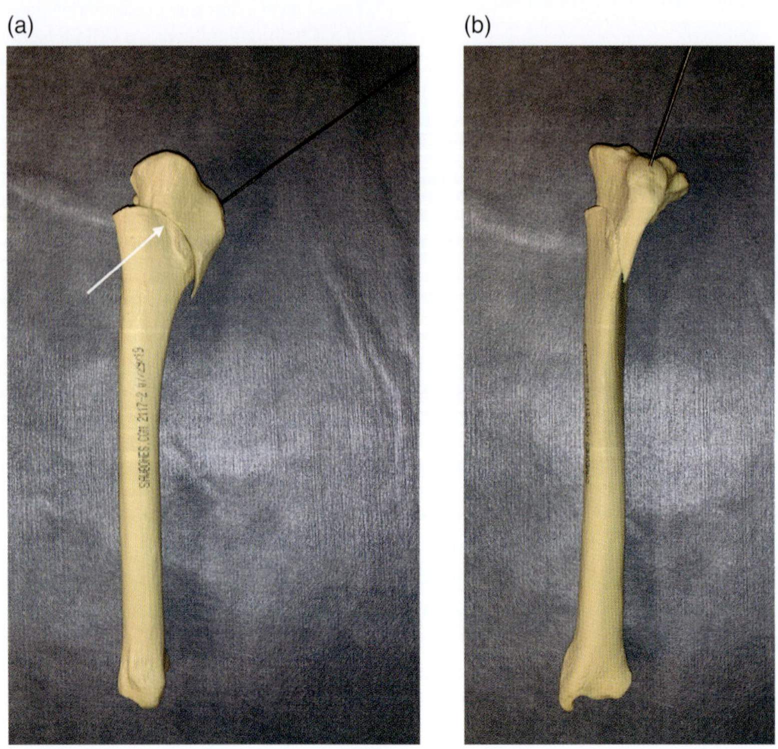

Figure 11.10 **(a)** Medial aspect of the tibia of a bone model demonstrating lack of the lateral step of the distal segment (white arrow). In this situation, the medial cortices of both segments are lined up. **(b)** Frontal view of the tibia of a bone model revealing inappropriate joint alignment of the proximal and distal tibial articular surfaces following rotation. This should be avoided by ensuring a lateral step of the distal segment.

aspect of the tibia is narrower than the disto-caudal aspect of the distal segment. With the CBLO, the cranial rotation will result in a lateral step of the distal segment (Figure 11.9). This is due to the fact that the proximo-caudal aspect of the proximal segment is wider than the disto-cranial aspect of the distal segment. It is important that one does not try to line up the osteotomy of the proximal and distal segments; doing so can result in a translational effect of the proximal segment or induction of proximal tibial varus or valgus (Figure 11.10).

To minimize this complication, it is imperative that a TPLO jig be used. The jig is applied in the same fashion as when used for the TPLO. Briefly, a 25 G needle is used to locate the caudo-proximal aspect of the stifle joint. The proximal jig pin is placed about 3–4 mm distal to the joint surface and caudal to the medial collateral ligament. The proximal jig pin should be driven parallel to the joint surface and perpendicular to the sagittal plane. The distal jig pin is inserted in the distal tibial diaphysis/metaphysis and driven parallel to the proximal jig pin and perpendicular to the sagittal plane.

11.4 Tips to Minimize Complications

Laceration of the cranial tibial artery has been noted in patients undergoing TPLO, and methods to control hemorrhaging following a TPLO have been described [8]. To date, no method has been described to control hemorrhaging following a CBLO but the same techniques used to control bleeding following a TPLO can likely be used [8]. To minimize damage to the vessel, the authors recommend elevation of the popliteal muscle from the caudal tibial cortex along with packing of the area with gauze during the osteotomy. To help maintenance of gauze position as well as tissue retraction, the authors recommend using a single moistened gauze placed between the popliteal muscle and caudal tibial cortex. The most proximal and distal aspects of the gauze are marked and held in place using two 18 G hypodermic needles. Once the osteotomy is complete, the gauze should be removed prior to rotation.

It could be argued that protection of the artery is more important with a CBLO over a TPLO because the rotation of the CBLO is cranial as opposed to caudal with a TPLO. Pozzi et al. proposed that in cases of mild hemorrhaging, the caudal rotation of the TPLO can compress the cranial tibial artery and minimize bleeding [9]. Currently, no investigation has been performed looking at the vascular trauma following a CBLO.

Another consideration is avoidance of the compression screw when placing the plate screws. It is recommended that preoperative planning be completed (Figure 11.11) prior to placing any implants to ensure there will be no implant conflict. Using a cannulated headless compression screw can aid in plate placement. Leaving the K-wire in the headless compression screw allows one to visualize the trajectory of the compression screw to help avoid conflict when placing the plate screws. As noted earlier, from a biomechanical standpoint it is not known what means of fixation is needed to counteract the pull of the quadriceps. Currently, in an unpublished study by one of the authors (DLD), *in vitro* data reveal the best resistance to the pull of the quadriceps mechanism is

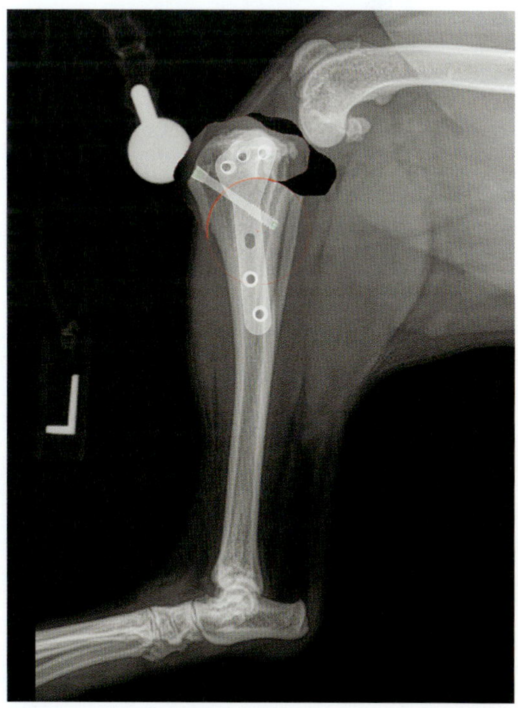

Figure 11.11 Preoperative planning radiograph to ensure that plate placement will not interfere with the headless compression screw.

through adding a tension band fixation along with the compression screw and CBLO plate. Radiographically, it has been shown that quicker healing is achieved with the addition of a tension band fixation along with the compression screw and plate [4]. Therefore, the current recommendation for biomechanical strength is utilization of a tension band fixation, headless compression screw, and CBLO plate. Preoperative and intraoperative planning of the plate placement is needed to ensure that the tension band hole is not at or in the cranial tibial cortex. In some situations, this may necessitate the use of a smaller plate.

As with any procedure, catastrophic failure can occur following a CBLO. This can be the result of uncontrolled excessive activity in the 2–4 weeks following surgery. Alternatively, it can be the result of the attending surgeon making poor decisions or technical errors. An example of poor decision making is exemplified in Figure 11.12. In this case, a standard 3.5 plate was used to stabilize the osteotomy in a 170 lb dog. The fixation failed within 10 days following surgery (Figure 11.8). Revision surgery is achieved with removal of failed implants and stabilization with medial and cranial locking plates (Figure 11.13).

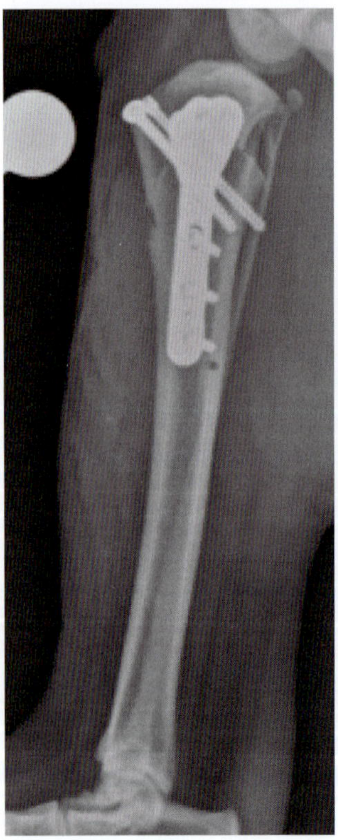

Figure 11.12 Immediate postoperative lateral radiograph of a 170 lb dog following a CBLO. The osteotomy was stabilized with a standard 3.5 mm CBLO plate, one headless compression screw, and one positional cortical screw. In a dog of this size, while radiographs may appear appropriate, the osteotomy is not stable. Ideally, a 3.5 mm broad CBLO plate or a double plating technique should have been used.

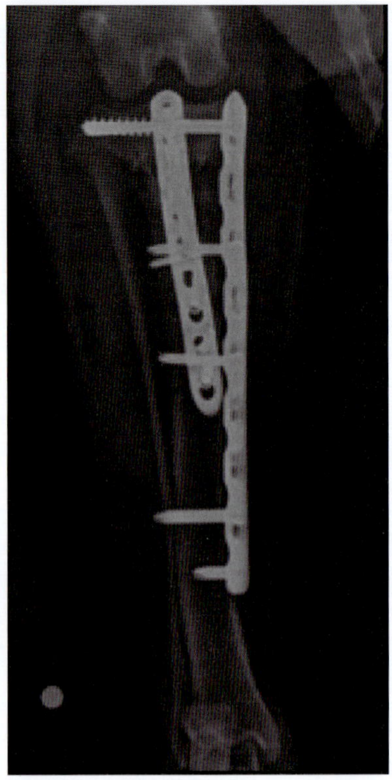

Figure 11.13 Immediate cranio-caudal postoperative view following revision surgery of the dog in Figure 11.12. The CBLO plate and screws were removed and the osteotomy was reduced and stabilized by using two 3.5 mm plates, one cranially and one medially.

References

1. Hulse, D., Beale, B., and Kowaleski, M. (2010). CORA based leveling osteotomy for the treatment of the CCL deficient stifle (abstract). In: *Proceedings of the World Orthopaedic Veterinary Congress. Bologna, Italy*, 120–121.

2. Hulse, D., Beale, B., and Kowaleski, M. (2010). CORA based leveling osteotomy for the treatment of the CCL deficient stifle (abstract). In: *Proceedings of the American College of Veterinary Surgeons Symposium. Seattle, WA*, 516–518.
3. Raske, M., Hulse, D., Beale, B. et al. (2013). Stabilization of the CORA based leveling osteotomy for treatment of cranial cruciate ligament injury using a bone plate augmented with a headless compression screw. *Vet. Surg.* 42: 759–764.
4. Johnson, T., Hulse, D., Peycke, L. et al. (2018). Radiographic healing following stabilization of cranial cruciate ligament deficient stifles with a CORA based leveling osteotomy, bone plate/headless compression screw, augmented with a tension band (abstract). *Vet. Comp. Orthop. Traumatol.* 31 (S02): A1–A25.
5. Vasquez, B., Hule, D., Beale, B. et al. (2018). Second-look arthroscopic findings after CORA-based leveling osteotomy. *Vet. Surg.* 47: 261–266.
6. McDougall, R., Dycus, D.L., Peycke, L. et al. (2018). Evaluating the feasibility and long-term outcome of the CORA-based leveling osteotomy in juvenile dogs (abstract). *Vet. Surg.* 47: E1–E69.
7. Kishi, E. and Hulse, D. (2016). Owner evaluation of a CORA-based leveling osteotomy for treatment of cranial cruiate ligament injury in dogs. *Vet. Surg.* 45: 507–514.
8. Matres-Lorenzo, L., McAlinden, A., Bernarde, A. et al. (2018). Control of hemorrhage through the osteotomy gap during tibial plateau leveling osteotomy: 9 cases. *Vet. Surg.* 47: 60–65.
9. Pozzi, A., Samii, V., and Horodyski, M.B. (2011). Evaluation of vascular trauma after tibial plateau leveling osteotomy with or without gauze protection. *Vet. Comp. Orthop. Traumatol.* 24: 266–271.

12 Complications Associated with Tibial Tuberosity Advancement

Matthew D. Barnhart

12.1 Introduction

Tibial tuberosity advancement (TTA) is a well-accepted, extensively published, and proven surgical technique for treating the lameness associated with canine cranial cruciate ligament (CCL) disease. Since it was first reported in 2002 by Montavan, numerous descriptions of other similar procedures have been published [1]. Despite variations in the techniques and implants used, the modified Maquet and tibial tuberosity advancement rapid (TTA-R) procedures are very similar to the original TTA in principle. All attempt to neutralize the cranial tibiofemoral shear force generated in the CCL-deficient stifle by cranially advancing a longitudinal frontal plane osteotomy of the tibial crest until the attached straight patella ligament insertion is approximately perpendicular to the tibial plateau. All then utilize procedure-specific implants to stabilize the osteotomy in the advanced position.

The TTA-R is a modification of the TTA in that it utilizes an osteotomy of the proximal tibia which is incomplete distally. As originally described, the osteotomy ends distally in a Maquet hole in order to minimize the chance of fissure formation; however, it is not always used [2, 3]. A single implant that functions as both an advancement wedge and a plate is used to stabilize the osteotomy (Figure 12.1). Between the two techniques, the original TTA has been the subject of the majority of published studies to date. The frequency of reported complications for both surgeries is similar to that of other tibial osteotomy-based stifle procedures [4–8]. This chapter will focus on complications associated with the TTA and TTA-R while the modified Maquet technique will be the focus of Chapter 13.

Tibial tuberosity advancement surgery not only has the potential for development of general surgical complications but also those associated with an osteotomy and internal fixation and those unique to the technique itself. Numerous reports exist describing complications associated with TTA surgery. Making direct comparisons between these studies is difficult because how the complications are reported relative to type, timing, and classification varies considerably among publications. Table 12.1 provides a comprehensive list of the studies that report complications with TTA and TTA-R surgery. The complications are generally divided relative to timing (intraoperative and postoperative) and further divided into

Complications in Canine Cranial Cruciate Ligament Surgery, First Edition. Edited by Ron Ben-Amotz and David L. Dycus.

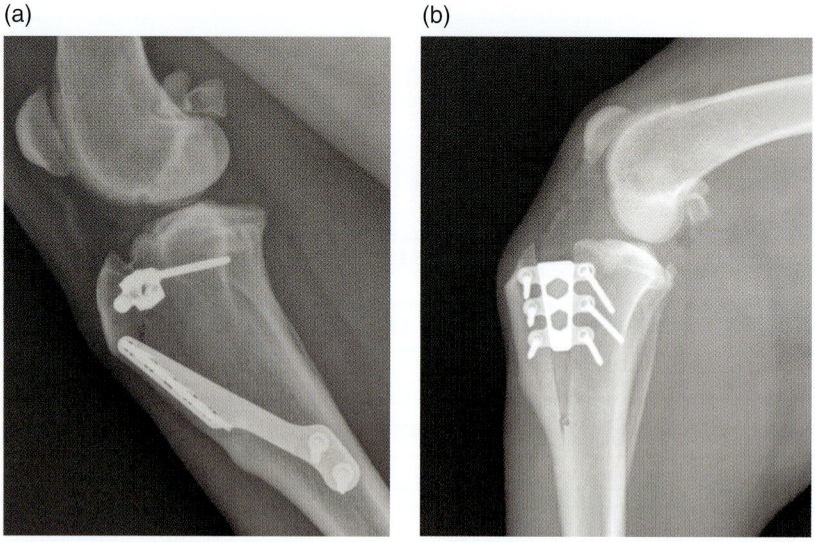

Figure 12.1 Medio-lateral postoperative radiographs of the (a) original TTA and (b) TTA-rapid procedures. Source: Image (b) courtesy of Dr Justin Harper.

severity (major and minor). The greatest variability exists with the latter, with some studies not distinguishing between major and minor, others use different criteria for classification inclusion and still others report on only one type of complication (i.e., major only). While rates vary among the 21 studies, the types of intraoperative and postoperative complications described are similar.

12.2 Intraoperative Complications

Intraoperative complications are only sporadically included in TTA and TTA-R studies. When evaluated as part of TTA study objectives, they either did not occur [9, 10] or were both rare and minor (0.4–3.1%) [11–14]. Intraoperative TTA complications included trans cortical chip fractures, screws stripping, breakage of cage flanges, intraarticular screw placement, nondisplaced tibial fracture, broken drill bits and screws, etc. One study described a tibial tuberosity fracture that was remedied by modifying the plate size and position [15]. Hoffmann et al. reported an inadvertent transection of the long digital extensor tendon during the osteotomy. It was not repaired and did not appear to affect patient recovery [12].

Compared to TTA, TTA-R has a higher incidence of reported intraoperative complications ranging from 2% to 8.3% [3, 16]. Among the four studies that documented TTA-R intraoperative complication occurrence, the most common (75%, 9/12) were fractures/fissures at the level of the Maquet hole and/or distal tibial crest, three of which were classified as major complications [2, 3, 16, 17]. These findings have prompted some surgeons to debate the value of the Maquet hole and discontinue its use in TTA-R surgery [3]. This is discussed further in Chapter 13.

Only a single study exists which directly compares short-term outcomes and complications between two types of TTA: the original TTA and a modified Maquet-tibial tuberosity advancement (mTTA) technique [9]. No intraoperative complications were reported in the 35 TTA cases compared to 5/35 (14.2%) of mTTA cases that developed fractures at the Maquet hole. The latter required no treatment and were deemed of questionable clinical significance after the 8-week postoperative follow-up was completed.

The reported low incidence of intraoperative TTA complications is consistent with this author's experience; they are rare and when they do occur, require either no or only minor treatment. Difficulty closing fascia and the aponeurosis of the gracilis, semimembranosus, and semitendinosus muscles (pes anserinus) over the TTA osteotomy gap and implants is, in my experience, the most commonly encountered intraoperative TTA challenge yet is not mentioned in the literature. This difficulty is not surprising given that one is attempting to reappose a minimally compliant tissue over a newly widened proximal tibia with a large defect (i.e., osteotomy gap). Excessive tension of this closure can lead to early dehiscence, seroma formation, and a transient increase in lameness. If necessary, the tension can be relieved by making a releasing incision through the pes anserinus and caudal aspect of the tibial fascia under which there are no implants or osteotomy.

Implant placement complications were common during the early learning phase of the TTA technique, particularly when attempting to ensure the fork engaged properly with the multiple tibial tuberosity drill holes and the plate. Incomplete fork–bone tunnel engagement and/or bent fork tines were a source of challenge. The creation of a TTA plate that secures the plate to the tibial crest using bone screws alleviated these issues entirely and is a proven alternative to the fork-based plate (Figure 12.2) [9, 15, 18]. Broken cage flanges are usually a result of overzealous countering. The flanges (aka "wings") are small and not very stiff and will actually self-contour as the screw engages the bone, so precise contouring is not necessary. Trans cortical chip fractures are most often incidental findings on postoperative radiographs and in the author's experience do not require specific treatment as long as the applied screw in question has engaged the bone well. Additionally, the author has found that the cranial cage screw can be more prone to stripping if applied perpendicular to the bone. This is particularly true if the medial to lateral tibial tuberosity osteotomy is directed slightly cranially. This may cause that screw to only engage the cis cortex if driven perpendicularly (Figure 12.3). Routinely angling this screw cranially will help to prevent this regardless of osteotomy obliquity.

Many of the intraoperative complications associated with tibial plateau leveling osteotomy (TPLO), such as fibula fracture, popliteal, or cranial tibial artery laceration, retained surgical sponges and jig pin fractures, are not reported or expected during TTA because of the technical differences between the two surgeries [6, 8]. Additionally, inadvertent intrarticular screw placement, while documented with TTA, is far less likely to occur during TTA than TPLO. However, to avoid the latter, caudal cage screws should be angled in a slightly distal direction.

12.3 Postoperative Complications – Overall Frequency

"Overall complication rates" are perhaps the most referenced and discussed form of documented complications for any given surgery and are often used as an indirect indicator of procedure success. However, they are the most difficult to compare between studies because of methodology variations and should therefore be considered cautiously. As stated by Cook et al. regarding the veterinary literature, "This lack of standardization limits our abilities to communicate study results in a consistent manner, interpret data appropriately, and compare results across studies, centers, and techniques" [19]. Reports on TTA complications are no exception. As stated earlier, there is considerable variation among TTA studies relative to how and what complications are reported. Additionally, many of the studies are hampered by low sample populations and thus prone to type II error. Nonetheless, Table 12.1 includes an extensive list of the different published TTA and TTA-R complication rates, either as directly reported by the study or as extrapolated by this author. For the purpose of this discussion, overall complication rate includes intraoperative and postoperative complications (major and minor).

Of the 17 TTA studies in Table 12.1, only six provide enough information to determine an overall rate. Rates range from 8.6% to 59% (mean = 25.4%) for TTA and 11.8% to 61.5% (mean = 34%) for TTA-R. All of these studies were retrospective. The highest rate of 59% was reported by Hoffmann et al. who included any observed perioperative abnormality as a complication including inappetance, diarrhea, vomiting, lethargy, etc. [12]. The lowest rate of 8.6% came from a study of 35 dogs, the smallest sample size of any of the six TTA studies included [9]. By contrast, the single largest TTA study to provide an overall complication included 501 stifles and reported a rate of 19% [14]. An overall rate can be determined for all four of the TTA-R studies. The highest rate reported for TTA-R was 61.5%, which included a very small sample population of 13 dogs [17]. A much larger sample population of 152 stifles, the largest published TTA-R study to date, provided a much lower rate of 11.8% [16].

As with any complicated surgical technique, surgeon experience plays an understated but key

Table 12.1 Summary of publications which report complications associated with tibial tuberosity advancement (TTA) and tibial tuberosity advancement-rapid (TTA-R).

Author (year) Sample Population	Objectives	Intraoperative (IOP) Complications	Major / Minor Postoperative (PO) Complication Rate	Overall Complication Rate	Major Postoperative Complications (n)	Minor Postoperative Complications (n)	Risk Factors Identified	Mensical Release Done? Protective ?	Postoperative Antibiotic? Protective?
Bisgard, et al (2011) 125 dogs	Retrospective study of TTA plate type and graft effect on postoperative complications	Not evaluated	3/125 (2.4%) 1 0/125 (8%)	13/125 10.4% (major + minor PO)	Fractures (3)	Fractures (6) Implant loosening (4)	No risk factors for complications indentified	Yes Not evaluated	Yes Not evaluated
Butterworth, et al (2017) 152 stifles	Retrospective study of TTA Rapid short- and medium-term outcome	3/152 2%	Not differentiated* (15/152 PO)	18/152 11.8% (IOP + PO*)	Meniscal tear (9)* Fissures/ Fractures (3)* Infection (3)*		Not evaluated	Not reported	Not reported
Calvo, et al (2014) 200 stifles	Retrospective study of tibial tuberosity fracture as a complication of TTA	Not evaluated	4/200 (2%) 6/200 (3%)	10/200 5% (major + minor PO)	Fractures (4)	Fractures (7)	Not evaluated	Not evaluated	Not evaluated
Costa, et al (2017) 1613 dogs	Retrospective study of major TTA complications	Not evaluated	216/1613 13.4% Not reported	216/1613 13.4% (major PO)	Infection (112) Patella luxation (20) Implant failure (17) Fractures (16) Meniscal tear (4)		No risk factors for complications indentified	Yes Yes	Yes Not evaluated
de Lima Dantas et al (2016) 307 stifles	Retrospective study of TTA complication incidence in Boxer vs. to non Boxer dogs	6/307 2%	51/307 (16.6%) 12/307 (3.9%)	69/307 22.5% (IOP+ major + minor PO)	Infection (18) Mensical tear (4) Fractures (3) Patella luxation (2)	Fractures (4) Patellar desmitis (2) Implant loosening (2) Seroma (1) Swelling (2) Lick granuloma (1)	Risk factor: Boxer breed	Yes (n=3) Not evaluated	Yes (n=176) No
Dymond, et al (2010)[a]	Retrospective study of TTA outcomes and complications	Not reported	6/92 (6.5%) 27/92 (29.3%)	33/92 35.8% (major + minor PO)	Meniscal tear (4) Fractures (2)	Incision bruising & swelling (13) Infection (8)	Not evaluated	No	Yes (n=15) Not evaluated
Dyall, et al (2017) 92 stifles	Prospective evaluation of TTA Rapid in small dogs: complications and outcomes	4/48 8.3%	5/48 (10.4%) 1/48 (2.1%)	10/48 20.8% (IOP + major + minor PO)	Fissures/Fractures (2) Meniscal tear (2) Infection (1)	Incisional swelling (1)	Not evaluated	Not reported	Not reported
Edwards et al (2016) 438 stifles	Retrospective study of major complications with fork- and screw-based TTA implants	5/438 1.1%	46/438 (10.5%) Not evaluated	49/438 11.6% (major PO and IOP)	Meniscal tear (13) Implant loosening (11) Infection (9) Patella luxation (5) Implant failure (3) Fractures (2)		No risk factors for complications indentified	Yes (n=124) Not evaluated	Not reported
Ferreira, et al (2019)[b] 35 stifles	Prospective study of TTA in small breed dogs	Not reported	2/35 (5.7%) None	2/35 5.7% (major + minor PO)	Incision dehiscence (1) Implant loosening (1)		Not evaluated	No	Yes Not evaluated
Ferrell et al (2019) 1768 stifles	Retrospective study of antibiotic impact on TTA infection rates and implant removal	Not evaluated	Not differentiated*	82/1768 4.6% (infection only*)	Infection (82)*		Postop antibiotic use associated with oxacillin-resistant infection	Not evaluated	Yes No
Hans, et al (2017) 91 stifles (TTAs)	Retrospective study of TPLO and TTA postoperative complications in dogs >50kg	Not evaluated	TTAs only 18/91 (19.8%) 13/91 (14.3%)	31/91 (TTA) 34.1% (major + minor PO)	Infection (14) Fracture (4)	Seroma (7) Fracture (3) Patellar desmitis (1) Implant failure (1) Partial incision dehiscence (1)	High bodyweight	Yes Not evaluated	Yes Yes

Author (year) Sample Population	Objectives	Intraoperative (IOP) Complications	Major / Minor Postoperative (PO) Complication Rate	Overall Complication Rate	Major Postoperative Complications (n)	Minor Postoperative Complications (n)	Risk Factors Identified	Mensical Release Done? Protective ?	Postoperative Antibiotic? Protective?
Hoffmann, et al (2006) 65 stifles	Retrospective study of TTAs (included ANY postop abnormality as a complication-inappetance, etc.)	2/65 3.1%	Not differentiated*	38/65 59% (IOP + PO*)	Incision bruising & swelling (21)* Infection (4)* Implant failure (4)* Meniscal tear (3)* Patella luxation (1)* Fractures (1)*		Not evaluated	No	No
Lafaver, et al (2007) 114 stifles	Retrospective study of early TTA results and complications	1/114 0.9%	14/114 (12.3%) 22/114 (19.3%)	37/114 32.4% (IOP + major + minor PO)	Meniscal tear (7) Fractures (2) Lick granuloma (2) Implant failure (1) Infection (1) Poor performance (1)	Fractures (4) Suspected meniscal tear (3) Implant failure (3) Limb swelling (3) incision issues (4) Incomplete healing (3)	Not evaluated	Yes (n=22) Yes	Not reported
Livet, et al (2019) 13 dogs (TTAs)	Prospective study comparing outcomes between TPLO and TTA Rapid	1/13 (TTA-R) 7.7%	TTA-R only 4/13 (30.8%) 3/13 (23%)	8/13 (TTA-R) 61.5% (IOP + major + minor PO)	Meniscal tear (2) Patellar desmitis (1) Implant loosening (1)	Infection (2) Implant loosening (1)	Not evaluated	Not reported	No
Nutt, et al (2015) 254 stifles	Retrospective study of risk factors for tibial tuberosity fracture after TTA	Not evaluated	Not differentiated*	13/254 5.1% (PO*)	Fractures (13)*		Osteotomy shape, plate & cage position	Not evaluated	Not evaluated
Retallack, et al (2018) 70 dogs (35-mTTA, 35-TTA)	Modified Maquet (m) TTA compared to TTA: retrospective study of short term outcome and complications	5/35 (mTTA) 14.2% 0/35 (TTA) 0%	mTTA - 1/35 (2.9%) TTA- 1/35 (2.9%) mTTA- 3/35 (8.6%) TTA- 2/35 (5.7%)	9/35 (mTTA) 25.7% 3/35 (TTA) 8.6% (IOP + major + minor PO)	Wound dehiscence (1-mTTA, 1-TTA)	Fissures/ Fractures (2-mTTA) Infection (1-mTTA, 2-TTA)	Not evaluated	Yes Not evaluated	Not reported
Samoy, et al (2015) 50 dogs	Prospective study of TTA Rapid- technique and short term results	4/50 8%	2/50 (4%) 15/50 (30%)	21/50 42% (IOP + major + minor PO)	Fractures (2)	Patellar tendon thickening (12) Fractures (4)	Not evaluated	Yes Not evaluated	Yes Not evaluated
Stein, et al (2008) 70 stifles	Retrospective study of short term and 8-12 month results of TTA	Not reported	12/70 (17.1%) Not reported	12/70 17.1% (major PO)	Meniscal tear (6) Fractures (3) Incision dehiscence (1) 2nd look arthroscopy required (2)		Not evaluated	No	No
Steinberg, et al (2011) 193 stifles	Retrospective study to describe TTA complications and risk factors	0/193 0%	Not differentiated* (21/193 PO)	21/193 11% (IOP + PO*)	Meniscal tear (10)* Implant failure (2)* Fracture (2)* Patella luxation (1)* Infection (1)*		Increasing bodyweight, small cage size	Yes (n=2) Not evaluated	Not reported
Wolf, et al (2012) 501 stifles	Retrospective study of TTA surgical and postoperative complications	2/501 0.4%	57/501 (11.4%) 38/501 (17.6%)	97/501 19% (IOP + major + minor PO)	Fracture (21) Meniscal tear (17) Implant failure (10) Incision closure (3) Implant removal (3) Patella luxation (2)	Incision infection (33) Seroma (3) Patellar tendonitis (2)	High body weight, preoperative patella tendon angle	Yes Yes	Varied Not evaluted
Yap, et al (2015) 224 stifles	Retrospective study of TTA perioperative risk factors for SSI	Not evaluated	Not differentiated*	12/224 5.3% (infection only*)	Infection (12)		Increased surgical & anesthesia time	Not evaluated	Yes No

[a]Major and minor complications were not differentiated in the manuscript.

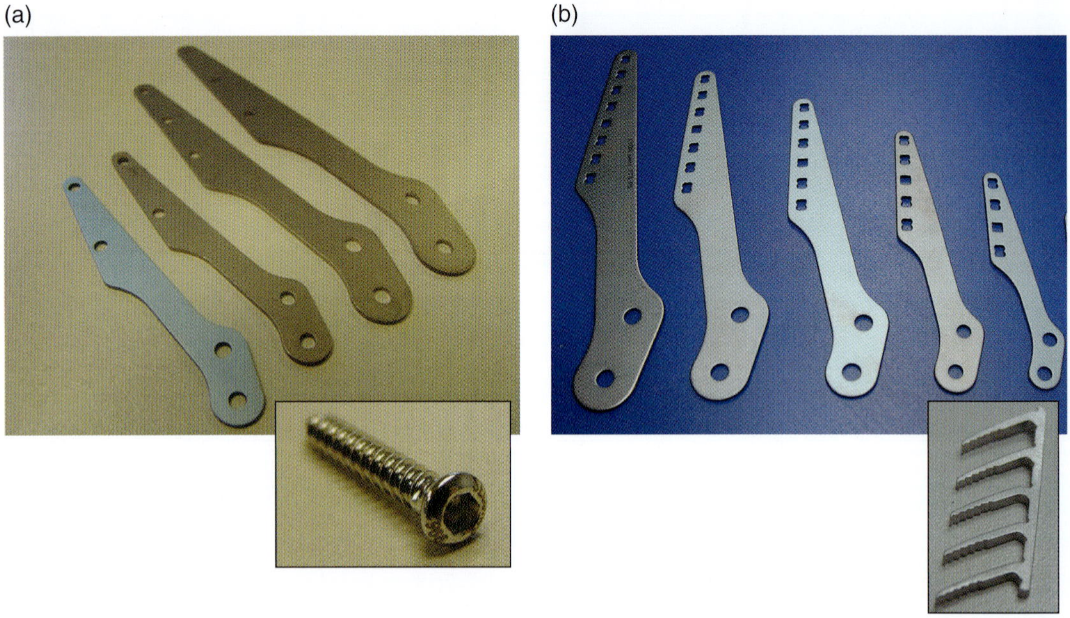

Figure 12.2 (a) Screw and (b) fork-based TTA plates.

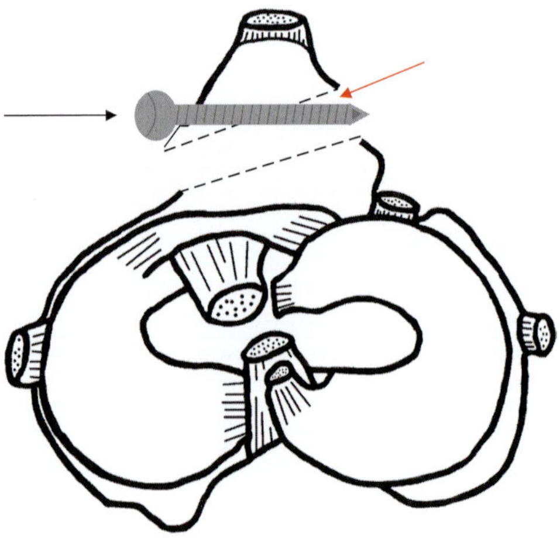

Figure 12.3 A proximodistal view of the articular surface of the tibia. A cranially directed osteotomy (dotted black lines) creates a segment of bone with more available cis than trans cortex. A screw driven perpendicular (black arrow) will not engage the trans cortex (red arrow), resulting in monocortical screw placement that is prone to stripping.

role in TTA outcomes and complication rates. Multiple reports have documented the impact that increasing surgical experience with TTA has on reducing complications [13, 20, 21]. Performing a clinical audit for TTA using the cumulative summation technique, Proot and Corr determined that the learning curve for an experienced general practitioner to reach complication rates within published ranges is 22 procedures [21].

12.4 Postoperative Complications – Minor

Minor postoperative complications are included less frequently in TTA studies compared to major complications. Of the 17 TTA studies that report on postoperative complications, only nine differentiate them as minor or major compared to three of four TTA-R studies. The mean minor TTA complication rate from these studies is 11.2% (range 0–29.3%) and for TTA-R 18.4% (range 2.7–30%). It is worth noting that if minor complications were defined as those not requiring *any* additional surgical or medical treatment to resolve, many of those listed in Table 12.1 would be reclassified as major [19]. This is particularly true of the "minor" surgical site infections (SSIs) because they often required antibiotic therapy for resolution.

Interestingly, postoperative tibial fractures, which might be presumed to be a more severe complication, are a commonly reported articular complication in many TTA and TTA-R studies [2, 4, 11, 13, 18, 22]. They are often discovered

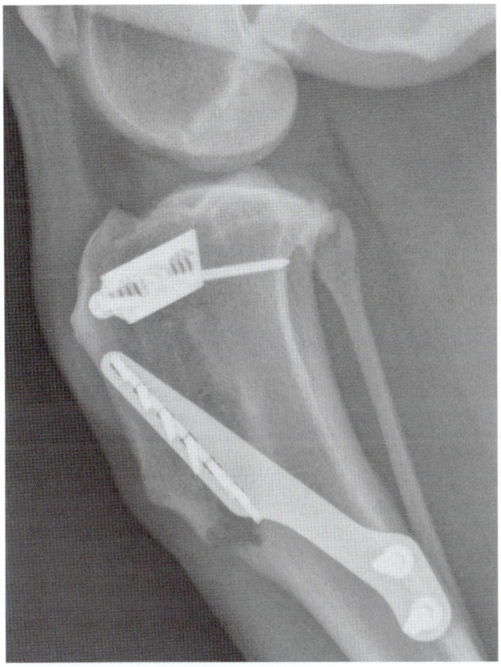

Figure 12.4 A distal tibial tuberosity avulsion fracture involving the fork tines and subsequent partial loss of internal fixation found incidentally on scheduled 8-week postoperative reevaluation radiographs. It was deemed a minor postoperative complication because no treatment was required for a satisfactory outcome. Note the nearly complete osetotomy healing despite the complication occurrence. The technical error that likely lead to this fracture was poor distal plate position.

as incidental findings on scheduled postoperative radiographs with no clinical history or physical findings supportive of an impactful complication. This author's experience is consistent with these reports (Figure 12.4).

The decision of how to proceed with a tibial fracture following TTA should be based on the severity of the clinical signs, degree of radiographic healing, and postoperative timing versus fracture configuration and degree of displacement [22]. These recommendations are consistent with this author's experience in that many seemingly severe postoperative fractures can be managed successfully without surgery. This is particularly true when the patella mechanism appears unaffected by the fracture (Figure 12.5). However, fractures that produce morbidity and/or are expected to negatively impact long-term outcomes are not minor and should not be considered candidates for conservative management.

12.5 Postoperative Complications – Major

In contrast to minor complication rates, the majority of TTA studies provide information on major postoperative complications. The largest sample population TTA study to date of 1613

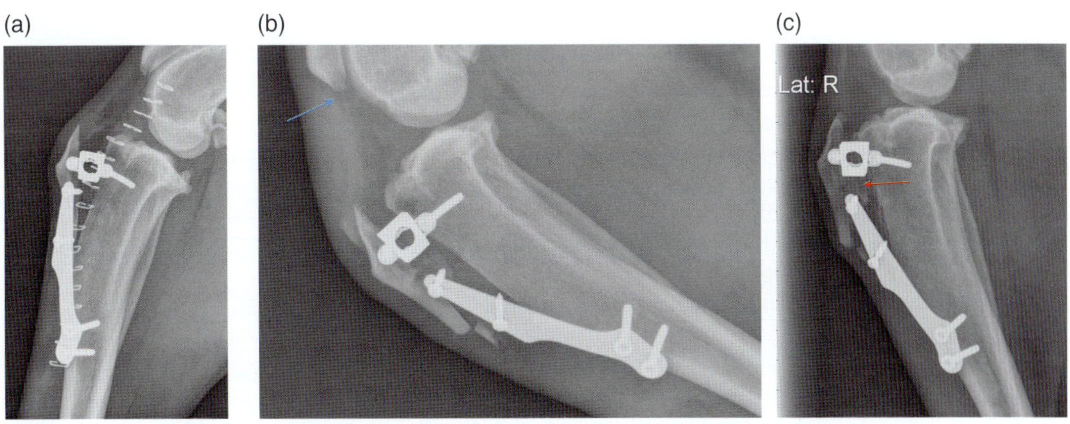

Figure 12.5 **(a)** Mediolateral radiograph of an immediate postoperative stifle. Note the technical errors present including a very thin osteotomy and a distally placed cage. **(b)** The thin osteotomy has resulted in tuberosity fracture, partial loss of internal stabilization, and cranial tipping of the tuberosity. While the initial impulse might be to surgically address these issues, the very thin fractured tuberosity would be challenging to effectively engage with implants, especially if the goal is to attempt to maintain the TTA. Fortunately, the patella position is unchanged (blue arrow) when compared to the immediate postoperative radiographs. Additionally, the patella tendon angle still measures close to 90° despite the tuberosity tipping. **(c)** Progressive bridging callus formation (red arrow) is present and the implants are static following 4 weeks of external coaptation with a full limb cast and the original goal of the TTA has been accomplished.

dogs actually focuses only on major complications [23]. Unlike with minor complications, if major complications are defined as those that require surgical or medical treatment to resolve, then the majority of studies are consistent in this "major" designation [19]. The mean reported TTA major complication rate is 10.1% (range 2–19.8%) and for TTA-R 15.1% (range 4–30.8%). The two largest TTA studies to date of 1613 dogs and 501 stifles report similar major complication rates of 13.4% and 11.4% respectively [14, 23].

Similar to TPLOs, the most commonly reported major TTA postoperative complications include meniscal injury, tibial fracture, infection, and implant-related issues.

12.5.1 Meniscal Injury

Postoperative meniscal tears are a commonly reported major postoperative TTA complication as with other surgical techniques used to treat canine CCL disease. In those TTA studies that provided information on postoperative meniscal tears, they accounted for an average of 13.7% (range 0.5–50%) of all major complications and were the most common reason for additional surgery. Three of the four TTA-R studies report postliminary meniscal injury as the most common major complication, accounting for an average of 50% (range 40–60%) of all major postoperative complications encountered and also the most common cause for a required second procedure.

Since Slocum first described it in 1993 as a means of minimizing the chance of meniscal injury following TPLO surgery, meniscal release has been a source of considerable debate [24]. This chapter will focus on meniscal release only as it relates to the TTA technique. Chapter 18 provides greater detail regarding the technical data and general evidence for and against meniscal release use.

Medial meniscal release has been used since some of the earliest published reports of the TTA technique and its use has been primarily dictated by surgeon preference. Thirteen TTA and one TTA-R report(s) listed in Table 12.1 provided information as to whether or not a meniscal release was performed. Eight of the 13 (61%) TTA studies utilized meniscal release, but in 50% (4/8) of these it was performed in only a minority of the subjects. Only three (38%) of the eight studies evaluated its effectiveness as a prophylactic means of preventing meniscal injury. Of the three TTA studies that evaluated whether or not release was protective, all confirmed its benefit at preventing medial meniscal injury [13, 14, 23]. The largest sequential TTA case series published found that dogs who did not have a meniscal release were significantly more likely to develop a postliminary tears that required surgical treatment [23]. Over 10% of the dogs with a normal medial meniscus at the time of TTA surgery that were not released subsequently developed tears compared to only 0.5% of dogs that had a meniscal release performed. Making these differences even more meaningful is the fact that a much larger number of dogs were released (n = 694) than were not (n = 264).

Wolf et al. released the largest percentage of normal menisci (84%) in 501 stifles and reported that it lowered postoperative tear incidence from 27% to 2.5% [14]. Interestingly, Lafaver et al. did not perform a meniscal release during their first series of 68 TTAs but did so in their second series of 22 stifles because of a deemed unacceptable postoperative meniscal injury rate of 14.7% in the first series [13]. No postoperative meniscal injuries developed in dogs in the second series. The one TTA-R study that reported meniscal release being performed did not evaluate its impact on postoperative injury [2].

While this discussion will by no means settle this controversial issue, the preponderance of published TTA data supports meniscal release as an effective means of preventing postoperative meniscal injury. Therefore, at least in TTA surgery, the proven benefit of meniscal release should be considered strongly against its potential known and theoretical detrimental effects.

12.5.2 Tibial Fractures

Postoperative tibial fractures are a commonly reported potential complication following both TTA and TTA-R surgery and they can range in severity from minor to catastrophic. Eighty six percent (12/14) of applicable TTA and 75% (3/4) of TTA-R studies reported the occurrence of postoperative tibial fractures. Of the seven TTA studies that differentiated between major and minor tibial fracture complications, five (71%) encountered them as both and two (29%)

experienced them only as major complications. All fractures were classified as major in the TTA-R studies. Overall, fractures occur in 1–14% of TTA patients [20]. Fracture configurations and locations vary but they can divided into tibial tuberosity (crest) and tibia (diaphyseal and metaphyseal) fractures, with the former being by far the most common. Unlike some postoperative complications, fractures are most often a direct result of technical error and are therefore quite preventable.

Nutt et al. compared a control group of 212 dogs that did not have tibial tuberosity fractures following TTA to 12 dogs that developed 13 fractures [20]. They evaluated 15 features on immediate postoperative radiographs for predictors of outcome and potential fracture risk factors. A partial list of these features included cage position, distal contact between the osteotomy and tibia, osteotomy width, fork plate position, and osteotomy shape (straight or curved). They determined that only poor distal osteotomy width (<25% of the common tibial shaft width), poor fork plate position (proximal pole ≥5 mm and distal pole ≥3 mm from the cranial edge), and poor cage position (>3 mm distal to the tibial plateau) were significantly associated with fracture development (Figure 12.6). To help prevent tibial tuberosity fracture, the goal should be to make the widest tibial tuberosity osteotomy possible. The most proximal extent of the osteotomy should be immediately cranial to the articular surface and extend through the most distal aspect of the tibial tuberosity (Figure 12.7). However, the skeletal landmarks for the latter can be difficult to discern as the morphology of the proximal tibia varies considerably among dogs (Figure 12.8). For this reason, rather than use skeletal features, the author recommends using for a landmark a thin band of fascia that conspicuously indicates the most distal aspect of the tibial tuberosity regardless of tibia shape (Figure 12.9). Note that it does not matter whether the osteotomy is started or ends proximally or distally.

Creating a properly "shaped" osteotomy is also important in order to prevent tibial fractures. The ideal osteotomy is either straight or gently curved but *not* angled as it courses distally (Figure 12.10). Angled osteotomies must be avoided as they are a predictable cause of tibial fissures or fractures (Figure 12.11). Since the angled portion of the osteotomy can be

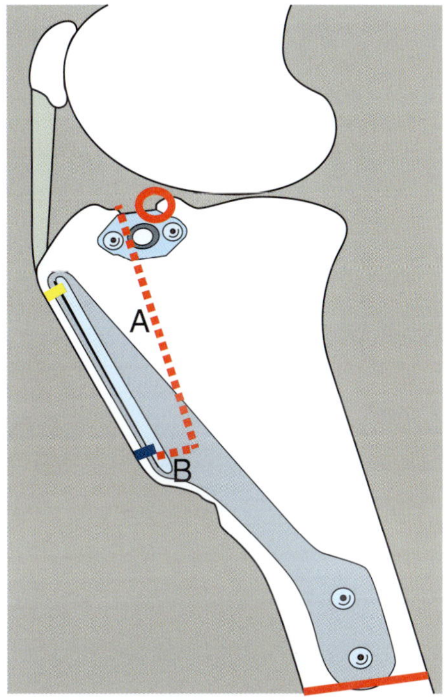

Figure 12.6 Correct TTA implant application principles and osteotomy characteristics can help to minimize the chances of tibial fracture. The distal osteotomy width (red dotted line B) should be >25% of the tibial diaphysis width (solid red line). This can be determined by drawing a line along the cranial edge of the osteotomy (dotted red line A) and then making line B perpendicular to it at the level of the central portion of the most distal fork tine. Ideal fork plate position is where the most proximal tine is ≤5 mm from the cranial edge of the tuberosity (yellow line) and the most distal tine is ≤3 mm (blue line) from the same edge. The proximal caudal edge of the cage should be <3 mm below the tibial plateau (red circle). Source: Based on Nutt et al. [20].

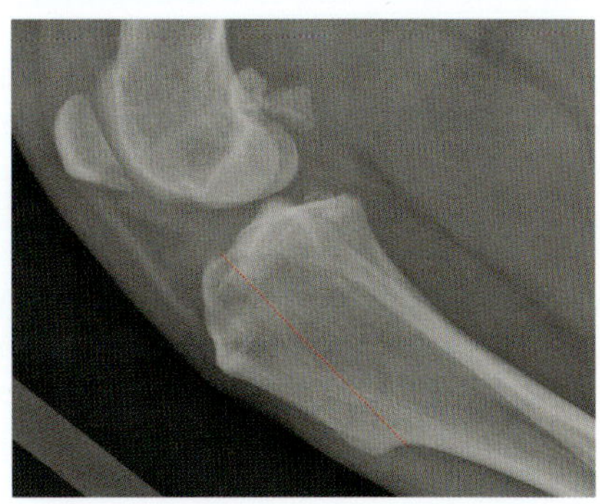

Figure 12.7 Mediolateral radiograph of a stifle illustrating an ideal tibial tuberosity osteotomy (red dotted line). The most proximal extent of the osteotomy is immediately cranial to the tibial articular surface and extends through the most distal aspect of the tuberosity.

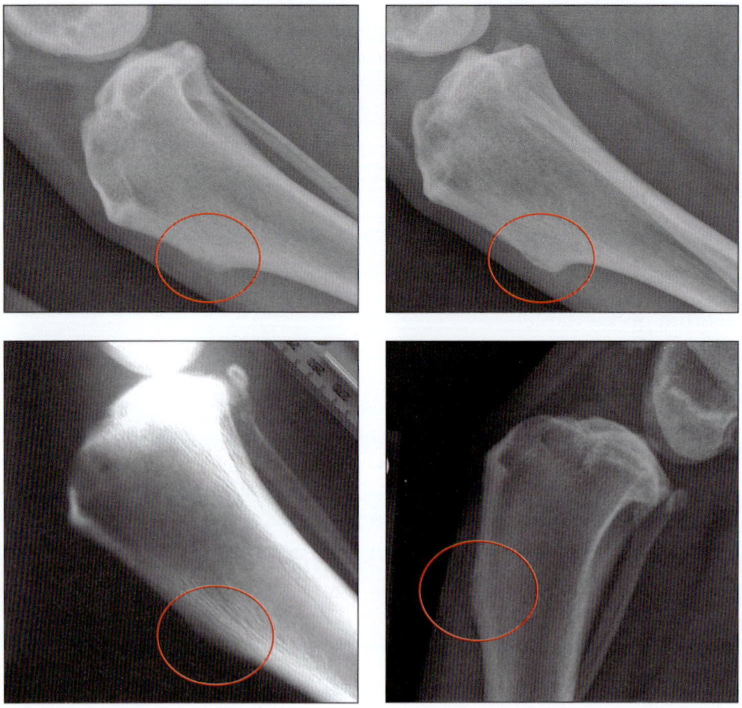

Figure 12.8 Multiple mediolateral stifle radiographs demonstrating the variability in the skeletal landmarks of the most distal extent of the tibial tuberosity (red circles). Some dogs have robust prominences while others do not.

obscured by the TTA plate, it may not be appreciated on immediate postoperative radiographs so intraoperative awareness is critical. In the author's experience, angled cuts are often due to a lack of attention being paid to where the saw is directed as it travels distally. This results in the need for an acute, cranially directed osteotomy correction in order to end it at the distal extent of the tibial crest.

Multiple studies have found that TTA plates that utilize screws in the tuberosity are either the same as or better than fork-based plates relative to complications [15, 19, 25]. Screw-based plates have similar technical guidelines for application and avoiding tibial tuberosity fracture as those previously described for fork-based plates, with a few differences worth reviewing. Unlike fork-based plates which necessitate using the largest implant possible in order to maximize the numbers of tines engaging the bone, plate size is far less important when screws are used in the tuberosity. Given the differences in how screws engage bone versus fork tines, no more than two (smaller plates) to three (large plates) screws are required in the tuberosity. Using a smaller plate ensures that the most proximal tuberosity and

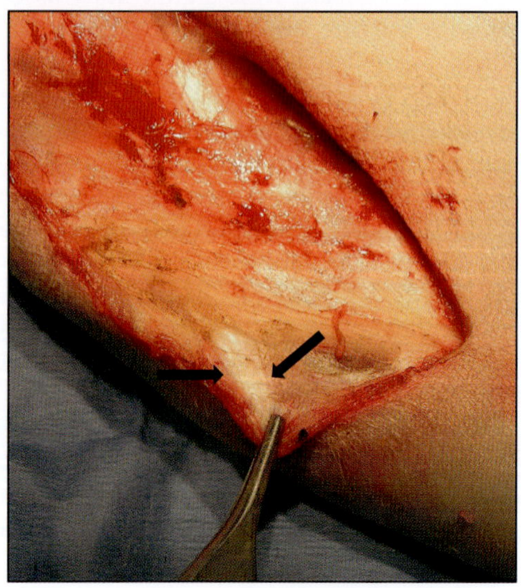

Figure 12.9 Intraoperative view of the proximal medial tibia showing the thin band of fascia that marks the most distal aspect of the tibial tuberosity (black arrows).

cranial cage screws "straddle" the straight patellar ligament insertion (Figure 12.12). These screws should be at least 1 cm apart because if they encroach upon the insertion, they may

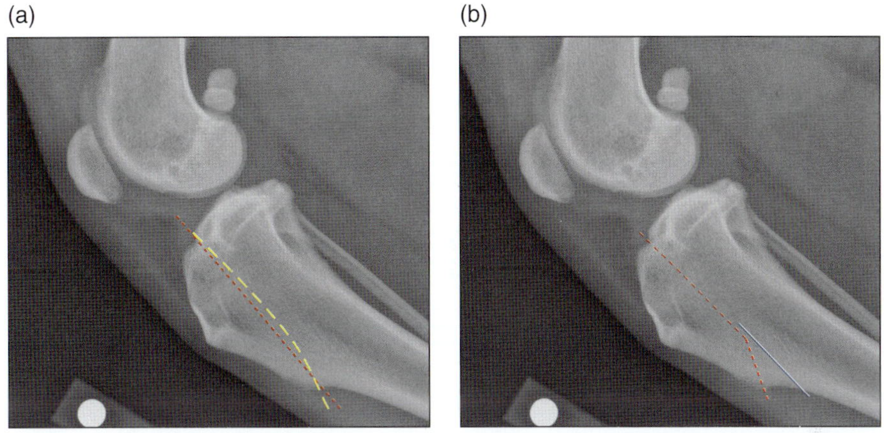

Figure 12.10 (a) Mediolateral radiograph of a stifle showing proper straight (red dotted line) and curved (yellow dotted line) osteotomy orientations. (b) Angled osteotomies may lead to fractures.

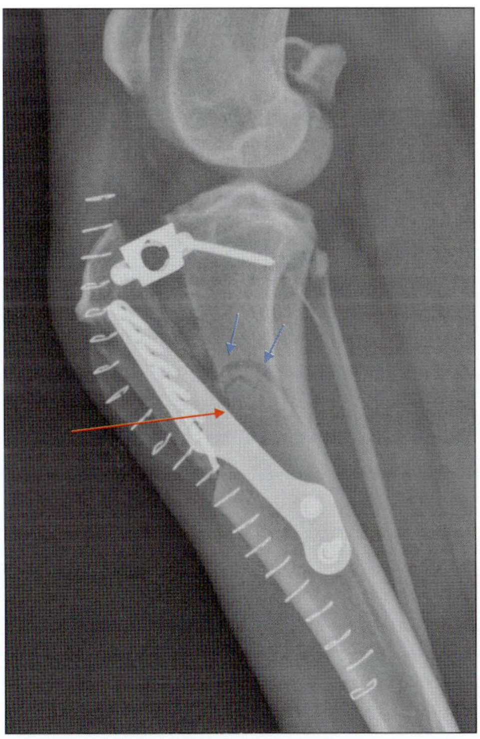

Figure 12.11 Mediolateral radiograph of a postoperative stifle revealing fissure formation (blue arrows) at the level of the excessively angled osteotomy (red arrow). Note it is difficult to appreciate the degree of angulation because of the proximity of the radiopaque plate.

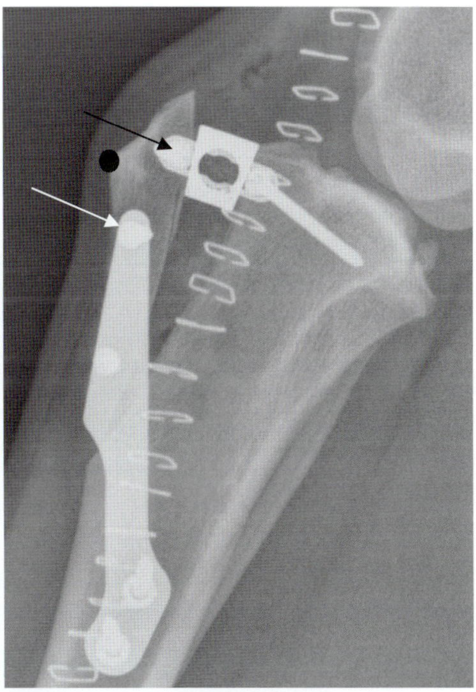

Figure 12.12 Mediolateral radiograph of an immediate postoperative stifle illustrating proper "straddling" of the straight patellar ligament insertion (black dot) by the cranial cage screw (black arrow) and the most proximal tibial crest plate screw (white arrow). The more these screws converge on the straight patellar ligament insertion, the greater the risk for tuberosity fracture.

create stress risers that predispose to tuberosity fracture (Figure 12.13). This further supports the need for proper cage location as recommended by Nutt et al. [20].

While the guidelines described above for fork plate position on the tuberosity can be followed when using screw-based plates, the author has not experienced the same fracture

(a) (b)

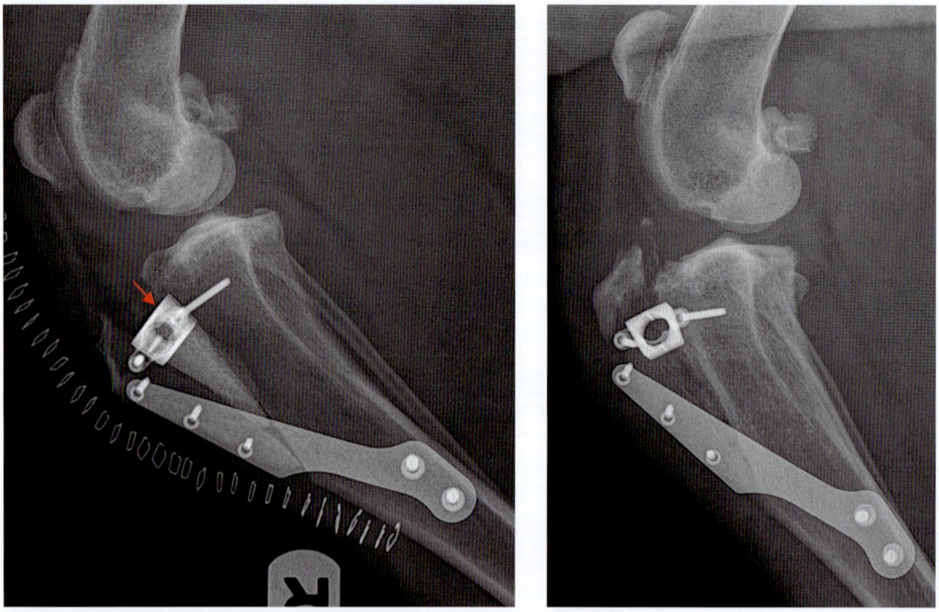

Figure 12.13 **(a)** The distal placement of the cage (red arrow) has brought the cranial cage screw to a distance less than 1 cm from the proximal plate screw. **(b)** The close proximity of the screw holes to the straight patellar ligament insertion resulted in a tibial tuberosity fracture. Note the proximal displacement of the patella as well.

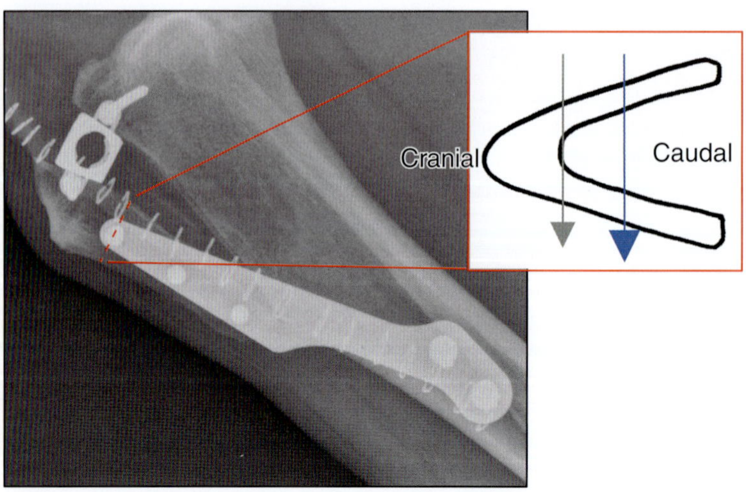

Figure 12.14 Mediolateral radiograph of an immediate postoperative stifle illustrating a properly applied screw-based TTA plate. The triangular cross-section of the tibial tuberosity (dotted red line) as viewed proximo-dorsal reveals the difference in satisfactory screw (blue arrow) vs fork tine (gray arrow) position. Screws can still engage an adequate amount of bone when placed in a more caudal location. Also note the well-spaced proximal plate and cranial cage screws on either side of the straight patellar ligament insertion.

consequences reported for a more caudally located plate on the tuberosity. This is likely a result of the superior purchase of screws in the thinner cortical bone present caudally compared to fork tines (Figure 12.14).

No TTA or TTA-R studies have classified any postoperative fractures or other complications as catastrophic – a complication that causes permanent unacceptable function, is directly related to death, or is cause for euthanasia [19].

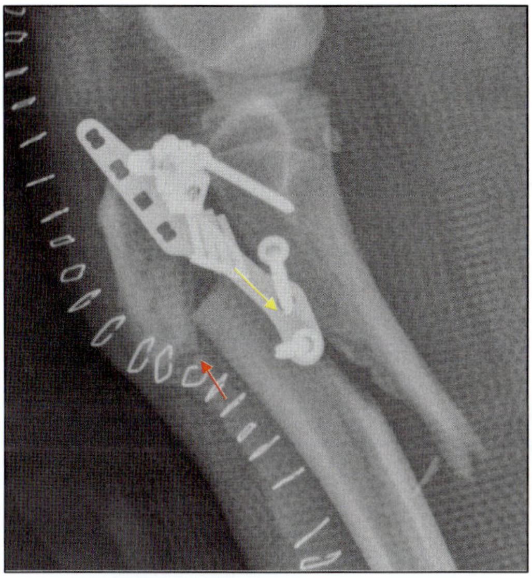

Figure 12.15 A mediolateral radiograph of a potentially catastrophic complication following TTA surgery. This radiograph again illustrates the importance of not making a sharply angled osteotomy. Note the nearly 90° angle of the distal extent of the osteotomy (red arrow). This created a stress riser in conjunction with the distal plate screw holes (yellow arrow) that lead to the tibial diaphyseal fracture and complete loss of internal stabilization.

However, all reports discussing complications and the TTA "learning curve" reviewed procedures being performed by board-certified surgeons or experienced general practitioners. In the author's experience, it is in the hands of veterinarians who lack practical experience with internal fixation and osteotomy techniques as well as a comprehension of TTA principles in which catastrophic complications can and do occur (Figure 12.15). As such, TTA and TTA-R should never be viewed as technically "simple" or "less complicated" procedures in order to broaden their appeal to a wider audience.

When revision surgery is required to address tibia fracture(s) following TTA, the first goal is to preserve the tibia and the patella mechanism. The former should not be sacrificed in an attempt to preserve the TTA. Reducing the tibial tuberosity back to its pre-TTA position in order to reestablish the patella mechanism and/or the weight-bearing axis of the tibia may be necessary (Figure 12.16). Only once the fracture has healed sufficiently should consideration be given to how best to manage the original CCL disease. By contrast, some fracture configurations are amenable to preservation of the TTA surgery while also addressing the complication (Figure 12.17).

12.5.3 Surgical Site Infections

As with other surgical techniques used to treat CCL disease, postoperative SSIs are one of the most common and potentially challenging of postoperative TTA complications. The focus of this chapter will be on SSI as it specifically relates to TTA techniques. For a more thorough discussion of SSI in general, please refer to Chapters 2 and 3.

Reported TTA SSI rates vary widely among studies. If only the four largest sample population TTA studies to date are considered, rates are as follows: 4.6% (1768 stifles [27]), 5.3% (224 stifles [26]), 6.6% (501 stifles [14]), and 8.1% (1613 dogs [23]). The reported incidence of TTA-R SSI ranges from 0% to 15.4%, which is derived from much smaller sample populations [2, 17]. Identified risk factors for TTA SSI include increases in body weight, anesthesia, and surgery durations, which are similar to those reported with TPLO [4, 26].

As with TPLO and other clean orthopedic procedures, conflicting information exists as to the value of prophylactic postoperative antibiotic (PPA) use in TTA patients for the prevention of SSI. Some TTA studies do not provide information on the use of antibiotics in their sample populations while for others there is variation on how the use of PPA is reported (Table 12.1). Only one TTA-R study reported the use of PPA but did not evaluate their impact relative to SSI. Of the four TTA studies that did analyze the effect of PPA use, three reported no benefit in the prevention of SSI. Ferrell et al. also found that the use of PPA was a significant risk factor for the development of oxacillin-resistant bacteria infections in TTA patients [27]. Furthermore, such infections were more likely to require implant removal in order to achieve resolution when compared to nonoxacillin-resistant bacteria. By contrast, in a study comparing TPLO and TTA postoperative complications in dogs >50 kg body weight, the use of PPA did significantly reduce the risk of SSI occurrence in both groups [4]. This finding is consistent with other TPLO studies that found PPA to be

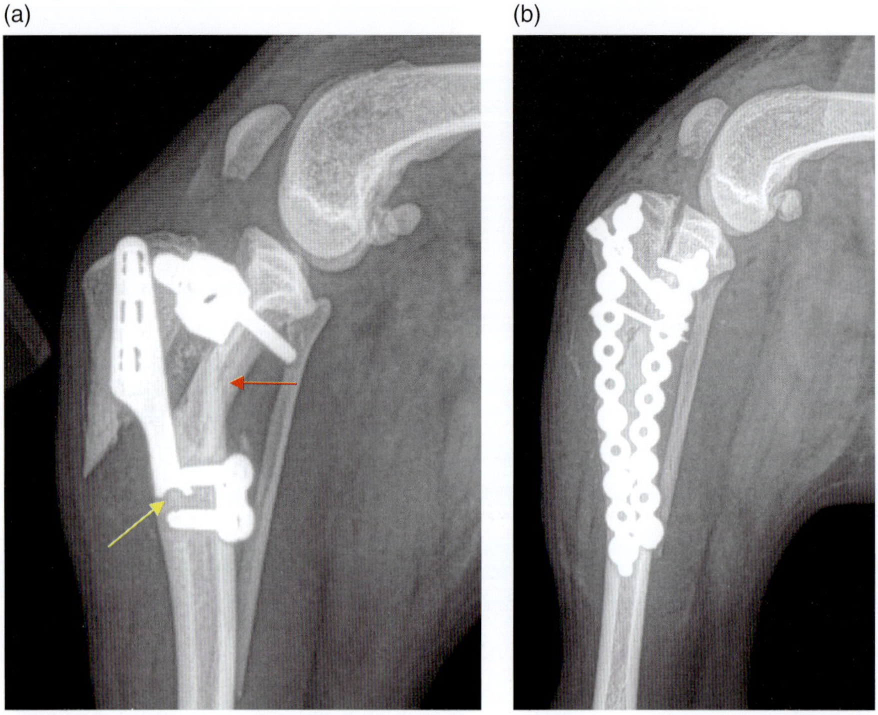

Figure 12.16 **(a)** Mediolateral radiograph of a potentially catastrophic complication following TTA surgery. The tibial tuberosity osteotomy was excessively wide and appears to violate the cranial articular surface. This incorrect osteotomy resulted in a very narrow proximal tibial diaphysis which subsequently fractured (red arrow). The TTA plate broke (yellow arrow) as a result of excessive load following the fracture. **(b)** Immediate post-revision medio-lateral radiograph showing the tibial tuberosity reduced to its pre-TTA position. The osteotomy and the diaphyseal fracture were stabilized with a combination of string-of-pearls (SOP) plates, headless compression screw, and pin. Source: Courtesy of Dr David L. Dycus.

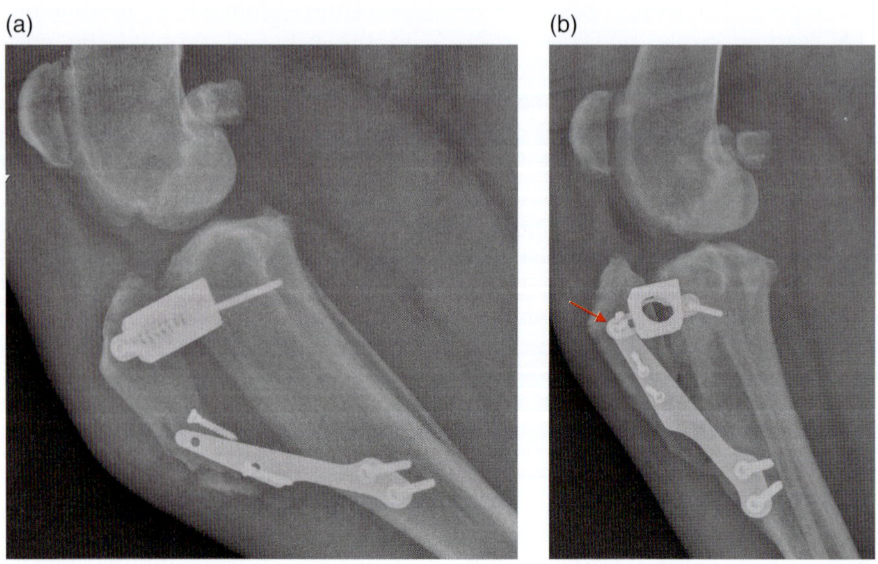

Figure 12.17 **(a)** Mediolateral radiograph revealing a cranially displaced tibial tuberosity fracture with complete loss of TTA plate fixation. This plate was applied too cranially on the tuberosity, resulting in a fracture of the cortex. This plate was also small, however, a larger plate could also have failed if applied in a similar position. **(b)** Six-week post-revision medio-lateral radiograph; the fracture configuration allowed for preservation of the TTA while reestablishing internal fixation of the osteotomy. The original TTA plate was removed and the TTA reduced distally. A larger three-hole screw-based plate was applied more proximally so as to share the cranial cage screw (red arrow) in order to completely bridge the fracture site. Note the large amount of mineralized bone present within the osteotomy gap.

protective against SSI but is the only TTA study to demonstrate this. Based on the preponderance of the data, the routine use of PPA in TTA patients cannot be supported except perhaps in very large and giant-breed dogs.

The reported overall requirement for TTA implant removal ranges from 0% to 1.8%. However, it is a much higher 39% in stifles that develop SSI [12, 13, 23, 27, 28]. While TTA plate removal is simple and expected to be without complications, cage removal is not. The overall requirement for cage removal is reported to be very low (0.5%; 9/1768 stifles) [27]. However, the mere thought of this potential undertaking is enough to cause stress in even the most experienced surgeon. Since the majority of the TTA cage resides within the proximal tibia and is designed to facilitate osseous ingrowth, extracting it is not only difficult but also associated with a high postoperative complication rate of 40% [29]. Fortunately, its removal is often not required to achieve SSI resolution. Ferrell et al. reported that 62.5% of SSI resolved by plate removal alone with the cages left in situ [27]. Of the 23 stifles in which the cage was left in place in the presence of a SSI, only three ultimately required removal. We propose only performing initial removal of the cage if radiographs demonstrate periimplant lucency and/or a wound/draining tract is present directly over the cage.

An exception to this recommendation is in the case when biocomposite cages are used. Varying amounts of periimplant lucency can be normal long term as bone ingrowth lags behind biocomposite hydrolysis and degradation, producing small voids around the implant as it slowly resorbs [30]. As such, these cages may not require removal even if lucency is noted on radiographs (Figure 12.18).

Based on the above findings and the challenges that complicate cage removal, the author does not typically remove a cage unless there is an obvious indication to do so.

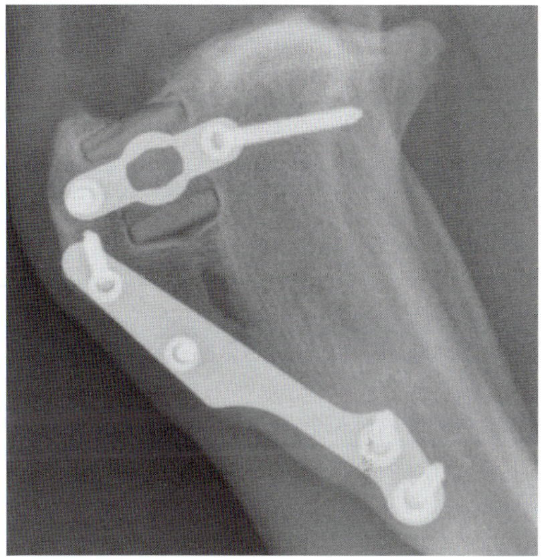

Figure 12.18 Mediolateral radiograph of the proximal tibia illustrating the appearance of a biocomposite cage approximately 6 months following implantation. Note the periimplant lucency which is within normal limits for this type of implant.

12.5.4 Patella Luxation

Medial patella luxation (MPL) is a rare but potentially major complication following TTA surgery. Four studies reported a combined MPL occurrence of 28 in 2551 total cases (1.1%), the majority of which required surgical correction [10, 11, 15, 23]. It has not been reported following TTA-R surgery. Boudrieu proposed three potential mechanisms for postoperative MPL occurrence including a decrease in retropatellar pressure, performing an oblique (vs transverse) osteotomy, and poor plate contouring [31]. Lateral patella luxation has not been reported.

The Maquet procedure advances the tibial tuberosity in order to decrease retropatellar pressure in humans suffering from patellofemoral pain. Given that TTA in canines is a modification of the Maquet procedure, it is not surprising that a decrease in retropatellar forces also occurs [32]. Since this pressure change is expected to occur in every dog undergoing TTA surgery, it alone is unlikely to be a major contributing cause given how rarely MPL occurs. However, in the presence of other predisposing factors (patella alta, osteotomy angle, shallow trochlear groove), it may be enough to bring about this complication.

Tibial tuberosity advancement occurs perpendicular to the plane of the osteotomy because a rigid rectangular-shaped cage is inserted within it. If the osteotomy is made obliquely in a medial

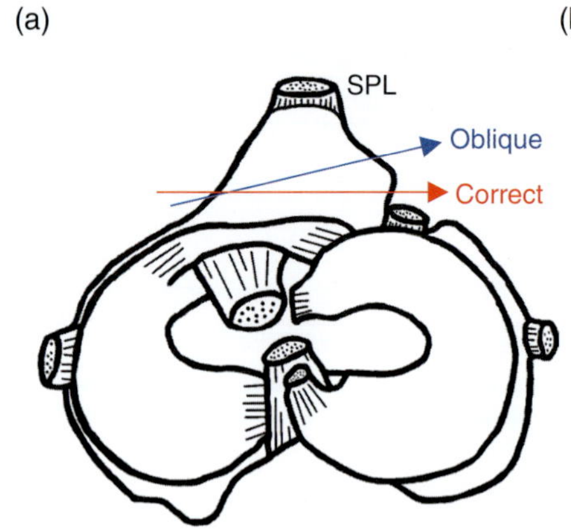

Figure 12.19 A proximodistal view of the tibia. **(a)** The oblique tibial osteotomy (blue line) contrasts the correctly oriented transverse osteotomy (red line). **(b)** Tibial tuberosity advancement (black arrows) occurs perpendicular to the osteotomy plane, which results in medial transposition of the straight patellar ligament insertion (SPL) when an oblique osteotomy is made.

orientation, then medialization of the tibial tuberosity will occur [31] (Figure 12.19). Similar to the retropatellar force changes, this alone is not likely to produce an MPL but when combined with other stifle abnormalities or technical errors, it may contribute to the complication occurring. Overcontouring the plate to produce lateral transposition of the tibial tuberosity while performing a TTA has been described as a method for addressing concomitant MPL and CCL insufficiency [33]. Therefore, if inadvertent excessive contouring of the plate occurs in the medial direction, the resultant medial tibial tuberosity transposition could potentially predispose to an MPL.

Whether to address a postoperative MPL surgically or not depends on whether it is associated with clinical signs. A low-grade MPL may be appreciated on physical examination yet not be a source of dysfunction. If lameness is attributed to the MPL then surgical intervention is warranted. Well-described procedures that deepen the trochlear groove combined with medial retinacular release and lateral retinacular imbrication would be expected to effective. If patella mechanism realignment is deemed necessary, tibial tuberosity transposition is highly problematic following a TTA because of the presence of the cage. A recently performed TTA in which the osteotomy has not yet healed may be amenable to revision and performing a lateral tuberosity transposition. However, if the TTA ostectomy has healed, a corrective distal femoral ostectomy is preferable to disturbing the tibial tuberosity and the cage.

12.6 Risk Factors for Postoperative Complications

A minority of TTA studies that provided information on postoperative complications also evaluated for the risk factors associated with them. Ten TTA studies have attempted to identify a variety of risk factors potentially associated with reported complications while no TTA-R studies have done so to date. Six of these 10 studies focused only on risk factors for a specific type of complication (e.g., tibial fractures, SSI, etc.) or in a particular sample population (large dogs only). Overall, three studies failed to find any significant correlation between their analyzed factors and the occurrence of postoperative complications [15, 19, 23]. The largest study to consider a variety of potential risk factors found a complication association with high body weight and preoperative patella tendon angle [14]. This is consistent with the findings in two other reports that also determined increasing body weight to be a significant risk factor for complication development [4, 10]. By contrast, Costa et al. found no such complication association with body weight in the largest sample population TTA study [23]. A summary of identified risk factors is provided in Table 12.1.

12.7 Conclusion

In conclusion, TTA and TTA-R have the potential for developing complications with similar frequency as that of other osteotomy-based procedures. Many of these complications can be avoided by adhering to established technical guidelines and are reduced with increasing surgeon experience.

12.7.1 Disclosure Statement

The author has performed thousands of TTAs and TPLOs but has no personal experience performing TTA-R. I am a paid lecturer for Securos and received royalties from the sales of some Securos and Everost products.

References

1. Montavan, PM., Tepic, S. (2002). Advancement of the tibial tuberosity for treatment of the cranial cruciate deficit canine stifle. Proceedings of the 1st World Orthopedic Veterinary Congress, Munch, Germany, September 5–8.
2. Samoy, Y., Verhoven, G., Bosmans, T. et al. (2015). TTA rapid: description of the technique and short term clinical trial results of the first 50 cases. *Vet. Surg.* 44: 474–484.
3. Dyall, B. and Schmoekel, H. (2017). Tibial tuberosity advancement in small-breed dogs using TTA rapid implants: complications and outcome. *J. Small Anim. Pract.* 58: 314–322.
4. Hans, E.C., Barnhart, M.D., Kennedy, S.C. et al. (2017). Comparison of complications following tibial tuberosity advancement and tibial plateau leveling osteotomy in very large and giant dogs 50 kg or more in body weight. *Vet. Comp. Orthop. Traumatol.* 30: 299–305.
5. Ness, M.G. (2016). The modified Maquet procedure (MMP) in dogs: technical development and initial clinical experience. *J. Am. Anim. Hosp. Assoc.* 52: 242–250.
6. Pacchiana, P.D., Morris, E., Gilkings, S.L. et al. (2003). Surgical and post-operative complications associated with tibial plateau leveling osteotomy in dogs with cranial cruciate ligament rupture: 397 cases (1998–2001). *J. Am. Vet. Med. Assoc.* 222: 184–193.
7. Ramirez, J., Barthelemy, N., Noel, S. et al. (2015). Complications and outcome of a new modified Maquet technique for treatment of cranial cruciate rupture on 82 dogs. *Vet. Comp. Orthop. Traumatol.* 5: 339–346.
8. Stauffer, K.D., Tuttle, T.A., Elkins, A.D. et al. (2006). Complications associated with 696 tibial plateau leveling osteotomies (2001–2003). *J. Am. Anim. Hosp. Assoc.* 42: 44–50.
9. Retallack, L.M. and Daye, R.M. (2018). A modified Maquet-tibial tuberosity advancement technique for treatment of canine cranial cruciate ligament disease: short-term outcome and complications. *Vet. Surg.* 47: 44–51.
10. Steinberg, E.J., Prata, R.G., Palazzini, K. et al. (2011). Tibial tuberosity advancement for treatment of CrCL injury: complications and owner satisfaction. *J. Am. Anim. Hosp. Assoc.* 47: 250–257.
11. De Lima Dantes, B., Sul, R., Parkin, T. et al. (2016). Incidence of complications associated with tibial tuberosity advancement in boxer dogs. *Vet. Comp. Orthop. Traumatol.* 1: 39–45.
12. Hoffmann, D.E., Miller, J.M., Ober, C.P. et al. (2006). Tibial tuberosity advancement in 65 stifles. *Vet. Comp. Orthop. Traumatol.* 5: 219–227.
13. Lafaver, S., Miller, N.A., Stubbs, W.P. et al. (2007). Tibial tuberosity advancement for stabilization of the canine cruciate ligament-deficient stifle joint: surgical technique, early results and complications in 101 dogs. *Vet. Surg.* 36: 573–586.
14. Wolf, R.E., Scavelli, T.D., Hoelzler, M.G. et al. (2012). Surgical and postoperative complications associated with tibial tuberosity advancement for cranial cruciate ligament rupture in dogs: 458 case (2007–2009). *J. Am. Vet. Med. Assoc.* 240: 1481–1487.
15. Edwards, G.A., Hosgood, G., Hancock, R.B. et al. (2016). Major complications associated with fork-based and screw-based tibial tuberosity advancement implants: 438 cases. *Can. Vet. J.* 57: 415–420.
16. Butterworth, S.J. and Kyudd, D.M. (2017). TTA-rapid in the treatment of the canine cruciate deficient stifle: short- and medium-term outcome. *J. Small Anim. Pract.* 58: 35–41.
17. Livet, V., Baldinger, A., Viguier, E. et al. (2019). Comparison of outcomes associated with tibial plateau leveling osteotomy and a modified tibial tuberosity advancement for treatment of cranial cruciate ligament disease in dogs: a randomized clinical study. *Vet. Comp. Orthop. Traumatol.* 32: 314–323.
18. Bisgard, S.K., Barnhart, M.D., Shiroma, J. et al. (2011). The effect of cancellous autograft and novel plate design in radiographic healing and postoperative complications in tibial tuberosity advancement for cranial cruciate-deficient canine stifles. *Vet. Surg.* 40: 402–407.
19. Cook, J.L., Evans, R., Conzemius, M.G. et al. (2010). Proposed definitions and criteria for reporting time frame, outcome, and complications for clinical orthopedic studies in veterinary medicine. *Vet. Surg.* 39: 905–908.

20. Nutt, A.E., Garcia-Fernandez, P., San Roman, F. et al. (2015). Risk factors for tibial tuberosity fracture after tibial tuberosity advancement in dogs. *Vet. Comp. Orthop. Traumatol.* 28: 116–123.
21. Proot, L.J.L. and Corr, S.A. (2013). Clinical audit of the tibial tuberosity advancement. *Vet. Comp. Orthop. Traumatol.* 4: 280–284.
22. Calvo, I., Aisa, J., Chae, D. et al. (2014). Tibial tuberosity fracture as a complication of tibial tuberosity. *Vet. Comp. Orthop. Traumatol.* 2: 148–154.
23. Costa, M.C., Craig, D., Cambridge, T. et al. (2017). Major complications of tibial tuberosity advancement in 1613 dogs. *Vet. Surg.* 46: 494–500.
24. Slocum, B. and Slocum, T.D. (1993). Tibial plateau leveling osteotomy for repair of cruciate ligament rupture in the canine. *Vet. Clin. North Am. Small Anim. Pract.* 23: 777–795.
25. Danielson, B., Barnhart, M.D., Kennedy, S.C. et al. (2016). Results of single-session bilateral tibial tuberosity advancements as a treatment for bilaterally ruptured cranial cruciate ligaments in dogs: 90 cases (2006–2010). *J. Am. Anim. Hosp. Assoc.* 52: 109–114.
26. Yap, F.W., Calvo, Smith, K.D. et al. (2015). Perioperative risk factors for surgical site infection in tibial tuberosity advancement: 224 stifles. *Vet. Comp. Orthop. Traumatol.* 28: 199–206.
27. Ferrell, C.L., Barnhart, M.D., and Herman, E. (2019). Impact of postoperative antibiotics on rates of infection and implant removal after tibial tuberosity advancement in 1,768 canine stifles. *Vet. Surg.* 48: 694–699.
28. Stein, S. and Schmoekel, H. (2008). Short-term and eight and 12 month results of a tibial tuberosity advancement as treatment of canine cranial cruciate ligament damage. *J. Small Anim. Pract.* 49: 398–404.
29. Serratore, V.R. and Barnhart, M.D. (2018). Results and complications after removal of tibial tuberosity advancement for treatment of surgical site infections: a retrospective study. *Vet. Surg.* 47: 768–773.
30. Ferrell, C.L., Barnhart, M.D., Watson, A. et al. (2019). Long-term radiographic appearance of a bioabsorbable biocomposite tibial tuberosity advancement cage implant. *Aust. Vet. J.* 98: 30–34.
31. Boudrieu, R. (2011). Patella luxation after TTA. Proceedings of the European Society of Veterinary Orthopaedics and Traumatology. Lyon, France, October 20–22.
32. Hoffman, D.E., Kowaleski, M.P., Johnson, K.A. et al. (2011). ex vivo biomechanical evaluation of the canine cranial cruciate ligament-deficient stifle with varying angles if stifle joint flexion and axial loads after tibial tuberosity advancement. *Vet. Surg.* 40: 311–320.
33. Yeadon, R., Fitzpatrick, N., and Kowaleski, M.P. (2011). Tibial tuberosity transposition-advancement for treatment of patellar luxation and concomitant cranial cruciate ligament disease in the dog. *Vet. Comp. Orthop. Traumatol.* 1: 18–26.
34. Dymond, N.L., Goldsmid, S.E., and Simpson, D.J. (2010). Tibial tuberosity advancement in 92 canine stifles: initial results, clinical outcome and owner evaluation. *Aust Vet J* 88: 381–385.
35. Ferreira, A.J.A., Bom, R.M., and Tavaers, S.O. (2019). Tibial tuberosity advancement technique in small breed dogs: study of 30 consecutive dogs (35 stifles). *J Small Anim Pract* 60: 305–312.

13 Complications Associated with the Modified Maquet Technique

Marc H. Balligand

13.1 History

In the 1970s, Paul Maquet developed a technique dedicated to treat patello-femoral chondromalacia in human patients (Figure 13.1) [1]. Patello-femoral chondromalacia is suspected to be the consequence of excessive pressure in the patello-femoral joint upon contraction of the quadriceps musculature during mobilization of the knee joint. Maquet logically deduced that the quadriceps muscle could take advantage of an increased lever arm to reduce its force exerting the same effect on the knee joint. This resultant increased lever arm in return reduced the patello-femoral compressive force [2].

The technique designed by Maquet to increase the quadriceps lever arm consisted of performing an incomplete axial osteotomy of the tibial crest, allowing its distocranial rotation around a bony hinge. The displacement was maintained by interposing between the tibial crest and the proximal tibial metaphysis an autologous cortical graft harvested from the ilium (Figure 13.1). Altough esthetically questionable, the technique, referred to as the Maquet technique, appeared to be effective. When Maquet reported his original technique, it was noted that this procedure had another biomechanical effect: the directional change of the quadriceps musclature force reduced tibial thrust upon knee loading [3].

In 2002, Montavon and Tepic, inspired by the Maquet technique, described a new surgical procedure (referred to as the tibial tuberosity advancement technique or TTA) to stabilize the canine cranial cruciate ligament (CCL)-deficient stifle joint [4]. More in-depth information about the biomechanics and theory of the TTA can be found elsewhere [5, 6]. In a general sense, the TTA limits cranial tibial translation by increasing the lever arm of the quadriceps. Montavon and Tepic proposed to osteotomize the tibial crest (including the tibial tuberosity [TT]) and to displace it cranially so the resultant angle between the patella tendon and the tibia plateau would be 90°. In order to circumvent the need for an autologous cortical graft as Maquet used to do, they designed a spacer in the form of a titanium cage to place into the osteotomy gap. The required advancement of the tibial tuberosity, allowing the patella tendon to become perpendicular to the tibial plateau, was determined using a transparent layout (Kyon, Zurich, Switzerland) on a lateral radiograph of the stifle joint, positioned as it would be during

Complications in Canine Cranial Cruciate Ligament Surgery, First Edition. Edited by Ron Ben-Amotz and David L. Dycus.

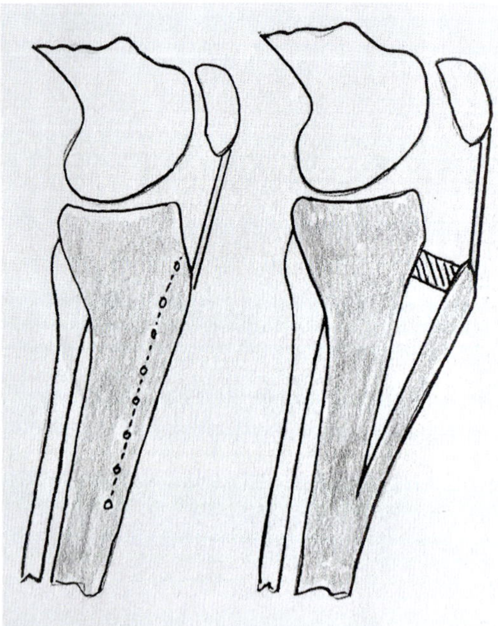

Figure 13.1 Original design and rationale of the Maquet technique. Source: Redrawn from Maquet [1].

stance phase (around 135°) and with the tibia in a physiological position (cranial subluxation reduced) (Figure 13.2a). In contrast to Maquet, Montavon and Tepic opted to completely free the tibial crest from the tibia, allowing the patella to remain in a physiological position but requiring the use of implants to secure the crest to the tibial shaft.

In 2010, Balligand and collaborators performed an incomplete longitudinal osteotomy of the tibial crest, preserving a distal bone hinge and therefore avoiding the need for implants other than the cage. In this procedure, named the modified Maquet technique or MMT, a cage was used as a spacer. Based on a growing series of clinical cases, the technique has been progressively refined. Initially, the osteotomy length was equal to the tibial crest length and a hole was drilled in the distal extent of the osteotomy (called the Maquet hole by certain authors) to act as a stress reducer. This hole was supposed to prevent the occurrence of fissures or even fractures upon advancement. The hole was rapidly abandoned, and the osteotomy length created was close to twice or even longer than the length of the tibial crest. This most recent version of the MMT was recognized as the new MMT or N-MMT [7] (Figure 13.2b,c).

It was also recognized that opening the osteotomy angle above 9–10° (the angle created at the distal osteotomy) would increase the incidence of perioperative fissure or fracture of the hinge. Therefore, a recommendation was made to stay below 10° and to calculate the length of the osteotomy according to the required advancement via a simple trigonometric method. In the equation:

$$y = x/tg\ \alpha$$

x is the required advancement, α is set at 9° (or possibly lower), and y corresponds to the length of the osteotomy. Based on these calculations, the length (mm) of the osteotomy grossly equals 7.5 (7–8) times the width of the cage (mm), thus making the osteotomy lengths range from 25 to 105 mm corresponding to cage widths ranging from 3 to 15 mm (Table 13.1).

To further refine the osteotomy, Brunel et al. developed an equation to reduce hinge fractures based as a function of the patient's body weight (BW) [8]. The objective is to resist loads at the distal cortical hinge up to six times the dog's body weight (in kilograms). Applying this assumption leads to a recommended thickness of the distal hinge between 1 and 7 mm for dogs weighing between 2 and 70 kg (Table 13.2). Finally, taking into account the viscoelasticity of the bone as a material, the author recommends to rotate the tibial crest around the distal bone hinge gradually and *slowly*, thus reducing even further the incidence of fissure/fracture.

Although the cage used by the author is still the one initially designed by Tepic and Montavon (TTA, Kyon), various other types of cages/spacers made of various materials have been used with good to excellent clinical outcome (TTA-2 [9]; TTA-rapid [10]; titanium foam, modified Maquet *procedure* (MMP) [11]; β-tricalcium phosphate [12]; bioabsorbable material [13]). A few surgeons proposed using K-wires, as in the MMP [10], or absorbable sutures, as in the TTA-2 [8], at the bone hinge in order to increase the ultimate tensile strength of the bone.

In past years, the MMT has been reported also in cats with good clinical outcome, although the biomechanics of the cat's stifle might differ from the dog [14, 15]. Further information on complications of CCL stabilization in the cat can be found in Chapter 16.

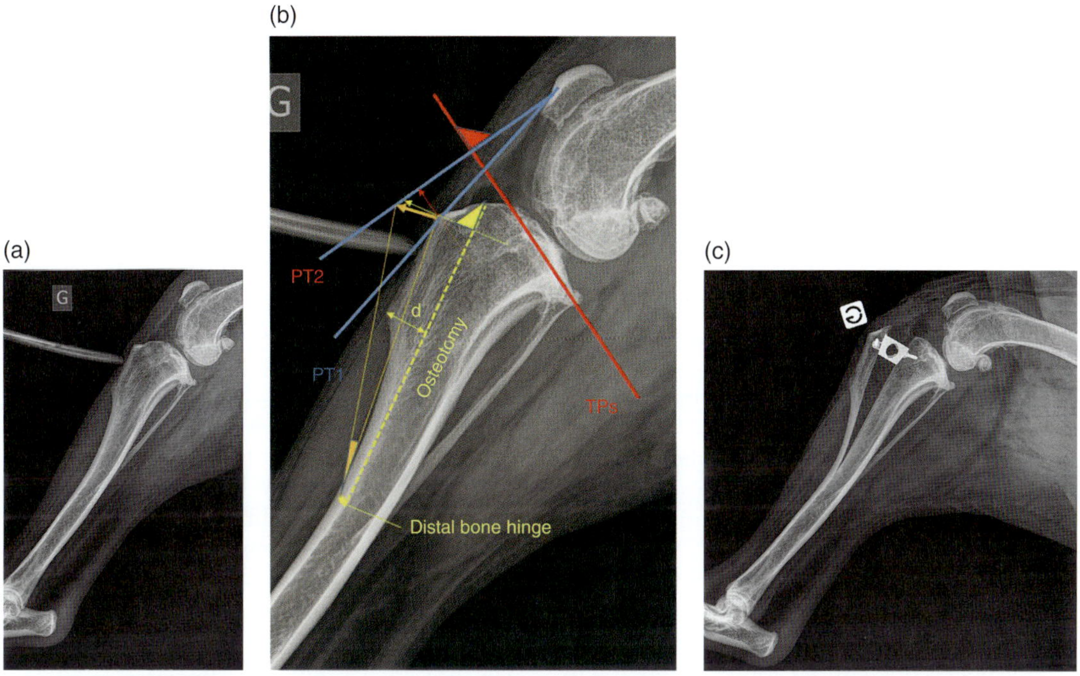

Figure 13.2 (a) Radiograph of the stifle joint in an appropriate position to measure the desired tibial tuberosity advancement (TTA). Note that the stifle is in close to maximal extension (>135°), the tibia is reduced in relation to the femur (a stick is seen to reduce the tibial translation). Neglecting to completely reduce the tibial subluxation leads inevitably to suboptimal advancement of the tibial tuberosity. (b) Method used by the author to determine the desired TTA: red line = tibial plateau slope (TPs), blue line PT1 = patellar tendon (PT) direction before advancement; blue line PT2 = desired PT direction after desired TTA (PT2 is now perpendicular to TPs); thin bright yellow arrow = TTA if TT is advanced perpendicularly to the osteotomy line; orange arrow = final desired TTA (gives the size of the cage) as TT is indeed rotated around the bone distal hinge (note that the difference between yellow and orange arrows is negligible). Dashed yellow line = tibial osteotomy, passing 1 cm (d) parallel and caudal to the cranial border of the tibial crest and joining a distal point along the cranial tibial cortex, several mm caudal to the cranial tibial border according to patient body weight (the hinge). (c) Immediate postoperative radiograph showing the cage in place (15 mm in this case) and a long rectilinear osteotomy.

Table 13.1 Calculation of the osteotomy length in function of the desired TTA.

Width of cage (mm)	Length of osteotomy (mm)
3	25
6	45
9	65
12	85
15	105

The objective is to keep the opening angle of the osteotomy gap under 10°, a scenario that has been shown to limit the risk of hinge fracture upon advancement. A simple trigonometric function, $y = x/tg\ \alpha$, is applied where x is the desired TTA, α (opening angle) is set at 9° (or possibly lower) and y corresponds to the osteotomy length. Calculations indicate that the osteotomy length grossly equals 7–8 times the width of the cage, meaning the osteotomy lengths range from 25 to 105 mm for cage widths ranging from 3 to 15 mm.

Table 13.2 Calculation of bone hinge thickness in function of patient body weight (BW).

BW (kg)	Hinge thickness (mm)	BW (kg)	Hinge thickness (mm)
1	0.91	15	2.10
5	1.25	20	2.52
6	1.33	30	3.37
7	1.42	40	4.22
8	1.50	50	5.07
9	1.59	60	5.92
10	1.67	70	6.77

The objective is to keep enough bone to resist a tension up to six times BW, a force that a dog could apply to the patella tendon upon jumping over a height. The following equation is applied: Thickness (mm) × 508.116 = (6× BW (N) + 417.561) − (15.68 × BW) (kg) [8]; calculations indicate thicknesses ranging from 1 to 7 mm for dogs with BW ranging from 2 to 70 kg.

13.2 Guidelines to Perform a Modified Maquet Technique

13.2.1 Preoperative

An adequate TTA measurement on the preoperative radiograph is a major prerequisite for successful surgery. Several strict conditions must be considered (Figure 13.2; Tables 13.1 and 13.2).

- The stifle radiograph must be in an appropriate position (≥135°; lateral view) in order to determine the tibial plateau slope (Figure 13.2a). This ideally corresponds to stifle extension at the beginning of the stance phase (Figure 13.3).
- The tibia should be reduced into its physiological place underneath the femur (subluxation must be reduced) (Figure 13.2a). If the tibia is not reduced appropriately, it will lead to a decrease of the angle between the patella tendon and the tibial plateau.
- As a reminder, the TTA means advancement of the *tibial tuberosity*, which is the point of insertion of the patella tendon on the tibial crest. It is not the upper limit of the tibial crest nor any point located in between. Desired TTA should therefore indicate the width of the upper border of the cage to be used.
- TTA is to be measured in a direction perpendicular to the osteotomy plane, not in a direction parallel to the tibial plateau (light yellow arrow, Figure 13.2b).
- Length of the osteotomy is determined according to the desired TTA, allowing the opening of the osteotomy to stay below 10°. Use Table 13.1 to make the process easier and faster.
- The BW of the patient determines the width of the distal bone hinge. A safety factor of at least six times BW is recommended. Use Table 13.2 to assist in this process.

13.2.2 Intraoperative

The decision to evaluate the meniscus is surgeon dependent with multiple factors that need to be considered. Additional information on meniscal decision making can be found in Chapter 18.

- A routine medial parapatellar approach is made.
- The infrapatellar fat pad is gently dissected in order to expose the medial margin of the

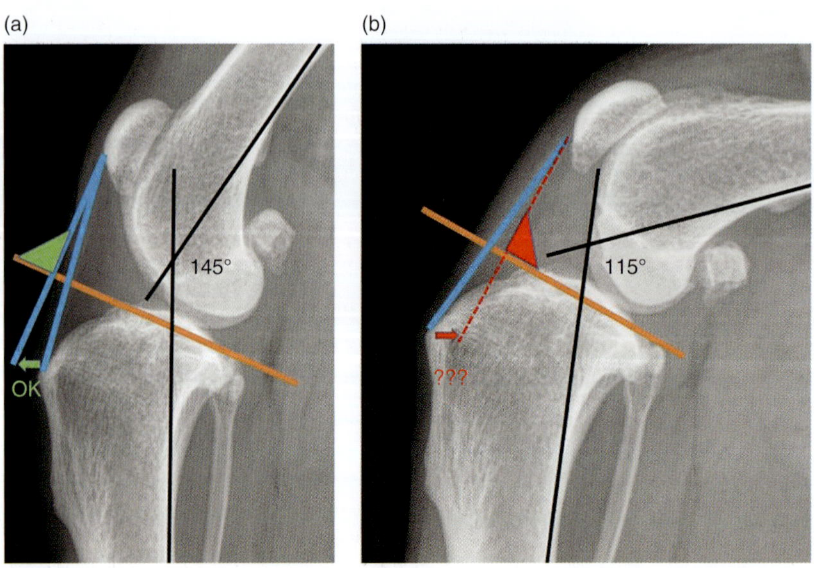

Figure 13.3 Major effect of stifle extension angle on measurement of desired TTA. **(a)** The stifle is extended 145° and the desired TTA (green arrow) can be measured. **(b)** The *same* stifle is only extended 115° and the measurement indicates a desired caudal crest transposition which cannot be performed (red triangle). Neglecting to sufficiently extend the stifle (even beyond 135°) when the preoperative radiograph is taken to measure the desired TTA is a major cause of suboptimal TTA.

patella tendon and the proximal medial margin of the tibial crest. This will allow visualization of the proximal exit of the oscillating saw blade.

- The tibial periosteum is incised longitudinally and elevated from mid tibia to the upper margin of the tibial crest. This allows marking of the osteotomy and secure placement of the saw blade to the bone. At the level of the bone hinge, the anterior border of the tibia should be clearly exposed, allowing precise measurement of the width of the hinge with a ruler. This is a critical point to insure adequate thickness of the hinge. According to the author's personal experience, the calculated thickness of the bone hinge (Table 13.2) can be rounded upwards but should never exceed 30% of the diaphyseal tibial diameter.
- The tibial osteotomy should be carried out very precisely, following a quasirectilinear line marked on the bone with a sterile dermatological pen or an electrocautery. The line should run distally and parallel to the cranial rim of the tibial crest, around 1 cm caudal to it, to join distally a point along the tibial diaphysis, several millimeters caudal to the cranial rim of the tibial diaphysis (according to the calculated thickness of the hinge) (Figure 13.2b). The saw blade should be tilted around 20° from the plane perpendicular to the tibia (going in a caudo-medial to cranio-lateral direction). Because of the triangular shape of the diaphysis, if the blade stays perpendicular to the medial tibial cortex, the thickness of the transcortex will be significantly larger than the cis cortex. If this occurs, the hinge will be stiffer than expected, and therefore more prone to intraoperative fissure/fracture upon advancement (Figure 13.4). The author recommends to first cut through just the cis cortex for the entire osteotomy line before continuing with the trans cortex. Both cuts (cis and trans cortex) should have the same length. The tibial crest will become movable only when the cis and trans cortex have been fully cut through. It is very important to visualize the osteotomy line through the cutting process (continuous irrigation and suction is recommended).
- The tibial crest should be *slowly* cranially advanced, progressing by successive steps of 3 mm, changing one spacer to the next larger one until the desired advancement is reached (Figure 13.5). In cases with a larger advancement (for example, 12–15 mm), the whole process should take more time, up to 3–5 minutes.
- The final spacer should be replaced by the cage, and the cage secured to the tibia with two small bicortical self-tapping 1.8 mm screws (Kyon). When placing the cage

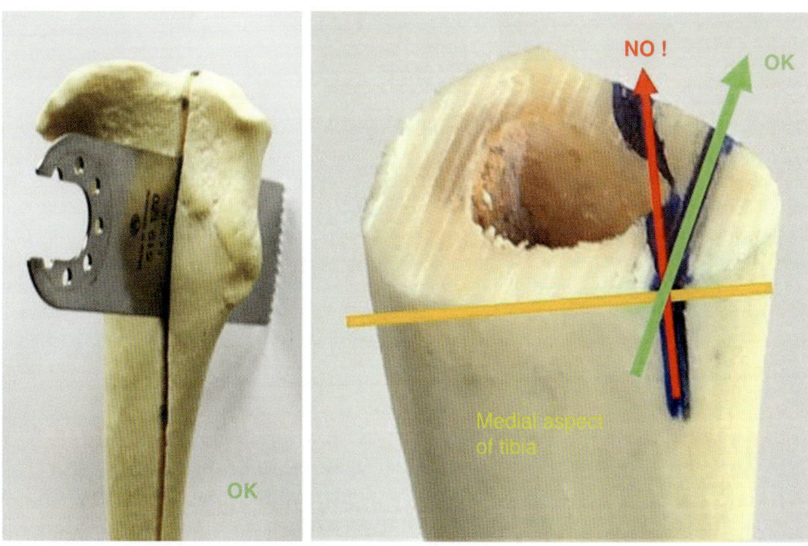

Figure 13.4 Illustration of the approximate 20° tilt of the oscillating saw blade when tibial osteotomy is performed. Neglecting to do so leads to widening of the hinge on the lateral side of the tibia (that has a triangular shape) which makes the hinge stiffer and more prone to fissure or even breakage upon advancement.

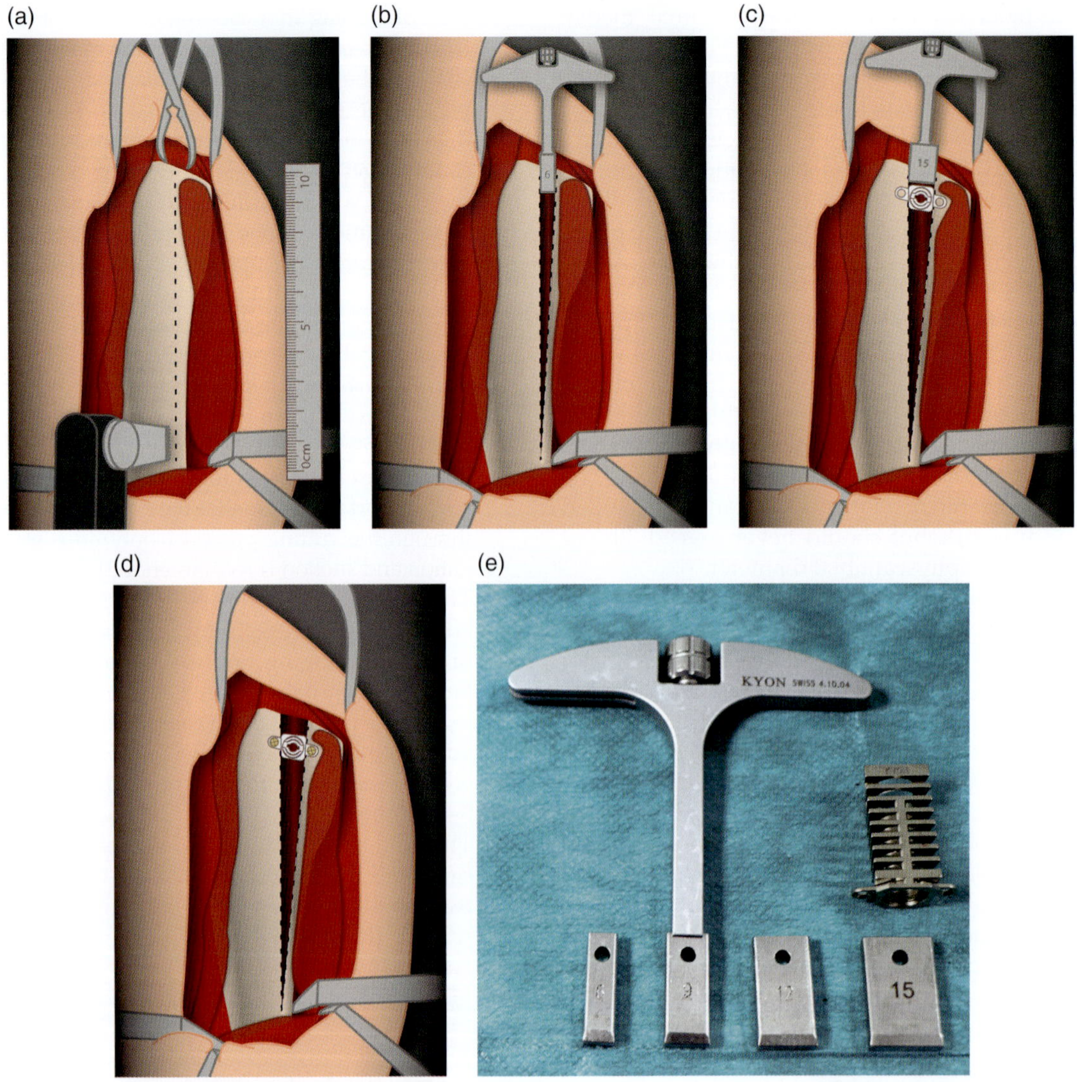

Figure 13.5 Successive steps of the modified Maquet technique (MMT). **(a)** The osteotomy line is rectilinear with the medial side of the tibia parallel to the operating table and the oscillating saw blade slightly tilted by about 20° in a caudo-medial to cranio-lateral direction. The length of the osteotomy is determined preoperatively according to the desired TTA in order to stay equal to or under 10° of opening (Table 13.1). The width of the distal bone hinge is determined preoperatively according to the body weight of the patient (Table 13.2). **(b,c)** The opening of the osteotomy gap is slowly (over 3–5 minutes) increased by introducing successive spacers of 3, 6, 9, 12, and 15 mm (6 and 15 mm in the illustrated case). **(d)** The cage is secured to the tibia with two self-tapping 1.8 mm screws at a divergent angle. The osteotomy gap is not grafted. Soft tissues are routinely closed. **(e)** The different spacers (Kyon) are fixed to a T-handle; spacers are introduced in the gap on their narrow border and then slowly twisted 90° to spread the gap.

screws, attempts should be made to ensure that these screws are bicortical. Since the "ears" of the cage are small and very close to the osteotomy plane, the direction of the screws should be divergent. The upper border of the cage should be aligned with the tibial tuberosity (Figure 13.6).

- It is the author's preference not to graft the osteotomy gap although this is surgeon dependent. If a graft is used, it can be

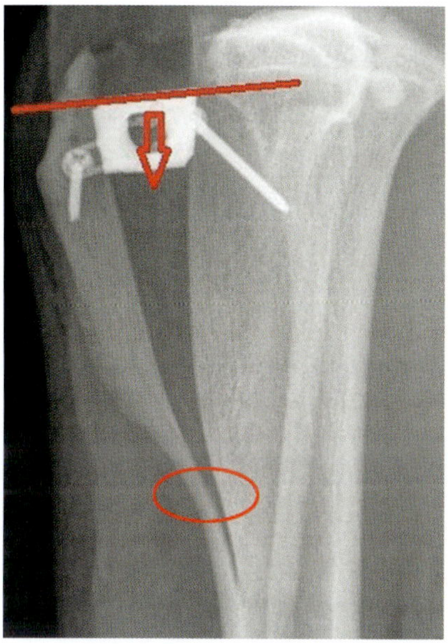

Figure 13.6 Illustration of an isthmus (within red ellipse) along the cranial part of the tibia. This narrowing should be avoided as it creates a stress riser, possibly leading to fracture. Note also the inappropriate position of the cage, placed too high in the osteotomy gap, hence possibly not delivering the expected stabilizing effect due to lack of sufficient advancement.

obtained from the proximal tibial metaphysis through the osteotomy. If a graft is not used, it is advised to "leave" the formed hematoma in the osteotomy gap.

- Once the procedure has been completed, the subcutaneous tissues and skin are closed routinely. Use caution when closing the distal aspect of the arthrotomy especially in cases of a large advancement (12–15 mm) as it can be challenging to suture. There should be no clinical impact if capsular closure is not feasible

13.2.3 Postoperative

- A modified Robert-Jones bandage can be applied to the leg for several days to prevent edema and protect the surgical wound (surgeon preference).
- Nonsteroidal antiinflammatories, analgesic medications, and antibiotics are generally prescribed according to surgeon preference.
- Exercise restriction of the patient is required for the first 4–6 weeks. Over the course of 6 weeks the lameness should be minimal or completely resolved. Progressive return in 2–4 weeks to normal activity can begin once signs of bone consolidation are observed (Figure 13.7a). However, it should be noted that the gap may never be completely filled in with bone (Figure 13.7b).
- In some situations, even with a well-executed procedure (i.e., there is appropriate advancement of the tuberosity, with adequate 90° angle between the patella tendon and tibial plateau), lameness may persists after the first 4–6 weeks. In these cases physical rehabilitation therapy is recommended to allow adaptation to normal weight bearing, with adequate quadriceps muscle contraction. This is important for the overalll patello-femoral mechanisam.
- If persistent lameness is observed, underadvancement, infection, implant failure, or a postliminary meniscal tear should be considered and closely evaluated.

13.3 Specific Complications

13.3.1 Postliminary Medial Meniscal Tear

13.3.1.1 Definition

Although absent at the time of initial surgery, meniscal lesions (bucket handle tear, etc.) can occur in the postoperative period, affecting mainly the medial meniscus. The rate of occurrence is comparable to other techniques (tibial plateau leveling osteotomy [TPLO], TTA). As such, the rate of postliminary meniscal injury following the MMT is around 5% when the technique is correctly performed [7].

13.3.1.2 Risk Factors

- Lack of cranio-caudal stifle joint stability after ineffective MMT due to technical errors such as imprecise estimation of the required advancement, incorrect choice of spacer width, incorrect placement of the cage within the osteotomy gap (see below).

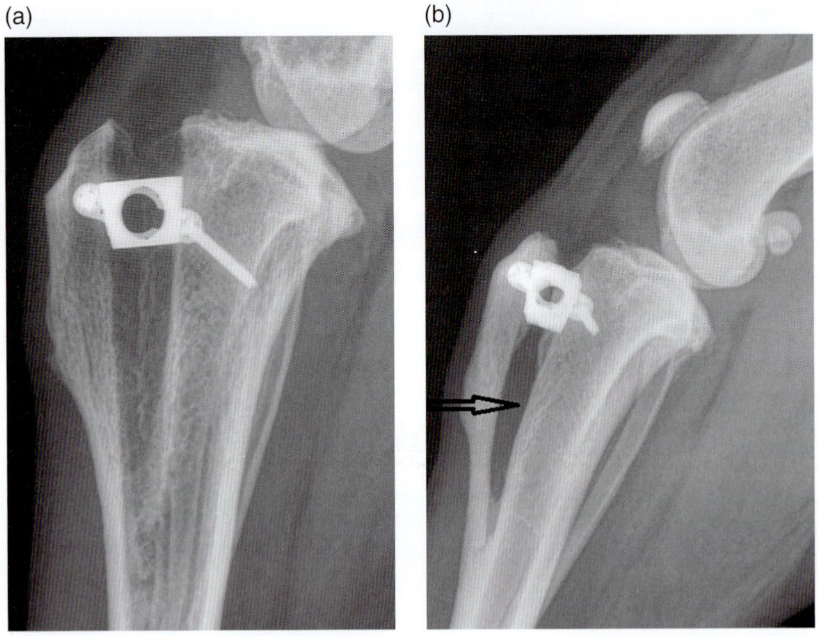

Figure 13.7 (a) Appropriate osteotomy gap healing 8 weeks post surgery. Note the appropriate cage height and screw position. At this stage, the patient's exercise restriction can be lifted and normal physical activity can be progressively resumed over 2–3 weeks. (b) Persistent incomplete osteotomy gap healing 4 months after MMT (black arrow) with good limb function. In this patient, the osteotomy had not been grafted. Given the lack of difference in outcome, the author does not recommend routine grafting of the osteotomy site.

13.3.1.3 Diagnosis

Treatment varies according to the suspected origin of the problem.

- Persistence of lameness beyond expected time of osteotomy healing/functional recovery.
- Meniscal click upon knee mobilization (28% of cases) [17].
- Ultrasonography, arthroscopy, and magnetic resonance imaging (MRI) can be conclusive [18].

13.3.1.4 Treatment

Treatment varies according to the suspected origin of the problem.

- If persistence of rotational instability after TTA is noted [16], the use of an antirotational suture should be considered. Persistence of lameness beyond expected time of osteotomy healing/functional recovery.
- If persistence of rotational instability after MMT is noted, the use of antirotational suture should be considered. In cases of a suboptimal tuberosity advancement, revision surgery (Figure 13.8) using a TPLO, extracapsular or intracapsular stabilization procedure can be undertaken. The author has no personal experience with repeating MMT (increasing the advancement via a second surgery) although it could be feasible in some cases.
- If a torn portion of the meniscus is identified during stifle exploratory procedure, it is advised to remove the torn portion.
- In some cases, rehabilitation therapy can greatly improve the joint stability by increasing thigh muscle mass and restoring good proprioception [5, 19].

13.3.1.5 Outcome

- Favorable once stifle joint stability is achieved.
- Favorable once clinically significant meniscal tears have been addressed.

13.3.2 Underestimation of Required Tibial Tuberosity Advancement

13.3.2.1 Definition

Numerous methods using either overlay or software (tibial plateau method, modified

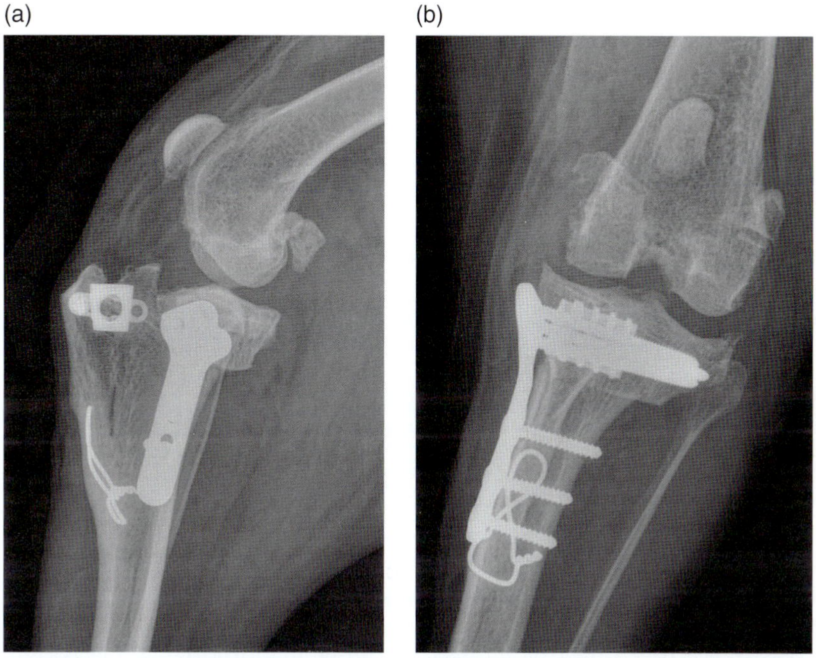

Figure 13.8 (a,b) Medio-lateral and cranio-caudal radiographs of a dog in which a TPLO was performed to improve limb function 2 years after initial unsuccessful MMT. The caudal screw of the TTA cage had to be removed to allow the TPLO blade to cut through the bone. Function was considerably improved after the TPLO procedure, indicating that the MMT had not delivered the expected stifle stability, possibly due to a technical error (underadvancement). Note the presence of a tension band wire that was placed at the end of the first surgery as fracture of the hinge had occurred.

tuberosity advancement method, common tangent method, Orthomed [Sound-Eklin™, Carslbad, CA, USA], Orthoplan™, Pillard et al. method [20]) have been proposed to estimate the required TTA, which unfortunately do not always deliver identical results [21, 22]. Since suboptimal advancement seems to be the main cause of persistent instability, it is advisable to go for the highest value measured on the preoperatrive radiographs.

It should be emphasized, however, that the MMT relies on the theoretical statement that the femoro-tibial joint force is parallel to the patellar tendon; therefore meticulous (within 1 mm) calculation of the required advancement based on a predetermined angulation of the stifle joint (≥135°) remains questionable as a patient might have several ways to restore stifle joint stability via specific voluntary muscle activation and/or slight change of joint angulation during the stance phase. This could explain why, sometimes, dogs do well despite technical mistakes whereas others, although operated strictly by the rules, may not immediately respond as expected.

13.3.2.2 Risk Factors

- Nondiagnostic radiographs (lack of definition, incorrect joint position).
- Stifle insufficiently extended (at least 135° required) (Figure 13.3).
- The tibia is not reduced in relation to the femur such that cranial translation of the tibia in relation to the femur is noted. Specific instruments such as a wooden spoon can be used to help reduce the tibia when taking radiographs (Figure 13.2a).
- Osteoarthritis (OA) makes anatomical landmarks difficult to identify.

Precision of measurement is based on the described technique (Figure 13.2b).

13.3.3 Inadequate Choice (Width) of Cage

13.3.3.1 Definition

The width of the selected cage can be indequate if measurement of the desired displacement is underestimated or not appropriately calculated. As a general rule, the larger the patient, the greater the desired advancement and the need for a wider cage.

13.3.3.2 *Risk Factors*

- Lack of attention to radiographic landmarks and surgical templating guidelines.
- Shortage of available cage sizes in one's inventory.

13.3.3.3 *Diagnosis*

- Postoperative radiographs are indicative of underadvancement of the tibial tuberosity. The surgeon should measure on the postoperative radiographs the angle achieved between the patella tendon and the tibia plateau. Underadvancement will likely increase the incidence of continued stifle instability.
- Possible persistence of a direct or indirect cranial drawer sign at the end of the surgical procedure does not necessarily indicate a suboptimal advancement as gravitational, ground reaction and muscle forces are required to stabilize the tibia (rationale of MMT) which are inactivated during anesthesia. In other cases, crest advancement results in tension of the surrounding soft tissues, thus masking potential instability [23].

13.3.3.4 *Treatment*

- If underadvancement is identified on the immediate postsurgical radiographs, the cage should be changed to a larger size. As an alternative solution, the cage can be moved distally in the osteotomy gap. Care should be taken if this technique is chosen (the cage is placed below the patella insertion point) as placement of the cage in this position can increase the incidence of tuberosity fracture (excessive bending moment). At a more advanced stage (e.g., at recheck radiographs), it is not recommended to try and remove the cage. Other stabilizing procedures should be considered (TPLO, extra/intracapsular stabilization) (Figure 13.8).
- Physcial rehabilitation therapy can be considered as muscle forces are major contributors to stifle stability. Goals of physical rehabilitation should include increasing thigh muscle mass (quadriceps included), improving proprioception, and decreasing patient BW to help restore joint stability [7, 19, 24; author's personal observations].

13.3.3.5 *Outcome*

Favorable after correction.

13.3.3.6 *Prevention*

Relevant choice of cage' width is based on appropriately positioned radiographs, sound understanding of the measuring techniques, and good surgical technique.

13.3.4 Incorrect Cage Placement

13.3.4.1 *Definition*

Even with appropriate size selection, the cage can be inappropriately placed within the osteotomy gap (Figure 13.6). The upper limit of the cage should be aligned with the tibial tuberosity (point of insertion of the patella tendon) which in some cases can be several millimeters lower than the upper margin of the tibial crest. Placing the cage only 2–5 mm underneath the proximal margin of the tibial bone (crest), in order to decrease the risk of tibial tuberosity fracture/avulsion, can lead to suboptimal advancement of the tuberosity.

13.3.4.2 *Diagnosis*

- Checking the placement of the cage intraoperatively to ensure it is at the correct position.
- Postoperative radiographs are conclusive to determine incorrect cage placement (Figure 13.6).
- Persistent clinical signs of limping and palpation of joint instability can be associated with incorrect cage placment.

13.3.5 Fissure/Fracture of the Tibia at the Bone Hinge; Fracture of the Tibial Shaft

13.3.5.1 *Risk Factors*

- Advancement of the tibial tuberosity too quickly can result in fissuring of the cranial distal cortex. Advancement should be

gradual and slow. Advancement of the tibial crest should ideally take several minutes (3–5 minutes), going progressively, step by step, changing one spacer to the next larger one until the desired advancement is reached and the cage can eventually be placed (Figure 13.5a–d).
- Having an osteotomy length that is too short will increase the risk for fissuring of the bone distal to the osteotomy. Ideally, the osteotomy length (in mm) should approximately equal 7.5 times the width (in mm) of the cage in order to keep the opening angle of the osteotomy gap underneath 10° (Figure 13.2b,c; Table 13.1).
- If the bone hinge is too wide (Figure 13.9b), its strength will increase and thus its flexibility will decrease accordingly. Using Table 13.2 can help with estimating the desired bone hinge thickness.
- Age of the patient has a significant negative impact [7] likely because aged bone is more brittle.
- A spacer that is too wide or placed too low within the osteotomy gap can lead to fissuring.
- Any combination of the above risk factors can contribute to fissures/fractures.
- When the crest is moved in a cranial and lateral direction (when concurrent medial patella luxation is addressed), this puts the distal hinge under both bending and torsional stress.

13.3.5.2 Diagnosis

- Visually noting a fissure during surgery; in some situations dissection of the periosteum is needed to visualize a fissure.
- A cracking sound upon advancement can indicate a fissure.
- Sudden loss of resistance when the crest is advanced cranially.
- Postoperative radiographs are conclusive with particular attention to the distal aspect of the osteotomy (Figure 13.9b).

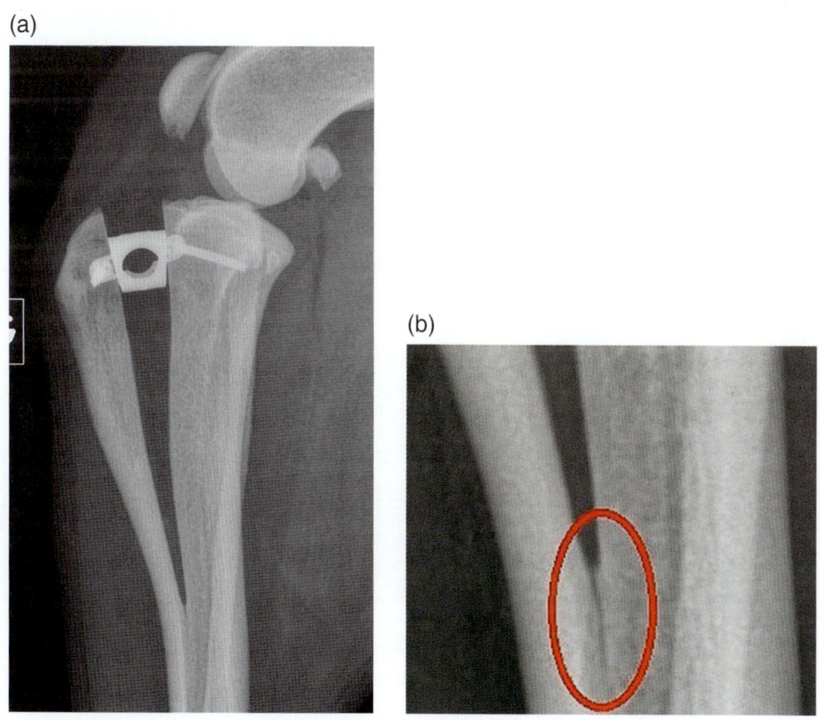

Figure 13.9 (a) Postoperative radiograph of a MMT; note that a fissure can be seen extending distally beyond the osteotomy. (b) A magnified image of the fissure (red circle) noted to be extending beyond the distal aspect of the osteotomy. Fissures are regularly observed when the bone hinge is too wide and hence too stiff and/or the osteotomy length is too short. A fissure aligned with the osteotomy as in this case would not require any additional attention in most cases.

- In any case where acute lameness develops, immediate radiographic investigation is warranted.

13.3.5.3 *Treatment*

- If the fissure stays well aligned with the osteotomy line, no particular treatment is recommended (Figure 13.9).
- If the fissure diverges from the osteotomy line (Figure 13.10a,b), and the width of bone hinge is reduced, then adjunct fixation should be used (Kirschner wires, cerclage wires) (Figure 13.10c). Care must be taken to place the wire in a drilled hole that is located distal and caudal to the tip of the osteotomy.
- If the fissure engages the tibial shaft, risk of a diaphyseal fracture increases under bending or torsional stress (Figure 13.11a). A plate spanning the fissure/fracture line should be applied to the tibia (Figure 13.11b,c), or a splint could be placed and maintained for several weeks (Figure 13.11d–g) while strict patient confinement is implemented.

13.3.5.4 *Outcome*

- Favorable when appropriate measures are taken to prevent a fissure from propagating into a tibial diaphyseal fracture, or immediate measures are taken when the fractures are identified.

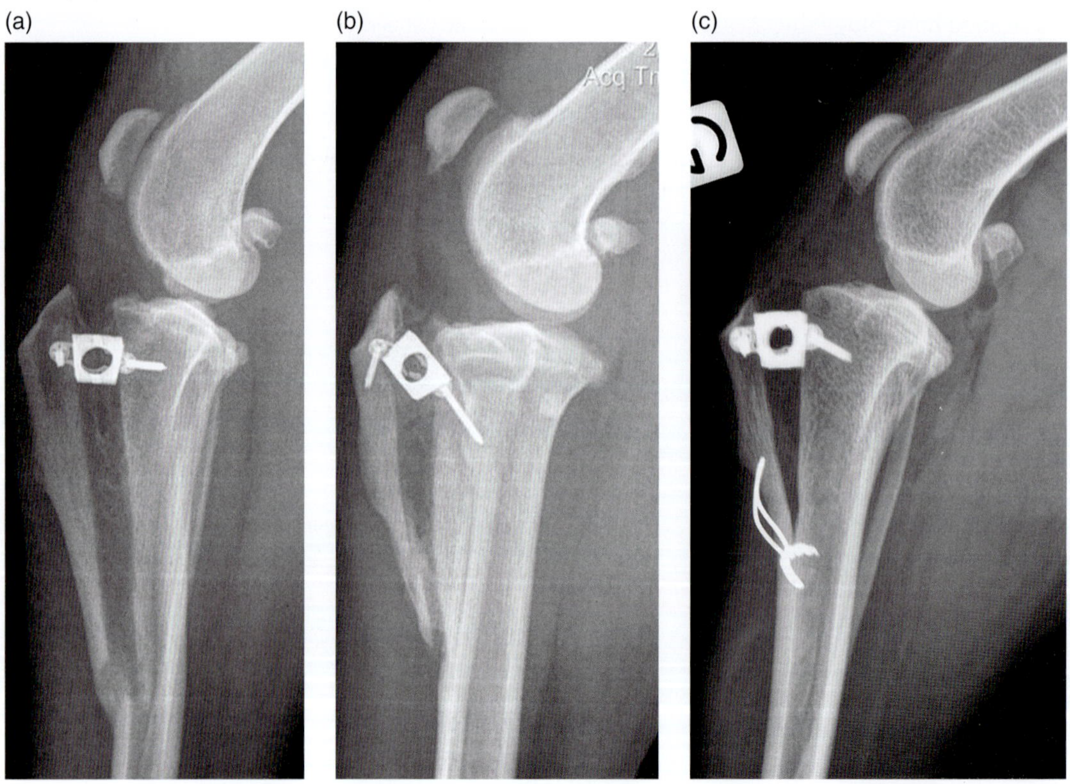

Figure 13.10 (a) A fracture of the distal aspect of the osteotomy resulting in mild proximal displacement of the tibial crest. In this case, since the displacment was mild with no instability of the stifle noted, the patient was managed conservatively and the bone went on to heal uneventfully. (b) A fracture of the distal aspect of the osteotomy resulting in moderate proximal displacement of the tibial crest. This displacement led to stifle instability. A hinge that was too thin was likely the cause of this fracture. As can be seen by the radiograph, healing is occurring at the fracture site. (c) Immediate postoperative radiograph of a figure of eight wire placed intraoperatively in a prophylactic manner to prevent fissuring/fracturing of the hinge. The thickness of the hinge was probably excessive, making the hinge too stiff. A longer osteotomy would decrease the bending stress on the hinge.

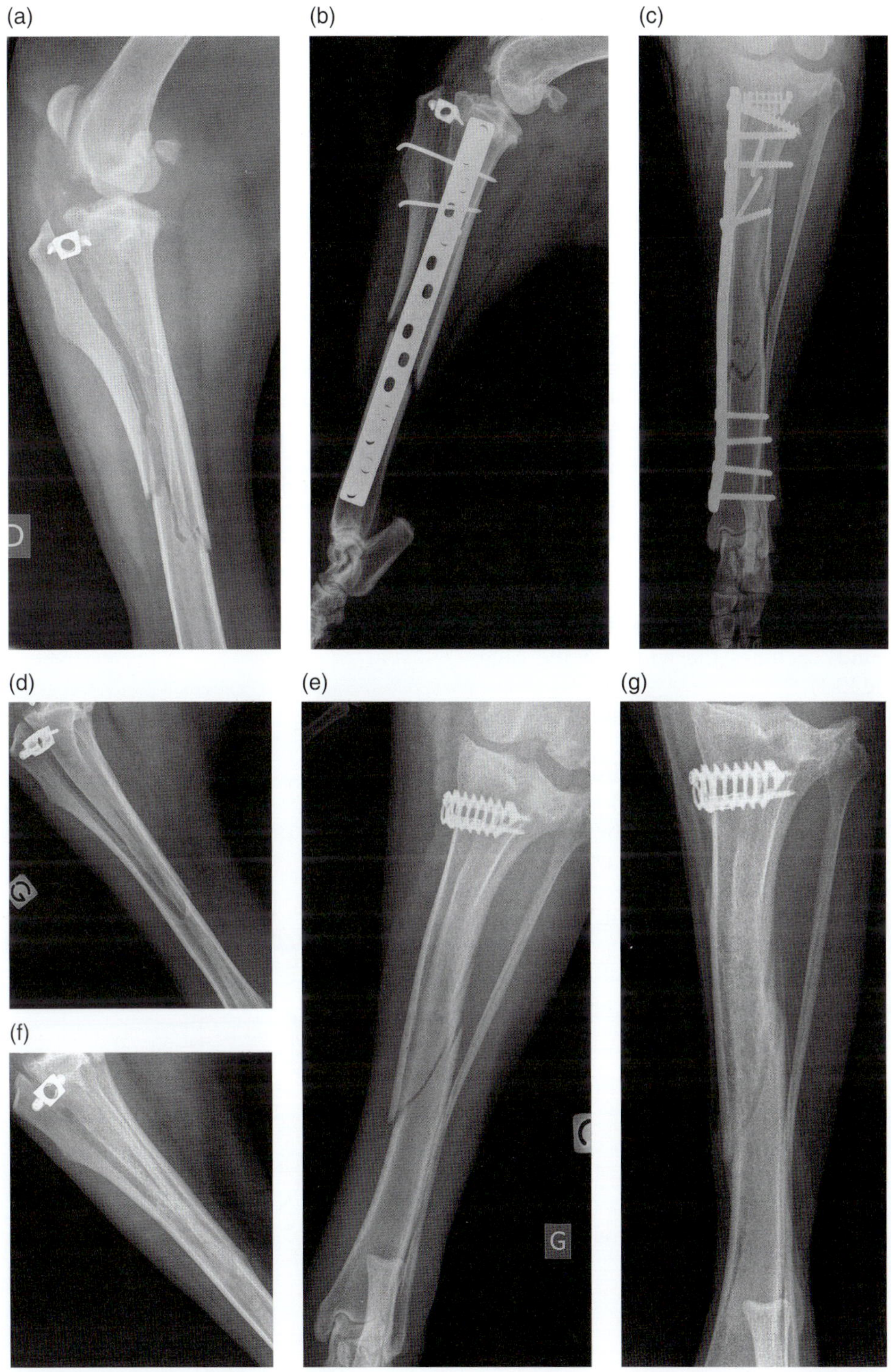

Figure 13.11 Fractures of the tibial shaft following an MMT procedure. Case 1 (a–c): Bernese Mountain Dog, 79 kg; the tibia fractured within 24 hours postoperative; the hinge thickness was too large and the osteotomy was irregular (multiple planes). Two K-wires were first used to secure the crest to the caudal proximal tibia segment. A 3.5 mm broad dynamic compression plate was applied on the medial tibia extending from the proximal to the distal tibia spanning the fracture. Recovery was uneventful. Case 2 (d–g): Bouvier des Flandres, 52 kg; a long fissure had already occurred during surgery and the tibial shaft fractured within 5 days postoperative. The hinge was too thick, especially on the lateral side of the tibia (trans cortex), probably because the saw blade had not been adequately tilted during the osteotomy. Given that the fibula was intact, it was elected to manage this with immobilization using a modified Robert-Jones bandage followed by strict confinement for 6 weeks. This resulted in acceptable bone healing and a good functional recovery.

- Nondisplaced tibia shaft fractures with an intact fibula can be managed conservatively with cage rest and splintage.
- If the hinge fracture results in a slightly cranially displaced tibial crest, while the cage is intact, the tibial tuberosity will maintain its advanced position, with no negative effect on stifle stability. The preserved soft tissues surrounding the proximal tibia probably contribute to this scenario. If this is observed during surgery, a figure eight wire, K-wire or plate application should be used to avoid further displacement.

13.3.5.5 Prevention

- Slow and progressive advancement of the tibial tuberosity (proceed by 3 mm increments in 3–5 minutes).
- The osteotomy should be long enough (around 7.5 times the width of the cage; Table 13.1).
- Adequate width of the bone hinge (2–8 mm according to BW; Table 13.2).
- Using a cage of adequate width (according to TPA and size of the patient).
- Follow the guidelines for the osteotomy directions (caudo-medial to cranio-lateral 20° to the sagittal plane).
- Score and cut the cis cortex first. Use a sharp blade for the osteotomy.
- Open an osteotomy angle of <10°.
- Creating a hole in the distal osteotomy is no longer recommended.

13.3.6 Patella Baja

13.3.6.1 Definition

Patella baja refers to a distalized (lower than normal) position of the patella in relation to the femoral trochlear groove.

13.3.6.2 Risk Factors

- The MMT pulls the patella downwards several millimeters as the tibial tuberosity is cranio-ventrally rotated around its distal bone hinge.
- The larger the advancement, the higher the magnitude of patella baja [25].

13.3.6.3 Diagnosis

Radiographs are definitive whereas palpation may not be clear. Different ratios have been proposed to assess the patella height from digital radiography: Insall–Salvati, Blackburne–Peel, and Caton–Deschamps [26].

13.3.6.4 Treatment

Patella baja, following MMT, does not seem to be of clinical relevance, hence no treatment is indicated (Figure 13.12).

13.3.7 Patella Luxation

13.3.7.1 Definition

Medial or lateral displacement of the patella.

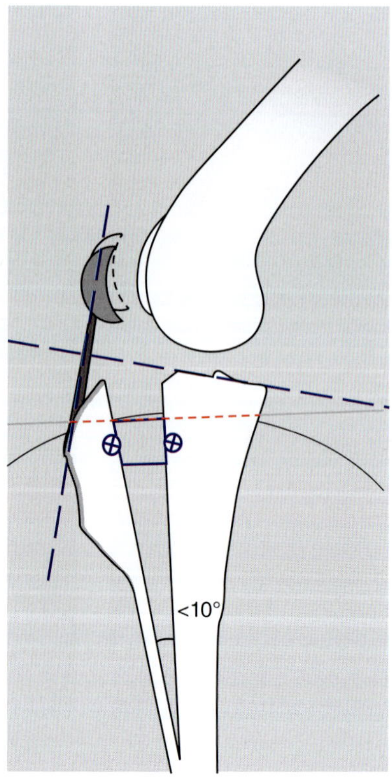

Figure 13.12 This drawing illustrates patella baja expected after application of a large TTA cage. The change in the patella position typically does not have any negative clinical impact.

13.3.7.2 *Risk Factors*

- Poor surgical technique leading to uncontrolled displacement of the tibial crest. This is possibly due to incorrect placement of the spacer within the osteotomy gap or incorrect osteotomy with unequal thickness between cis and trans cortex of the bone hinge (Figure 13.4). Uncontrolled displacment of the tibial crest is more likely to occur if the bone hinge breaks during advancement. This will allow the tibial crest to easily move in any direction, and as such could lead to unanticipated medial or lateral transpostion of the tibial crest.
- Although the MMT, like any other tuberostiy advancement procedure, decreases the force exerted by the quadriceps mechanism by reducing the force pushing the patella against the femoral trochlea, this does not seem to increase the risk of patella luxation.

13.3.7.3 *Diagnosis*

- Persistent or intermittent lameness consistent with patella luxation.
- Palpation will reveal the luxation direction (medial versus lateral).
- Radiographs are helpful to evaluate the osteotomy as well as other predisposing pathologies associated with patella luxation such as distal femoral varus.

13.3.7.4 *Treatment*

If diagnosis is made once the cage is positioned within the osteotomy gap, the cage should be removed, allowing correct realignment of the tibial tuberosity with the tibial shaft and repositioning of the cage. In case of later diagnosis when bone healing has already taken place, revision surgery becomes more complex as cage extraction from its bony environment can be tedious. The cage can be removed by using small chisels lightly disrupting the osteointegration between the bone and the cage, and the osteotomy should be revised to allow crest movement in either the lateral or medial plane (according to the luxation). Care must be taken to control for collapse of the previously measured crest advancement.

13.3.7.5 *Outcome*

- A positive outcome can be expected in acute cases where early identification and revision are considered.
- In chronic cases, the functional prognosis might be less favorable.

13.3.7.6 *Prevention*

- Minimize the incidence of distal bone hinge breakage by strictly following technical recommendations.
- In case of distal bone hinge breakage, check the alignment of the tibial crest with the tibial shaft and patella position before securing the cage with screws and restabilizing the tibial crest.

13.3.8 Incomplete Bone Healing (Filling) of the Osteotomy Gap

13.3.8.1 *Definition*

In some rare cases, the osteotomy gap never entirely fills in with new bone (Figure 13.7b). Typically, there is complete or nearly complete healing of bone within the osteotomy gap (Figure 13.7a).

13.3.8.2 *Risk Factors*

- Absence of graft during the surgical procedure.
- Possibly in a construct where stiffness is too great, the minimum interfragmentary effective strain theoretically required to trigger new bone formation can not be reached, hence no new bone is laid down.

13.3.8.3 *Diagnosis*

- Radiographs are conclusive.
- There seem to be no clinical signs associated with it.

13.3.8.4 *Treatment*

No treatment is usually recommended as the situation does not seem to cause any functional problem. Some surgeons do not feel confortable with leaving the osteotomy gap unfilled, hence they systematically graft the area using an autologous cancellous bone graft harvested locally at the proximal tibial metaphysis.

13.3.8.5 *Outcome*

Favorable.

13.3.8.6 *Prevention*

Grafting of the osteotomy site with cancellous autogenous bone graft should prevent this from occurring. However, given that lack of new bone production into the osteotomy site does not result in a negative consequence, it can be argued that bone grafting is not needed. The author does not routinely graft the osteotomy gap.

13.4 Relevant Literature

The MMT has been largely inspired by what Maquet developed 40 years ago and used throughout the world to treat chondromalacia of the femoro-patellar joint in humans [2, 3, 27, 28]. Publications reporting complications after TTA performed with maintenance of a distal bone hinge, as Maquet initially designed, are still scarce in veterinary orthopedics [7, 19, 28–33]. The technique of advancing the tibial tuberosity to achieve stifle joint stability while maintaining the distal bone hinge is still relatively new in the veterinary field, In other techniques inspired by Maquet like the TTA-Rapid [10] and the MMP [11], the osteotomy does not extend distal to the tibial crest and a hole (called a Maquet hole by some authors) is drilled through the tibia at the tip of the osteotomy to serve as a stress reducer, likely easing the tibial crest advancement while decreasing the risk of fissure or fracture. Only the TTA-2 technique, designed by Tepic and Hopmans in 2004 [9], prolongs the osteotomy far below the tibial crest to extend into the tibial diaphysis as Maquet did [2] and as the MMT does.

The original TTA technique has moved from a rather small cage of the first generation affixed to the bone with two small self-tapping screws to a longer cage (TTA-2), better filling the osteomy gap and avoiding the two screws thanks to a serrated profile. Furthemore, TTA-2 is a very standardized operative procedure, nicely designed and supported by specific hardware (an articulated sawing guide and a very fine spreader), recommended to strengthen the tibial crest attachment with a suture. This author, driven by the desire to spare the soft tissues and to keep the procedure as simple as possible yet making it safe and effective, favors a more patient-specific approach where, after progressive refinement from an experimental trial, length of the osteotomy now varies according to the desired advancement and the width of the bone hinge varies with the weight of the patient. All of these elements aim at decreasing to a minimum the risk of fissure and fractures of the tibial crest and tibial diaphysis [7, 8, 12, 19, 34–37].

Although possible persistence of stifle joint instability has been an issue (likely caused by insufficient cranial advancement of the tibial tuberosity with postliminary meniscal tears as a consequence) since the MMT has been used in clinics, this complication is not by any means specific to the MMT as it can affect all types of TTA techniques. A possible negative impact of the so-called Maquet hole, distally limiting the osteotomy, is no longer an issue with the MMT, as the author does not recommend it [7] and even advises against it.

Conversely, what is specific to the MMT (and related techniques like the MMP and TTA-2) is the development of patella baja. Although the absence of proximal translation of the tibial tuberosity upon advancement contributes to increasing by several degrees (2–4° according to the measuring method) the patellar tendon angle (PTA) with the tibial plateau slope or the common tangent, the clinical implication is unknown and likely irrelevant as the 90° PTA target is not very strict. Apelt et al. [6] have indeed demonstrated that neutralization of tibio-femoral shearing forces occurred at a PTA of 90.3 +/− 9°, hence from 81° to 99°. Furthemore, the vertical position of the patella decreases only by 3–4 mm in 30 kg dogs [25] and even less in small-breed dogs. As the position of the patella already changes throughout the physiological stifle range of motion and as every dog has its own particular physiological range throughout the stance phase, a change of only a few millimeters in the vertical position has, not surprinsingly, little clinical relevance, if any.

References

1. Maquet, P. (1984). *Biomechanics of the Knee*, 2e. Cham: Springer Verlag.
2. Maquet, P. (1976). Advancement of the tibial tuberosity. *Clin. Orthop. Relat. Res.* 115 (1): 223–227.
3. Rappoport, L.H., Browne, M.G., and Wickiewicz, T.L. (1992). The Maquet osteotomy. *Orthop. Clin. North Am.* 4: 645–656.
4. Montavon, P.M., Damur, D.M., and Tepic, S. (2002). Advancement of the tibial tuberosity for the treatment of carnial cruciate deficient canine stifle. In: *Proceedings of the First World Orthopaedics Veterinary Congress*, 152. Munich.
5. Tepic, S., Damur, D.M., and Montavon, P.M. (2002). Biomechanics of the stifle joint. In: *Proceedings of the First World Orthopaedics Veterinary Congress*, 189–190. Munich.
6. Apelt, D., Kowaleski, M., and Boudrieau, R. (2007). Effect of tibial tuberosity advancement on cranial tibial subluxation in canine cranial cruciate-deficient stifle joints: an in vitro experimental study. *Vet. Surg.* 36 (2): 170–177.
7. Ramirez, J., Barthelemy, N., Noël, S. et al. (2015). Complications and outcome of a new modified Maquet technique for treatment of cranial cruciate ligament rupture in 82 dogs. *Vet. Comp. Orthop. Traumatol.* 28 (5): 339–346.
8. Brunel, L., Etchepareborde, S., Barthélémy, N. et al. (2013). Mechanical testing of a new osteotomy design for tibial tuberosity advancement using the modified Maquet technique. *Vet. Comp. Orthop. Traumatol.* 26 (1): 47–53.
9. Tepic, S. and Hopmans, J. (2016). *TTA-2 Instruction Manual*. Zurich: Kyon.
10. Samoy, Y., Verhoeven, G., Bosmans, T. et al. (2015). TTA rapid: description of the technique and short term clinical trial results of the first 50 cases. *Vet. Surg.* 44 (4): 474–484.
11. Ness, M.G. (2016). The modified Maquet procedure (MMP) in dogs: technical development and initial clinical experience. *J. Am. Anim. Hosp. Assoc.* 52 (4): 242–250.
12. Etchepareborde, S., Barthelemy, N., Brunel, L. et al. (2014). Biomechanical testing of a β-tricalcium phosphate wedge for advancement of the tibial tunerosity. *Vet. Comp. Orthop. Traumatol.* 1: 14–19.
13. Barnhart, M.D., Watson, A.T., Thatcher, L.G. et al. (2016). Prospective randomized clinical and radiographic evaluation of a novel bioabsorbable biocomposite tibial tuberosity advancement cage implant. *Vet. Surg.* 45 (5): 651–658.
14. Allan, R.M. (2014). A modified Maquet technique for management of cranial cruciate avulsion in a cat. *J. Small Anim. Pract.* 55: 52–56.
15. Retournard, M., Bilmont, A., Asimus, E. et al. (2016). Effect of tibial tuberosity advancement on cranial tibial subluxation in the feline cranial cruciate deficient stifle joint: an ex vivo experimental study. *Res. Vet. Sci.* 107: 240–245.
16. Brown, N., Bertocci, G., and Marcellin-Little, D. (2015). Canine stifle biomechanics associated with tibial tuberosity advancement predicted using a computer model. *Vet. Surg.* 44 (7): 866–873.
17. Case, J.B., Hulse, D., Kerwin, S.C. et al. (2008). Meniscal injury following cranial cruciate ligament stabilization surgery in 26 dogs (29 stifles). *Vet. Comp. Orthop. Traumatol.* 21 (4): 365–367.
18. Blond, L., Thrall, D.E., Roe, S.C. et al. (2008). Diagnostic accuracy of magnetic resonance imaging for meniscal tears in dogs affected with naturally Occuring cranial cruciate ligament rupture. *Vet. Radiol. Ultrasound* 49 (5): 425–431.
19. Lefebvre, M., Broux, O., Barthélémy, N. et al. (2018). Risk factors for tibial damage associated with the modified Maquet technique in 174 stifles. *Vet. Surg.* 47 (1): 30–35.
20. Pillard, P., Livet, V., Cabon, Q. et al. (2017). Evaluation of a new method to determine the tibial tuberosity advancement distance required to reduce the patellar tendon-tibial plateau angle to 90° with the modified Maquet technique in dogs. *Am. J. Vet. Res.* 78 (4): 517–528.
21. Millet, M., Bismuth, C., Labrunie, A. et al. (2013). Measurement of the patellar tendon-tibial plateau angle and tuberosity advancement in dogs with cranial cruciate ligament rupture. Reliability of the common tangent and tibial plateau methods of measurement. *Vet. Comp. Orthop. Traumatol.* 26: 469–478.
22. Cadmus, J., Palmer, R.H., and Duncan, C. (2014). The effect of preoperative planning method on recommended tibial tuberosity advancement cage size. *Vet. Surg.* 43: 995–1000.
23. Ober, C.A., Factor, G., Meiner, Y. et al. (2019). Influence of tibial plateau leveling osteotomy and tibial tuberosity advancement on passive laxity of the cranial cruciate deficient stifle in dogs. *Vet. Surg.* 48: 401–407.
24. Ramirez, J., Lefebvre, M., Böhme, B. et al. (2015). Preactivation of the quadriceps muscle could limit cranial tibial translation in a cranial cruciate ligament deficient canine stifle. *Res. Vet. Sci.* 98: 115–120.
25. Neville-Towle, J., Makara, M., Johnson, K., and Voss, K. (2017). Effect of proximal translation of the osteotomized tibial tuberosity during tibial tuberosity advancement on patellar position and patellar ligament angle. *BMC Vet. Res.* 13 (1): 18.
26. Blackburne, J.S. and Peel, T. (1977). A new method of measuring patella height. *J. Bone Joint Surg.* 59-B: 241–242.
27. Mendes, D.G., Soudry, M., and Iusim, M. (1987). Clinical assessment of Maquet tibial tuberosity advancement. *Clin. Orthop. Relat. Res.* 222: 228–238.

28. Bessette, G.C. and Hunter, G.E. (1988). The Maquet procedure. A retrospective review. *Clin. Orthop. Relat. Res.* 232: 159–167.
29. Marques, D.R.C. and Ibanez, J.F. (2017). Complications associated with the Maquet procedure – two case reports in dogs. *SOJ Vet. Sci.* 3 (1): 1–3.
30. Retallack, L. and Daye, R.M. (2018). A modified Maquet-tibial tuberosity advancement technique for treatment of canine cranial cruciate ligament disease: short term outcome and complications. *Vet. Surg.* 47 (1): 44–51.
31. Crovace, A.M., Staffieri, F., Monopoli, D. et al. (2020). Role of tibial tuberosity fracture/fissure through the Maquet hole in stifle osteoarthritis after porous tibial tuberosity advancement in dogs at mid-term follow-up. *Vet. Sci.* 7: 1.
32. De Sousa, R., Egan, P., Parsons, K. et al. (2017). Treatment of tibial diaphyseal fractures following plateless tibial tuberosity advancement to manage cranial cruciate disease. *J. Small Anim. Pract.* 58: 372–379.
33. Costa, M., Craig, D., Cambridge, T. et al. (2017). Major complications of tibial tuberosity advancement in 1613 dogs. *Vet. Surg.* 46 (4): 494–500.
34. Etchepareborde, S., Mills, J., Busoni, V. et al. (2011). Theoretical discrepancy between cage size and efficient tibial tuberosity advancement in dogs treated for cranial cruciate ligament rupture. *Vet. Comp. Orthop. Traumatol.* 24 (1): 27–31.
35. Etchepareborde, S., Brunel, L., Bollen, G., and Balligand, M. (2011). Preliminary experience of a modified Maquet technique for repair of cranial cruciate ligament rupture in dogs. *Vet. Comp. Orthop. Traumatol.* 24 (3): 223–227.
36. Etchepareborde, S., Barthelemy, N., Mills, J. et al. (2010). Mechanical testing of a modified stabilisation method for tibial tuberosity advancement. *Vet. Comp. Orthop. Traumatol.* 6: 400–405.
37. Barthelemy N, Brunel L, Laurent C, and Farnir F, Balligand M. (2013). Mechanical torsional properties of tibiae following modified maquet technique or tibial tuberosity advancement. *Proceedings of the Fourth VOS Annual Meeting.*

Section V

Nonsurgical Management and Physical Rehabilitation

14 Complications Associated with Stifle Orthotics

Bryan T. Torres and Steven C. Budsberg

14.1 Introduction

The use of stifle orthoses in dogs with cruciate pathology is gaining popularity in both preoperative and postoperative patients as well as those that are unable to undergo surgery. While significant numbers of orthoses are being recommended and prescribed in lieu of surgery, no clinical data exist to support the efficacy of these orthotics as a replacement for surgical repair [1, 2]. Additionally, our understanding of the impact of orthoses on joint function in companion animals is limited, with very few studies focused on the dog stifle. The majority of information available to clinicians on orthoses is limited to other joints [3–7] or review articles [2, 8].

Critical evaluation of the effects on stifle function following orthoses application is limited to two studies that assessed the joint motion and one study that evaluated paw pressure before and after orthosis application. The first study utilized a computerized simulation to assess the impact of an orthosis on virtual joint motion [9]. The second study evaluated joint motion and other temporospatial variables in a group of normal dogs with and without a stifle orthosis [10]. Finally, a small retrospective case series evaluated paw pressure in dogs wearing stifle orthoses but did not evaluate joint function specifically [11].

Unfortunately, there is even less information available on complications experienced by dogs wearing stifle orthoses. One recent survey examined owner satisfaction with orthoses and did document some common complications [12], the vast majority of which involved skin lesions as a result of wearing the orthosis. However, complications that have not been addressed previously are the potentially unintended impact of stifle orthosis use on the adjacent joints and associated soft tissues [10].

In this chapter we will explore the available evidence for the use of stifle orthoses in dogs, paying particular attention to their impact on the restoration of joint motion, clinical use in injured limbs, and associated complications.

14.2 Stifle Orthoses Construction

The construction of orthoses is important and depending on changes in the components and/or composition, it can impart varying degrees of stability to the underlying joint. Orthosis can vary from rigid to semi-rigid, and flexible.

Complications in Canine Cranial Cruciate Ligament Surgery, First Edition. Edited by Ron Ben-Amotz and David L. Dycus.

These varying degrees of stability can be affected by the material from which the body of the orthosis (i.e., "frame") is made as well as the type of moveable joint (hinge) or in some cases the absence of a moveable joint [2, 9].

14.2.1 Stifle Orthosis Frame

The majority of stifle orthoses frames used in dogs are made from a rigid material and are custom designed from a cast or mold to fit an individual limb. These frames are formed using various materials, including thermosetting plastics that are molded into a permanent shape after heating or various forms of thermoforming plastics (e.g., thermoplastic) which soften when heated, harden when cooled, and can be reheated and reshaped numerous times (Figure 14.1) [13]. Orthoses can be made without a moveable joint to restrict motion or more commonly with some form of hinge joint to allow varying degrees of joint motion. The fabrication of a custom orthosis can require a period of weeks before it is available for patient use. However, these orthoses are designed to an individual patient's specifications. The currently available clinical data on stifle orthosis function in dogs are centered around custom-fit orthoses [9–11].

Alternatively, off-the-shelf stifle orthoses are also available. The frames of these types of orthoses are prefabricated and produced in select sizes (small, medium, large, etc.). This can allow an in-hospital and semicustomizable fit due to the integration of heat-moldable material and other adjustable components within the orthosis frame (Figure 14.1). Off-the-shelf orthoses have the benefit of allowing quick and repeated frame customization and may prove beneficial for those patients who experience changes in limb size (e.g., during the postsurgical and rehabilitation period). However, in the authors' experience, off-the-shelf orthoses often require more extensive in-hospital adjustments to provide adequate fit and function, as compared to custom orthoses, and this may lead to more complications, especially skin issues. Unfortunately, most veterinarians have limited experience and/or expertise in orthosis fitting and adjustment, making it challenging to obtain the level of fit that a custom-made orthotic can provide.

To date, a comparison between custom-made and off-the-shelf stifle orthoses in dogs has not been performed. Therefore, for those patients

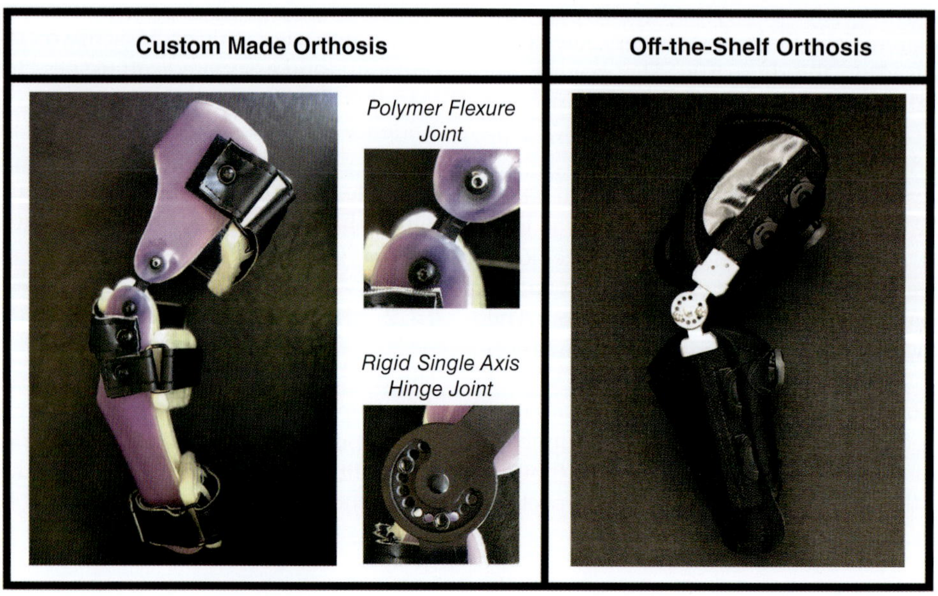

Figure 14.1 Examples of a custom-made and an off-the-shelf stifle orthosis for use in dogs. Source: Bryan T. Torres.

where optimal orthosis fit and function is required, a custom-made orthosis represents the best available option.

14.2.2 Moveable Joint Options with Stifle Orthoses

Orthosis movement is achieved with the placement of a joint between the thigh frame (i.e., femoral component) and the crus frame (i.e., tibial component). Various types of moveable joints have been utilized in stifle orthoses. The two most common types of joints are a rigid single-axis hinge joint and a more "rubberized" flexible joint often referred to as a polymer flexure joint (Figure 14.2). The type of joint present in an orthosis directly impacts the overall support imparted to the braced joint and thus its range of motion (ROM). Additionally, rigid single-axis hinge joints may have adjustable stops that allow clinicians to selectively restrict joint flexion and extension and flexible joints are available in varying degrees of stiffness.

The available research regarding the impact of joint type on stifle orthosis motion is limited. A small unpublished kinematic study evaluating normal dogs wearing two different stifle orthoses with differing joints (metal hinge joint versus flexible joint) found differences in overall orthosis motion (Figure 14.2). While flexion and extension of the orthosis were similar, a more profound difference was seen in the other planes of motion (internal/external rotation and abduction/adduction). A notable difference occurred during internal/external rotation of the orthosis, with more profound internal rotation during maximum joint flexion, corresponding with the typical screw-home mechanism of the femoral-tibial joint. Similar findings were reported in a recent computerized simulation [9]. That study found that hinge stiffness impacted internal rotation, with stiffer hinges allowing less internal rotation and less stiff hinges allowing more.

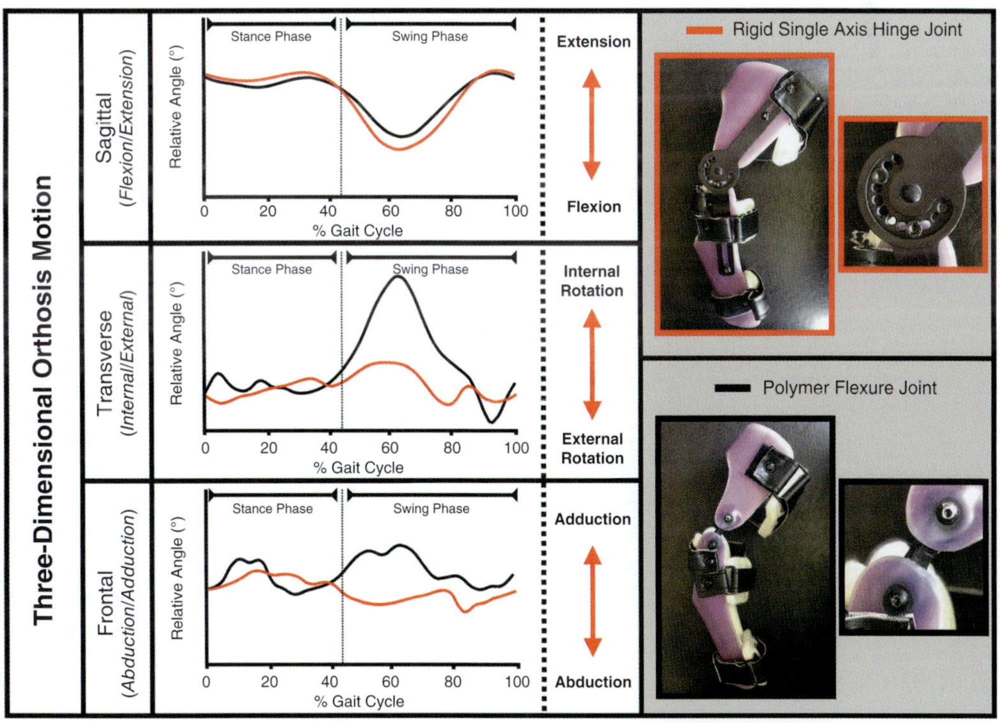

Figure 14.2 Three-dimensional orthosis motion during a trotting gait. Data were obtained from a single dog wearing custom-fit orthoses manufactured with differing joints. For ease of comparison, the graph waveforms have been produced to illustrate relative angular orthosis joint motion. The red lines represent the orthosis with a rigid single-axis hinge joint and the black lines represent the orthosis with a polymer flexure joint. Source: Bryan T. Torres.

It is possible that cranial cruciate ligament-deficient dogs with more profound rotational instability (e.g., "pivot shift") either before or after surgery may benefit from an orthosis with increased stiffness, especially to internal rotation. Unfortunately, the ideal hinge stiffness for a cranial cruciate-insufficient dog using an orthosis in lieu of surgery or post surgery is unknown.

14.3 Stifle Orthoses and Owner Perception

According to a recent survey-based study, the perception of owners of dogs who had orthoses to manage cranial cruciate ligament (CCL) rupture was good and indicated that they may provide some benefit [12]. That study found that 85% of owners who chose an orthosis as the primary treatment for CCL rupture in their dogs were satisfied with that decision and would make the same choice again. Interestingly, this was similar to those who chose surgical treatment with tibial plateau leveling osteotomy (TPLO) as indicated by a 90% satisfaction rate. However, those who chose surgery with TPLO were significantly more likely to rate that treatment as "excellent, very good, or good" compared to those owners who chose to use an orthosis as the primary means of joint stabilization. Additionally, owners of dogs who underwent surgical stabilization were more likely to report that their dogs had "mild or no lameness" following treatment. An additional study found that the three most common reasons for owners electing an orthosis in lieu of surgery in dogs with CCL rupture were: (i) dislike the idea of the surgery/too invasive; (ii) age of the dog; (iii) cost of surgery [1].

Overall, owner perception of orthoses as a treatment for CCL rupture is good, but the clinical results are inferior to TPLO. Most owners who choose orthoses over surgical correction do so based on patient-related concerns or for financial reasons [1].

14.4 Stifle Orthoses and Weight Bearing

Limited information is available regarding the impact of stifle orthoses on weight bearing in dogs with CCL rupture. Currently, there is only one study that has evaluated dynamic weight bearing in dogs with CCL rupture and treated with orthoses [11]. In that study, 10 dogs with unilateral CCL rupture were treated with orthoses and evaluated after 90 days or more of orthosis usage. The findings of this study demonstrated a small increase (3–5%) in weight bearing in dogs with CCL rupture fitted with custom orthoses. That is significantly less than the >18% increase reported in dogs with CCL rupture only 2 months after TPLO surgery [14]. Therefore, it is difficult to assess the benefits of wearing an orthosis in a cruciate-deficient stifle at this time. These findings appear to show that the positive subjective owner perceptions of orthosis usage and success are divergent from the objective data available and may be explained in part by the caregiver placebo effect [15]. Thus, this raises the question as to whether the clinical complications seen with orthoses are outweighed by the small clinical improvements documented.

14.5 Stifle Orthoses and Cranial-Caudal Translation

The ability of stifle orthoses to reduce or eliminate cranial-caudal translation in dogs with CCL rupture is unclear. Previous work has demonstrated that dogs with intact CCLs have <1 mm of passive joint laxity. However, dogs with CCL loss have significant passive cranial displacement and instability of approximately 11 mm [16]. These findings are more profound during active limb use (i.e., walking) [16, 17]. Thus, a primary goal of treating CCL injuries utilizing stifle orthoses should be the restoration of normal cranial-caudal joint stability.

Unfortunately, research regarding the ability of a stifle orthosis to impart cranial-caudal joint stability is limited. A recent computer simulation predicted that a stifle orthosis would reduce but not completely eliminate tibial translation in a dog with CCL rupture after the application of a stifle orthosis (Figure 14.3a) [9]. It is possible that this computer-predicted reduction in tibial translation after orthosis application would benefit dogs with CCL rupture who are not candidates for surgical stabilization. However, how this translates to clinical patients is unknown and the impact of orthosis

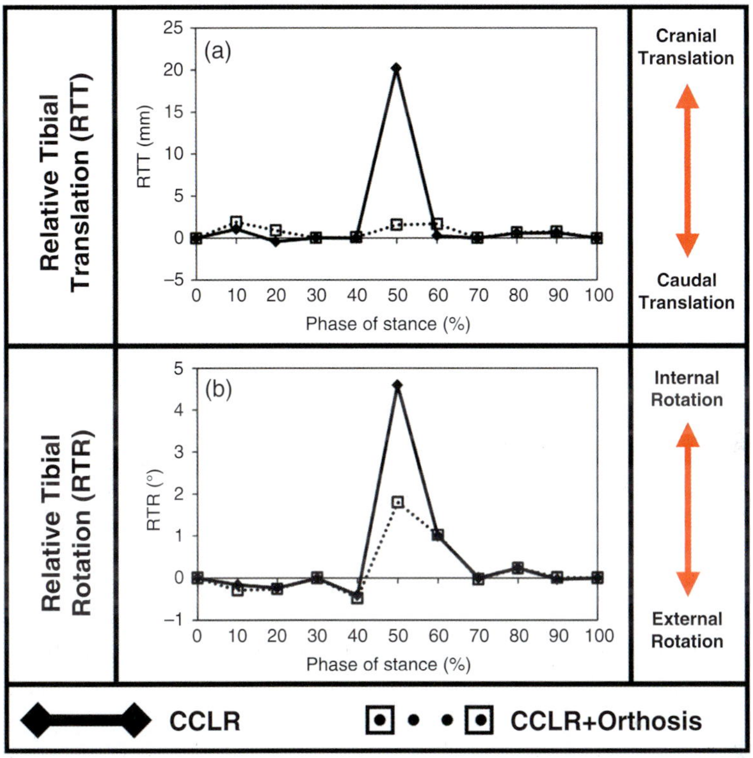

Figure 14.3 Computer-simulated relative tibial translation (RTT) (a) and relative tibial rotation (RTR) (b) throughout the stance phase. The solid line with black diamonds represents relative motion in a cranial cruciate-deficient stifle compared to a normal stifle. The dotted line with white squares represents relative motion in an orthosis-managed cranial cruciate-deficient stifle joint compared to a normal stifle. Lines connecting each 10% discrete interval of the stance phase are for visual purposes only and do not represent values obtained by use of the computer simulation. Source: Data in this figure have been adapted from a publication by Bertocci et al. [9].

use in stabilizing cranial-caudal instability *in vivo* has not been demonstrated. Therefore, the clinical utility and/or ability of stifle orthoses to provide cranial-caudal joint stability in dogs with CCL injury is uncertain. It is this lack of demonstrated ability of stifle orthoses to improve cranial-caudal stifle joint stability that may ultimately lead to continued or increasing osteoarthritis in the affected joint.

14.6 Stifle Orthoses and Joint Rotation

The reestablishment of normal joint motion is critical in dogs with CCL injuries. Treatment with orthoses that are too restrictive or allow excessive motion has the potential for deleterious effects on the recovering joint and long-term joint health. Currently, our understanding of how a stifle orthosis impacts joint rotation in dogs is limited to the information gleaned from two studies.

The first is a computer-based CCL rupture simulation model developed from a single dog that predicted relative internal-external rotation of the tibia with and without orthosis application [9]. In this study, internal tibial rotation was predicted to be reduced, but not completely eliminated, with orthosis application (Figure 14.3b). Additionally, changes in hinge stiffness affected internal/external tibial rotation, with stiffer hinges reducing rotation and less stiff hinges increasing rotation. Unfortunately, the degree to which an orthosis should restrict tibial rotation in a dog with a CCL injury is unclear. Previous studies have demonstrated the stifle to have a normal amount of internal tibial rotation during dynamic motion, most significant during stifle flexion [18–20]. This is termed the "screw-home mechanism." In cranial cruciate-deficient dogs, a recent study found a significant increase in internal tibial rotation during stance phase in clinically affected dogs [21]. These data correlate with the clinical findings in those cases where veterinarians find cruciate ligament-deficient dogs that have palpably excessive internal tibial rotation. Thus, it is possible that a more rotationally restrictive orthosis may prove beneficial and conversely, those orthoses that cannot restrict rotational instability may again contribute to continued joint degeneration.

The second study involved clinically normal dogs and reported on 3D joint motion of the pelvic limb with and without a stifle orthosis [10]. This study found that joint motion (flexion/extension, internal/external rotation, and abduction/adduction) was altered with the use of stifle orthoses at both a walk and trot. Interestingly, joint ROM was most profoundly affected at the end of the stance phase and led to a reduction in stifle extension during this time (Figure 14.4). Additionally, when complete joint and orthosis motion was evaluated, it was found that the relative stiffness of the orthosis was not fully translated to the underlying joint. This is highlighted by the more limited motion

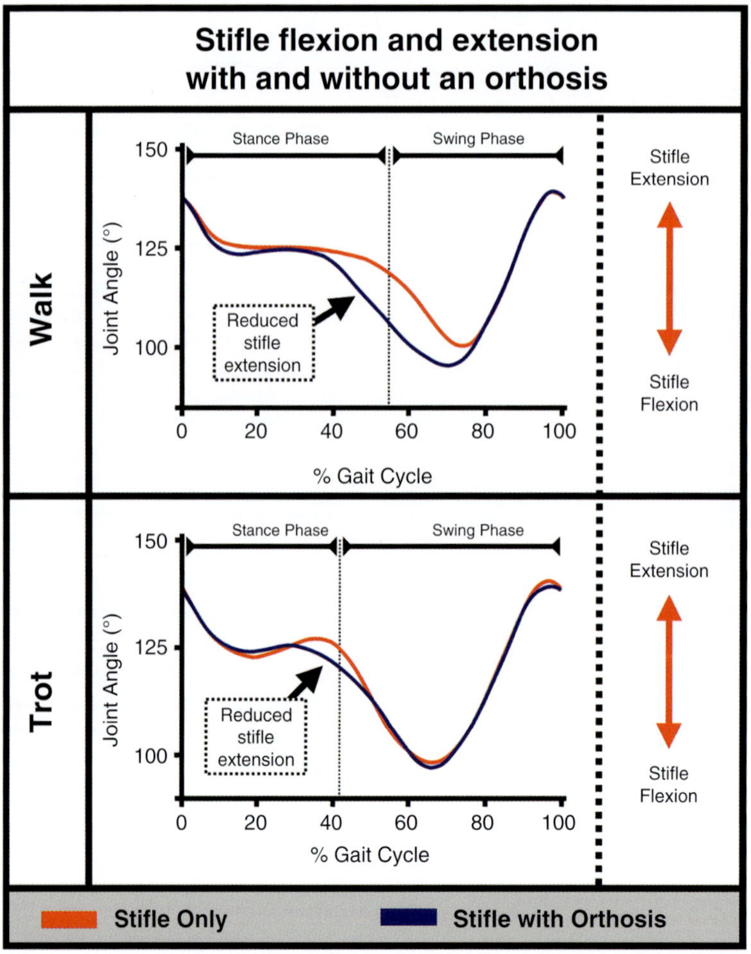

Figure 14.4 Stifle motion (flexion and extension) with and without an orthosis at a walk and trot. The red lines represent the stifle and the blue lines represent the braced stifle. The black arrows highlight the reduction in stifle extension at the end of stance phase. Source: Data in this figure have been adapted from a publication by Torres et al. [10].

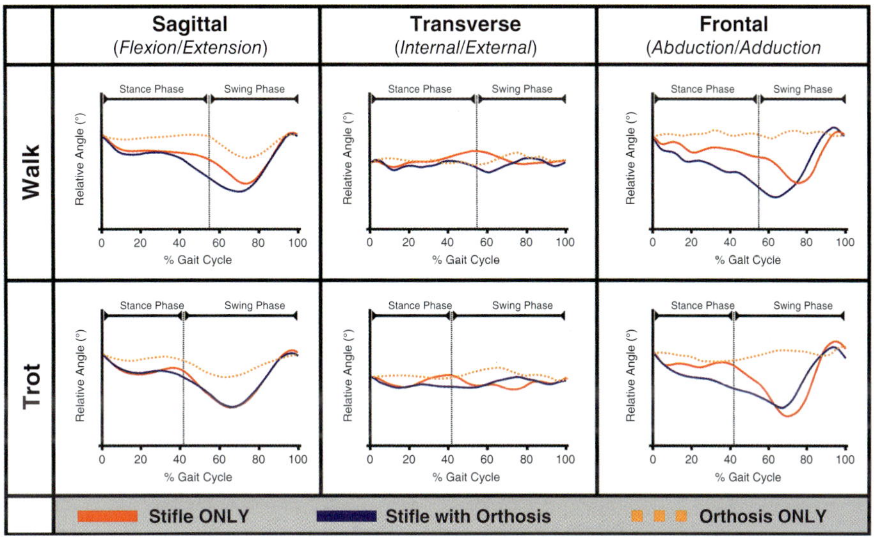

Figure 14.5 Three-dimensional stifle motion with and without an orthosis at a walk and trot. The graphs illustrate the mean stifle and orthosis angles from dogs with and without a stifle orthosis applied to the limb. For ease of comparison, the graph waveforms have been produced to illustrate relative angular joint motion for the three values. The red lines represent the stifle, the blue lines represent the stifle with orthosis, and the orange dotted line represents the orthosis alone. Source: Data in this figure have been adapted from a publication by Torres et al. [10].

of the orthosis compared to the underlying stifle joint (Figure 14.5). In this way, the orthosis failed to produce a significant "bracing" effect on the stifle.

14.7 Stifle Orthoses and the Impact on Adjacent Joints

An unexpected complication associated with stifle orthosis usage may be a negative impact on the adjacent joints. In humans, it has been shown that bracing of a lower limb extremity can impact adjacent joints during various activities [22, 23]. However, similar information is limited in dogs. Kinematic data from normal dogs with and without a stifle orthosis found that the application of a stifle orthosis resulted in concurrent changes to adjacent joint ROM, with a general reduction in hip motion and more profoundly tarsal motion (Figure 14.6) [10]. It is possible that changes in orthosis design and joint stiffness may influence the degree of impact a stifle orthosis has on adjacent joint motion. It is important that clinicians are aware of the potential to influence adjacent joints, especially in animals with polyarthropathies.

14.8 Clinical Complications during Orthotic Usage

As with all externally captive devices, stifle orthotics in dogs can lead to various complications. In humans, orthoses have been reported to result in both physical and psychosocial complications [13]. In animals, the most recognized complications are physical and can include skin and local tissue irritation, compression of local neurovascular structures, and pressure necrosis. Many of these complications are related to improper fit and/or function of the orthosis. Additionally, patient acceptance of the orthosis may also be a considerable factor and preclude usage.

14.8.1 Skin Irritation

This is the most commonly reported complication [12] and occurs secondary to abnormal interface or improper fit between the orthosis and the limb. Similar to other forms of external coaptation, this is a result of abnormal pressure or movement of the orthosis over the skin and is frequently seen in areas of maximal

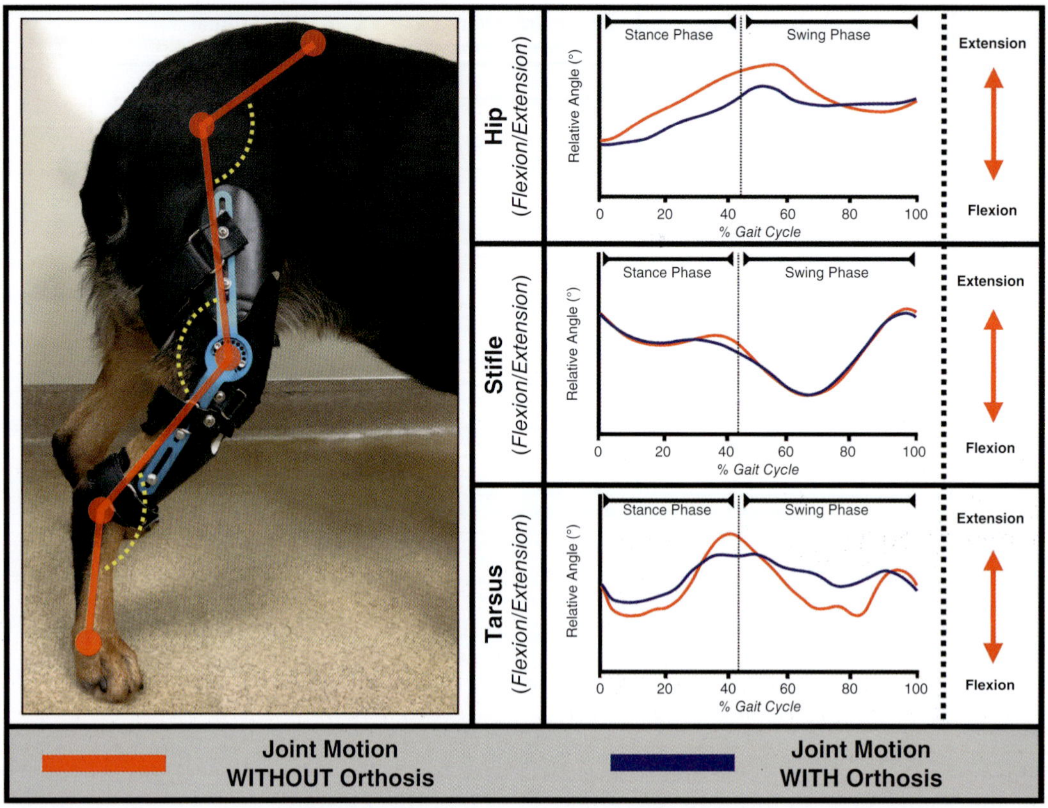

Figure 14.6 Pelvic limb joint motion (flexion and extension) with and without an orthosis at a trot. For ease of comparison, the graph waveforms have been produced to illustrate relative angular joint motion. The red lines represent joint motion without the stifle orthosis applied to the limb and the blue lines represent joint motion with the stifle orthosis applied to the limb. Source: Data in this figure have been adapted from a publication by Torres et al. [10].

orthosis/skin contact (Figure 14.7). Establishing a proper fit and enhancing padding in those areas are beneficial in addressing these issues. In some cases, major adjustments to the orthosis may be required and medical treatment of the lesion may be necessary to the point of limiting usage of the orthosis. If a brace is chosen as a primary treatment option, it is advised to slowly introduce the patient to its use. Currently, structured recommended guidelines for the introduction of orthosis usage are not available. However, daily usage is limited for the first week with a gradual increase in daily wear time. The owner should document any device problem (e.g., slippage, ease of donning or doffing, recognizing pressure sores, etc.) in order to be able to address any concerns. In addition, frequent rechecks with a veterinarian are encouraged to ensure proper fit of the orthosis.

14.8.2 Compression Phenomenon

Compression of local neurovascular structures can occur when the orthosis results in abnormal limb compression on the limb. This can lead to secondary pain, changes in local circulation resulting in impaired vascular supply, and/or limb edema [13]. Clinically, this can occur when either applied too tightly or when limb swelling is not appropriately anticipated, especially in the postoperative patient. The end-result of these two situations is similar (i.e., neurovascular compression) but the initial clinical situation and recognition differ.

When an orthosis is applied too tightly to a limb where swelling is not anticipated (i.e., "tourniquet effect"), the initial recognition of clinical signs can be related to peroneal nerve neuropraxia (drooped tarsus, toes are "dragged"

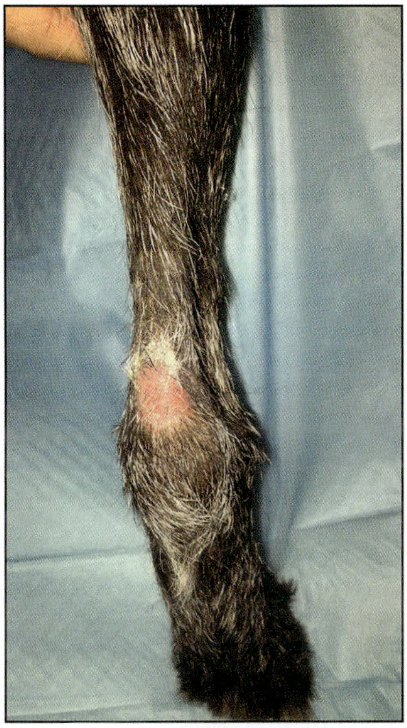

Figure 14.7 Image of skin lesion caused by an orthosis. Hair loss and skin irritation can be seen and, in many cases, may require medical care as well as orthosis adjustment. Source: Bryan T. Torres.

when the patient walks) or local vascular compromise as first recognized by distal limb swelling and a change in temperature (cold). In patients who have had surgery, normal postoperative swelling may be restricted by the orthosis, resulting in neurovascular compression (i.e., "compartment syndrome"). In these cases, clinicians may see excessive swelling of the braced limb accompanied by significant pain on limb/joint palpation with reluctance to bear weight. In the authors' experience, incisional dehiscence often occurs in these situations. Regardless, if any of these findings are recognized, the brace should be immediately removed in order to prevent irreversible damage.

Unfortunately, while orthosis use in the immediate postoperative patient may prove beneficial, the ideal postoperative time for orthosis application to reduce the chance of this complication is unknown. However, in cases where postoperative orthoses are to be used, the authors frequently apply standard external coaptation for a minimum of 2 weeks and then consider transition to a custom orthotic when applicable.

14.8.3 Localized Pressure Necrosis

Pressure necrosis can occur in localized areas due to abnormal forces distributed at the interface between the orthosis and the limb. This may be most pronounced in areas where orthosis–limb interaction occurs over a bony prominence or areas with limited soft tissue coverage. To reduce the chances of pressure necrosis related to orthosis application, clinicians should pay careful attention to optimizing orthosis contouring and fit, proper mechanical design to reduce forces placed on the skin, and ample padding over all contact areas [13].

14.9 Conclusion

Overall, there are very limited data to help guide clinical decision making regarding the use of orthoses for dogs with CCL injuries. Complications can result from numerous sources, including an inability to properly stabilize an unstable joint as well as improper orthosis design and fit. Currently, the available evidence supports surgical correction over the use of orthoses. However, for those patients where surgical correction is not possible, the use of a properly designed and fitted stifle orthosis may provide some benefit.

References

1. Bertocci, G.E., Brown, N.P., and Mich, P.M. (2017). Why owners choose an orthosis over stifle surgery for canine cranial cruciate ligament deficiency. *Top. Companion Anim. Med.* 32 (4): 130–138.
2. Marcellin-Little, D.J., Drum, M.G., Levine, D., and McDonald, S.S. (2015). Orthoses and exoprostheses for companion animals. *Vet. Clin. North Am. Small Anim. Pract.* 45 (1): 167–183.
3. Case, J.B., Palmer, R., Valdes-Martinez, A. et al. (2013). Gastrocnemius tendon strain in a dog treated with autologous mesenchymal stem cells and a custom orthosis. *Vet. Surg.* 42 (4): 355–360.
4. Hardie, R.J. and Lewallen, J.T. (2013). Use of a custom orthotic boot for management of distal extremity and pad wounds in three dogs. *Vet. Surg.* 42 (6): 678–682.
5. Levine, J.M. and Fitch, R.B. (2003). Use of an ankle-foot orthosis in a dog with traumatic sciatic neuropathy. *J. Small Anim. Pract.* 44 (5): 236–268.

6. Swiderski, J., Fitch, R.B., Staatz, A., and Lowery, J. (2005). Sonographic assisted diagnosis and treatment of bilateral gastrocnemius tendon rupture in a Labrador retriever repaired with fascia lata and polypropylene mesh. *Vet. Comp. Orthop. Traumatol.* 18 (4): 258–263.
7. Tomlinson, J.E. and Manfredi, J.M. (2014). Evaluation of application of a carpal brace as a treatment for carpal ligament instability in dogs: 14 cases (2008–2011). *J. Am. Vet. Med. Assoc.* 244 (4): 438–443.
8. Mich, P.M. (2014). The emerging role of veterinary orthotics and prosthetics (V-OP) in small animal rehabilitation and pain management. *Top. Companion Anim. Med.* 29 (1): 10–19.
9. Bertocci, G.E., Brown, N.P., and Mich, P.M. (2017). Biomechanics of an orthosis-managed cranial cruciate ligament-deficient canine stifle joint predicted by use of a computer model. *Am. J. Vet. Res.* 78 (1): 27–35.
10. Torres, B.T., Fu, Y.C., Sandberg, G.S., and Budsberg, S.C. (2017). Pelvic limb kinematics in the dog with and without a stifle orthosis. *Vet. Surg.* 46 (5): 642–652.
11. Carr, B.J., Canapp, S.O., Meilleur, S. et al. (2016). The use of canine stifle orthotics for cranial cruciate ligament insufficiency. *Vet. Evid.* 1 (1): 1–13.
12. Hart, J.L., May, K.D., Kieves, N.R. et al. (2016). Comparison of owner satisfaction between stifle joint orthoses and tibial plateau leveling osteotomy for the management of cranial cruciate ligament disease in dogs. *J. Am. Vet. Med. Assoc.* 249 (4): 391–398.
13. Ramachandran, M. (2018). *Basic Orthopaedic Sciences*. Boca Raton, FL: CRC Press.
14. Conzemius, M.G., Evans, R.B., Besancon, M.F. et al. (2005). Effect of surgical technique on limb function after surgery for rupture of the cranial cruciate ligament in dogs. *J. Am. Vet. Med. Assoc.* 226 (2): 232–236.
15. Conzemius, M.G. and Evans, R.B. (2012). Caregiver placebo effect for dogs with lameness from osteoarthritis. *J. Am. Vet. Med. Assoc.* 241 (10): 1314–1319.
16. Korvick, D.L., Pijanowski, G.J., and Schaeffer, D.J. (1994). Three-dimensional kinematics of the intact and cranial cruciate ligament-deficient stifle of dogs. *J. Biomech.* 27 (1): 77–87.
17. Tinga, S., Kim, S.E., Banks, S.A. et al. (2018). Femorotibial kinematics in dogs with cranial cruciate ligament insufficiency: a three-dimensional in-vivo fluoroscopic analysis during walking. *BMC Vet. Res.* 14 (1): 85.
18. Kim, S.E., Jones, S.C., Lewis, D.D. et al. (2015). In-vivo three-dimensional knee kinematics during daily activities in dogs. *J. Orthop. Res.* 33 (11): 1603–1610.
19. Vasseur, P. and Arnoczky, S. (1981). Collateral ligaments of the canine stifle joint: anatomic and functional analysis. *Am. J. Vet. Res.* 42 (7): 1133–1137.
20. Arnoczky, S. and Marshall, J. (1977). The cruciate ligaments of the canine stifle: an anatomical and functional analysis. *Am. J. Vet. Res.* 38 (11): 1807–1814.
21. Tinga, S., Kim, S.E., Banks, S.A. et al. (2020). Femorotibial kinematics in dogs treated with tibial plateau leveling osteotomy for cranial cruciate ligament insufficiency: an in vivo fluoroscopic analysis during walking. *Vet. Surg.* 49 (1): 187–199.
22. Ewing, K.A., Begg, R.K., Galea, M.P., and Lee, P.V. (2016). Effects of prophylactic knee bracing on lower limb kinematics, kinetics, and energetics during double-leg drop landing at 2 heights. *Am. J. Sports Med.* 44 (7): 1753–1761.
23. Simpson, K.J., Yom, J.P., Fu, Y.-C. et al. (2013). Does wearing a prophylactic ankle brace during drop landings affect lower extremity kinematics and ground reaction forces? *J. Appl. Biomech.* 29 (2): 205–213.

15 Complications from Cranial Cruciate Ligament Surgery: Rehabilitation Considerations

Matthew W. Brunke, David Levine, David L. Dycus, and Denis J. Marcellin-Little

15.1 Introduction

The field of veterinary rehabilitation has expanded as veterinarians have realized the importance of optimizing oversight and postoperative care and managing patients with a variety of conditions without surgery [1]. Rehabilitation therapy uses a number of techniques such as manual therapy physical modalities, and therapeutic exercises. The overarching goal of rehabilitation is to return patients to the best possible level of function as pets or working dogs, while improving their quality of life.

Pathology of the cranial cruciate ligament (CCL) has received attention from a rehabilitation perspective both following surgical stabilization and as part of a conservative approach to CCL injuries [2]. The benefits of surgical stabilization for CCL ruptures have been widely investigated [3]. By comparison, the benefits of rehabilitation following CCL surgery have only been reported in a limited number of studies [4, 5]. Several therapeutic steps used in rehabilitation after CCL surgery have been shown to be beneficial, including cold compression therapy [6], neuromuscular electrical stimulation (NMES) [7], and extracorporeal shockwave therapy [8, 9].

A recent survey reported that 71% of the veterinarians who replied consistently recommended postoperative rehabilitation following CCL surgery [10]. Of those surveyed, 39% recommended rehabilitation for all cases postoperatively and 16% recommended that patients receive a consultation with a rehabilitation practitioner. Individuals were more likely to recommend rehabilitation therapy in geriatric, inactive, sporting and working dogs, and in cases with severe muscle atrophy or with decreased range of motion of the stifle or tarsus. The recommendations for rehabilitation therapy appeared to be based on what individuals were taught during veterinary school or during their residency training and, to a lesser extent, on published evidence or information learned at a conference. Most (92%) reported that guidelines for rehabilitation therapy in dogs after CCL surgery are helpful.

While individuals are generally familiar with rehabilitation following CCL surgery and often recommend rehabilitation, a need for specific guidelines remains. Also, several factors may deter individuals from recommending

Complications in Canine Cranial Cruciate Ligament Surgery, First Edition. Edited by Ron Ben-Amotz and David L. Dycus.

rehabilitation, such as its cost, the availability or distance to rehabilitation facilities, and the required time commitment [10]. In addition, some individuals may be under the impression that rehabilitation could increase likelihood of complications (Table 15.1), and therefore could hesitate to recommend rehabilitation.

One study evaluated the safety of a formal rehabilitation protocol following tibial plateau leveling osteotomy (TPLO) [2]. One treatment group underwent a formal rehabilitation plan and the other group underwent a traditional postoperative management protocol consisting of cage confinement and controlled leash walks. Perioperative complications and functional outcomes 8 weeks, 6 months, and 1 year after surgery were evaluated. The overall complication rate with both groups (26%) was consistent with complication rates reported in other studies. There was no difference in the complication rate in both groups, suggesting that formal rehabilitation does not increase the risk of complications. Further, at the 8-week time point, dogs in the formal rehabilitation plan were 1.9 times more likely to have returned to full function while dogs in the traditional postoperative plan were 2.9 times more likely to have unacceptable function.

The fear of complications resulting from rehabilitation exists in human medicine, where a subset of orthopedic surgeons reportedly have concerns related to the fact that rehabilitation professionals do not always possess sufficient knowledge of tissue healing times and postsurgical limitations [11]. Veterinarians could have similar concerns. Interprofessional communication can ensure that all caregivers are well informed and in agreement with regard to activity levels. The preferred communication methods vary among clinicians [12].

While the literature suggests that formal rehabilitation after CCL surgery is safe and efficacious, rehabilitation can also be used to help identify complications or prevent the progression of minor complications to major complications. One of the key advantages of formal rehabilitation is the frequent face-to-face evaluation of the patient by the rehabilitation practitioner. In most situations, patients are undergoing rehabilitation therapy once or twice a week. This gives the practitioner the ability to observe patients often and learn characteristics of their gait, limb use, and functional abilities throughout the postoperative period. The rehabilitation practitioner can use objective and subjective measures to ensure appropriate recovery and that a complication is not present. For example, evaluation of gait, palpation of the surgical limb (to assess for the presence of patellar ligament desmitis, for example), measurement of joint angles (goniometry), and measurement of thigh circumference provide information that informs clinicians of the potential presence of a complication.

15.2 Gait Evaluation

The evaluation of gait is an important aspect of recovery. Most patients recover in predictable fashion after CCL surgery but the rate of increase in limb use varies based on signalment, chronicity, and type of surgical intervention. Patients undergoing extracapsular stabilization often are nonweight bearing for the first few days after surgery. They tend to remain nonweight bearing for a longer period of time and take longer to regain full limb usage than patients undergoing TPLO or other osteotomies. After 3–5 days, they often are toe-touching and slowly progress to a weight-bearing lameness by the second week after surgery. Patients undergoing osteotomy-based procedures tend to be toe-touching at a slow speed the morning following surgery. Three to 5 days later, they bear weight consistently at a walk but still display a moderate lameness during weight bearing. By the second week, their lameness is commonly mild.

It is important that the rehabilitation practitioner and the veterinarian have an appreciation for the recovery of gait following any surgical procedure. The appreciation of differences in recovery rate and the regular observation of patients facilitate early detection of complications. Any deviation from anticipated limb use and setbacks in limb use during recovery should raise suspicion of a potential complication and trigger patient reevaluation. In some situations, delays in recovery or limb use setbacks represent a minor complication that requires no further intervention, beyond rest. In other situations, delays in recovery may represent early signs of a major complication where an intervention is warranted.

Table 15.1 Complications after surgical stabilization of cranial cruciate ligament injury in dogs.

Surgical procedure	Complications	Potential causes
Extracapsular stabilization or Tightrope® procedure	Cranial drawer sign	Failure of fixation (line breakage, fabellar displacement)
	Excessive internal rotation	Failure of fixation
	Lack of stifle extension	Tibial tunnel is excessively distal Excessive (caudal) articular or periarticular fibrosis
	Lack of stifle flexion	Excessive joint effusion Quadriceps muscle changes Excessive (cranial) articular or periarticular fibrosis Suture line not isometric (Tightrope™ procedure)
	Limb disuse	Lack of isometric suture placement Failure of fixation Infection Meniscal tear
Tibial tuberosity advancement	Cranial thrust	Crest is not sufficiently advanced Failure of fixation
	Excessive internal rotation	Preoperative torsional instability of the stifle
	Limb disuse	Infection Failure of fixation Meniscal tear
Tibial plateau leveling procedure	Cranial thrust	Tibial plateau is not sufficiently rotated Failure of fixation (plateau rollback)
	Excessive internal rotation	Preoperative torsional instability of the stifle
	Valgus or varus angulation	Preexisting angular deformity of the tibia or femur Failure of fixation Plateau osteotomy or reduction is oblique
	Limb disuse	Infection Failure of fixation, fibular fracture Meniscal tear Patellar tendonitis, patellar or tibial crest fracture

Several subjective scales and objective parameters can be used for gait evaluation. Various subjective numerical scales ranging from 1 to 4, 1 to 5 (Table 15.2), or 1 to 6 or a visual analog scale (VAS) can be used [13]. For both subjective numerical scales and VAS, the same examiner should evaluate the gait of the patient at each visit and document it in the medical record. The same scale should be used for all evaluations. Objective gait evaluation provides more precise information related to patient recovery and is more reliable than subjective gait evaluation, particularly when the lameness is mild. The agreement between numerical scales, VAS, and objective force plate analysis is low, suggesting that numeric scales and VAS are flawed for the assessment of lameness in dogs [14].

Table 15.2 Example of a 0–V numerical rating scale for subjective assessment of grading canine lameness.

Grade 0	Normal gait, no lameness
Grade I	Weight shifting, mild lameness noted at the trot, sound at the walk
Grade II	Mild weight-bearing lameness at the walk as noted by an experienced observer
Grade III	Weight-bearing lameness at the walk
Grade IV	Severe weight-bearing to toe-touching lameness at the walk
Grade V	Nonweight-bearing lameness

Source: Adapted from Carr and Dycus [13].

Kinematic gait analysis objectively describes gait by quantifying joint motion, limb segment velocity, acceleration, and deceleration, and angles of structures in space and time. Patients are often fitted with reflective markers and high-speed cameras are used to capture motion. Kinetic gait analysis involves the use of a force plate to measure ground reaction forces, in particular the peak vertical force (pVF, the largest vertical forced resisted by each limb) and vertical impulse (VI, the product of force and time during each stride for each limb). Both kinematic and kinetic gait analysis are mostly used in research settings and are uncommonly used for clinical evaluation. However, smartphone applications with 2D analysis are becoming more available to calculate joint angles passively (Figure 15.1) and during gait [15].

Pressure-sensing walkways and weight distribution platforms are emerging as objective tools for patient assessment (Figure 15.2). Pressure-sensing walkways have been studied to determine normal and abnormal gaits in dogs of various dog breeds [16–20]. Walkways use sensors to calculate velocity, stance time, swing time, stride length, step length, and the total pressure index (TPI). Pressure-sensitive walkways along with kinematic and kinetic evaluations rely on dynamic weight distribution to detect abnormalities during the gait. More recently, weight distribution platforms have been used to evaluate gait abnormalities in a static manner, when dogs are standing in place. Patients alter their static weight distribution as a result of pain. Even less is known about the shifts in weight distribution that result from limb pain in standing dogs compared to walking or trotting dogs. Weight distribution platforms collect measurements that are as accurate and repeatable as static standing on a pressure-sensitive walkway [21]. The sensitivity and specificity of weight distribution platforms for the detection of orthopedic lameness have been evaluated in clinical patients, making this method of objective evaluation an emerging consideration during postoperative recovery [22].

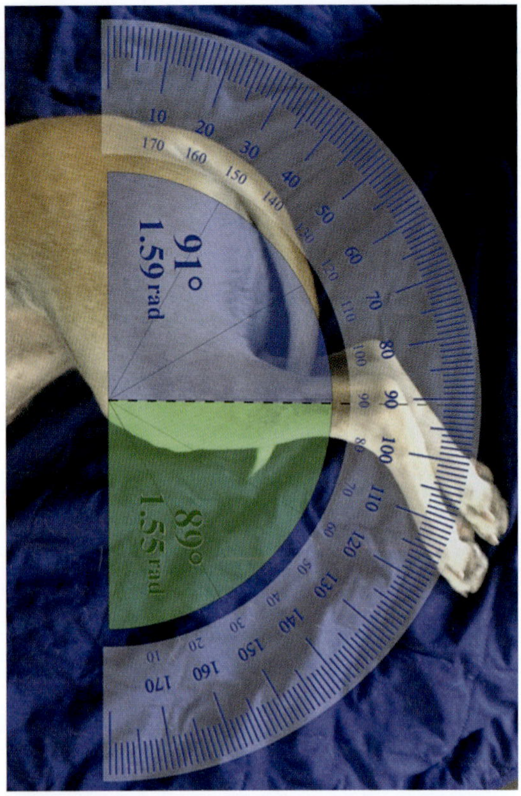

Figure 15.1 Screen capture of a goniometric measurement collected using a phone-based application (Protractor, Kewl.com, Kewlsoft, London, UK). The baseline of the goniometer is oriented along the femoral shaft and the moving arm is oriented along the tibial shaft. The application indicates that the stifle joint has a 91° angle.

The use of objective measures of gait can be incorporated into the postoperative evaluations to confirm continued improvement. While little information is known regarding the range in gains in pressure-sensitive walkway or weight distribution platforms after various CCL sur-

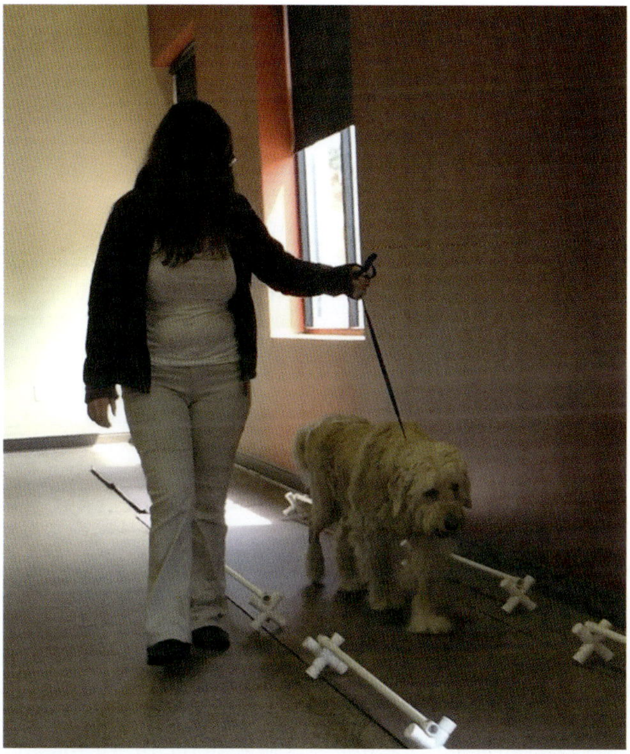

Figure 15.2 Screen capture of a video of a dog walking on a pressure-sensitive walkway. The handler is walking the dog at a constant speed. The dog is controlled by a leash. There is no tension on the leash to avoid artifacts. Also, the dog is walking in a straight line and is looking forward.

geries, rehabilitation clinicians who examine gait and limb use regularly are well prepared to detect a lack of progress in limb use or delayed progress during the recovery period. For dogs enrolled in a formal rehabilitation program, abnormal progress is often suggestive of the presence of a complication.

15.3 Surgical Limb Evaluation

Palpation of the surgical limb is also critical to the detection of potential complications. In the early postoperative period, particular attention is paid to the surgical incision to ensure appropriate healing with no evidence of excessive inflammation, infection, or seroma formation. Variations in surgical technique and intraoperative tissue trauma lead to differences in surgical wound inflammation. Any incision that appears inconsistent with common standards is reported to the group that performed the surgery. A conversation between the rehabilitation practitioner and the veterinarian who did the surgery optimizes subsequent management.

15.4 Range of Motion Evaluation

The rehabilitation clinician should evaluate the range of motion of the stifle joint, the presence of a pain response to flexion and extension, and the craniocaudal and torsional stability of the joint. For example, extracapsular stabilization of a CCL-deficient stifle joint can fail, resulting in the reoccurrence of stifle instability, detected through a decrease in limb use and the presence of a cranial drawer sign. In contrast, a decrease in limb use in a patient after an osteotomy can result from a failure of plate fixation and tibial plateau rollback. For a patient recovering from an osteotomy, the presence of cranial drawer is expected during the recovery period.

Joint motion is critical to limb use. Therefore, monitoring the motion of the stifle joint throughout recovery provides valuation information. Rehabilitation clinicians should monitor joint motion quantitatively by measuring maximal motion using goniometry and qualitatively by evaluating the pain response to joint motion and the feel at the end of motion (the end feel). Goniometry has been validated in several dog breeds (Table 15.3) [26]. Breed differences likely result from the variability in bone and joint geometry among dog breeds. Because the motions of adjacent joints are linked and because the presence of an orthopedic problem in the hip or tarsus influences limb use after CCL surgery, the motion of the hip and tarsus should also be measured. The contralateral limb should also be evaluated. Comorbidities in the stifle region and other regions will influence goniometric measurements. Since joint motion changes as a result of the presence of osteoarthritis [28] and because most dogs presenting with CCL injuries have osteoarthritis [29], the objective evaluation of stifle joint motion using a goniometer before surgery provides valuable information. Also, since surgery may impact the motion of the stifle joint (Figure 15.3), the evaluation of stifle joint motion after surgery also provides valuable information. A decrease in joint motion, particularly flexion, is expected in the early postoperative period because of the presence of edema.

Joint motion is likely to increase during recovery. While little is known about the long-term motion of the stifle joint in dogs undergoing extracapsular stabilization, the motion of the stifle joint in the long term after TPLO is near normal in most dogs and a lack of improvement or loss of stifle joint motion often indicates the presence of a complication [30]. It is therefore important to collect and record goniometric measurements at regular intervals during the recovery process. Those measurements can occur every few weeks or once a dog reaches a milestone during recovery, before they transition to more strenuous activity.

The quality of joint motion is also evaluated. The joint is evaluated for the presence of crepitus. In humans, the presence of knee crepitus is associated with a loss of strength [31]. Little is known about crepitus in dogs with CCL injury. Subjectively, while the absence of crepitus is a poor predictor for the absence of joint disease, the presence of crepitus is a good predictor for the presence of severe joint disease. Crepitus can be associated with bone-on-bone contact in meniscus-deficient joints or in joints with severe cranial displacement of the tibia. Crepitus also

Table 15.3 Mean ± standard deviation flexion and extension of the stifle joint in several dog breeds, listed in alphabetical order.

Breed	Stifle flexion	Stifle extension	References
Belgian Shepherd (Malinois)	29° ± 2°	156° ± 2°	Sabanci and Ocal [23]
Boxer	39° ± 9°	159° ± 4°	Sabanci and Ocal [23]
Doberman Pinscher	30° ± 2°	164° ± 6°	Sabanci and Ocal [23]
French Bulldog	59°[a]	173°[a]	Formenton et al. [24]
German Shepherd Dog	33° ± 7°	153° ± 4°	Thomas et al. [25]
	34° ± 2°	151° ± 5°	Sabanci and Ocal [23]
Golden Retriever	34° ± 3°	156° ± 4°	Sabanci and Ocal [23]
Labrador Retriever	42° ± 2°	162° ± 3°	Jaegger et al. [26]
	38° ± 4°	157° ± 6°	Sabanci and Ocal [23]
Rottweiler	34° ± 4°	154° ± 3°	Sabanci and Ocal [23]
	45° ± 7°	161° ± 7°	Mendonça [27]

[a] Standard deviations not available.

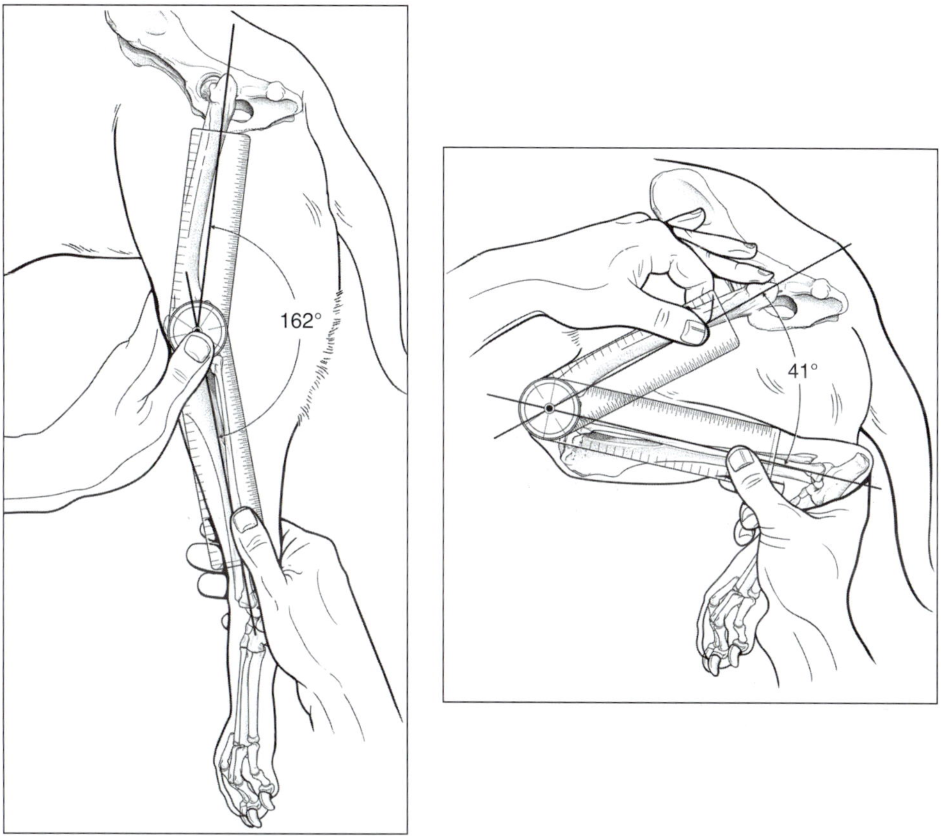

Figure 15.3 The evaluation of stifle joint motion using a goniometer provides valuable information before CCL stabilization surgery and during recovery after surgery. Goniometry is most often performed using a plastic goniometer whose arms are aligned along anatomical landmarks. The femoral arm is aligned along the line formed by the greater trochanter and the craniocaudal midpoint of the distal aspect of the femur, defined by the patella and lateral fabella. The tibial arm is aligned along the line formed by the craniocaudal midpoint of the proximal aspect of the tibia, defined by the tibial tubercle and the fibular head and the lateral malleolus. A lack of extension of the stifle before surgery suggests the presence of articular or periarticular fibrosis. A lack of extension of the stifle after extracapsular stabilization surgery may be related to suboptimal placement of the bone tunnel or anchor.

results from the presence of large osteophytes, a sign of severe osteoarthritis.

The pain response to joint flexion and extension is also evaluated throughout the recovery period. The pain response decreases over time, particularly after the end of the inflammatory phase of healing, typically 10–14 days after surgery. Persistent pain response to flexion or extension is likely to be associated with the presence of a complication, for example, an undiagnosed meniscal tear, low-grade infection, or persistent chronic pain. While little is known about the prevalence and predisposing factors to persistent pain in dogs with CCL, a subset of humans with knee OA have persistent pain, with predisposing factors linked to gender, race, and age [32]. In the arthritic dog hip, mechanical sensory thresholds are decreased and return to normal 3 months after joint replacement [33]. Mechanical sensory thresholds appear impaired in response to stifle joint osteoarthritis [34]. The physiology of recovery after CCL injury and surgery is likely similar. More subtle characteristics of joint motion such as glides, rolls, spins, distraction, and compression are sometimes used to manage dogs with osteoarthritis of the stifle joint [35]. These specialized mobilizations are beyond the scope of this chapter.

15.5 Meniscal Evaluation

Meniscal tears occur following CCL surgery at rates ranging from 3% to 17% [36]. A dog who fails to progress after CCL surgery could have had a meniscal tear that was not diagnosed at the time of surgery. Alternatively, a dog who progresses well in the early postoperative period and then has a clear decrease in limb use could have a late-onset meniscal tear.

The confirmation of a meniscal tear on physical examination is challenging. It lacks both sensitivity and specificity. While meniscal clicks are strongly predictive of meniscal injury [37], they are inconsistent and transient. A pain response to flexion and a change in joint end feel from a soft tissue end feel to a rubbery or hard end feel [38] suggest the presence of a meniscal injury. A loss of pain-free flexion can also be present. Such a change would also be detectable if changes in joint motion during the recovery period were monitored using goniometry. An increase in joint effusion in the stifle joint is also a potential sign of intraarticular inflammation. Therefore, it is important for the rehabilitation practitioner to perform regular evaluations at the onset and throughout the rehabilitation process.

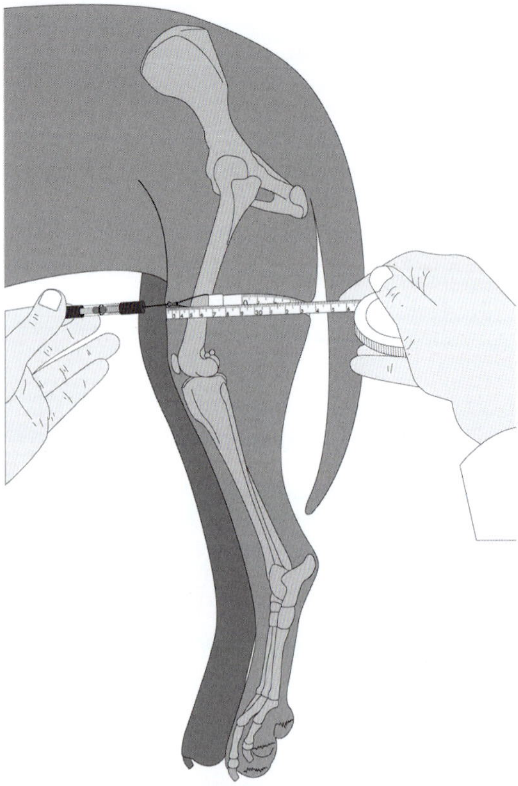

Figure 15.4 The evaluation of muscle mass is usually performed using a tape measure wrapped around the thigh. To maximize consistency, the tape measure is placed at a repeatable level. The level of measurement is usually relatively distal along the thigh to avoid interfering with the flank fold. In the illustration, the distance between the greater trochanter and lateral fabella has been measured and a point at 70% of that distance from the greater trochanter was used for the measurement.

15.6 Muscle Strength Evaluation

In humans, several tests are performed to determine the response to anterior cruciate ligament (ACL) reconstruction. These typically evaluate joint stability, joint motion, pain, muscle strength, and function [39]. Validated clinical tests evaluating muscle strength in the dog pelvic limb are lacking and little is known about the loss of strength after CCL rupture and the recovery of strength after surgery. CCL injuries and surgery, however, lead to a loss of muscle mass of the quadriceps and biceps femoris [40]. Presumably, that loss of muscle mass is associated with a loss of muscle strength and recovery of muscle mass will result in recovery of strength. It is therefore useful to measure thigh circumference initially and throughout the recovery process (Figure 15.4) [41]. A lack of increase in muscle mass of the thigh after CCL surgery, particularly for the biceps and quadriceps femoris muscles, suggests the presence of a complication. Deficits in strength that continue in the long term, especially in the quadriceps femoris muscle, are considered to be a complication following ACL reconstruction in humans as they can contribute to decreased function and future injuries to the limb [42, 43]. These deficits can be minimized with appropriate strength training and rehabilitation techniques.

15.7 Choice of Modalities

The choice of therapeutic modalities for dogs recovering from surgery to manage CCL injuries is complex. It is influenced by the medical problem (chronicity, severity), the dog (demeanor, training), and the owner (home care versus outpatient or inpatient rehabilitation, willingness and ability to deliver care). Viewed simply, rehabilitation relies on electrophysical modalities, manual therapy, therapeutic exercises, ergonomics, and patient/owner education. To an extent, each of those can be of benefit during recovery from CCL surgery.

In the first few days, emphasis is placed on cryotherapy, passive range of motion (PROM), and standing weight-bearing exercises. In the first few weeks that follow, exercises at a walk are introduced. Cryotherapy is sometimes used after exercise. Dogs that show signs of limb disuse may benefit from analgesic measures such as a massage or PROM, or electrical stimulation (ES) to either decrease pain or help strengthen muscles. Dogs that lack joint motion may benefit from stretching. After a few weeks, therapy consists mostly of therapeutic exercises. Ergonomics is particularly important when dog mobility is compromised, early after surgery for all patients and beyond in several affected patients and patients with comorbidities. Patient and owner education is also particularly important early after surgery and in severely affected patients.

15.7.1 Thermal Medicine

Cryotherapy, with or without compression, is widely used in the early postoperative period that follows surgery to manage CCL injuries. Cold and compression have been shown to increase weight bearing in the early postoperative period [6, 44]. The positive influence on cold and compression may result from pain relief: cold compression therapy increases pressure pain thresholds [45] and decreases nociception velocity [46]. It also limits periarticular swelling [47]. Cryotherapy is often applied to the operated area immediately after surgery for a period of 10–20 minutes. In addition, it is often used for a few days after surgery for 10–20 minutes 2–3 times daily. Some clinicians continue to recommend the use of cryotherapy after periods of rehabilitation and throughout the dog's recovery to decrease pain and postexercise inflammation. In one dog study, the focal application of ice compresses did not lower core temperature [48]. In humans, adverse events after cold therapy are exceedingly rare [49] and none have been reported in dogs.

Heat is used less frequently than cold for dogs recovering from stifle joint surgery. Clinicians use moist heat to elevate tissue temperature before stretching sessions in dogs with loss of range of motion of the stifle joint [50]. Stretching preheated tissues is safer and more effective than stretching nonheated tissues [51]. For dogs who need stretching, heat can be delivered superficially using a moist heat pack or more deeply using therapeutic ultrasound. Burns can occur after heat therapy [52], especially if commercial heating pads are used. Close oversight of the temperature and duration of exposure to heat is therefore warranted. Low-level tissue heating is sometimes used to promote relaxation and normalize blood flow. The benefits of low-level heat for dogs recovering from stifle joint surgery are not known.

15.7.2 Therapeutic Exercise

Rehabilitation for cruciate ligament injuries should focus on improving stifle extension and increasing muscle mass of the quadriceps femoris, semimembranosus, and biceps femoris [53]. Once proper pain management has been initiated, the focus should be on maintaining joint motion. It is important to return stifle motion to normal values by 2 weeks after surgery to regain full stifle extension [54]. Starting after surgery when the patient is conscious, PROM can be done 3–4 times a day. This is accomplished with the patient in lateral recumbency and should be a low-amplitude movement without reaching any resistance. Ten to fifteen gentle repetitions per set every 8 hours can reduce pain and minimize unwanted fibrosis. Care should be taken to avoid excessive flexion or extension, as this can lead to pain or even failure of fixation. PROM is often done at the beginning of a rehab session to prepare for weight-bearing activities. A warm compress can be applied a few minutes prior to PROM to improve tissue extensibility.

Moving toward therapeutic exercises must be done with an understanding of the surgical repair and level of tissue healing [55]. Once PROM and time result in the ability to bear weight, static weight bearing is introduced, usually on a nonslip surface and possibly with a sling or harness as needed. Active limb movement exercises follow this and include leash walks and other activities. Because a lack of extension negatively impacts the ability to bear weight when walking and trotting, the focus of rehabilitation is generally on regaining extension rather than flexion. Since swimming improves stifle joint flexion but not extension [4], it is generally avoided at that stage of rehabilitation. Similarly, other activities that promote flexion, including jumping, running, stair climbing [56], or walking in a crouched position, are also avoided.

Proper spacing and height of Cavaletti rails is important in the recovery of the CCL patient. Grouping the rails too close together can induce jumping, causing excessive flexion and increased stress from landing. Having the rails too high (at or above the stifle) will also trigger excessive flexion. Sit to stand exercises result in nearly twice as much flexion of the stifle compared to walking [57]. Therefore, this exercise should be incorporated once full normal range of motion has been achieved.

Underwater treadmill walking is introduced in most instances after the skin incision has healed, approximately 10 days after surgery. Underwater treadmill walking will provide a safe, contained environment and allow for stifle extension, weight bearing, and muscle building. Care should be taken not to exceed normal walking stride until the tissues have healed, including the tibia if osteotomy has been performed.

Walking the dog with the forelimbs raised off the ground is named dancing. This activity alters motion of the rear limb joints. When safely done, it challenges proprioception, coordination, and strength. The amount of pVF placed on the rear limbs is slightly greater than what would occur at a trot, so this exercise is avoided during the early stage of rehabilitation.

15.7.3 Electrical Stimulation

Electrical stimulation (ES) can be used in the rehabilitation of patients with CCL injuries. Electrical stimulation can be broadly used for two major purposes: strengthening, which is commonly termed neuromuscular electrical stimulation (NMES), and for pain control. While there is a large body of evidence for the use of NMES in humans who have undergone surgical ACL reconstruction, only a few studies have looked at CCL injury [7, 54]. One study reported the optimal pulse durations for individual muscles in dogs undergoing NMES [58]. As NMES has the potential to be painful, and requires a trained operator, it tends to be reserved for cases that are more complicated such as long-standing atrophy or the unwillingness to use the limb actively despite satisfactory surgical repair. In this case, electrodes may be placed on the clipped and cleaned skin over muscles that have atrophied (commonly the cranial and caudal thigh muscles) and used to cause a contraction to build strength. Electrical stimulation for pain control, while well established in people to decrease pain [59, 60], has little to no evidence for use in dogs following postoperative stabilization of the CCL.

15.8 Communication to Minimize Complications

During recovery from CCL surgery, interprofessional collaboration and communication are essential to optimize patient outcomes. Conversely, suboptimal interprofessional communication has been shown to negatively impact patient care [61]. Communication and documentation between caregivers (the veterinarian, the referring veterinarian if applicable, the person responsible for the physical rehabilitation, and in some cases the owner) are critical. Patient forms are a convenient way to enhance communication [62]. Patient medical records should be updated after each physical rehabilitation treatment.

References

1. McGonagle, L., Blythe, L., and Levine, D. (2014). History of canine physical therapy. In: *Canine*

Rehabilitation and Physical Therapy (eds. D.L. Millis and D. Levine), 1–7. Philadelphia, PA: Elsevier.

2. Romano, L.S. and Cook, J.L. (2015). Safety and functional outcomes associated with short-term rehabilitation therapy in the post-operative management of tibial plateau leveling osteotomy. *Can. Vet. J.* 56 (9): 942–946.
3. Bergh, M.S., Sullivan, C., Ferrell, C.L. et al. (2014). Systematic review of surgical treatments for cranial cruciate ligament disease in dogs. *J. Am. Anim. Hosp. Assoc.* 50 (5): 315–321.
4. Marsolais, G.S., Dvorak, G., and Conzemius, M.G. (2002). Effects of postoperative rehabilitation on limb function after cranial cruciate ligament repair in dogs. *J. Am. Vet. Med. Assoc.* 220 (9): 1325–1330.
5. Monk, M.L., Preston, C.A., and McGowan, C.M. (2006). Effects of early intensive postoperative physiotherapy on limb function after tibial plateau leveling osteotomy in dogs with deficiency of the cranial cruciate ligament. *J. Am. Vet. Med. Assoc.* 228 (5): 725.
6. Drygas, K.A., McClure, S.R., Goring, R.L. et al. (2011). Effect of cold compression therapy on postoperative pain, swelling, range of motion, and lameness after tibial plateau leveling osteotomy in dogs. *J. Am. Vet. Med. Assoc.* 238 (10): 1284–1291.
7. Johnson, J.M., Johnson, A.L., Pijanowski, G.J. et al. (1997). Rehabilitation of dogs with surgically treated cranial cruciate ligament-deficient stifles by use of electrical stimulation of muscles. *Am. J. Vet. Res.* 58 (12): 1473–1478.
8. Gallagher, A., Cross, A.R., and Sepulveda, G. (2012). The effect of shock wave therapy on patellar ligament desmitis after tibial plateau leveling osteotomy. *Vet. Surg.* 41 (4): 482–485.
9. Kieves, N.R., MacKay, C.S., Adducci, K. et al. (2015). High energy focused shock wave therapy accelerates bone healing. A blinded, prospective, randomized canine clinical trial. *Vet. Comp. Orthop. Traumatol.* 28 (6): 425–432.
10. Eiermann, J., Kirkby-Shaw, K., Evans, R.B. et al. (2020). Recommendations for rehabilitation after surgical treatment of cranial cruciate ligament disease in dogs: a 2017 survey of veterinary practitioners. *Vet. Surg.* 49 (1): 80–87.
11. Archer, K.R., MacKenzie, E.J., Bosse, M.J. et al. (2009). Factors associated with surgeon referral for physical therapy in patients with traumatic lower-extremity injury: results of a national survey of orthopedic trauma surgeons. *Phys. Ther.* 89 (9): 893–905.
12. Longstaffe, R., Slade Shantz, J., Leiter, J., and Peeler, J. (2015). Surgeon–therapist communication: do all members see eye-to-eye? *Phys. Sportsmed.* 43 (4): 381–387.
13. Carr, B.J. and Dycus, D.L. (2016). Canine gait analysis. *Today Vet. Pract.* 6: 93–100.
14. Quinn, M.M., Keuler, N.S., Lu, Y. et al. (2007). Evaluation of agreement between numerical rating scales, visual analogue scoring scales, and force plate gait analysis in dogs. *Vet. Surg.* 36 (4): 360–367.
15. Mourcou, Q., Fleury, A., Diot, B. et al. (2015). Mobile phone-based joint angle measurement for functional assessment and rehabilitation of proprioception. *Biomed. Res. Int.* 2015: 328142.
16. Light, V.A., Steiss, J.E., Montgomery, R.D. et al. (2010). Temporal-spatial gait analysis by use of a portable walkway system in healthy Labrador retrievers at a walk. *Am. J. Vet. Res.* 71 (9): 997–1002.
17. Besancon, M.F., Conzemius, M.G., Derrick, T.R., and Ritter, M.J. (2003). Comparison of vertical forces in normal greyhounds between force platform and pressure walkway measurement systems. *Vet. Comp. Orthop. Traumatol.* 16 (3): 153–157.
18. Lascelles, B.D., Roe, S.C., Smith, E. et al. (2006). Evaluation of a pressure walkway system for measurement of vertical limb forces in clinically normal dogs. *Am. J. Vet. Res.* 67 (2): 277–282.
19. Webster, K.E., Wittwer, J.E., and Feller, J.A. (2005). Validity of the GAITRite walkway system for the measurement of averaged and individual step parameters of gait. *Gait Posture* 22 (4): 317–321.
20. Gordon-Evans, W.J., Evans, R.B., and Conzemius, M.G. (2009). Accuracy of spatiotemporal variables in gait analysis of neurologic dogs. *J. Neurotrauma* 26 (7): 1055–1060.
21. Bosscher, G., Tomas, A., Roe, S.C. et al. (2017). Repeatability and accuracy testing of a weight distribution platform and comparison to a pressure sensitive walkway to assess static weight distribution. *Vet. Comp. Orthop. Traumatol.* 30 (2): 160–164.
22. Clough, W.T., Canapp, S.O. Jr., Taboada, L. et al. (2018). Sensitivity and specificity of a weight distribution platform for the detection of objective lameness and orthopaedic disease. *Vet. Comp. Orthop. Traumatol.* 31 (6): 391–395.
23. Sabanci, S.S. and Ocal, M.K. (2016). Comparison of goniometric measurements of the stifle joint in seven breeds of normal dogs. *Vet. Comp. Orthop. Traumatol.* 29 (3): 214–219.
24. Formenton, M.R., de Lima, L.G., Vassalo, F.G. et al. (2019). Goniometric assessment in French bulldogs. *Front. Vet. Sci.* 6: 424.
25. Thomas, T.M., Marcellin-Little, D.J., Roe, S.C. et al. (2006). Comparison of measurements obtained by use of an electrogoniometer and a universal plastic goniometer for the assessment of joint motion in dogs. *Am. J. Vet. Res.* 67 (12): 1974–1979.
26. Jaegger, G., Marcellin-Little, D.J., and Levine, D. (2002). Reliability of goniometry in Labrador retrievers. *Am. J. Vet. Res.* 63 (7): 979–986.

27. Mendonça, G.B.N. (2009). *Goniometria em cães de raça Rottweiler*. Brazil: Universade Federal de Goiás.
28. Greene, L.M., Marcellin-Little, D.J., and Lascelles, B.D. (2013). Associations among exercise duration, lameness severity, and hip joint range of motion in Labrador retrievers with hip dysplasia. *J. Am. Vet. Med. Assoc.* 242 (11): 1528–1533.
29. Gilbert, S., Langenbach, A., Marcellin-Little, D.J. et al. (2019). Stifle joint osteoarthritis at the time of diagnosis of cranial cruciate ligament injury is higher in boxers and in dogs weighing more than 35 kilograms. *Vet. Radiol. Ultrasound* 60: 280–288.
30. Jandi, A.S. and Schulman, A.J. (2007). Incidence of motion loss of the stifle joint in dogs with naturally occurring cranial cruciate ligament rupture surgically treated with tibial plateau leveling osteotomy: longitudinal clinical study of 412 cases. *Vet. Surg.* 36 (2): 114–121.
31. Pazzinatto, M.F., de Oliveira Silva, D., Faria, N.C. et al. (2019). What are the clinical implications of knee crepitus to individuals with knee osteoarthritis? An observational study with data from the osteoarthritis initiative. *Braz. J. Phys. Ther.* 23 (6): 491–496.
32. Carlesso, L.C., Segal, N.A., Frey-Law, L. et al. (2019). Pain susceptibility phenotypes in those free of knee pain with or at risk of knee osteoarthritis: the multicenter osteoarthritis study. *Arthritis Rheumatol.* 71 (4): 542–549.
33. Tomas, A., Marcellin-Little, D.J., Roe, S.C. et al. (2014). Relationship between mechanical thresholds and limb use in dogs with coxofemoral joint oa-associated pain and the modulating effects of pain alleviation from total hip replacement on mechanical thresholds. *Vet. Surg.* 43 (5): 542–548.
34. Harris, L.K., Whay, H.R., and Murrell, J.C. (2018). An investigation of mechanical nociceptive thresholds in dogs with hind limb joint pain compared to healthy control dogs. *Vet. J.* 234: 85–90.
35. Saunders, D.G., Walker, J.R., and Levine, D. (2005). Joint mobilization. *Vet. Clin. North Am. Small Anim. Pract.* 35 (6): 1287–1316.
36. Metelman, L.A., Schwarz, P.D., Salman, M., and Alvis, M.R. (1995). An evaluation of three different cranial cruciate ligament surgical stabilization procedures as they relate to postoperative meniscal injuries – a retrospective study of 665 stifles. *Vet. Comp. Orthop. Traumatol.* 8 (2): 118–123.
37. Neal, B.A., Ting, D., Bonczynski, J.J., and Yasuda, K. (2015). Evaluation of meniscal click for detecting meniscal tears in stifles with cranial cruciate ligament disease. *Vet. Surg.* 44 (2): 191–194.
38. Levine, D., Millis, D.L., and Marcellin-Little, D.J. (2005). Introduction to veterinary physical rehabilitation. *Vet. Clin. North Am. Small Anim. Pract.* 35 (6): 1247–1254.
39. Zebis, M.K., Warming, S., Pedersen, M.B. et al. (2019). Outcome measures after ACL injury in pediatric patients: a scoping review. *Orthop. J. Sports Med.* 7 (7):2325967119861803.
40. Dycus, D.L., Levine, D., and Marcellin-Little, D.J. (2017). Physical rehabilitation for the management of canine hip dysplasia. *Vet. Clin. North Am. Small Anim. Pract.* 47 (4): 823–850.
41. McCarthy, D.A., Millis, D.L., Levine, D., and Weigel, J.P. (2018). Variables affecting thigh girth measurement and observer reliability in dogs. *Front. Vet. Sci.* 5: 203.
42. Oberlander, K.D., Bruggemann, G.P., Hoher, J., and Karamanidis, K. (2013). Altered landing mechanics in ACL-reconstructed patients. *Med. Sci. Sports Exerc.* 45 (3): 506–513.
43. Schmitt, L.C., Paterno, M.V., Ford, K.R. et al. (2015). Strength asymmetry and landing mechanics at return to sport after anterior cruciate ligament reconstruction. *Med. Sci. Sports Exerc.* 47 (7): 1426–1434.
44. von Freeden, N., Duerr, F., Fehr, M. et al. (2017). Comparison of two cold compression therapy protocols after tibial plateau leveling osteotomy in dogs. *Tierarztl. Prax. Ausg. K Kleintiere Heimtiere* 45 (4): 226–233.
45. Tanaka, R., Umehara, T., Kawabata, Y., and Sakuda, T. (2018). Effect of continuous compression stimulation on pressure-pain threshold and muscle spasms in older adults with knee osteoarthritis: a randomized trial. *J. Manip. Physiol. Ther.* 41 (4): 315–322.
46. Algafly, A.A. and George, K.P. (2007). The effect of cryotherapy on nerve conduction velocity, pain threshold and pain tolerance. *Br. J. Sports Med.* 41 (6): 365–369.
47. Rexing, J., Dunning, D., Siegel, A.M. et al. (2010). Effects of cold compression, bandaging, and microcurrent electrical therapy after cranial cruciate ligament repair in dogs. *Vet. Surg.* 39 (1): 54–58.
48. Bocobo, C., Fast, A., Kingery, W., and Kaplan, M. (1991). The effect of ice on intra-articular temperature in the knee of the dog. *Am. J. Phys. Med. Rehabil.* 70 (4): 181–185.
49. Song, M., Sun, X., Tian, X. et al. (2016). Compressive cryotherapy versus cryotherapy alone in patients undergoing knee surgery: a meta-analysis. *Springerplus* 5 (1): 1074.
50. Marcellin-Little, D.J. and Levine, D. (2015). Principles and application of range of motion and stretching in companion animals. *Vet. Clin. North Am. Small Anim. Pract.* 45 (1): 57–72.
51. Warren, C.G., Lehmann, J.F., and Koblanski, J.N. (1976). Heat and stretch procedures: an evaluation using rat tail tendon. *Arch. Phys. Med. Rehabil.* 57 (3): 122–126.
52. Nadler, S.F., Weingand, K., and Kruse, R.J. (2004). The physiologic basis and clinical applications of cryotherapy and thermotherapy for the pain practitioner. *Pain Physician* 7 (3): 395–399.

53. Francis, D.A., Millis, D.L., and Head, L.L. (2006). Bone and lean tissue changes following cranial cruciate ligament transection and stifle stabilization. *J. Am. Anim. Hosp. Assoc.* 42 (2): 127–135.
54. Millis, D.L. (1997). A preliminary study of early physical therapy following surgery for cranial cruciate ligament rupture in dogs. *Vet. Surg* 26 (5): 434.
55. Kirkby Shaw, K., Alvarez, L., Foster, S.A. et al. (2020). Fundamental principles of rehabilitation and musculoskeletal tissue healing. *Vet. Surg.* 49 (1): 22–32.
56. Durant, A.M., Millis, D.L., and Headrick, J.F. (2011). Kinematics of stair ascent in healthy dogs. *Vet. Comp. Orthop. Traumatol.* 24 (2): 99–105.
57. Feeney, L.C., Lin, C.F., Marcellin-Little, D.J. et al. (2007). Validation of two-dimensional kinematic analysis of walk and sit-to-stand motions in dogs. *Am. J. Vet. Res.* 68 (3): 277–282.
58. Sawaya, S.G., Combet, D., Chanoit, G. et al. (2008). Assessment of impulse duration thresholds for electrical stimulation of muscles (chronaxy) in dogs. *Am. J. Vet. Res.* 69 (10): 1305–1309.
59. Poitras, S. and Brosseau, L. (2008). Evidence-informed management of chronic low back pain with transcutaneous electrical nerve stimulation, interferential current, electrical muscle stimulation, ultrasound, and thermotherapy. *Spine J.* 8 (1): 226–233.
60. Rutjes, A.W., Nuesch, E., Sterchi, R. et al. (2009). Transcutaneous electrostimulation for osteoarthritis of the knee. *Cochrane Database Syst. Rev.* 4: CD002823.
61. Williams, R.G., Silverman, R., Schwind, C. et al. (2007). Surgeon information transfer and communication: factors affecting quality and efficiency of inpatient care. *Ann. Surg.* 245 (2): 159–169.
62. Henderson, A., Levine, D., Millis, D.L., and Drum, M. (2014). Appendix 1 - Protocol development and protocols. In: *Canine Rehabilitation and Physical Therapy*, 2e (eds. D.L. Millis and D. Levine), 669–729. Philadelphia, PA: Elsevier Saunders.

Section VI

Adjunctive Information

16 Complications Associated with Feline Cranial Cruciate Ligament Techniques

Sorrel J. Langley-Hobbs and Eva Schnabl-Feichter

16.1 Introduction

Cranial cruciate ligament (CCL) rupture in cats is much less common than it is in dogs. Both traumatic ruptures [1] and degenerative ruptures are suspected [2]. In the cat, most published reports describe or assume a traumatic etiology, but there is a subset of cats that parallels the older, overweight, canine patients in which degenerative rupture of the CCL is seen [3]. Bilateral degenerative rupture in the younger large-breed cat has also been recognized. Conservative management and surgery, most commonly extracapsular repair or tibial osteotomies, have been used to address this condition, with osteotomies being used with increasing frequency more recently, paralleling the situation in the dog.

16.2 Anatomy

The cruciate ligaments and the medial and lateral collateral ligament are the primary stabilizing structures of the feline stifle. Secondary stabilizers are the joint capsule, the menisci, and the muscles and tendons that span the joint [4].

The CCL prevents stifle hyperextension, excessive internal rotation, and cranial translation of the tibia. The caudal cruciate ligament prevents caudal translation of the tibia. The CCL is larger and stronger than the caudal cruciate ligament in cats which may preclude its rupture in the cat compared to the dog [4].

16.3 Cranial Cruciate Ligament Rupture

16.3.1 Etiopathogenesis

There are thought to be two main forms of cruciate ligament rupture in the cat: traumatic and degenerative. Seven of 50 cats developed bilateral rupture in an epidemiological study [2]. In another series of cases, the cats that had suffered cruciate ligament rupture were heavier than the general population of cats and it was purported that this injury parallels the degenerative CCL ruptures seen in overweight small-breed dogs [3]. Periarticular osteophytosis (Figure 16.1) may be present when the cat presents with an apparent acute onset of lameness, similar to the situation in dogs.

Complications in Canine Cranial Cruciate Ligament Surgery, First Edition. Edited by Ron Ben-Amotz and David L. Dycus.

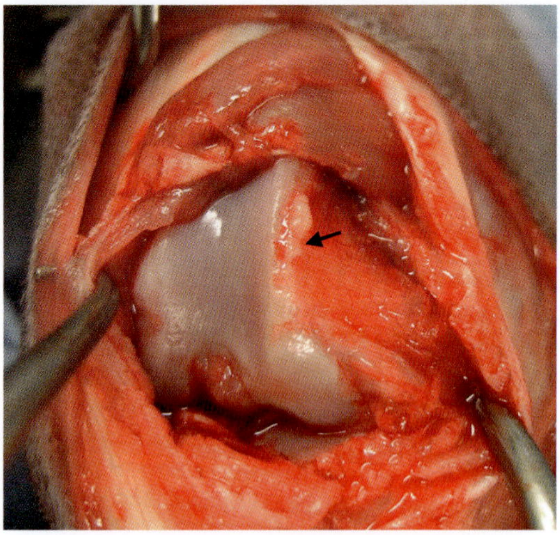

Figure 16.1 Intraoperative view of the stifle of a cat with a cranial cruciate ligament rupture showing osteophytosis along the abaxial trochlear ridge (arrow). Source: © Sorrel J. Langley-Hobbs.

Osteoarthritis was graded as moderate to severe in 10 of 11 stifle joints in cats with CCL rupture, a finding that does not support the assumption of acute traumatic CCL rupture and making a degenerative etiology more likely [5].

In the traumatic form, there may be an isolated CCL rupture but there can also be damage to other periarticular structures such as the collateral ligaments, menisci and caudal cruciate ligament, usually known as multiligamentous, disrupted or deranged injuries. In the most severely affected stifles, the femorotibial joint may be dislocated. It is very important to distinguish between an isolated CCL rupture and a deranged stifle with rupture of other ligaments as the treatment and prognosis are dramatically different between the two. Misdiagnosing a multiligamentous injured stifle as an isolated CCL rupture can have serious consequences for the outcome in the cat.

16.3.2 Clinical Signs

Cats with complete CCL ruptures will have hindlimb lameness and stifle joint swelling, and the cranial drawer test and tibial thrust test will be positive.

Partial cranial cruciate rupture has been seen in cats and in this situation the drawer test may be negative. A retrospective study evaluating 98 feline stifle joints with naturally occurring CCL disease identified 6% partial ruptures [6]. Only one partial CCL rupture was detected in another study [7] which might be due to a low incidence in cats, low case numbers, or the fact that the minimal clinical signs are not observed by owners.

Traumatic ruptures may be more sudden in onset and other conditions may be present such as rupture of other ligaments (medial or lateral collaterals and caudal cruciate), patella luxation or fractures and concurrent injuries elsewhere in the body. In a cadaveric study utilizing normal cats, CCL sectioning resulted in a cranial tibial translation of nearly 9 mm [8]. Instability in cats with traumatic rupture can be pronounced and the cranial drawer can be dramatic.

16.3.3 Diagnosis

The diagnosis of CCL rupture is made by a combination of the history and physical examination and radiographic changes (Algorithm 16.1). Radiographs are taken to confirm the suspected diagnosis and rule out other potential causes or comorbidities (Table 16.1). Affected stifles will show compression of the infrapatellar fat pad associated with a joint effusion. It can be more difficult to detect stifle joint effusion on a radiograph in a cat compared to a dog; good-quality radiographs and careful interpretation are required so compression of the intraarticular fat pad is not missed [9] (Figure 16.2).

Intraarticular mineralization may be present and this has commonly been associated with medial compartment degenerative joint disease [10], particularly if lesions are large [11]. Small discrete lesions are common, and these may be normal or incidental findings [12].

The cat should be sedated or anesthetized prior to performing testing for cruciate ligament integrity. Both the cranial drawer and tibial compression test should be conducted. Instability will be palpable with complete ruptures; this may be pronounced if the cat has a traumatic CCL rupture. The results of the tests may be inconclusive in the presence of partial ruptures.

Algorithm 16.1 Diagnosing CCL rupture in the cat.

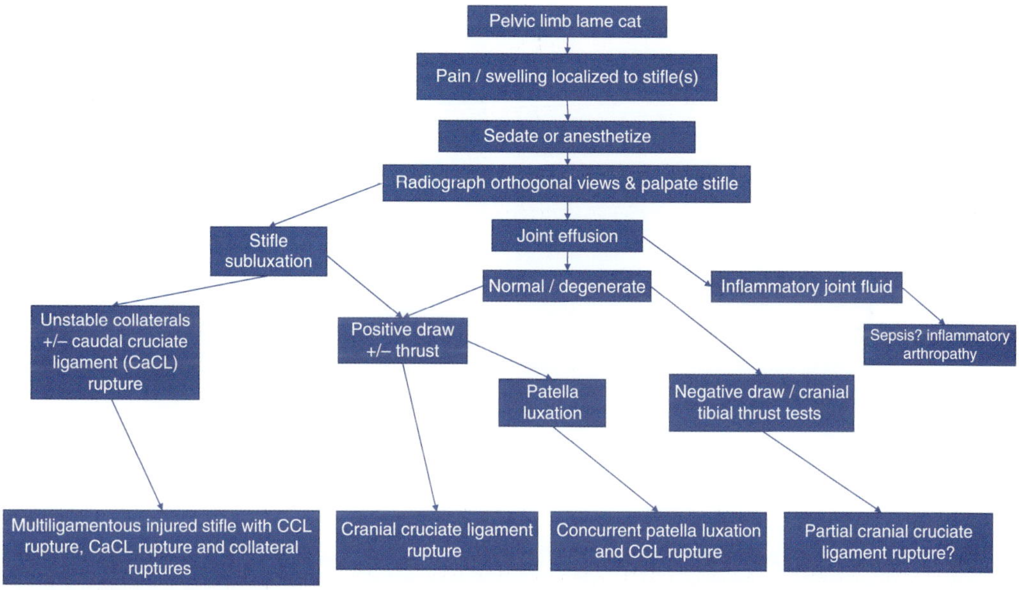

Table 16.1 Clinical and radiographic changes in cats with cranial cruciate ligament rupture.

Stifle pain on manipulation, particularly on extension
Periarticular thickening especially medially
Hindlimb muscle atrophy, particularly thigh muscles
Positive cranial drawer (partial rupture may be minimal or negative)
Positive tibial thrust or compression test (partial rupture may be minimal or negative)
Joint effusion
Periarticular osteophytosis
Enthesophytes
Distal displacement of the popliteal sesamoid bone on lateral radiographs
Intraarticular radiodense bodies and mineralization

It is important to diagnose the cat with a deranged, disrupted or multiligamentous rupture where in addition to a CCL rupture, there will be other ligamentous structures injured, most commonly the medial or lateral collateral ligament, caudal cruciate ligament, and medial meniscus. In multiligamentous injuries, there is usually significant displacement of the tibiofemoral joint or complete luxation. With the cat sedated or anesthetized, in addition to the cranial drawer and tibial compression tests, varus and valgus maneuvers should be performed to detect concurrent collateral ligament injury. However, it is worth noting that some cats with traumatic rupture of the CCL can have marked subluxation of the stifle without disruption of other ligaments (Figure 16.3).

16.4 Meniscal Injury

The incidence of meniscal injuries in feline CCL-deficient stifles has been reported to be between 18% and 67% [2, 6, 7]. In the largest retrospective study, meniscal tears were found in 67 of 100 cats [6]. Isolated medial meniscal injuries were found in most cases. There was no correlation between the presence of a meniscal injury and age, breed, sex, weight, duration of lameness, presence of concurrent medial patellar luxation, degree of degenerative joint disease, or presenting side of lameness.

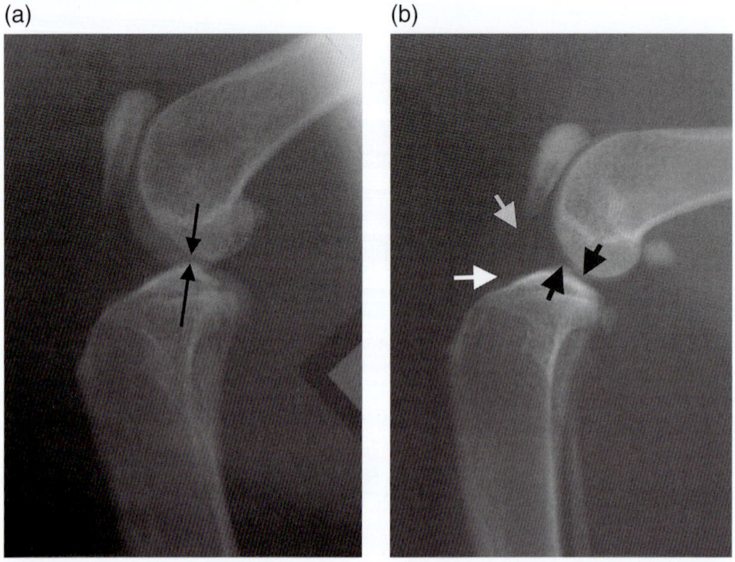

Figure 16.2 (a) A radiograph of a normal feline stifle; arrows indicate the normal relationship of the femoral condyle adjacent to the tibial eminences. (b) The contralateral stifle with cranial cruciate ligament rupture has a joint effusion (white arrows) and subluxation of the stifle (indicated by black arrows at the center of the femoral condyle and at the center of the weight-bearing axis at the level of the tibial eminences). Source: © Sorrel J. Langley-Hobbs.

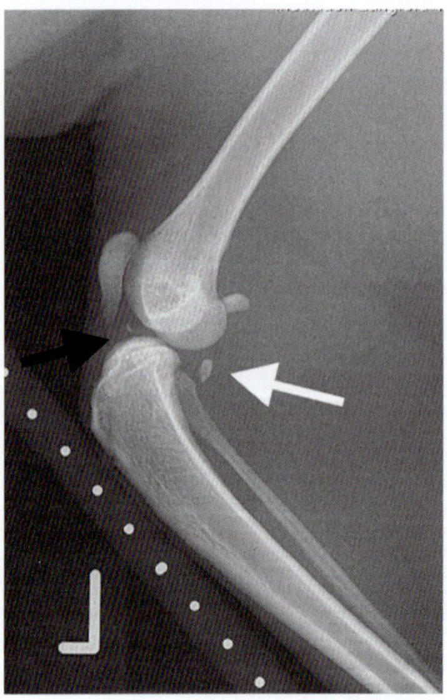

Figure 16.3 Lateral stifle radiograph from a MN 7 kg Bengal. The cat had an acute onset of lameness after a fall. There is an isolated rupture of the cranial cruciate ligament with no other ligamentous injuries although the degree of subluxation on the radiograph is marked. There is a small ossification in the stifle (black arrow), which is an incidental finding in many cats, although a likely differential diagnosis in this cat would be an avulsion fracture. The cat has displacement of the popliteal sesamoid (white arrow) which is common in cats with CCL rupture; additionally it only has one fabella, also a common finding in cats with the medial fabella often absent (unossified). Source: © Sorrel J. Langley-Hobbs.

16.4.1 Intraarticular and Meniscal Mineralization

Intraarticular or meniscal mineralization is a common finding in domestic cats [10–12]. The prevalence was reported as 46% in a population of 100 cats with the cats being significantly older and having a lower body condition score than those without stifle pathology [10]. Smaller meniscal ossifications in cats are suspected to represent a normal anatomical finding, a meniscal sesamoid bone also referred as lunula [12, 13] (Figure 16.4a). Meniscal ossicles have also been found frequently in large cats like lions, tigers and leopards older than 1 year. Those ossicles were found in the cranial horn of the medial menisci [10–12, 14].

Larger mineralizations in cats were found to be ossifications, commonly located in the joint capsule and fat pad [11], so not isolated to the meniscus (Figure 16.4b). In cats, it has been shown that larger mineralizations cause significantly more cartilage damage on the femur and tibia and therefore lead to the development of medial compartment disease [10, 11]. Interestingly, pain scores in cats with meniscal mineralization were not different to others [10, 15]. Larger meniscal calcifications have also been found in cats with cruciate disease [11] and might be connected to a traumatic event [13, 16].

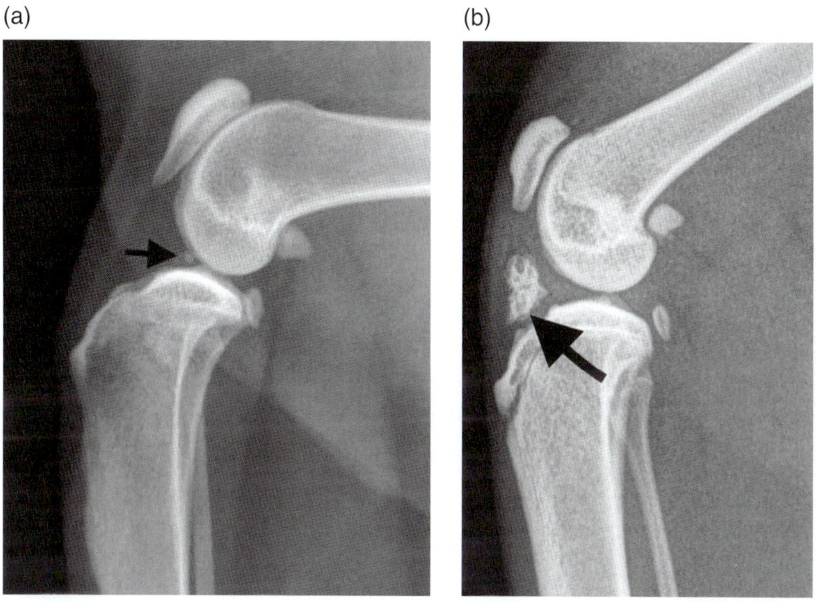

Figure 16.4 Intraarticular mineralization. (a) A small lesion is often a normal finding and incidental (arrow). (b) Larger lesions most likely affecting the fat pad and joint capsule. These large lesions (arrow) are often associated with degenerative joint disease and cranial cruciate ligament rupture and their careful dissection and removal should be considered. Source: © Sorrel J. Langley-Hobbs.

Histologically, the meniscus seems to undergo a process of ossification. It starts with a chondral to osseous transformation of the cartilage with ultimate mineral deposition. Finally, this organizes into cancellous bone and bone marrow structures [10].

16.5 Tibial Plateau Angle Measurement

Measuring the tibial plateau angle (TPA) in cats is done in a similar way as described in dogs (Figure 16.5) [17]. Overall, the medial tibial articular surface is less definable in cats compared to that in dogs [7, 18]. One study compared the TPA in cats with and without CCL rupture and found a significant difference in TPA measurements between inexperienced and experienced observers [18]. Possible causes were poor definition of the cranial and caudal bone landmarks; the amount of osteoarthritis present at the caudal point of the TPA can impede making correct measurements.

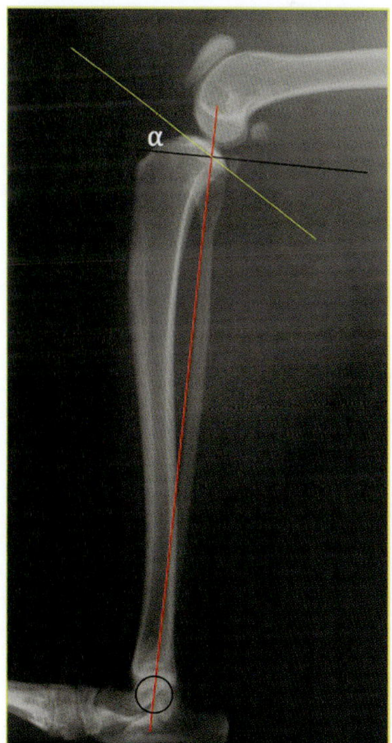

Figure 16.5 Preoperative measurement of tibial plateau angle (TPA) before performing a tibial plateau leveling osteotomy (TPLO) in a cat. Red line: tibial functional axis. Yellow line: tibial plateau slope. Black line: perpendicular line to the tibial functional axis. α = tibial plateau angle (TPA). Source: © Eva Schnabl-Feichter.

According to Schnabl et al. [18], cats with CCL rupture had a significantly greater mean TPA (24.7°) compared to those without any evidence of CCL injury (21.6°). The conclusion was that cats with CCL rupture have a

Table 16.2 Tibial plateau angle (TPA) measurements in the cat.

	Number of cats/stifles	Tibial plateau angle	Reference
Healthy/normal cats with no stifle disease	(50 cats, 100 stifles) (34 cats, 68 stifles)	24.84±4.05 (16–33) 21.6±3.7 (12–27)	[1] [18]
Mean angles		23.52 (12–33)	
Cats with CCLR	(25 cats, 25 stifles)	22.72±4.51 (13–30)	[1]
	(21 cats, 21 stifles)	24.7±4.5 (17–37)	[18]
Mean angles		23.62 (13–37)	

greater TPA, and this at least lends some credence to the possibility of higher TPA being a predisposing factor for cruciate injury in this species [18]. However, another study found no difference in the TPA when comparing 50 normal cats to 25 cats with CCL rupture [1]. The mean TPA in both normal cats and cats with CCL rupture in these two studies was between 23° and 24° [1, 18] (Table 16.2).

16.6 Management Considerations

Surgical management of CCL rupture in cats will give a quicker return to function and is the preferred choice in most circumstances. Conservative management is an alternative if surgical stabilization is not a viable option for an individual cat.

16.6.1 Conservative Management

There is limited published evidence about the effectiveness and outcome of conservative management of CCL rupture in cats. In one study from the 1980s where 18 cats were treated conservatively, they took an average of 5 weeks to regain gait that was considered normal by veterinarian observation [19]. The conservative management consisted of keeping the cats indoors in a room or cage for 4 weeks and then restricting activity indoors for a further 4–6 weeks, together with instigating weight loss when appropriate. A satisfactory outcome was defined as a clinically normal gait with little or no apparent muscle atrophy at the time of follow-up; this was considered to have been achieved in all cats in a mean duration of 4.8 weeks, with a range of 1–16 weeks.

Experimental transection of the CCL in cats [5] caused a distinct unloading of the deficient hindlimb when compared with the non-operated hindlimb, which persisted for about 16–18 weeks. A decrease in muscle mass was found from muscles of the experimental hindlimb compared to the mass of muscles from the contralateral hindlimb, which was largest at 4 weeks and smallest at 35 weeks post CCL transection [5]. There was a delayed appearance of osteophytes in this model compared with the dog, suggesting that cats may be better able to compensate for CCL deficiency. This may be associated with factors of loading, the smaller size of cats compared with dogs, or a better developed neuromuscular control system in the cat [5].

Complications with conservative management include persistent lameness [9]. Eighty percent of the cats in one study showed persistent cranial drawer motion and evidence of degenerative joint disease upon physical examination and radiography despite apparent resolution of the lameness [19]. In a study of 50 cats with CCL rupture, 28 were treated conservatively and they were found to experience less chronic pain at long-term follow-up, and better quality of life (QoL) on the feline musculoskeletal pain index (FMPI). However, one of the limitations of this study was a possible selection bias due to a clinical decision to treat less lame cats with less severe joint disease conservatively [2].

If lameness persists following conservative management then there are various options, including continuing conservative management for a longer period of time or opting for surgical management (Algorithm 16.2). The cat

Algorithm 16.2 Decision making when presented with a lame cat following conservative management of CCL rupture.

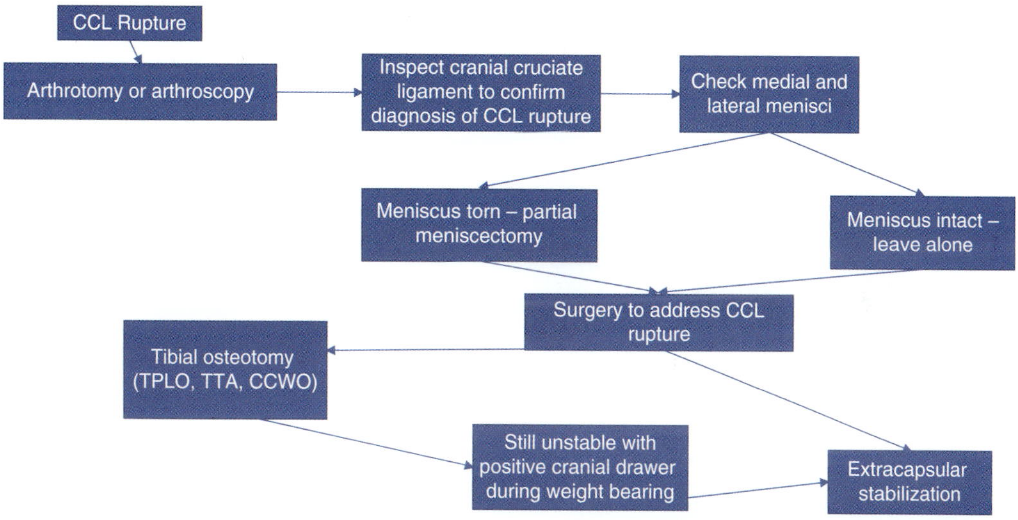

should be reassessed in case a multiligamentous injury has been missed or there is another cause for the lameness such as a meniscal tear which may require treatment.

16.6.2 Surgical Stabilization

Surgery is purported to give a quicker return to function and given the high rate of meniscal pathology in cats with CCL ruptures, exploratory surgery for meniscal assessment and concurrent stifle stabilization should be considered in feline patients [6].

In an experimental model of CCL transection, the medial meniscus was often reported as ragged at 12 weeks and in one cat it was visibly torn [5]. Treatment of meniscal injury (Figure 16.6) is by partial meniscectomy and careful removal of the damaged portion, preserving the intact remainder of the meniscus.

Treatment or removal of the small meniscal mineralizations is generally not recommended as they may be incidental findings and not pathological. Attempts at removal will cause damage to the meniscus. Nevertheless, due to the possibility of cartilage lesions secondary to or concurrent with the large intraarticular mineralizations

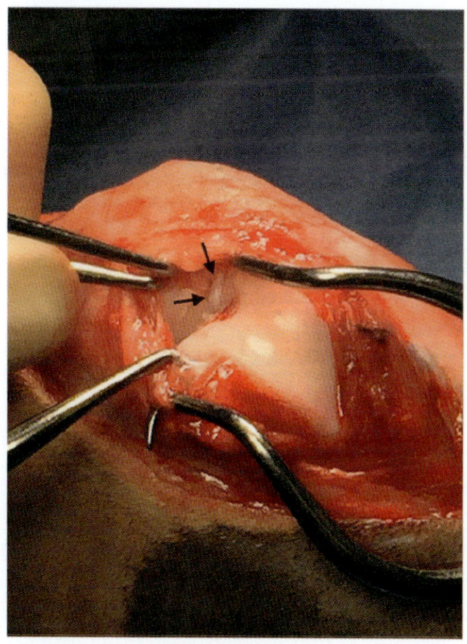

Figure 16.6 A medial meniscal bucket handle tear in a cat with the torn portion folded forward (arrowed). Source: © Sorrel J. Langley-Hobbs.

in the joint capsule or fat pad, excision can be performed if needed but taking care not to damage the meniscus or intermeniscal ligaments [10, 11].

Algorithm 16.3 Decision making for the cat with isolated CCL rupture.

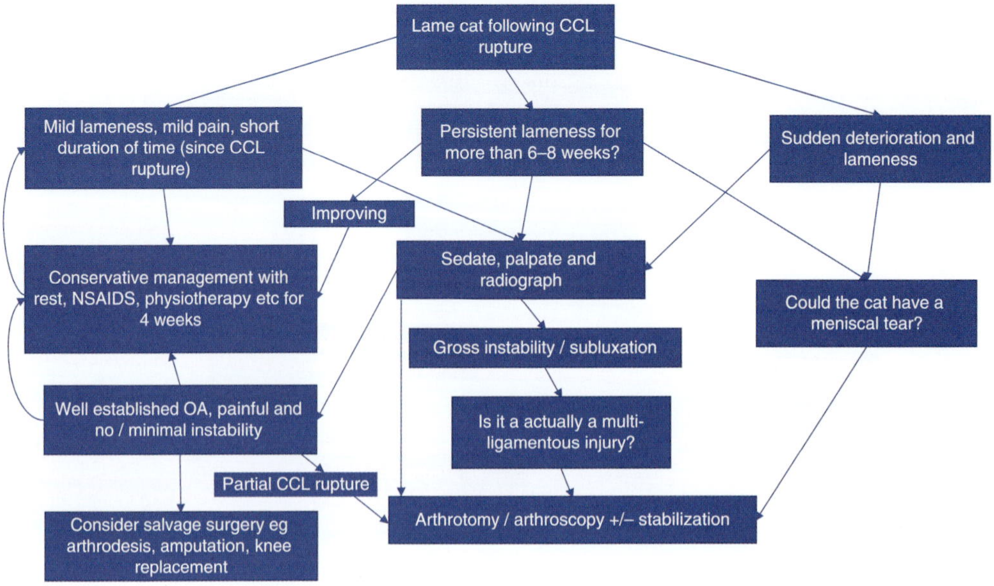

Following arthrotomy or arthroscopy, the different categories of surgical options in use in the cat are extracapsular stabilization and osteotomies including tibial plateau leveling osteotomy (TPLO), tibial tuberosity advancement (TTA) and cranial closing wedge ostectomy (CCWO). Intraarticular stabilization is another option that could be considered but there is very limited evidence to support the use of this technique.

Decision making in surgery can be aided by working through Algorithm 16.3.

16.7 Extracapsular Stabilization

Surgical management with extracapsular suture stabilization gives an apparent quicker return to function compared to conservative management [3]. Extracapsular stabilization techniques are commonly used in the cat.

The results of studies [20] showed that placing a suture between the fabella or through a suture screw close to the fabella to a hole through the tibia at the level of the insertion of the patellar ligament produced a suture that had minimal change in length during normal range of motion of the stifle and restored good function to a cadaveric stifle by elimination of cranial drawer [21]. Placement of the suture hole too far distal in the tibia is a common mistake that can result in failure of stabilization [9]. The femorofabellar ligament in the cat is fairly lax and clinically anchoring the suture around this ligament can produce a loose lateral suture. Placement of a suture through the eyelet of a suture anchor or suture screw in the femur adjacent to the lateral fabella may give better stability than placing the suture around the lateral fabella [21] and the use of suture anchors should be considered in clinical cases (Table 16.3).

Table 16.3 Tips for extracapsular stabilization surgery for CCL rupture in the cat.

Arthrotomy or arthroscopy to inspect meniscus and perform partial meniscectomy if torn
Suture placement – placing a suture between the femorofabellar ligament or through a suture anchor close to the fabella to a hole in the tibia at the level of the insertion of the patella ligament [20]
Material – large gauge [3] or 40 lb monofilament nylon, tightened at 20 N, produced favorable biomechanical stabilization of cruciate-related stifle instability directly after surgery in an *ex vivo* model [22]

16.7.1 Complications with Extracapsular Stabilization

In a retrospective study of 50 cats with CCL rupture, 22 had surgical stabilization with extracapsular sutures – the lateral fabellotibial suture (LFS) technique was used in all cats [2]. Arthrotomy was performed in 19/22 surgeries and a complete CCL rupture was noted in all 19 cats. Postoperative surgical complications were recorded in 6/22 cats (27%). Twelve surgeons with different levels of experience performed the procedures so it is possible that the low number of LFS surgeries per surgeon contributed to the complication risk. Notably multiligament stifle injuries were diagnosed in five surgically treated cats; four had collateral ligament damage and two of these had an additional complete rupture of the caudal cruciate ligament. The fifth cat had caudal cruciate ligament rupture but intact collateral ligaments. Two cats had one postoperative complication, while four cats had two. Three of the six cats with complications underwent a second surgery.

Complications following extracapsular stabilization and their possible solutions are listed in Table 16.4. They include neurological deficits, seroma, persistent instability, infection, persistent lameness, stiffness on rising, osteoarthritis (Figure 16.7) and late meniscal tear [2, 3]. Reduced range in motion of the stifle following CCL surgery can be seen and may be associated with the presence of osteoarthritis. Recurrence of instability may occur due to breakage or loosening of the suture or suture anchor pull-out. An algorithm is provided to aid in decision making about how to proceed with the different complications seen following surgery (Algorithm 16.4).

One of the main reasons for complications in cats is when the cat is misdiagnosed as having an isolated CCL rupture when in fact it has a multiligamentous injury (e.g., collateral ligament ruptures, caudal cruciate ligament and

Table 16.4 Complications following extracapsular stabilization in the cat, with initial, subsequent or other options for management.

Complication	Initial management	Subsequent or other options
Persistent lameness	Pain medication (NSAIDs), rest, possibly physical rehabilitation	Investigate for other causes of lameness such as multiligamentous injury, neoplasia or patella luxation; consider an alternative surgical strategy
Meniscal tear	Arthrotomy or arthroscopy and partial meniscectomy	Pain medication (NSAIDs), rest
Infection	Culture and sensitivity and antibiotics.	Revision surgery or an alternative surgical strategy may be required later on (e.g., different suture material, TPLO, TTA)
Osteoarthritis	Pain medication (NSAIDs), rest, nutraceuticals, weight loss, environmental adaption, possibly physical rehabilitation	Salvage surgery – amputation, arthrodesis, joint replacement
Reduction in range of motion	Pain medication, physical rehabilitation	Reevaluation of the stifle stability, extracapsular suture removal?
Neurological deficits	Gabapentin or amantadine	Removal of the extracapsular suture if concerned about the suture being around popliteal nerve
Seroma	Aspiration, bandage, heat	Explore and drain or resect seroma, culture and sensitivity, extracapsular suture removal
Instability persistent	Rest; if in pain – NSAID	Revision surgery or an alternative surgical strategy may be required (i.e., TPLO + extracapsular ligament repair)

NSAID, nonsteroidal antiinflammatory drug; TPLO, tibial plateau leveling osteotomy; TTA, tibial tuberosity advancement.

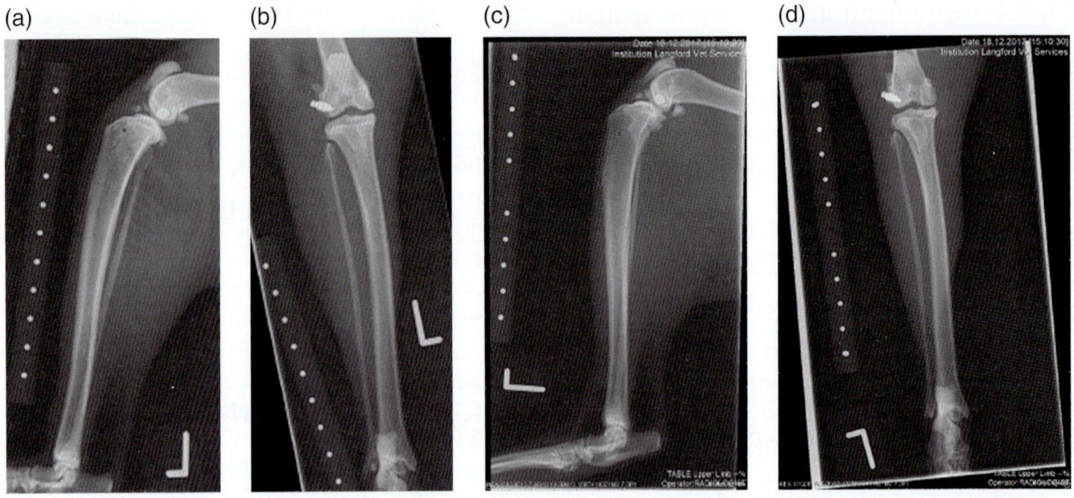

Figure 16.7 (a,b) A 6-year-old British Blue cat presented with left cranial cruciate ligament rupture which was treated with extracapsular stabilization. A suture was threaded through a suture anchor in the femur and then through two bone tunnels in the proximal tibia. (c,d) The cat was represented 18 months later with right cranial cruciate ligament rupture and radiographs of the left stifle at this time show progression of the osteoarthritis with more pronounced periarticular osteophytosis and intraarticular mineralization. The suture anchor is unchanged in position. Source: Images (a-c) © Sorrel J. Langley-Hobbs. Image (d) Institution Langford Vet Services.

Algorithm 16.4 Decision making when presented with a lame cat post surgical management of CCL rupture.

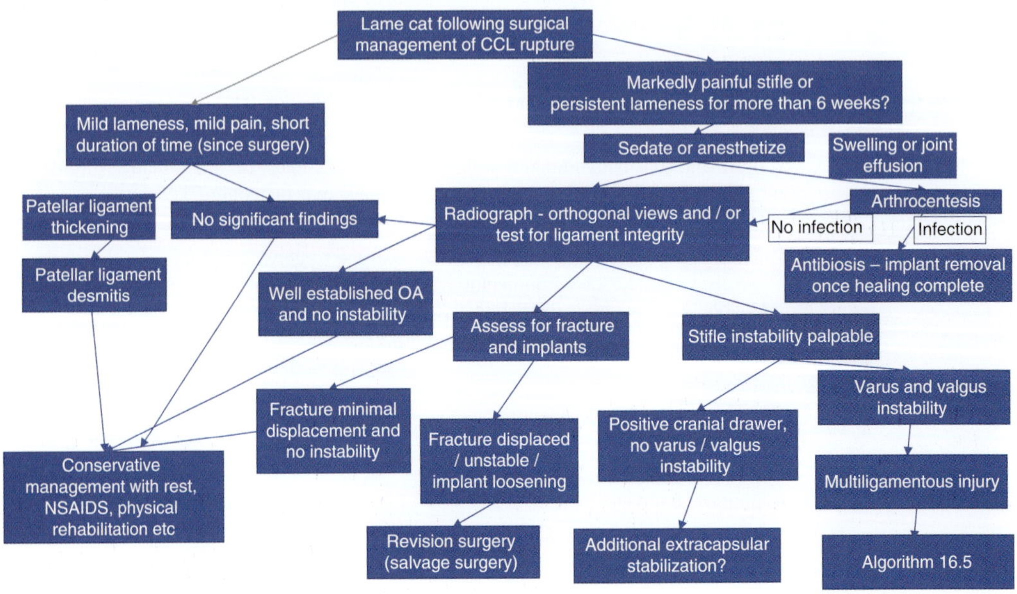

Algorithm 16.5 Treatment algorithm for multiligamentous injury of the feline stifle.

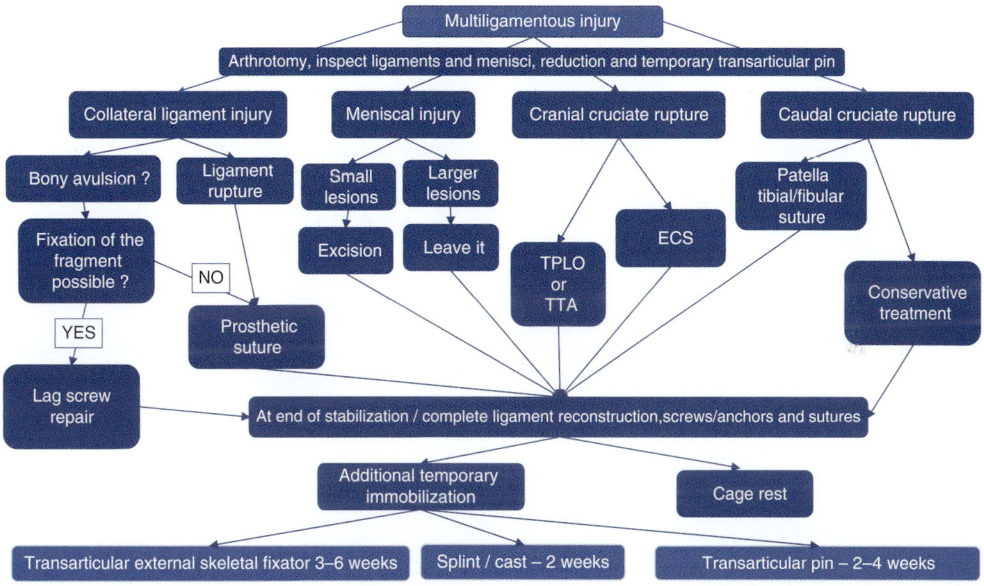

meniscal tears). These injuries are associated with a high complication rate, and treatment options and postoperative stabilization are very different (Algorithm 16.5).

16.8 Osteotomy for Cranial Cruciate Ligament Rupture in the Cat: Considerations

Traditionally, conservative management and extraarticular stabilization have been the treatment options used most commonly to manage cats with CCL rupture. More recently, case reports and small case series report success with osteotomy techniques, including TPLO and TTA techniques [7, 9, 23, 24]. However, cadaveric studies have not supported the use of osteotomies in cats to stabilize stifles following transection of the CCL [8, 25].

In the cadaveric models of the feline stance phase, CCL sectioning resulted in cranial tibial subluxation and internal tibial rotation, as observed in the dog [25]. The simple cadaveric model of the feline stifle failed to demonstrate a positive effect of TTA. Nor was stability improved by further advancement of the tibial tuberosity by 1 or 2mm. Even though the validity of the model can be questioned, the behavior of the feline stifle was different to that of the canine stifle under similar conditions. Transposing the TTA technique from the dog to the cat may not be as direct and simple as it might seem [25].

In a similar cadaveric model, cranial tibial subluxation and internal tibial rotation were not significantly altered after TPLO with a TPA of +5° [8]. Additional rotation of the tibial plateau to a TPA of 0° and −5° had no significant effect on cranial tibial subluxation and internal tibial rotation, although two out of 10 specimens were stabilized by a postoperative TPA of −5°. No stabilization of the CCL-deficient stifle was observed in this model of the feline stifle after TPLO [8]. Given that stabilization of the CCL-deficient stifle was not obtained in the model tested, simple transposition of the TPLO technique from the dog to the cat may not be appropriate [8]. More studies are required to evaluate the effect of TTA and TPLO in the feline stifle [8, 25].

Following tibial osteotomies for CCL rupture in the cat, strict exercise restriction is required

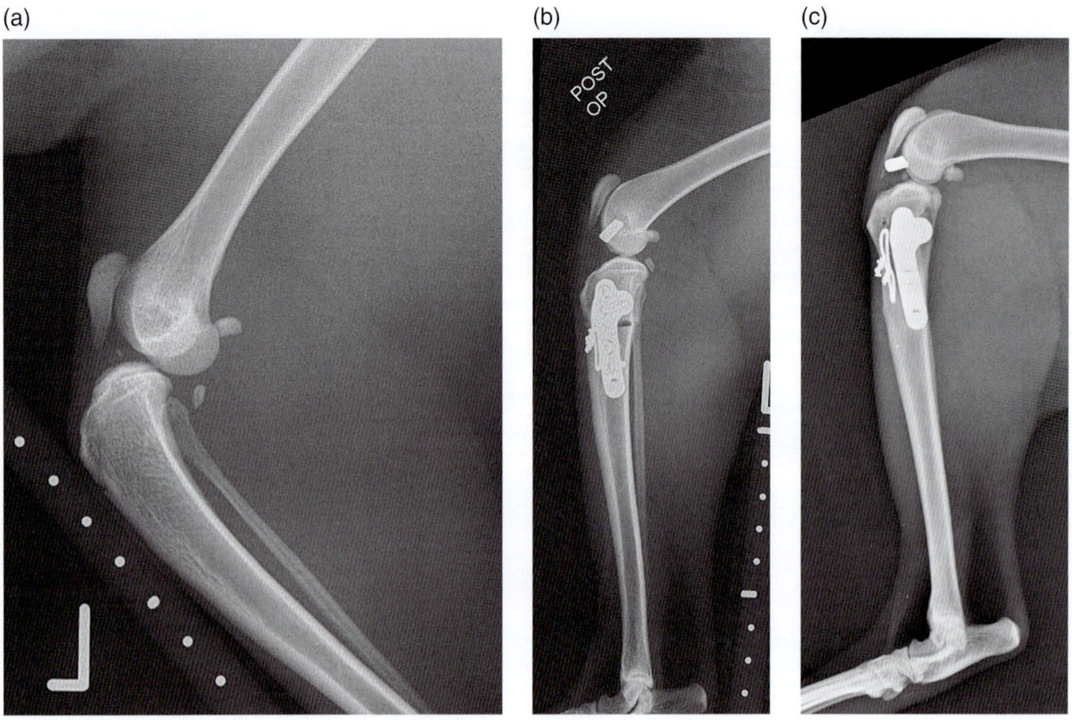

Figure 16.8 A combined technique of cranial closing wedge osteotomy and extracapsular suture was used in this 7 kg Burmese cat with pronounced stifle instability after sustaining a CCL rupture following a fall. **(a)** Preoperative view showing stifle subluxation. **(b)** Postoperative view following cranial closing wedge osteotomy and an additional lateral suture, needed to reduce subluxation and restore stifle stability as the CCWO alone was not sufficient in this cat with a traumatic CCL rupture. **(c)** Eighteen months postoperative radiograph showing the healed osteotomy. There is some mild periarticular osteophytosis and mineralization of the stifle joint. Source: All images © Sorrel J. Langley-Hobbs.

and cage rest is mandatory for a 4–6-week postoperative period. Failure of the owner to comply with these restriction will very often produce major complications like implant-associated complications or fracture of the tibia.

It is important in the cat, where traumatic rupture is more common, to consider whether osteotomies alone are sufficient to stabilize the joints (Algorithm 16.3). In some cases where instability is pronounced, an osteotomy combined with an extracapsular suture may be necessary to restore stability (Figure 16.8). This situation is occasionally also encountered in dogs with severe internal tibial rotation where osteotomies are combined with lateral sutures [26].

16.9 Tibial Plateau Leveling Osteotomy

The use of TPLO was first reported in one cat with a steep TPA; the procedure was combined with a cranial closing wedge to reduce the TPA [24]. An *in vitro* study on cadavers [8] concluded that TPLO was not able to neutralize cranial tibial thrust but the results of a clinical case series suggested that the procedure may be effective *in vivo* [7]. The recent prospective clinical study supported the use of TPLO in cats but commented that case numbers are still low, and a longer term follow-up is needed particularly with regard to evaluating the development and clinical relevance of osteoarthritis [7]. Eleven cats were operated on, eight had acute onset of lameness, three chronic, and one cat had two previous surgeries. Despite the reported acute onset of lameness in eight cats, osteoarthritis was graded as moderate to severe in 91% of the joints, a finding that does not support the assumption of acute traumatic CCL rupture and makes a degenerative etiology more likely [5]. Several considerations should be borne in mind when performing a TPLO in the cat (Figure 16.9) (Table 16.5).

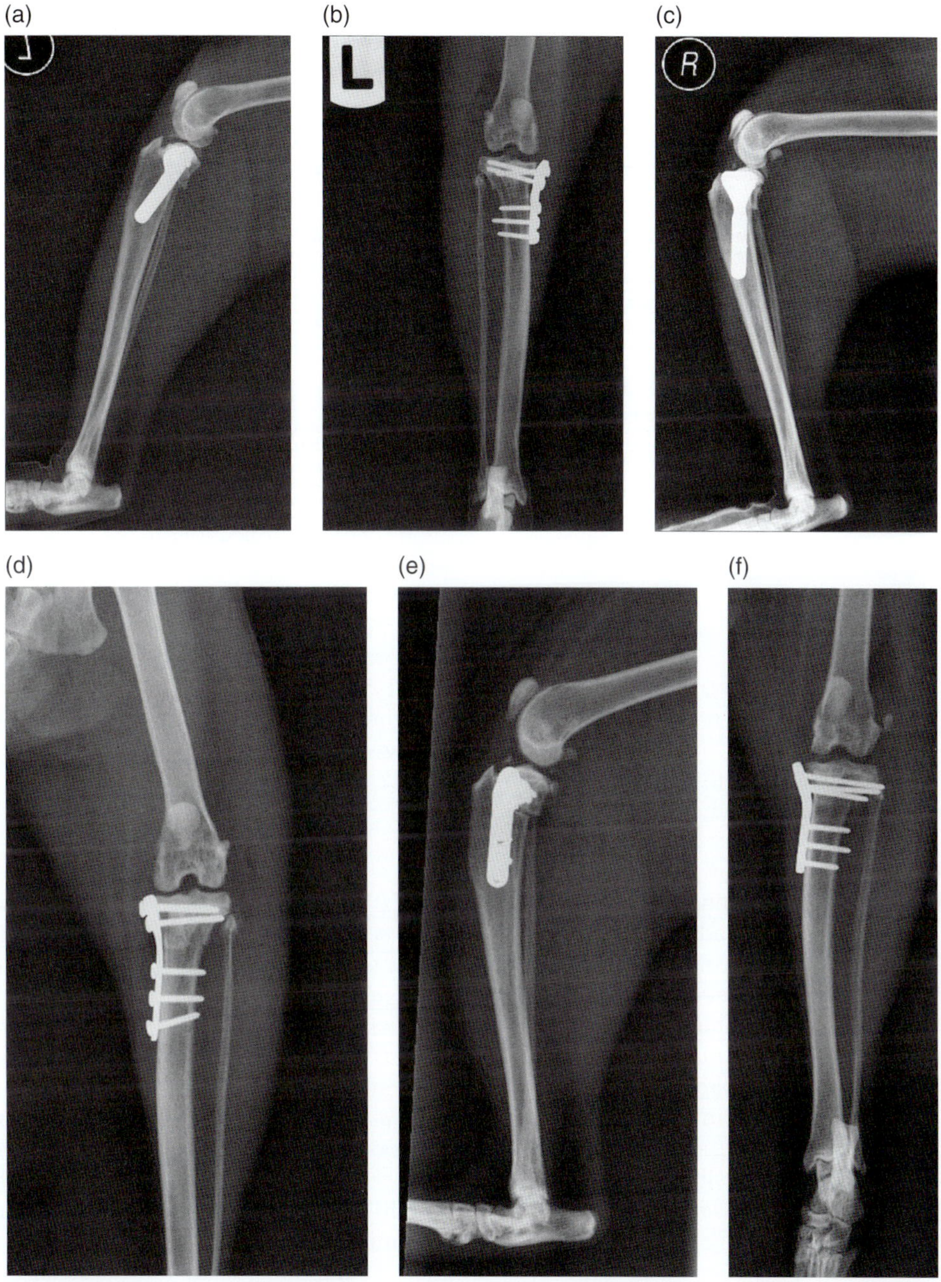

Figure 16.9 Different 2.0 mm plates which have been used for TPLO procedure. (a,b) DSH cat, TPLO with a 2.0 mm Slocum plate. Using the plate resulted in a caudocranial malposition of the plate. (c,d) DSH cat, TPLO with a 2.0 mm Orthomed plate. The plate is a very tight fit proximally, and there is a mild caudocranial malposition. (e,f) Persian, TPLO with a 2.0 mm Synthes locking plate. Due to the dedicated shape of the plate, it is a better fit to the tibial shape with the positioning more central on the tibia. Source: All images © Anicura, TK Hollabrunn.

Table 16.5 Tips for tibial plateau leveling osteotomy (TPLO) surgery for CCL rupture in the cat.

Measurement techniques for osteotomy positioning as described previously [17].
Arthrotomy or arthroscopy to inspect meniscus and perform partial meniscectomy if torn.
A 12 mm TPLO blade used in all cats [7].
Use of a caudally tilted TPLO plate (e.g., Synthes and Arthrex) that is better suited to the shape of the tibia avoids the distal end of the plate being placed too close to the cranial edge of the tibia (Figure 16.9).
Use a narrow 2.0 TPLO plate (the original 2 mm plate is quite broad) (a 2.4 mm plate was used in a 11 kg cat) [7].
Consider placing an additional antirotational suture if persistent instability post TPLO.
Enforce strict cage rest postoperatively.

16.9.1 Complications Following TPLO in Cats

Intra- and postoperative complications occurred in 5/11 cats in which TPLO was performed for CCL rupture [7]. Complications included infection, patellar ligament desmitis, suboptimal plate positioning, fibular fracture, osteotomy gap, under- and overcorrection of the TPA [7], persistent instability, and patella luxation.

Intraoperative complications included suboptimal positioning of the plate in three cats [7], although this did not impair the patients' outcome. An iatrogenic proximal fibular fracture occurred in one cat during drilling of a proximal screw hole and a visible osteotomy gap was present in another. Neither of these cats suffered delayed osteotomy healing or a worse clinical outcome [7]. Patellar desmitis occurred in two cats [7]. Possible causes are excessive patellar ligament retraction, heat development while sawing, or increased activity postoperatively. Larger case numbers are needed to evaluate whether or not this contributes to the development of patellar desmitis in the cat and what the long-term outcome is.

Careful preoperative TPA measurements are very important in order to prevent overcorrection, as can be seen in small dogs. Even small increments (in the angle measurement) in these small patients will result in undesirable results. Although the mean TPA in the 11 cats of 8° was close to the 5–6.5°, two cats had a postoperative TPA lower than 5° (−2° and 4°) [7]. However, despite these low postoperative TPAs, both cats recovered uneventfully, and a caudal cruciate ligament rupture was not observed during the short-term follow-up [7].

See Algorithm 16.4 for help in decision making following surgical complications.

16.9.2 Outcomes Following TPLO in Cats

None of the complications in the 11 cats required surgical intervention [7]. At 4–8 weeks postoperative, all cats were either sound or had mild intermittent lameness. Complete bony union was present radiographically within 4–12 weeks in all cases. Owners reported a high level of comfort and mobility in every cat at the final follow-up, despite a positive "sit test" in seven cats [7].

16.10 Tibial Tuberosity Advancement

An *ex vivo* experimental study did not find that TTA in cadaveric cats was effective [25]. This very simplified cadaveric model of the feline stifle (with no hamstring replacement) failed to demonstrate a positive effect of TTA and stability was also not improved by further advancement of the tibial tuberosity by 1 or 2 mm. The study involved making partial osteotomies (modified Maquet procedure) and during a preliminary study, an attempt was made to increase the transposition of the tibial tuberosity beyond +2 mm. This consistently led to catastrophic avulsion of the tibial tuberosity before stabilization of the CCL-deficient stifle could occur [25]. The behavior of the feline stifle was found to be different to that of the canine stifle under similar conditions so the conclusion from this study was that care should be taken when transposing the TTA technique from the dog to the cat. More studies may be useful for evaluation of the effect of TTA in the feline stifle.

Table 16.6 Tips for tibial tuberosity advancement (TTA) surgery for CCL rupture in the cat.

Standing angle of cat stifle (or contralateral stance angle if marked lameness on affected leg), e.g., 110–120° used for preoperative planning, as opposed to the 135° standing angle in the dog.
Arthrotomy or arthroscopy to inspect meniscus and perform partial meniscectomy if torn.
It is deemed important in cats to accurately gauge the compromise between where to make the osteotomy so there is a large enough tuberosity but not so large that there is risk of iatrogenic fracture of the tibia. Care to avoid creation of a narrow "isthmus" in the tibia caudal to the osteotomy, which might hypothetically predispose to fracture at this site (Figure 16.10a).
If planned advancement does not stabilize the cranial tibial thrust, then consider going up one cage size (maximum 1.5 mm bigger).
Autogenous cancellous bone graft or demineralized bone matrix is placed in the osteotomy gap caudal to the tuberosity.
Enforce strict cage rest postoperatively.

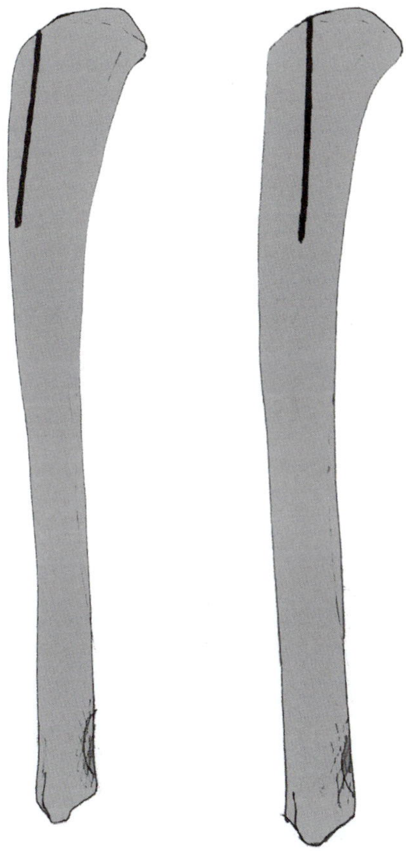

Figure 16.10 **(a)** An osteotomy performed for the modified Maquet procedure too far cranial, resulting in too small a tuberosity segment that may be prone to avulsion fracture. **(b)** The Modified Maquet procedure osteotomy is performed too far caudal, resulting in a stress riser in the tibia, making tibial diaphyseal fracture a likely complication.

Despite the negative results from cadaveric studies, both the traditional TTA and the modified Maquet technique (MMT) have been reported in very low numbers of cats. One cat with an isolated CCL rupture that stayed lame following conservative management, one with persistent lameness and instability following extracapsular stabilization [9], a cat with an avulsion of the CCL origin with failure to improve on conservative management [23] and one cat with a combined CCL rupture and medial patella luxation (MPL) [27] all resulted in good outcomes. Tips for planning and surgical technique can be found in Table 16.6.

16.10.1 Complications Following TTA in Cats

In cats, although the outcomes of the few reported cases in the literature are good, there were often implant-associated problems due to the size of the implants in relation to the size of cat bones [9, 23]. Postoperative radiography revealed suboptimal implant positioning for two cats [9]. Too cranial an osteotomy leads to difficulty in placing the cranial screw, while too caudal will raise the risk of iatrogenic fracture of the tibia (Figure 16.10b) [9, 23]. One cat suffered a tibial tuberosity fracture with preservation of the tuberosity advancement. It was treated by screw removal and conservative management as there was minimal displacement of the fracture fragment. Use of a smaller screw such as a 2.0 mm with a washer rather than a 2.4 mm screw, or not placing any screw in the cranial cage hole are options for avoiding this complication in future cases [9].

The two-fork plates for the traditional TTA appear to be more susceptible to failure (the forks specifically) and the small size of the tibial tuberosity fragment, the close proximity of the fork holes to the edges of the osteotomized fragment and the relatively narrow parent tibia may all be more susceptible to complications than following TTA in a dog with more ample bone stock (Figure 16.11a–c). One cat, although walking well, was seen to abduct the affected limb without full flexion when sitting on follow-up [9].

Postoperative exercise restriction following TTA in cats is strongly recommended. Complications often occur following an increase in exercise in the postoperative period.

Further information is needed before we can conclude that TTA is a safe procedure with a low enough complication rate to justify performance in the cat. It may have a place particularly for cats with concurrent CCL rupture and MPL, or for cats that fail to respond to either conservative management or ECS.

See Chapter 12 for help in decision making for surgical complications following TTA.

16.11 Multiligamentous Stifle Injuries/ Stifle Disruption

In cats with multiligament injuries of the stifle (Figure 16.12a) resulting in a severely unstable stifle joint, surgical stabilization is recommended. Rupture of the cranial and caudal cruciate concurrent with rupture of the medial or lateral collateral ligament is most common. Additionally, a complete peripheral avulsion of the medial and/or lateral meniscus is often seen in combination with the aforementioned injuries [28].

Due to the severity of the injury, cats show a nonweight-bearing lameness with marked soft tissue swelling [29]. In order to palpate the patient, sedation or anesthesia is mandatory in most cases and the drastic instability can then be detected and more precisely defined. The stifle should be palpated after manual reduction (if luxation is present) and cranial drawer, caudal drawer and valgus and varus maneuvers performed. A definitive diagnosis may still be difficult to determine and approaching the ligaments and viewing them at surgery may be necessary to make the definitive diagnosis. Stifle radiographs are taken to rule out further bony damage [29].

Surgical intervention is the main stem of treatment (Algorithm 16.5). During surgery, a temporary transarticular pin can be helpful if the correct position cannot be maintained easily by hand until the primary repairs are completed [30]. Unless the pin is large (Figure 16.13b), it should be removed and not left in at the completion of surgery, otherwise it is liable to break (Figure 16.12). In general, the injured tissues (cruciate ligaments and collateral ligaments) are primarily repaired and if necessary, additionally protected by temporary immobilization. Alternatively, a single transarticular pin can be used without primarily repairing individual ligaments (Figure 16.13). The most common form of immobilization after stifle disruption is a temporary transarticular external skeletal fixator (TESF) in a Type I frame configuration that is triangulated, with an additional bar placed between the most proximal and distal pins (Figure 16.13) [28]. Two fixation pins are placed in the femur and tibia. Fixation angles of 110–135° should be used. The fixator is left in place for 2–4 weeks.

16.11.1 Complications and Outcomes Following Multiligamentous Injuries in Cats

Despite the extent of damage in a case with a stifle disruption, the medium- to long-term outcome has been reported as good but with a complication rate of up to 30% leading to euthanasia or amputation in some cases [29] or requiring revision surgery. In one study [2], the FMPI results of five cats with multiligament injuries show that chronic pain could be expected in these cats, even after surgical correction. Complications include persistent instability, recurrent luxation or subluxation (Figure 16.14a–d), medial and lateral patella luxation and complications secondary to the temporary immobilization procedures such as fracture or osteomyelitis (Figure 16.14c–e).

Transarticular fixation with an ESF has deleterious effects on the joint and articular

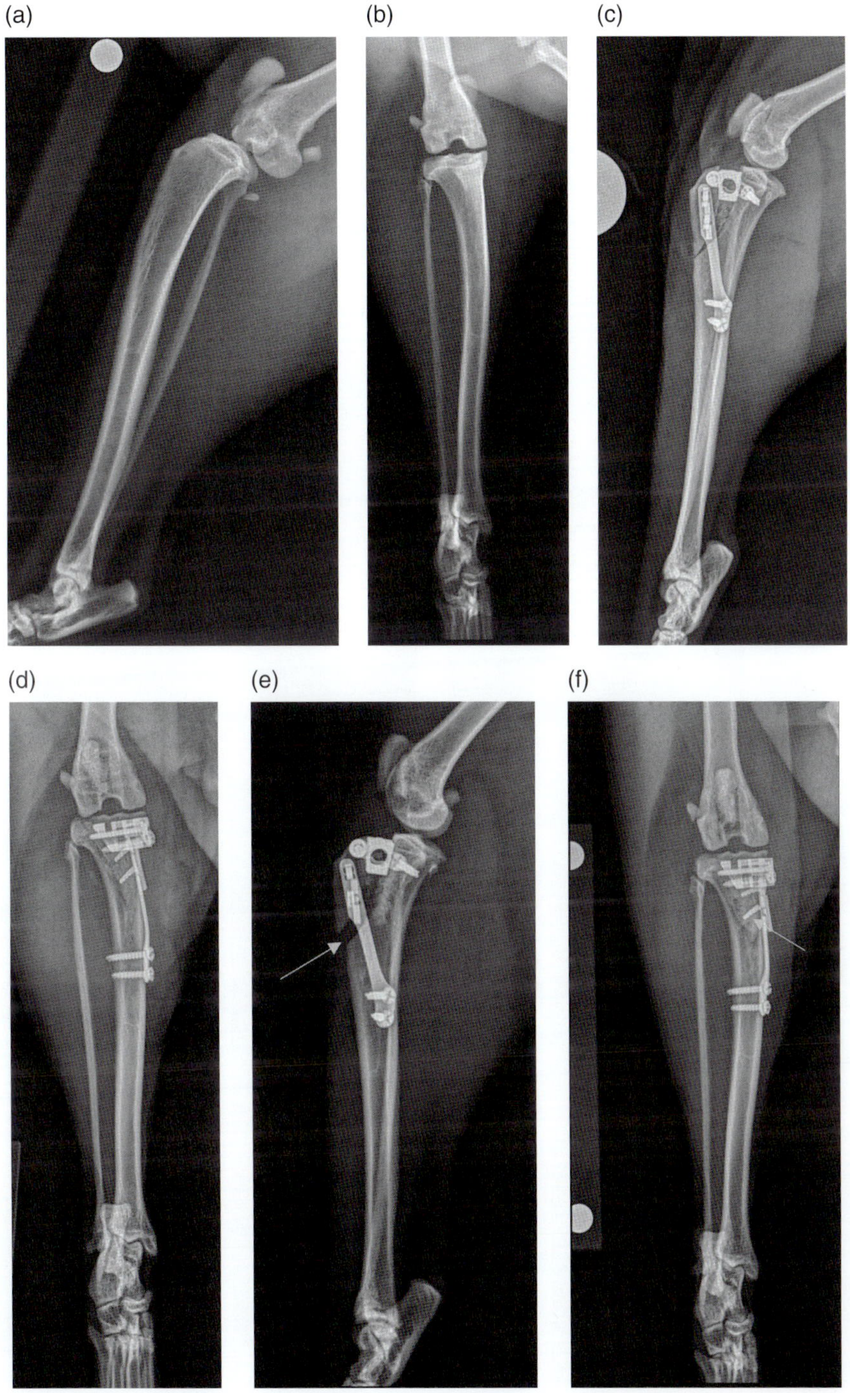

Figure 16.11 **(a)** Mediolateral and **(b)** craniocaudal preoperative views of a cat with concurrent CCL rupture and medial patella luxation. **(c)** Mediolateral and **(d)** craniocaudal immediate postoperative views following tibial tuberosity advancement (TTA). The implants used for this case were a Kyon two-fork plate and 6 mm cage. All screws were 2.4 mm except the one in the cranial ear of the cage which was a 2 mm screw with a washer. The cat had concurrent medial patella luxation treated with block recession and partial parasagittal patellectomy and lateral fascial imbrication. **(e)** Mediolateral and **(f)** craniocaudal radiographs taken 8 weeks postoperatively. The owners let the cat out of the cage 3 weeks postoperatively and then found him on the kitchen surface which he had jumped on to. He suffered a temporary mild deterioration in lameness for a few days. At recheck 8 weeks post-op, the distal fork had fractured (arrow) with loss of reduction of the tibial tuberosity distally (arrow). The stifle was still stable in cranial tibial thrust, the tibial tuberosity was palpably stable and the cat was not lame so no revision surgery was performed. Source: All images © Karen Perry.

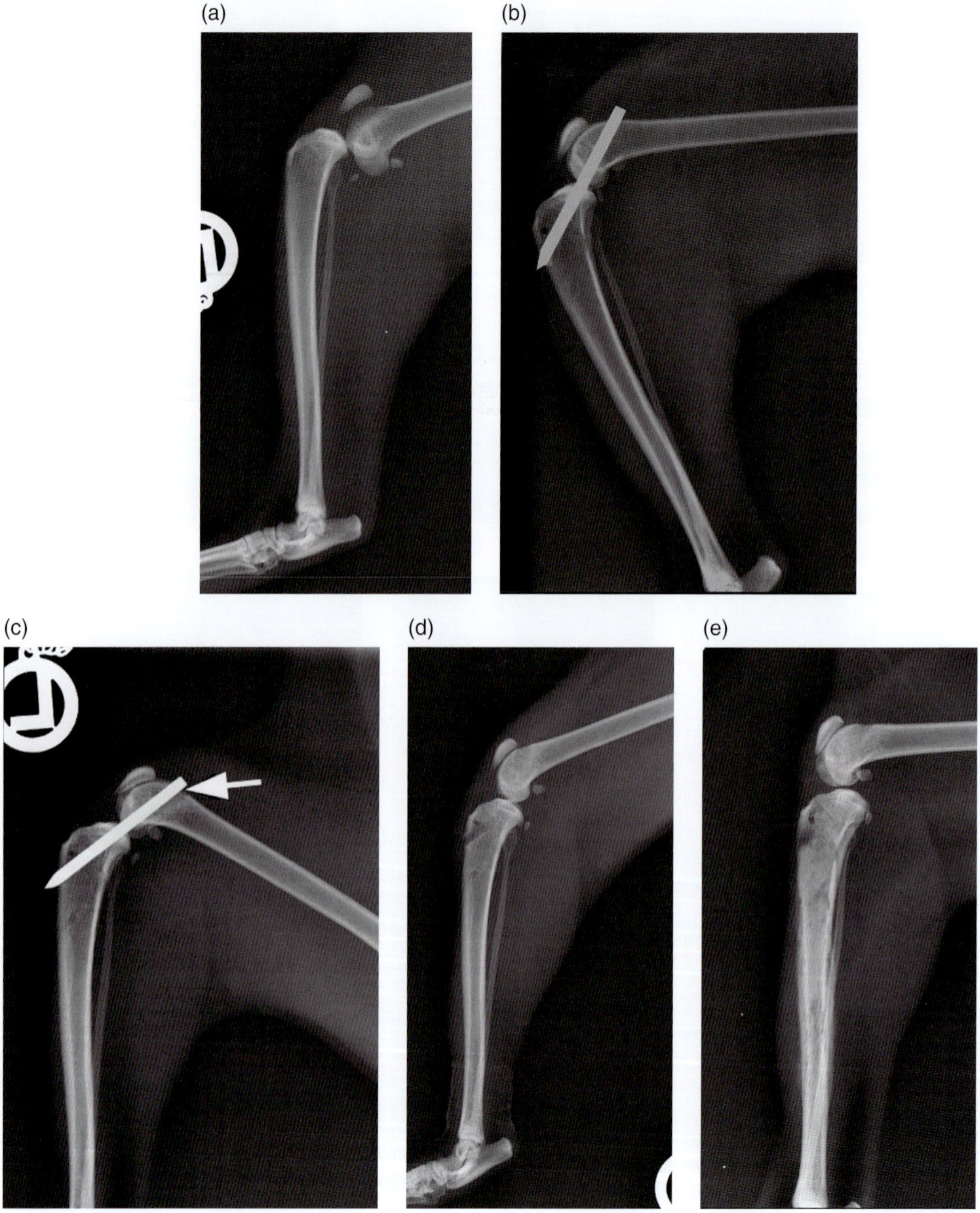

Figure 16.12 Osteomyelitis after transarticular pin placement. (a) A mediolateral radiograph of a cat that suffered a left multiligamentous stifle injury. (b) A single large transarticular pin was placed across this feline stifle without further reconstruction of the collateral ligaments. A hole is visible in the tibial tuberosity indicating the placement of an extracapsular suture for cranial cruciate ligament reconstruction. (c) Four-week postoperative radiograph reveals good implant position with subtle signs of pin loosening (arrow). (d) The surgery was relatively successful in maintaining reduction of the joint shown immediately post pin removal, although there is mild caudal displacement of the tibia. (e) The cat developed tibial osteomyelitis post implant removal and a more marked caudal subluxation of the stifle is evident. There is irregular bone architecture in the tibia with areas of increased and decreased bone density – changes compatible with osteomyelitis. The cat was treated with third-generation cephalosporins for 3 weeks and on clinical follow-up had a stable stifle in slight caudal drawer with reduced ROM. Source: All images © Anicura, TK Hollabrunn.

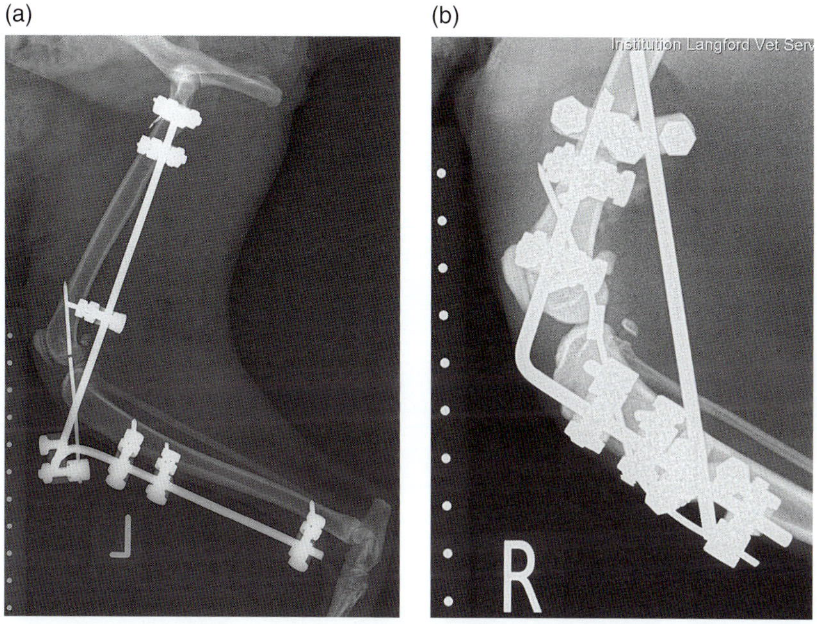

Figure 16.13 **(a)** A transarticular external skeletal fixator (TESF) placed to augment the repair for a multiligamentous injured stifle. The TESF extends from proximal femur to distal tibia which reduces the stress at the pin bone interface for the most proximal and distal pins and reduces the chance of fracture. A temporary transarticular pin was used to help maintain reduction of the joint while placing prosthetic ligaments; this was left in place but was found to have broken at the 6-week postoperative recheck. It is not recommended that these small temporary pins are left in place. **(b)** Triangulation of the TESF frame can add additional strength to the frame with addition of a bar extending from proximal to distal. Source: (a) © Sorrel J. Langley-Hobbs.

cartilage, especially if left in place for more than 4 weeks. The amount of time it is left in place is dependent on the severity of the original injury and is usually in the range of 3–6 weeks. Cats with severe instability or chronic problems prior to surgery may benefit from the longer period of temporary immobilization. Cartilage damage, stiffness, intraarticular adhesions, periarticular contractures, and osteoarthritis are all expected side effects of a transarticular external fixator. Complications from the ESF transosseous pins are also common and can include premature implant loosening or iatrogenic fracture of the femur or tibia [28, 31].

To decrease the likelihood of complications from the TESF, attempts should be made to place the pins in a far-near-near-far configuration, with pins at the proximal and distal ends of the femur and tibia as close to the joint as possible (e.g., in the distal femur and proximal tibia). Placement of TESF pins too close to the stifle can result in high stress at the pin–bone interface and the risk of diaphyseal fracture (Figure 16.15). Construction of a TESF that extends from proximal to distal on the hindlimb avoids this complication (Figure 16.13).

In order to avoid the potentially serious problems associated with use of temporary immobilization (cast, TESF), alternative primary internal reinforcements for the ruptured ligaments are under investigation (Mini TightRope® used for repair of the cranial cruciate ligament and PushLock® anchors loaded with FiberWire® to reconstruct the medial collateral ligaments). The aim is that these new techniques should be strong enough to avoid the need for temporary immobilization and therefore reduce the complication rate.

If complications are seen in cats with multiligamentous injury, a suggestion to help with determining treatment is shown in Algorithm 16.6.

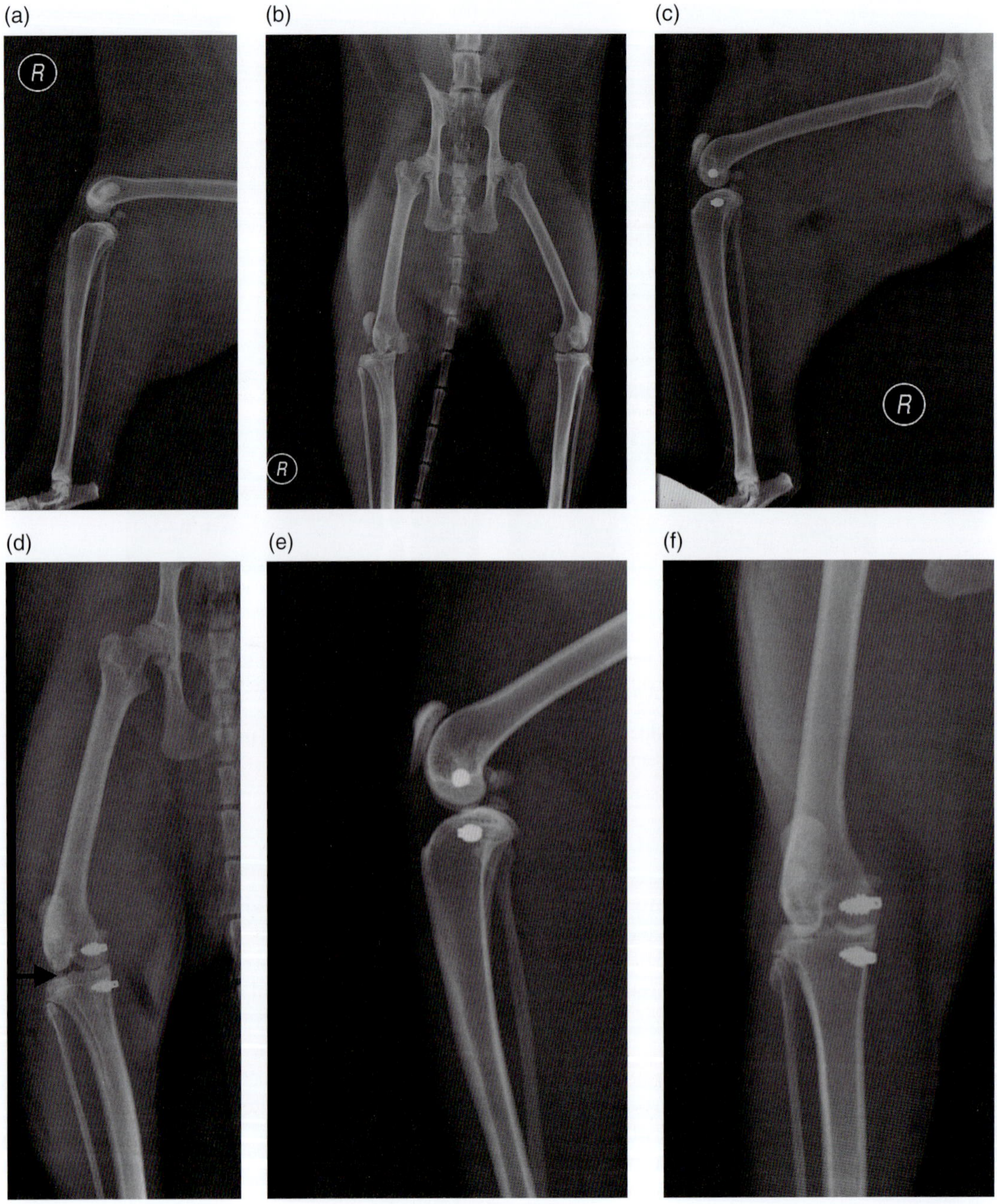

Figure 16.14 Subluxation following surgery for a multiligamentous injury in a cat. **(a)** Mediolateral and **(b)** craniocaudal radiographs of a cat that sustained a right stifle multiligamentous injury (ruptured cranial cruciate and medial collateral ligament) and concurrent patella luxation. **(c)** The stifle was stabilized with a lateral suture and a reconstruction of the medial collateral with bone anchors. No postoperative temporary immobilization device was used. Immediate postoperative radiographs show caudal subluxation and **(d)** a wide gap on the lateral aspect of the joint (arrow) suggestive of loss of lateral collateral ligament integrity. **(e,f)** Two weeks postoperatively the cat was still markedly lame and radiographs showed that there had been further subluxation of the joint and additional surgery was performed at this stage. A temporary transarticular pin was used to avoid overtensioning of the reconstructed ligaments. Caudal subluxation persists. Source: All images © Anicura, TK Hollabrunn.

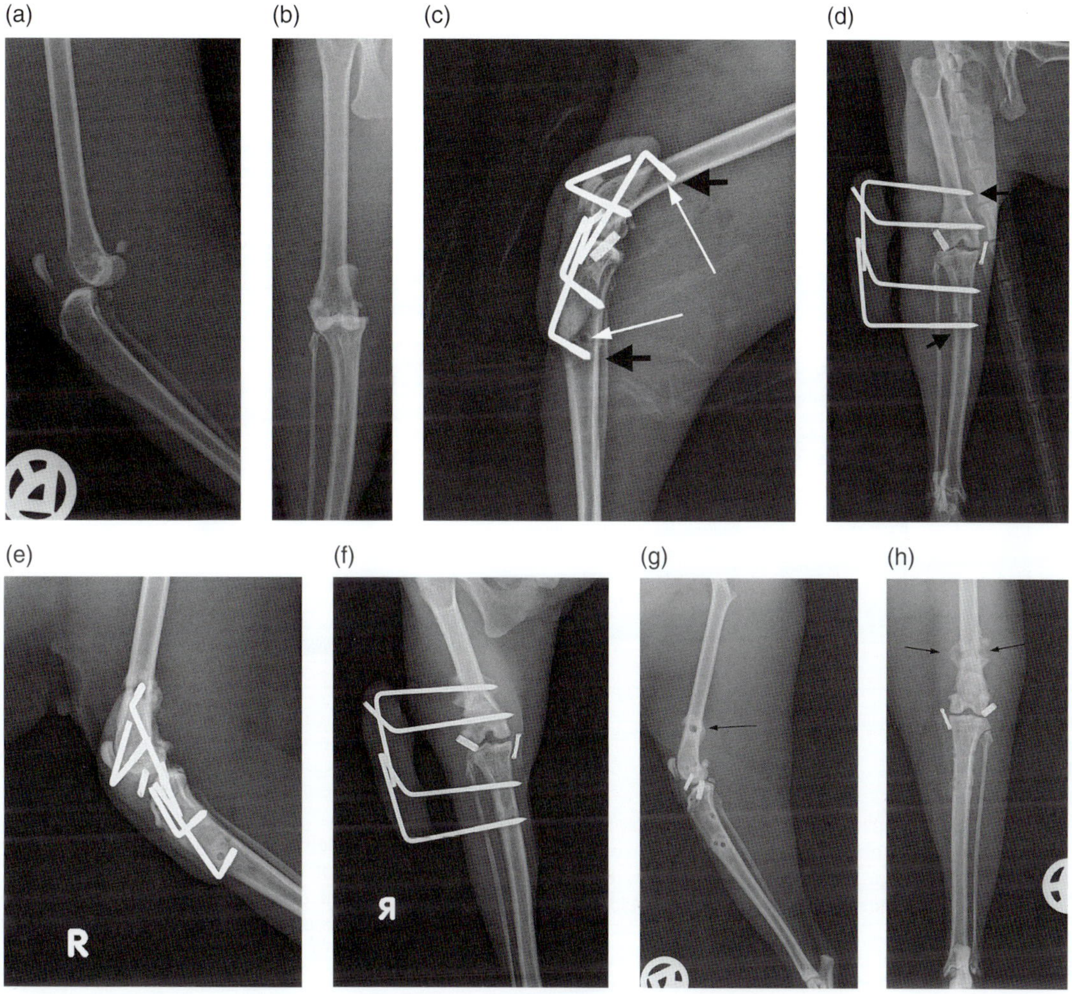

Figure 16.15 Pin tract infection and risk of fracture of the femur in a cat post TESF for a multiligamentous injured stifle. **(a)** Mediolateral and **(b)** caudocranial radiographs of a cat with multiligamentous injury of the stifle joint. **(c,d)** Postoperative views after reconstruction of the cranial and caudal cruciate ligaments with bilateral sutures and a short transarticular external skeletal fixator (TESF). This TESF has high pin bone stress forces at the proximal and distal pins in the femur and tibia (arrows). Additionally, there are some surgeon errors with the transosseous ESF pins missing the predrilled pin holes, resulting in empty holes in the bones that will increase stress risers further (white arrows). **(e,f)** Four weeks postoperative there is periosteal reaction around the proximal pin. **(g,h)** Following pin removal, the periosteal reaction around the most proximal pin hole in the femur is clearly obvious and there is risk of bone fracture at this site (arrows). Source: All images © Diagnostic Imaging, Vetmeduni Vienna.

Algorithm 16.6 Complications following surgery for multiligamentous stifle injury in the cat.

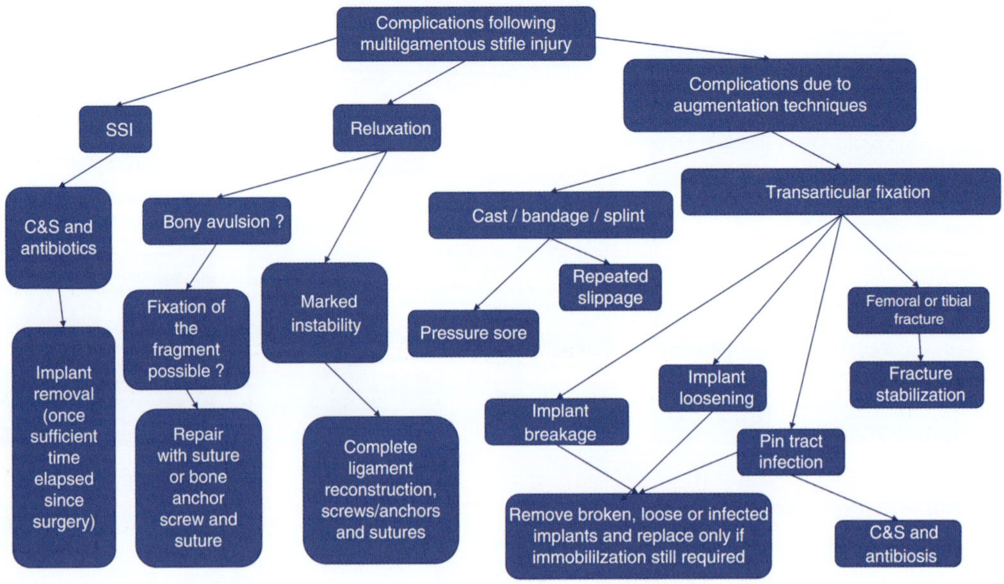

References

1. Arruda, A.F., Muzzi, L.A., Lacreta Jr, A.C. et al. (2018). Radiographic assessment of the proximal tibial angles in dogs and cats with and without cranial cruciate ligament rupture. *Pesqui. Vet. Bras.* 38 (6): 1190–1195.
2. Boge, G.S., Engdahl, K., Moldal, E.R., and Bergström, A. (2020). Cranial cruciate ligament disease in cats: an epidemiological retrospective study of 50 cats (2011–2016). *J. Feline Med. Surg.* 22 (4): 277–284.
3. Harasen, G.L. (2005). Feline cranial cruciate rupture. *Vet. Comp. Orthop. Traumatol.* 18 (04): 254–257.
4. Voss, K., Langley-Hobbs, S.J., and Montavon, P.M. (2009). Stifle joint. In: *Feline Orthopaedic Surgery and Musculoskeletal Disease* (eds. P.M. Montavon, K. Voss and S.J. Langley-Hobbs), 75–90. Edinburgh: Elsevier.
5. Herzog, W., Adams, M.E., Matyas, J.R. et al. (1993). Hindlimb loading, morphology and biochemistry of articular cartilage in the ACL-deficient cat knee. *Osteoarthritis Cartilage* 1: 243–251.
6. Ruthrauff, C.M., Glerum, L.E., and Gottfried, S.D. (2011). Incidence of meniscal injury in cats with cranial cruciate ligament ruptures. *Can. Vet. J.* 52: 1106–1110, 1110.
7. Mindner, J.K., Bielecki, M.J., Scharvogel, S., and Meiler, D. (2016). Tibial plateau levelling osteotomy in eleven cats with cranial cruciate ligament rupture. *Vet. Comp. Orthop. Traumatol.* 29 (6): 528–535.
8. Bilmont, A., Retournard, M., Asimus, E. et al. (2018). Effect of tibial plateau levelling osteotomy on cranial tibial subluxation in the feline cranial cruciate deficient stifle joint: an ex vivo experimental study. *Vet. Comp. Orthop. Traumatol.* 31 (4): 273–278.
9. Perry, K. and Fitzpatrick, N. (2010). Tibial tuberosity advancement in two cats with cranial cruciate ligament deficiency. *Vet. Comp. Orthop. Traumatol.* 23 (3): 196–202.
10. Freire, M., Brown, J., Robertson, I.D. et al. (2010). Meniscal mineralization in domestic cats. *Vet. Surg.* 39: 545–552.
11. Voss, K., Karli, P., Montavon, P.M., and Geyer, H. (2017). Association of mineralisations in the stifle joint of domestic cats with degenerative joint disease and cranial cruciate ligament pathology. *J. Feline Med. Surg.* 19 (1): 27–35.
12. Leijon, A., Ley, C.J., and Corin, A. (2017). Cartilage lesions in feline stifle joints – associations with articular mineralizations and implications for osteoarthritis. *Res. Vet. Sci.* 114: 186–193.
13. Whiting, P.G. and Pool, R.R. (1985). Intrameniscal calcification and ossification in the stifle joints of three domestic cats. *J. Am. Anim. Hosp. Assoc.* 21: 579–584.

14. Walker, M., Phalan, D., Jensen, J. et al. (2002). Meniscal ossicles in large non-domestic cats. *Vet. Radiol. Ultrasound* 43: 249–254.
15. Lascelles, B.D., Dong, Y.H., Marcellin-Little, D.J. et al. (2012). Relationship of orthopedic examination, goniometric measurements, and radiographic signs of degenerative joint disease in cats. *BMC Vet. Res.* 8 (1): 10.
16. Reinke, J. and Mughannam, A. (1994). Meniscal calcification and ossification in six cats and two dogs. *J. Am. Anim. Hosp. Assoc.* 30: 145–152.
17. Mossmann, H., von Pfeil, D.J.F., Nicholson, M. et al. (2015). Accuracy of three pre- and intraoperative measurement techniques for osteotomy positioning in the tibial plateau levelling procedure. *Vet. Comp. Orthop. Traumatol.* 4: 250–255.
18. Schnabl, E., Reese, S., Lorinson, K., and Lorinson, D. (2009). Measurement of the tibial plateau angle in cats with and without cranial cruciate ligament rupture. *Vet. Comp. Orthop. Traumatol.* 22 (2): 83–86.
19. Scavelli, T.D. and Schrader, S.C. (1987). Nonsurgical management of rupture of the cranial cruciate ligament in 18 cats. *J. Am. Anim. Hosp. Assoc.* 23: 337–340.
20. De Sousa, R.J., Knudsen, C.S., Holmes, M.A. et al. (2014). Quasi-isometric points for the technique of lateral suture placement in the feline stifle joint. *Vet. Surg.* 43 (2): 120–126.
21. De Sousa, R., Sutcliffe, M., Rousset, N. et al. (2015). Treatment of cranial cruciate ligament rupture in the feline stifle: biomechanical comparison of a standard fabella-tibial suture and lateral sutures placed between quasi-isometric points. *Vet. Comp. Orthop. Traumatol.* 28 (06): 401–408.
22. Kneifel, W., Borak, D., Bockstahler, B., and Schnabl-Feichter, E. (2018). Use of a custom-made limb-press model to assess intra-and extracapsular techniques for treating cranial cruciate ligament rupture in cats. *J. Feline Med. Surg.* 20 (4): 271–279.
23. Allan, R.M. (2014). A modified Maquet technique for management of cranial cruciate avulsion in a cat. *J. Small Anim. Pract.* 55 (1): 52–56.
24. Hoots, E.A. and Petersen, S.W. (2005). Tibial plateau leveling osteotomy and cranial closing wedge ostectomy in a cat with cranial cruciate ligament rupture. *J. Am. Anim. Hosp. Assoc.* 41 (6): 395–399.
25. Retournard, M., Bilmont, A., Asimus, E. et al. (2016). Effect of tibial tuberosity advancement on cranial tibial subluxation in the feline cranial cruciate deficient stifle joint: an ex vivo experimental study. *Res. Vet. Sci.* 107: 240–245.
26. Schaible, M., Ben-Amotz, R., Caceres, A. et al. (2017). Combined tibial plateau levelling osteotomy and lateral fabellotibial suture for cranial cruciate ligament rupture with severe rotational instability in dogs [published correction appears in *J. Small Anim Pract.* 2017; 58(5):303]. *J. Small Anim. Pract.* 58 (4): 219–226.
27. Moratalla, F. and Serra, A. (2018). Simultaneous treatment of rupture of the anterior cruciate ligament and medial dislocation of the patella in the feline species. *Argos-Informativo Veterinario* 202: 68–71.
28. Bruce, W.J. (1999). Stifle joint luxation in the cat: treatment using transarticular external skeletal fixation. *J. Small Anim. Pract.* 40: 482–428.
29. Addison, E. and Conte, A. (2019). Management of severe stifle trauma. 1. Stifle luxation. *J. Feline Med. Surg.* 21: 419–428.
30. Keeley, B., Glyde, M., Guerin, S. et al. (2007). Stifle joint luxation in the dog and cat: the use of temporary intraoperative transarticular pinning to facilitate joint reconstruction. *Vet. Comp. Orthop. Traumatol.* 20: 198–203.
31. Knudsen, C.S., Arthurs ,G.I., Hayes, G.M., and Langley-Hobbs ,S.J. (2012). Long bone fracture as a complication following external skeletal fixation: 11 cases. *J. Small Anim. Pract.* 53 (12): 687–692.

17 Complications Associated with Arthroscopic Evaluation of the Stifle and Decision Making

Brian S. Beale, Stephen C. Jones, and Selena Tinga

17.1 Introduction

Arthroscopic evaluation and treatment of joint disorders has become the gold standard in universities and veterinary specialty hospitals for small animals [1]. Arthroscopy provides a view of the joint under high magnification and illumination. This enhanced view can affect the decision-making process, not only during surgery but also after. Of particular importance is determining the condition of the cartilage, the severity and type of synovitis, and the integrity of the medial meniscus. Arthroscopic imaging gives the surgeon critical information to decide on the most appropriate intra- and postoperative management for each patient to improve long-term outcome and reduce insidious progression of osteoarthritis. Arthroscopic techniques can be challenging and are associated with a variety of complications and problems.

Complications can be acute and obvious in the perioperative period or they may be insidious and take months or years to appear. Complications of arthroscopy are typically not severe but significant morbidity can occur with poor execution. Complications may be self-limiting or may require intervention and treatment. When performing arthroscopy, the surgeon and their team should consider important factors preoperatively, intraoperatively, and postoperatively to avoid or reduce the occurrence and impact of complications.

17.2 Preoperative Considerations and Complications

Important factors to consider prior to surgery include correct patient positioning, adequate limb preparation, limb stabilization, and access to the surgical field. Patient positioning is important for several reasons. Arthroscopic evaluation requires accurate portal placement and the ability to manipulate the limb to certain positions to enhance the view of intraarticular anatomical structures. Technicians and nurses often position, prepare, and drape the patient. The staff should be trained to ensure proper surgical preparation so that portal sites are accessible for the surgeon. A common complication is inadequate clipping or draping of the surgical area. This can lead to compromised positioning of the egress, scope, or instrument portals, which in turn compromises ability to adequately evaluate or treat the joint. The patient should be positioned with a hanging leg

Complications in Canine Cranial Cruciate Ligament Surgery, First Edition. Edited by Ron Ben-Amotz and David L. Dycus.

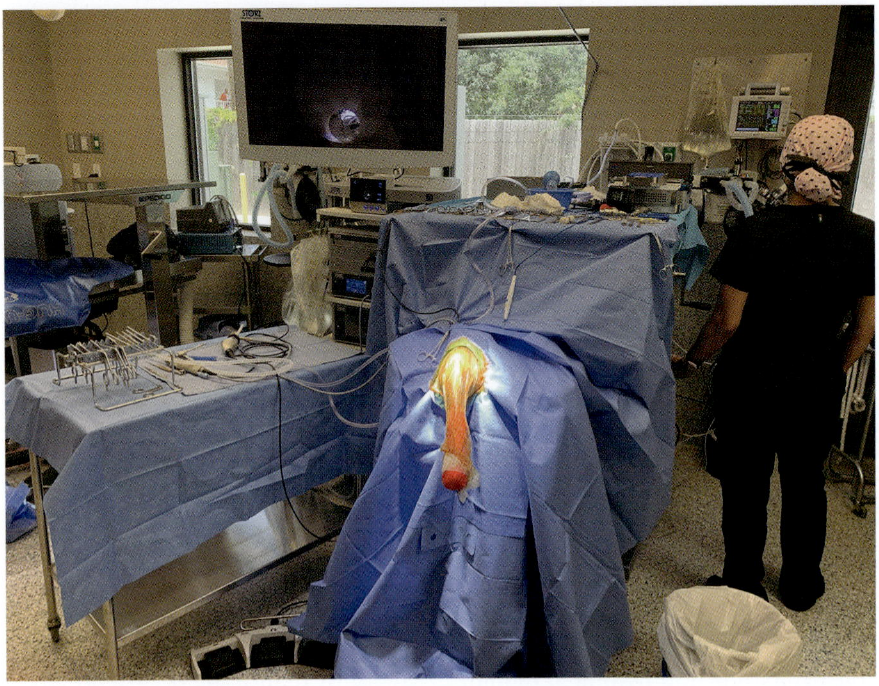

Figure 17.1 Recommended positioning for stifle arthroscopy with the patient in dorsal recumbency with the leg hanging off the back of the table.

preparation so that the entire limb is accessible in an aseptic field (Figure 17.1).

A routine aseptic surgical prep is recommended followed by a final application of iodine povacrylex (3M™ DuraPrep™ Surgical Solution [iodine povacrylex, 0.7% available iodine] and isopropyl alcohol, 74% w/w).The final prep should be allowed to dry completely, a minimum of 3 minutes. The leg is toweled and draped in routine fashion. A final adhesive antimicrobial incise drape is applied to the surgical site (3M Ioban 2™ Incise Drape) (Figure 17.2). This type of drape has been shown to reduce surgical site infections by providing a fluid-resistant barrier, immobilizing bacteria, and providing continuous antimicrobial activity [2].

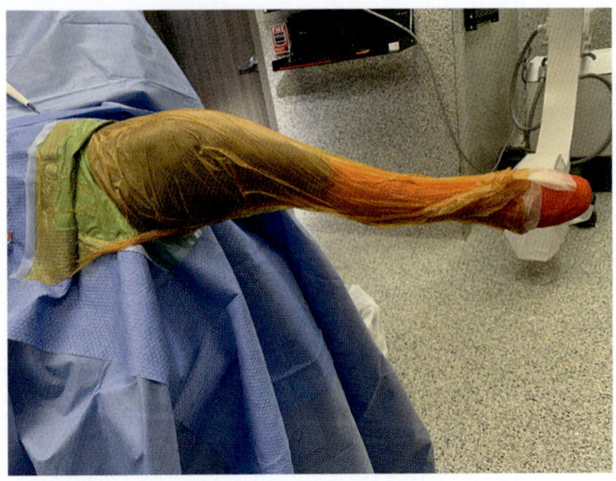

Figure 17.2 A final adhesive antimicrobial incise drape is applied to the surgical site, providing a waterproof barrier.

The surgeon should consider the likelihood of the need for stifle manipulation and movement throughout the procedure and this should be accounted for in limb preparation and draping. Optimal positioning of the patient for arthroscopy of the stifle has been previously described [3]. Some surgeons prefer a leg holding device [4], but most support the limb with sandbags or a positioning beanbag. The use of a holding device may allow surgeons to perform arthroscopy without an assistant and can be useful to position the leg at the surgeon's preference. The author does not routinely use a positioning device but prefers to have an assistant who can position the leg as needed to evaluate different areas of the joint. The assistant is particularly helpful to position the stifle appropriately to evaluate the menisci [3].

Surgical preparation of the patient may vary based on the experience and expertise of the surgeon. Novice arthroscopists may be more likely to convert an intended minimally invasive arthroscopic procedure into a traditional open surgical approach. The surgical nurses or assistants should consult with the lead surgeon prior to surgery to ensure adequate clipping of hair to accommodate the arthroscopic portals and the potential for a surgical incision.

17.3 Intraoperative Considerations and Complications

Complications during surgery include periarticular fluid extravasation, intraarticular hemorrhage, iatrogenic cartilage damage, inability to detect meniscal pathology, accidental trauma to joint structures, and instrument failure.

17.3.1 Extravasation of Fluid

A common intraoperative complication during arthroscopy is extravasation, which is the accumulation of arthroscopic fluid in the subcutaneous tissues (Figure 17.3). As fluid accumulates, edema and increased interstitial tissue pressure occur [5]. This increased pressure causes the joint capsule to collapse (Figure 17.4), compromising the ability to view the joint and complete the arthroscopic procedure. In addition, the tissue planes around the portals can shift in position and may close, making it difficult to insert instruments and manipulate the scope to obtain the desired arthroscopic view (Figure 17.5). Collapse of the joint capsule and/or loss of portal access are common causes for surgeons to convert to a miniarthrotomy or an open surgical approach to complete the procedure [6]. Extravasation is a common issue in stifle arthroscopy, particularly when the procedure is prolonged.

Extravasation occurs due to high intraarticular pressures and inability for fluids to exit adequately [5]. The surgeon should be cautious when performing arthroscopy to ensure adequate egress flow, especially when fluid inflow pressure is high. Egress can be provided by placement of an egress cannula [3], large gauge needle or creation of a large instrument portal. An egress cannula is the preferred method due to the multiple fenestrations in the cannula that help prevent obstruction (Figure 17.6). The surgeon needs to remember to reduce fluid inflow pressure after temporarily increasing it to distend the joint capsule or control hemorrhage. If extravasation occurs, the arthroscopic procedure can be continued in many patients if adequate egress flow can be reestablished. If significant extravasation is noted, it is important to make a conscious effort to maintain the scope in the joint while egress is reestablished. Loss of scope access in the face of extravasation and subsequent joint capsule collapse can make reentering the joint extremely difficult and often necessitates conversion to an arthrotomy.

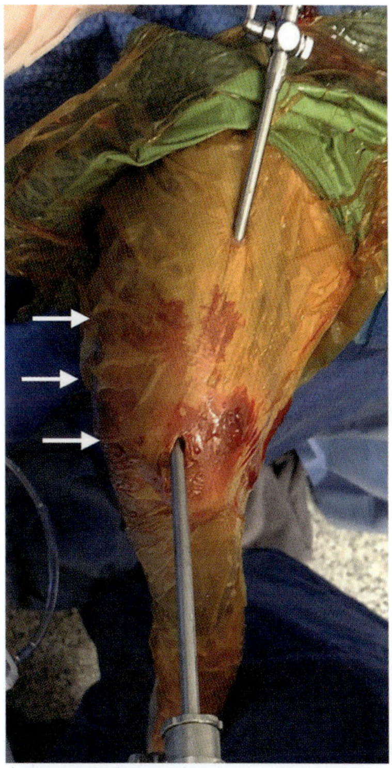

Figure 17.3 Extravasation is the accumulation of arthroscopic fluid in the lateral subcutaneous tissues adjacent to the scope portal (white arrows).

In addition to reestablishing fluid egress, massage of the leg in the area of extravasation can force fluid out of the portals, decreasing tissue swelling and pressure and, causing the joint capsule to collapse.

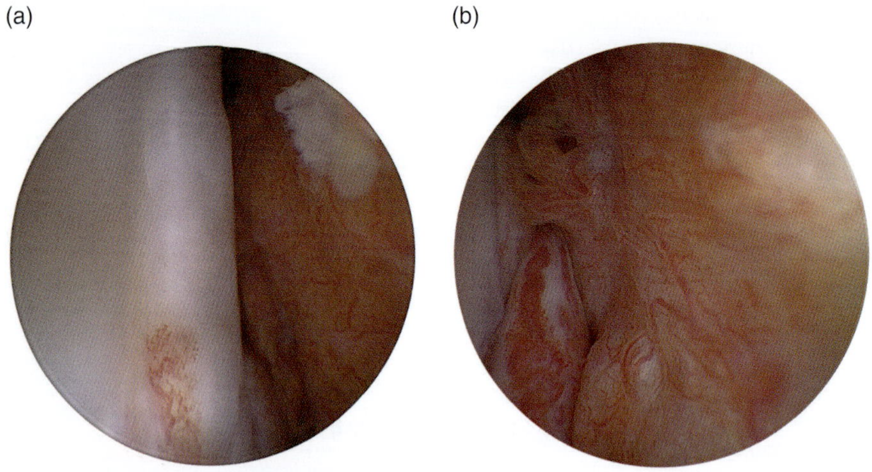

Figure 17.4 At the start of arthroscopy, the joint capsule is distended, enhancing the view of joint structures (a). Subcutaneous fluid extravastion leads to increased pressure, causing the joint capsule to collapse and compromising the ability to view the joint and complete the arthroscopic procedure (b).

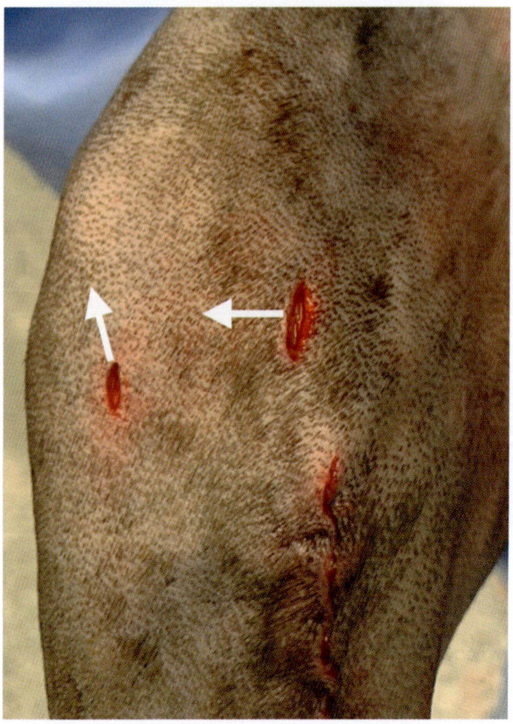

Figure 17.5 The scope and instrument portals can shift in position and may close, making it difficult to insert instruments and manipulate the scope to obtain the desired arthroscopic view.

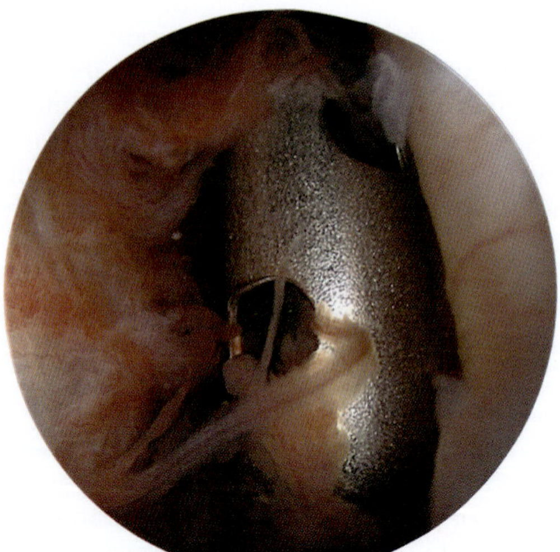

Figure 17.6 An egress cannula is the preferred method of egress due to the multiple fenestrations in the cannula that help prevent obstruction.

17.3.2 Intraarticular Hemorrhage

Intraoperative hemorrhage is a common problem that obscures the image, making diagnosis and treatment very difficult (Figure 17.7). A clear image is needed for accurate assessment of

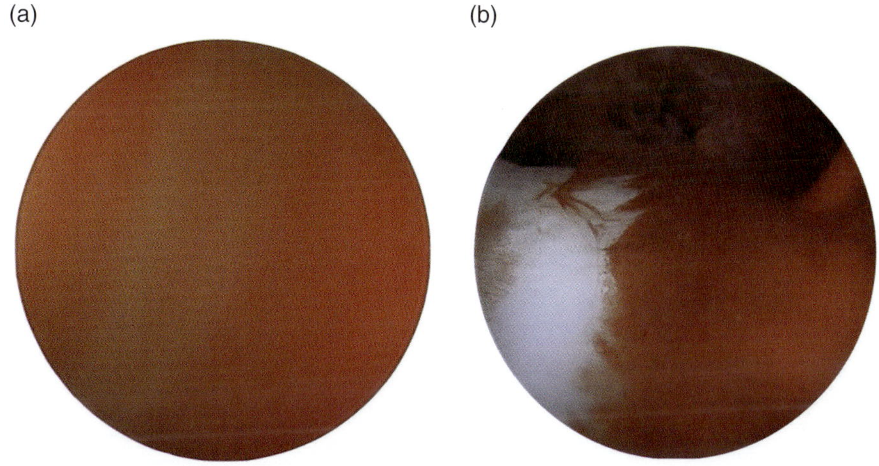

Figure 17.7 Intraoperative hemorrhage obscures the image, making diagnosis and treatment very difficult (a). Debridement of synovium should be limited to that required to obtain the necessary view to decrease the risk of hemorrhage. Bleeding can also result in thrombi that adhere to the joint structures, obscuring the surgeon's view (b). Fluid flow should be maintained in the joint to prevent thrombi formation.

intraarticular anatomy and precise treatment. Chronic injuries and conditions that have severe synovitis are more likely to have excessive intraarticular bleeding. The surgeon should be meticulous with portal placement and motorized shaving to lessen the chance of bleeding.

Excessive shaving disrupts more of the highly vascularized synovium, leading to bleeding. Shaving should be limited to that needed to provide an adequate view for diagnosis and treatment of the area of interest. One of the most frequent sources of hemorrhage in the stifle is a branch of the descending genicular artery that can be damaged when shaving or manipulating the infrapatellar fat pad. The surgeon is recommended to shave only that portion of the fat pad that obscures the field of interest. The inexperienced arthroscopist can spend much time and effort shaving and removing all visible fat pad. Not only does this increase surgery/anesthesia time and the potential for other complications, it also increases the risk of significant intraarticular hemorrhage.

Portal placement can also help in reducing the need for fat pad shaving. The more proximal the scope and instrument portals are placed, the less likely the fat pad will impede visualization and require debridement. In general, placement of these portals halfway between the patellar apex and the tibial tuberosity permits good visualization of the caudal poles of the menisci with minimal fat pad obstruction (Figure 17.8). The scope should be positioned to view the top of the intercondylar notch while the stifle is positioned in flexion. The shaver should be inserted just proximal to the fat pad into the roof of the intercondylar notch (Figure 17.9). Shaving of the fat pad from proximal to distal is performed until the cruciate ligaments and menisci are visible (Figure 17.10). Temporarily closing the egress cannula can improve visualization of the notch by increasing intraarticular pressure, thus compressing the fat pad. Fat pad shaving if performed as described above requires 3–5 minutes.

Some surgeons perform arthroscopy without shaving, but the authors would recommend shaving a small portion of the fat pad as described to enhance visualization, improve accuracy, and shorten arthroscopic time. Bleeding can be controlled using intraarticular cautery. Insulated cautery probes are available that function in a fluid environment to provide effective control of bleeding vessels. The surgeon can view the bleeding vessel arthroscopically while cauterizing the vessel under visualization (Figure 17.11). Caution most be exercised to prevent inadvertent thermal injury to the articular cartilage in proximity to the bleeding vessel. Hemorrhage can also be controlled by increasing intraarticular pressure by increasing the pressure of the fluid inflow and decreasing the egress flow. The increased

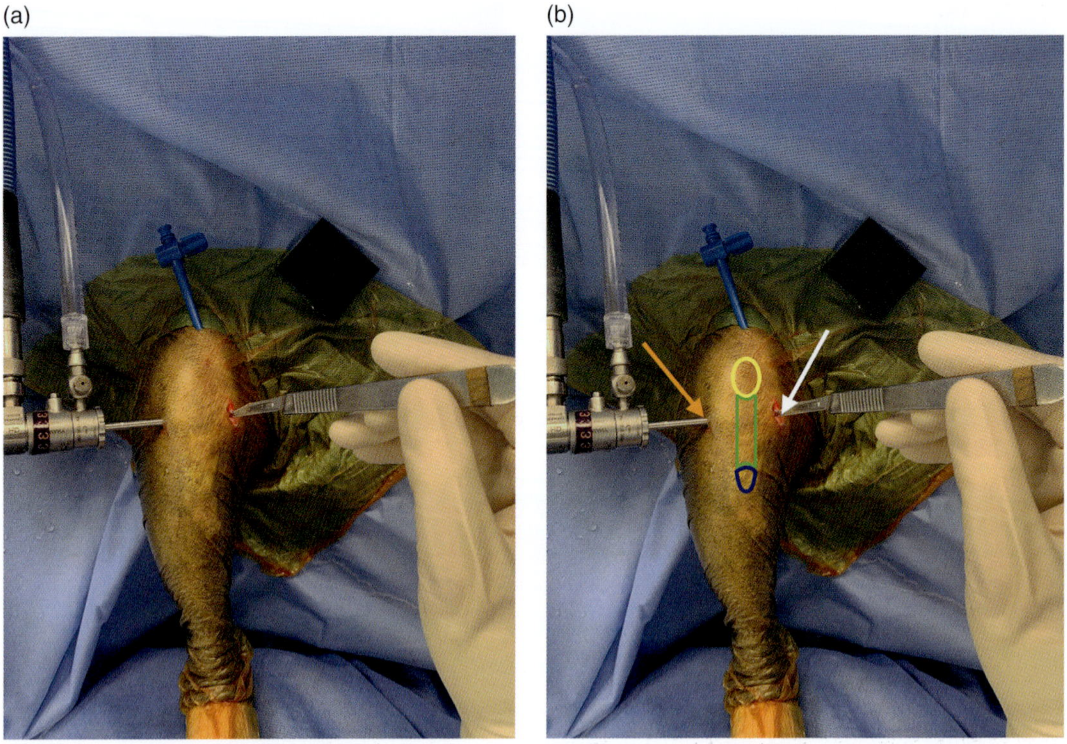

Figure 17.8 (a) Appropriate placement of the arthroscope, and egress cannula. A #11 blade is used for creation of the instrument portal. (b) The scope portal (orange arrow) is located lateral to the midpoint of the patellar tendon (green lines) which runs from the patella (yellow) to the tibial tuberosity (blue). The instrument portal (white arrow) is located medial to the patellar tendon at the same level as the scope portal.

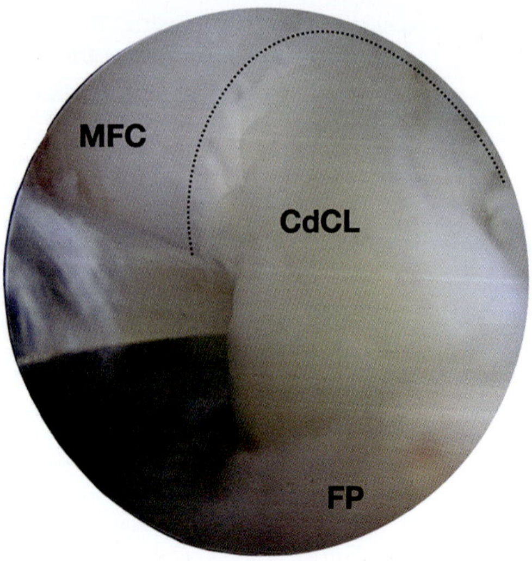

Figure 17.9 The scope should be positioned to view the top of the intercondylar notch while the stifle is positioned in flexion. The shaver should be inserted just proximal to the fat pad into the roof of the intercondylar notch. Minimal shaving is needed if the shaver is inserted in this position. MFC, medial femoral condyle; CdCL, caudal cruciate ligament; FP, fat pad

pressure will collapse small bleeding vessels, reducing hemorrhage.

The surgeon needs to be cautious of increasing intraarticular pressure too high or for too long because of the risk of fluid extravasation into the periarticular tissues. The inflow irrigation fluid pressure varies depending on the make of fluid pump, the elasticity of the joint capsule, and the extracapsular interstitial tissue pressure. The pump is often set to 30–35 mmHg when starting arthroscopy, but this setting may need to be adjusted higher to control bleeding and distend the joint capsule. It is not uncommon to raise the pressure up to 60 mmHg and occasionally a fluid pressure of over 100 mmHg may be used briefly to complete a procedure.

17.3.3 Iatrogenic Cartilage Damage

Another common intraoperative complication is iatrogenic cartilage damage [7]. Placement of the egress cannula is a common cause of this

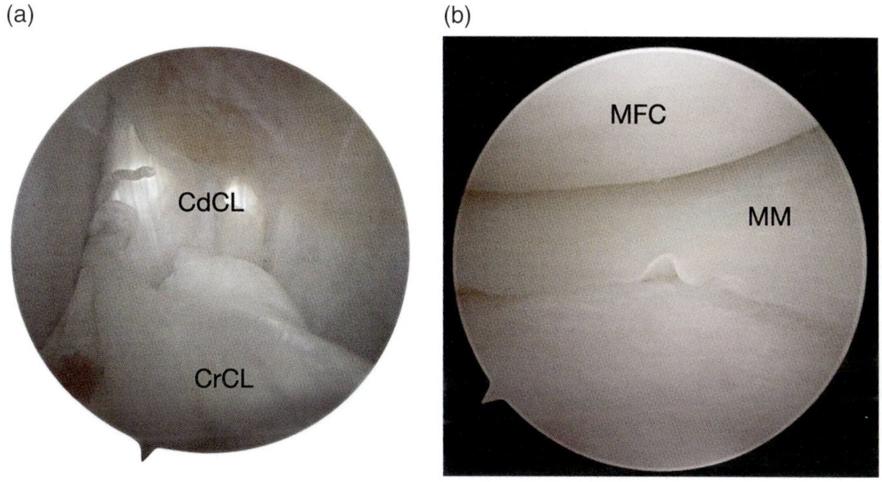

Figure 17.10 Shaving of the fat pad from proximal to distal is performed until the cruciate ligaments (a) and menisci (b) are visible. CrCL, cranial cruciate ligament; CdCL, caudal cruciate ligament; MFC, medial femoral condyle; MM, medial meniscus.

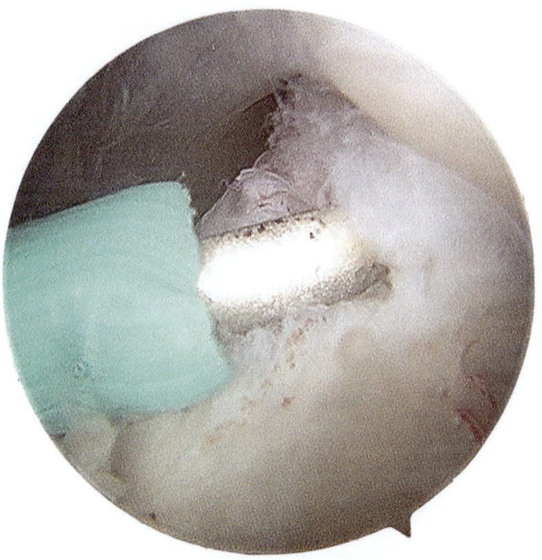

Figure 17.11 Cautery of bleeding vessels in the joint can be performed using a monopolar insulated electrode.

damage [8]. The egress cannula was first described to be placed using the scope portal under the patella in the trochlear notch due to ease of insertion [3]. The cannula should be inserted with the stifle positioned in relative extension to relax the tension on the patellar mechanism, thus creating more space to insert the obturator for the egress cannula (Figure 17.12). Direct placement into the medial compartment of the stifle in an effort to reduce the chance of iatrogenic cartilage damage has also been described but may be technically more challenging [8]. Flexible egress cannulas can also be used to reduce iatrogenic cartilage abrasion (Figure 17.13).

The surgeon should be careful to maintain good control of the arthroscope and instruments to prevent traumatic abrasion of cartilage surfaces and menisci (Figure 17.14). In addition, use of conical or blunt obturators (Figure 17.15) is recommended to avoid creating linear cartilage abrasions when inserting cannulas into the joint (Figure 17.16). Iatrogenic trauma is more common in patients with chronic joint disease due to the reduced ability to distend the fibrotic joint capsule and lever the joint space open. Forcing instruments between narrow joint spaces should be avoided. The joint space may be increased by having an assistant position the limb appropriately to distract the joint surfaces or by use of a joint distractor [3].

Iatrogenic cartilage damage is common in arthroscopy of all joints but is probably most common in the stifle [7]. Iatrogenic cartilage damage commonly occurs when trying to inspect the meniscus or when performing a partial meniscectomy due to the small space between the medial femoral condyle and the tibial plateau. The damage typically occurs when trying to force the scope cannula into a more caudal position in the joint. This action may cause the cannula to abrade the articular

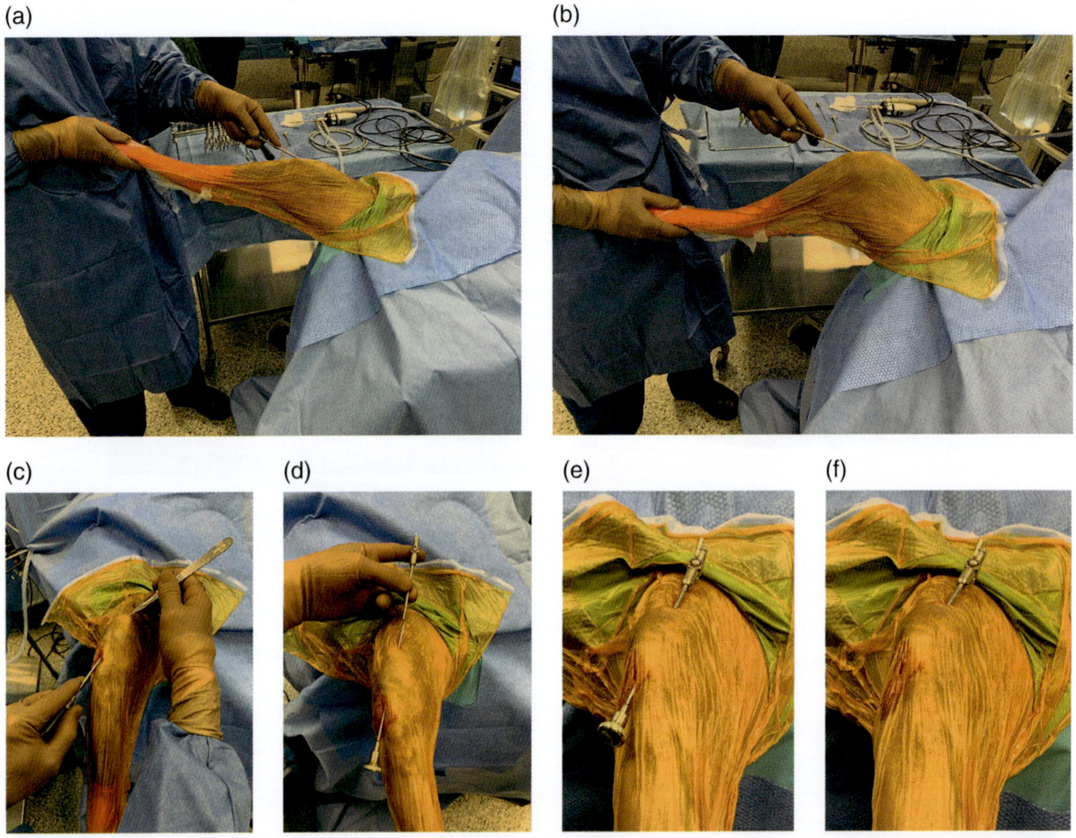

Figure 17.12 The egress cannula should be inserted with the stifle positioned in extension (a) to relax the tension on the patellar mechanism, thus creating more space to insert the obturator for the egress cannula. Placement of the cannula with the stifle held in flexion (b) increases the risk of iatrogenic damage to the articular cartilage. The egress cannula is inserted into the medial joint space over an obturator that is placed in the lateral scope portal and directed through the trochlear groove to exit at the medial aspect of the proximal joint pouch (c–f).

cartilage of the medial femoral condyle (Figure 17.17). The surgeon must caution the assistant to avoid flexing the stifle during this motion as this may increase the chance of impingement of the cannula on the femoral condyle. Another common cause of cartilage damage is instrument manipulation during partial meniscectomy. Damage to the articular cartilage of the femoral condyle or tibial plateau can occur when using graspers, punches, knives, and the shaver if not meticulous (Figure 17.18). On the other hand, proper technique can lead to a pristine partial meniscectomy with much less cartilage injury compared to open arthrotomy [3, 6, 9] (Figure 17.19).

The stifle can be positioned in slight flexion while externally rotating the foot and applying a valgus force to the stifle to increase this space [3]. A stifle distractor is commonly used to separate the joint surfaces of the stifle to allow better evaluation of the meniscus and perform partial meniscectomy if needed. There are two types of stifle distractors that can be used to increase joint space when viewing the joint with arthroscopy: hand-held intraarticular distractors and externally positioned self-retaining distractors (see Chapter 18). Hand-held distractors are placed through a second lateral instrument portal proximal to the scope portal in the intercondylar notch area to displace the caudal tibial plateau forward as an assistant levers on the handle (Figure 17.20). External self-retaining stifle distractors attach to pins inserted into the medial femoral condyle and medial tibial condyle and do not require an assistant (Figure 17.21).

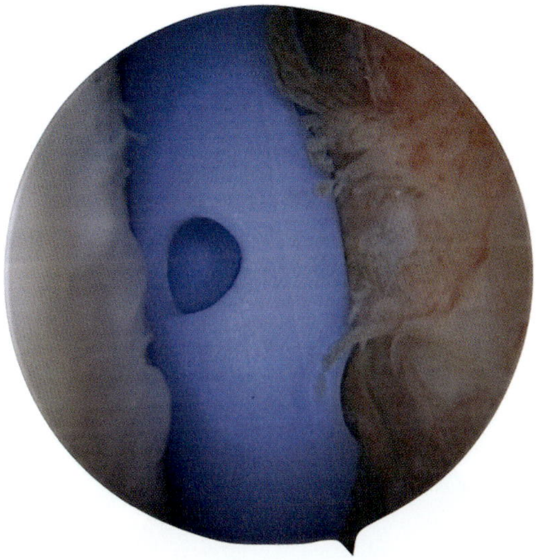

Figure 17.13 A flexible fenestrated egress cannula is preferred by some surgeons in an effort to decrease the risk of iatrogenic cartilage damage as stifle position changes during surgery.

17.3.4 Meniscal Identification

A common arthroscopic complication is the inability to identify meniscal tears. Meniscal tears are generally associated with an unstable stifle joint following partial or complete cranial cruciate ligament (CCL) injury. Arthroscopy has been found to be superior to arthrotomy for diagnosis of meniscal tears [10–12]. New stifle distractor devices and meniscal probes are important tools to assist accurate meniscal assessment [10, 11] (Figure 17.22). The prevalence of meniscal tears varies depends on the reference but they are a common comorbidity, necessitating careful meniscal examination at the time of surgery [9, 12].

Failure to detect a medial meniscal tear is generally due to incomplete inspection and probing of the caudal horn. There is a high probability that many meniscal tears diagnosed following tibial plateau leveling osteotomy (TPLO) surgery were actually present in a less severe form or in a nondisplaced position at the time of the original surgery. Likewise, failure to probe the remaining *in situ* caudal horn after removal of a bucket handle tear may result in failure to detect serial bucket handle tears of the medial meniscus (double bucket-handle tears)

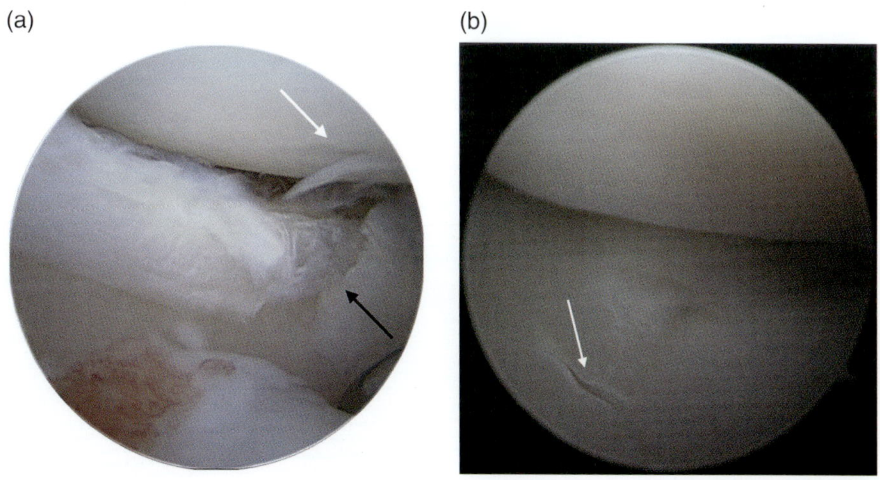

Figure 17.14 (a) Arthroscopic view of the caudal aspect of the medial stifle compartment. A full-thickness iatrogenic cartilage defect (white arrow) has been created in the medial femoral condyle during the process of transecting the caudal menisco-tibial ligament (black arrow) when performing a partial meniscectomy. (b) Arthroscopic view of the medial stifle compartment. An iatrogenic radial tear (white arrow) of the cranial pole of the medial meniscus occurred during creation of the arthroscope portal on the lateral aspect of the joint. The surgeon should make sure that the scalpel is not introduced too deeply during creation of the arthroscopic portals.

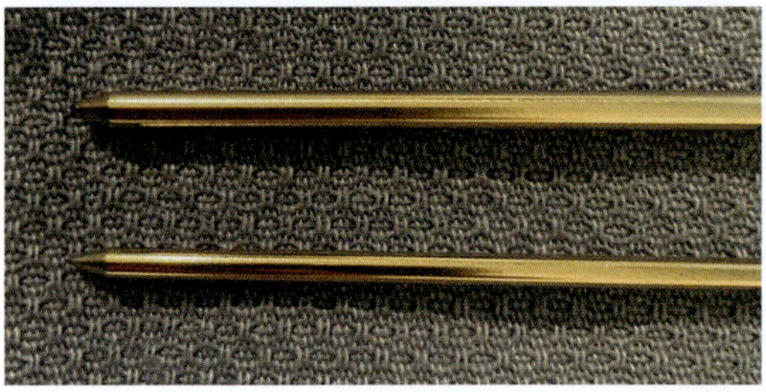

Figure 17.15 A blunt conical obturator is recommended when inserting scope, instruments, or egress cannulas to reduce the risk of iatrogenic cartilage damage. Source: Dr. David L. Dycus.

(Figure 17.23). The meniscus should also be carefully inspected for significant wear, even if no overt tear is present. The arthroscope provides magnification of the meniscus allowing the surgeon to assess meniscal integrity and the possibility of an impending tear. Significant weakening of the meniscus may affect decision making, causing the surgeon to perform a partial meniscectomy or medial meniscal release.

17.3.5 Surgical Trauma

An uncommon but important intraoperative complication is accidental transection of the cranial horn/body of the meniscus (Figure 17.24) or the long digital extensor (LDE) tendon when making a stab incision during creation of the

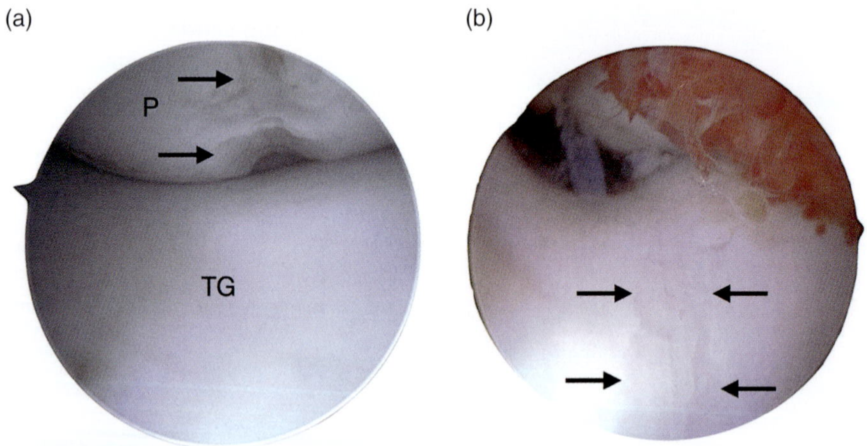

Figure 17.16 Iatrogenic damage to the articular cartilage of the patella (a) and trochlear groove (b) can occur with traumatic insertion of the egress cannula.

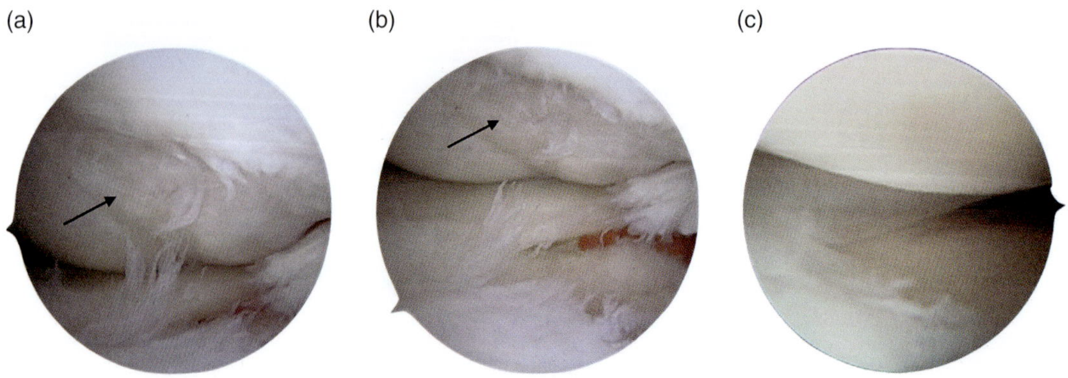

Figure 17.17 Iatrogenic cartilage damage occurred in these two patients (a,b) when positioning the scope cannula too close to the medial femoral condyle. Slight flexion of the stifle led to abrasion of the articular cartilage of the medial femoral condyle. Proper positioning of the scope cannula avoids this damage (c).

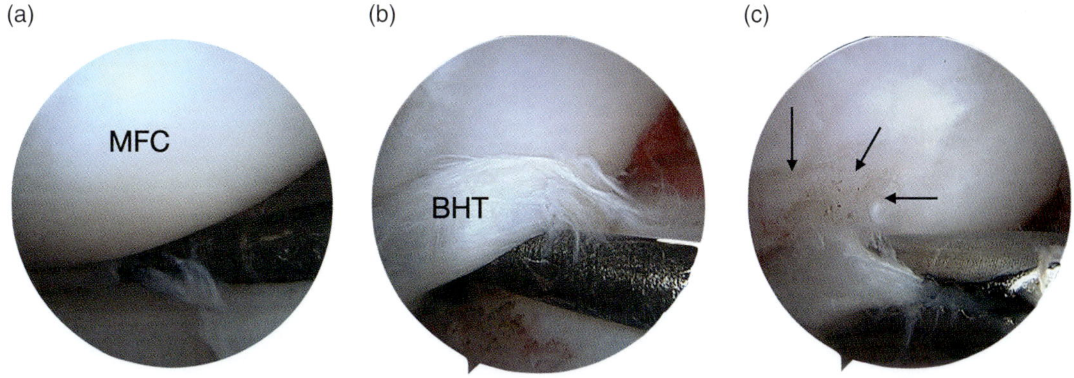

Figure 17.18 Cartilage damage can occur due to instrument manipulation during partial meniscectomy. The medial femoral condyle is seen to be normal (a) prior to grasping the bucket handle tear with graspers (b) and cutting the axial and abaxial attachments. Damage to the medial femoral condyle cartilage (black arrows) occurred due to impingement by the grasper (c). MFC, medial femoral condyle; BHT, bucket handle tear.

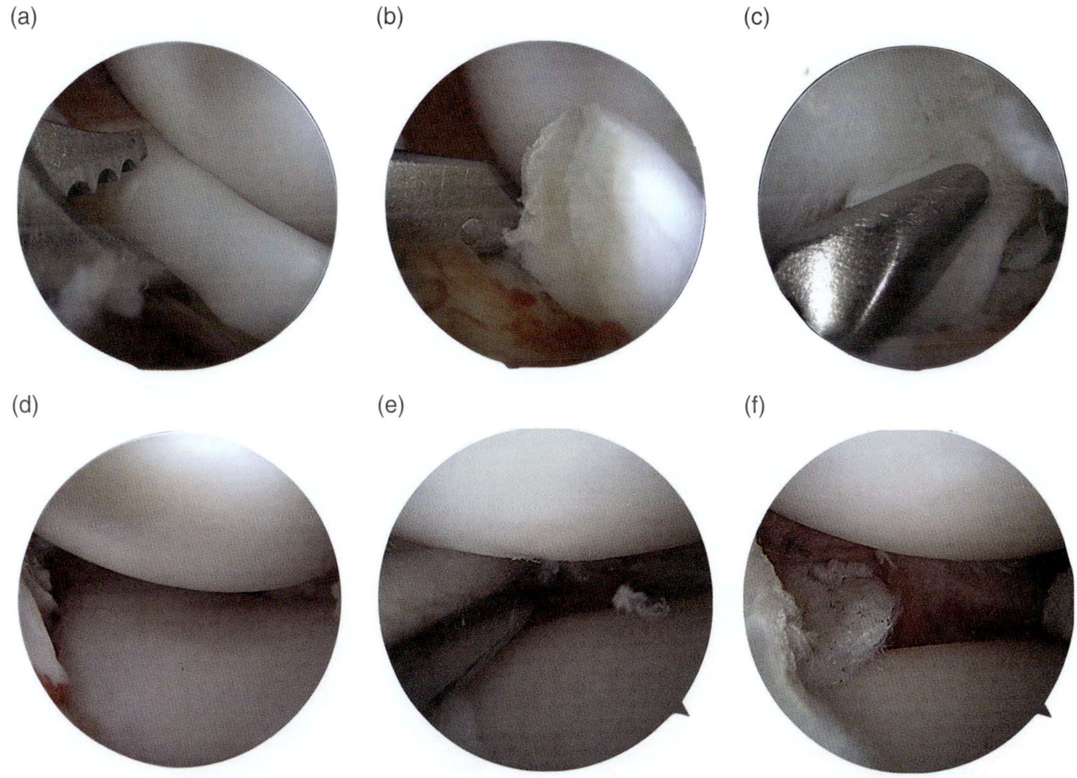

Figure 17.19 Meticulous handling of the arthroscopic instruments combined with appropriate positioning of the stifle to give adequate access to the medial compartment allows partial meniscectomy (a–c) without damage to the articular cartilage (d) in this patient. Use of the shaver is very helpful in removing residual torn fibers of the meniscus without cartilage damage because the cutting blade is shielded (e,f).

arthroscopic portal (Figure 17.25). Care should be taken to make the stab incision at the midpatellar region, immediately abaxial to the patellar ligament, to avoid this injury. The surgeon should also be careful to identify and protect the patellar ligament when making stab incisions for the arthroscope and instrument portal. The blade should be directed axially

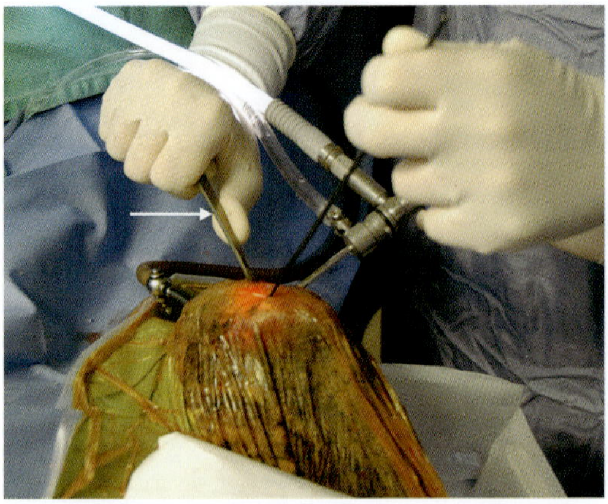

Figure 17.20 A second lateral instrument portal proximal to the scope portal was created to insert a hand-held stifle distractor into the joint. The tip of the distractor was inserted in the caudal aspect of the intercondylar notch to displace the caudal tibial plateau forward to give improved access to the caudal horn of the medial meniscus as an assistant levers on the handle.

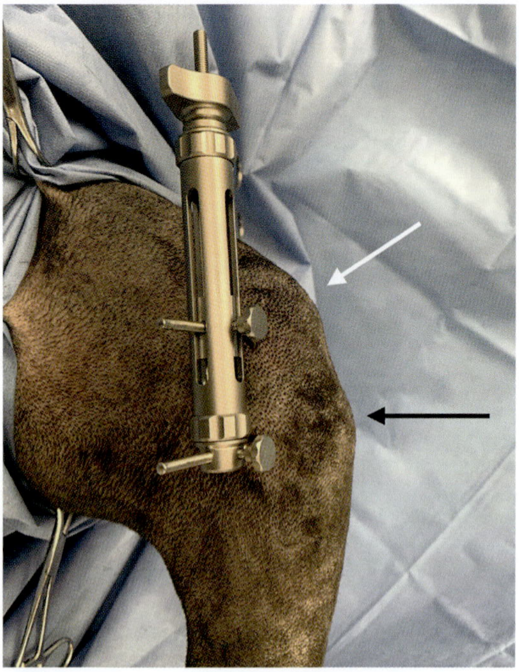

Figure 17.21 Leipzig stifle distractor. A negatively threaded pin (3 mm diameter) is percutaneously placed in the medial femoral condyle, perpendicular to the femoral long axis, halfway between the patellar apex (white arrow) and the medial fabella. A second similar pin is placed parallel to the first pin, at the most caudal aspect of the proximal tibia, at the level of the tibial tuberosity (black arrow). The distractor is placed over and secured to the pins before distraction is applied.

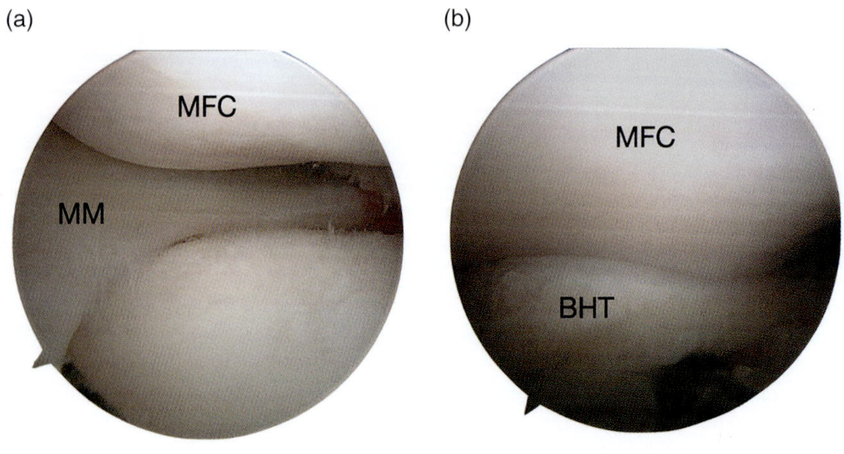

Figure 17.22 A common arthroscopic complication is the inability to identify meniscal tears. The meniscus should be carefully probed to detect nondisplaced tears of the caudal horn of the medial and lateral menisci. The medial meniscus in this patient initially appeared normal (a) but probing revealed a nondisplaced bucket handle tear (b).

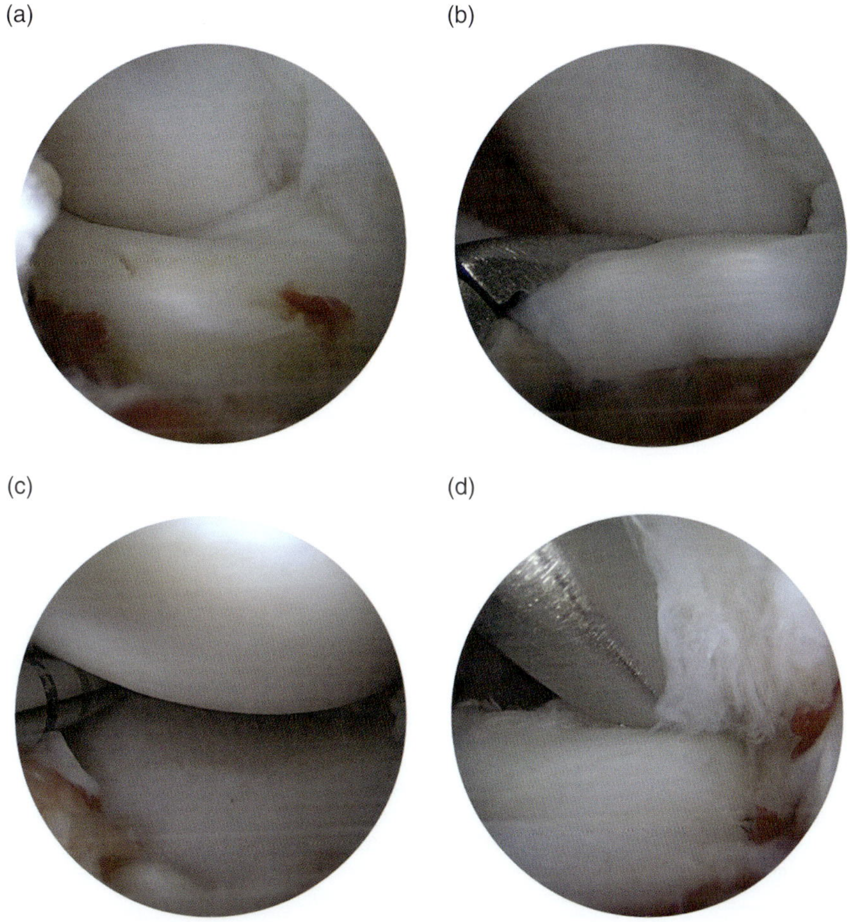

Figure 17.23 A partial meniscectomy was performed in this patient with a bucket handle tear of the medial meniscus (a,b). It is important to probe the caudal horn again after removal of a bucket handle tear to check for a second meniscal tear. A second bucket handle tear of the medial meniscus (double bucket handle tear) was found in this patient (c,d).

toward the top of the intercondylar notch and away from the femoral condyles and joint line to avoid iatrogenic injury to the LDE, menisci, or articular cartilage. Some surgeons will first make a shallow stab incision through the skin and subcutaneous tissues only. A conical obturator can then be used to enter the joint to complete the scope or instrument portal [3].

17.3.6 Instrument Failure

A less common complication is instrument failure during arthroscopic surgery. One common example is grasper failure when trying to remove large meniscal tears. The jaws of the grasper can break when applying too much pressure to a large piece of tissue when attempting to grasp and retract it from the joint (Figure 17.26). Occasionally, the jaw of the instrument can break off into the joint if grasped with too much force (Figure 17.27). This requires use of a second grasper to retrieve the intraarticular foreign body. Banana knives and scalpel blades can also break and dislodge within the joint if too much force is placed on them when performing a meniscectomy or meniscal release, for example.

If a broken instrument fragment cannot be removed arthroscopically, arthrotomy is recommended to remove the broken fragment. If the instrument fragment is inaccessible with arthrotomy and copious lavage, it may be necessary to leave the fragment behind and follow up regularly with patient examination and serial radiographic examination. If clinical signs of pain or lameness are seen, it may be necessary to attempt removal of the broken instrument fragment arthroscopically or via arthrotomy again.

17.4 Postoperative Considerations and Complications

Complications following surgery are generally mild and include postoperative swelling, infection, incisional issues, portal leakage, and

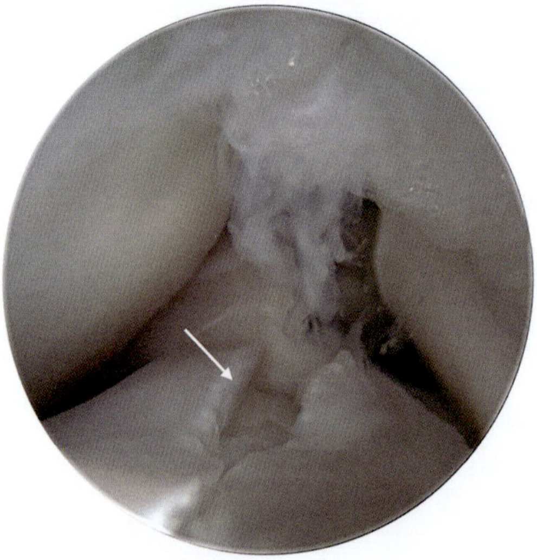

Figure 17.24 An uncommon but important intraoperative complication is accidental transection of the cranial horn/body of the meniscus (white arrow) during insertion of the scalpel to create the instrument portal.

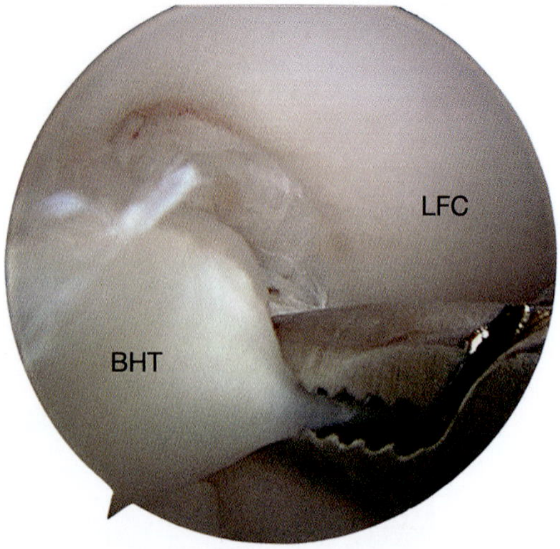

Figure 17.26 Care should be taken when using the grasper to remove a large meniscal fragment. The grasper can break when applying excessive pressure to a large piece of tissue or when twisting the instrument when retracting it from the joint.

(a)

(b)

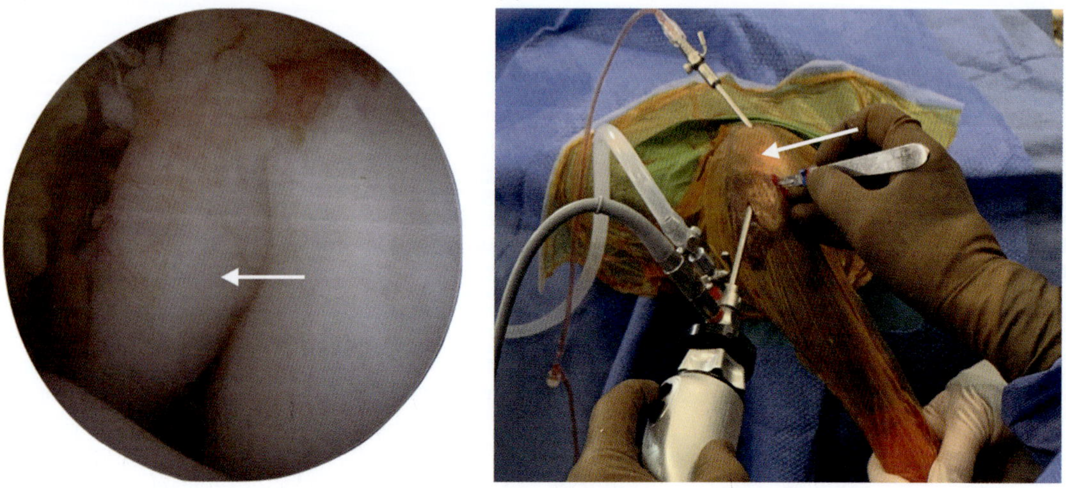

Figure 17.25 The long digital extensor tendon (white arrow) must be avoided when making a stab incision during creation of the arthroscopic portal (a). The scalpel blade should be inserted just lateral to the midportion of the patellar tendon and aimed toward the center of the intercondylar notch to avoid accidental transections of the tendon (b).

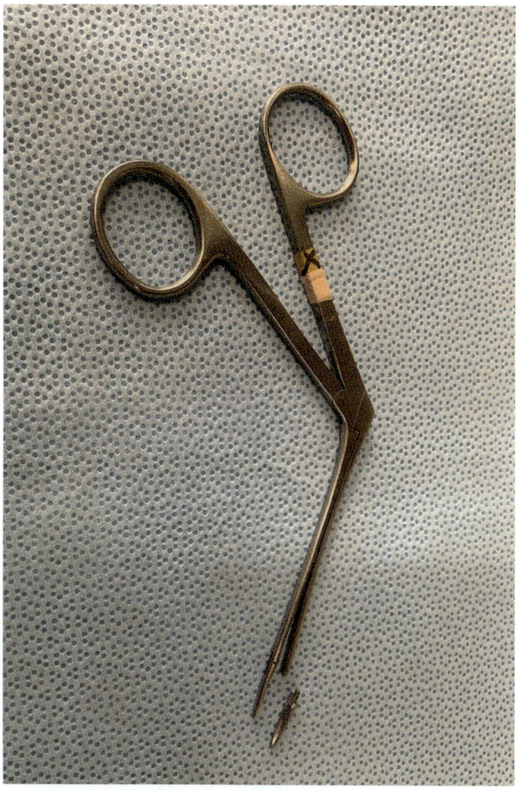

Figure 17.27 The jaw of this grasper broke during the arthroscopic procedure. The remnant of the grasper should be removed from the joint by arthroscopy or arthrotomy if possible.

bandage strike-through. Mild to moderate swelling can be controlled with cold therapy for 15–20 minutes every 4 hours. Activity should be limited, but short walks for 5–10 minutes every 4–6 hours are recommended to encourage lymphatic and venous drainage. If fluid extravasation occurs during the surgical procedure, massage can also be initiated. A soft padded bandage applied with mild pressure can also be used for 2–3 days to control swelling, but care must be taken to avoid bandage complications. If a padded bandage is used, strict activity restriction should be employed. Bandage wounds on the cranial aspect of the tarsus are particularly common. The majority of patients treated with arthroscopy do not require a soft padded bandage because of the minimally invasive nature of the surgery.

One of the hallmarks of arthroscopy is less morbidity compared to a traditional open surgical approach [13]. Infection can occur following arthroscopy, but the incidence appears to be less frequent compared to arthrotomy [3, 6, 13, 14]. A decreased infection rate could be due to the large amount of irrigation that occurs during arthroscopy or the decreased invasiveness of the procedure. Surgical incisions should be protected with a nonadherent adhesive bandage for the first 12–24 hours, to prevent environmental contamination. Although uncommon, portal leakage may be seen for 1–3 days after surgery. If present, portals should be covered with an absorbent adhesive bandage and changed as needed when strike-through occurs. This is critical to prevent ascending infection of the joint and surgical site.

17.5 Decision Making with Arthroscopy: Short-Term Implications

Arthroscopy gives the surgeon the necessary information to make important decisions on surgical treatment and postoperative management. Many veterinarians are aware of the reduced postoperative morbidity associated with arthroscopy, but the most important benefits are the illumination and magnification that provide enhanced examination of intraarticular structures in a fluid environment [3]. Enhanced visualization allows the surgeon to more accurately diagnose and precisely treat joint problems. Stifle arthroscopy has been shown to provide important information for diagnosis and treatment of partial CCL tears, meniscal tears, osteochondritis dissecans (OCD), and septic arthritis. The surgeon should be able to determine whether a tear is complete or partial. Partial CCL tears are often difficult to see without magnification [3] (Figure 17.28). Arthroscopy allows the surgeon to assess the integrity of the craniomedial and caudolateral bands of the CCL [3] (Figure 17.29). In addition, the surgeon can probe the remaining intact fibers of the CCL to determine if they are functional or nonfunctional [6] (Figure 17.30). If functional fibers persist many surgeons choose to perform a TPLO or CORA-based leveling osteotomy (CBLO) as these techniques have been shown to preserve remaining CCL fibers [9, 15, 16] (Figure 17.31). Preservation of functional fibers may preserve a degree of passive stifle stability and lessen the chance of future meniscal tears and osteoarthritis [15, 16].

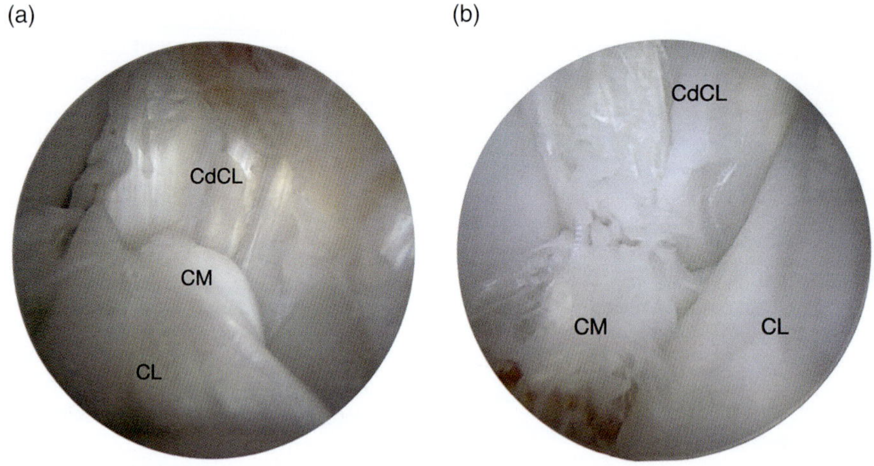

Figure 17.28 Diagnosis of early partial tears is greatly enhanced by the magnification provided by the arthroscope. These two patients with normal cranial drawer have early partial tears of the craniomedial band of the cranial cruciate ligament **(a,b)**. The caudolateral band is normal. CdCL, caudal cruciate ligament; CM, craniomedial band of the cranial cruciate ligament; CL, caudolateral band of the cranial cruciate ligament.

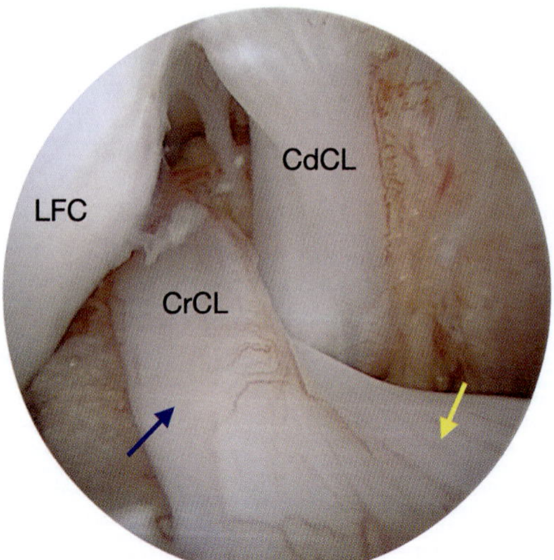

Figure 17.29 Arthroscopy allows the surgeon to assess the integrity of the craniomedial (yellow arrow) and caudolateral band (blue arrow) of the cranial cruciate ligament. CrCL, cranial cruciate ligament; CdCL, caudal cruciate ligament.

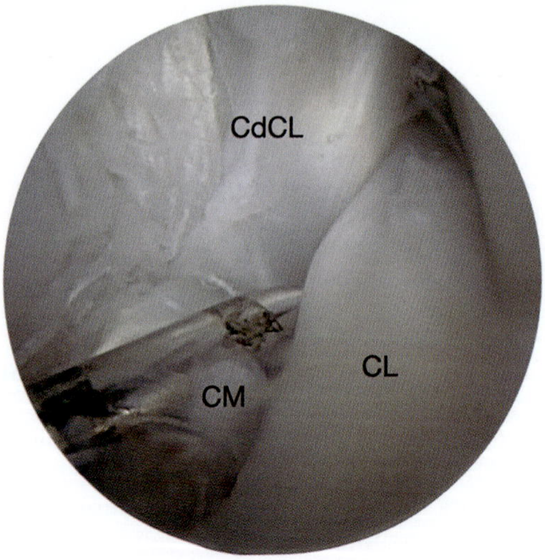

Figure 17.30 The remaining intact fibers of the CCL should be probed to determine if they are functional or nonfunctional. CdCL, caudal cruciate liagment; CM, craniomedial band of the cranial cruciate ligament; CL, caudolateral band of the cranial cruciate ligament.

17.6 Decision Making with Arthroscopy: Long-Term Implications

Arthroscopy provides an enhanced view of the condition of the articular cartilage and synovium compared to a traditional open approach. The grade of cartilage damage and severity of synovitis allow the surgeon to tailor long-term postoperative management to the individual patient rather than using the same treatment for every patient following surgery. In addition, the information gained using arthroscopy will help the surgeon better counsel the pet owner in regard to long-term prognosis and the importance of

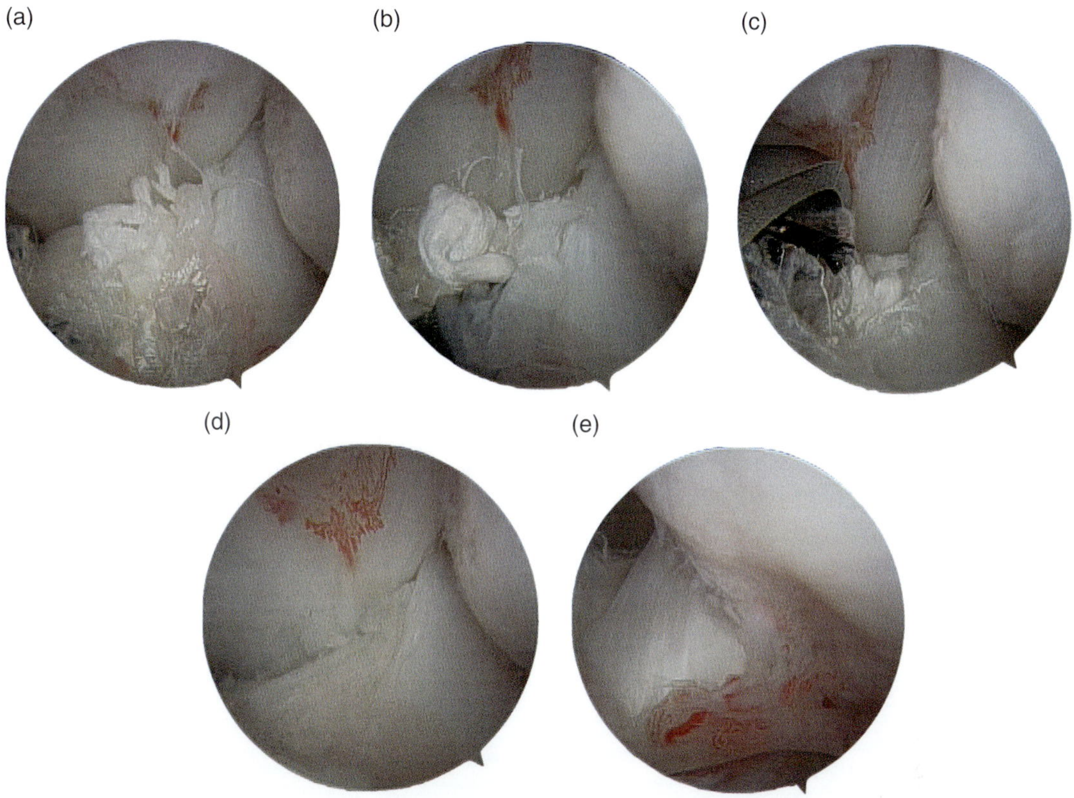

Figure 17.31 A partial tear of the craniomedial band of the cranial cruciate ligament is seen in this patient (a). Additional torn fibers are evident with probing (b). The torn fibers were debrided with a shaver (c), leaving the functional fibers of the CCL intact (d). A TPLO was performed. The remaining fibers of the CCL were observed to be intact and functional. (e) Two years later a second-look arthroscopic exam of the stifle was undertaken (at the time of a contralateral TPLO).

adhering to a long-term management plan. It does not make sense to manage a patient with mild acute synovitis and healthy cartilage in the same manner as a patient with severe cartilage wear and chronic severe synovitis (Figure 17.32).

Cartilage wear is best graded 0–5 using the Modified Mankin Scale [17]. In addition, it is helpful to assess if the synovitis is acute or chronic. Acute synovitis may have a better long-term outcome if properly managed because synovial changes may be reversible. On the other hand, chronic synovitis may have irreversible changes that can influence the surgeon's decision making on postoperative physical rehabilitation, medical treatment, and nutritional supplementation.

An example of how arthroscopy may influence decision making can be illustrated with treatment of CCL tear with TPLO. Chronic low-grade synovitis has been shown to occur commonly following previous TPLO surgery using second-look arthroscopy in almost all patients [9, 15] (Figure 17.33). Although the dog may clinically be functioning well, low-grade synovitis is present in most patients long term. The presence of significant synovitis and early cartilage wear may influence the surgeon to counsel the owner of the importance of suppressing background low-grade synovitis and providing nutritional factors to supplement cartilage metabolism. Chronic synovitis is thought to be a major factor in the insidious progression of osteoarthritis that has been identified in many papers assessing long-term outcome following CCL repair [9, 18]. Chronic inhibition of synovitis using

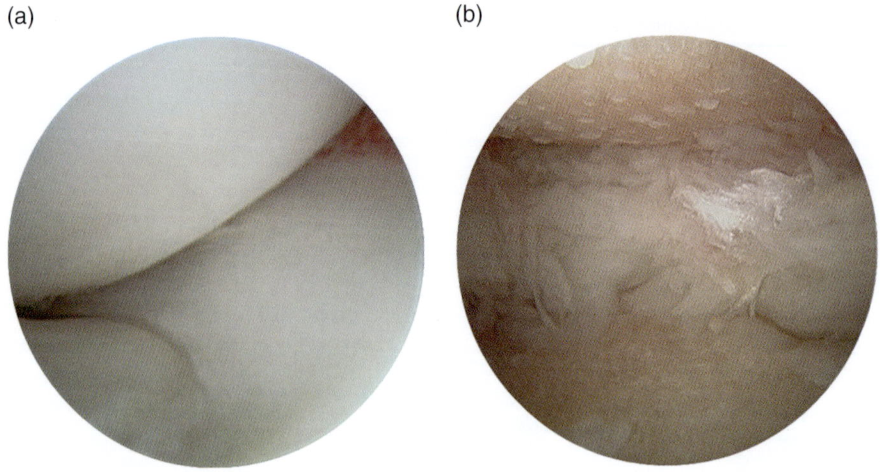

Figure 17.32 Arthroscopy provides an enhanced view of the condition of the articular cartilage and synovium compared to a traditional open approach. The grade of cartilage damage and severity of synovitis allow the surgeon to tailor long-term postoperative management to the individual patient rather than using the same treatment for every patient following surgery. Patients may have normal cartilage and minimal synovitis (a), while others may have severe cartilage erosion and chronic synovitis (b).

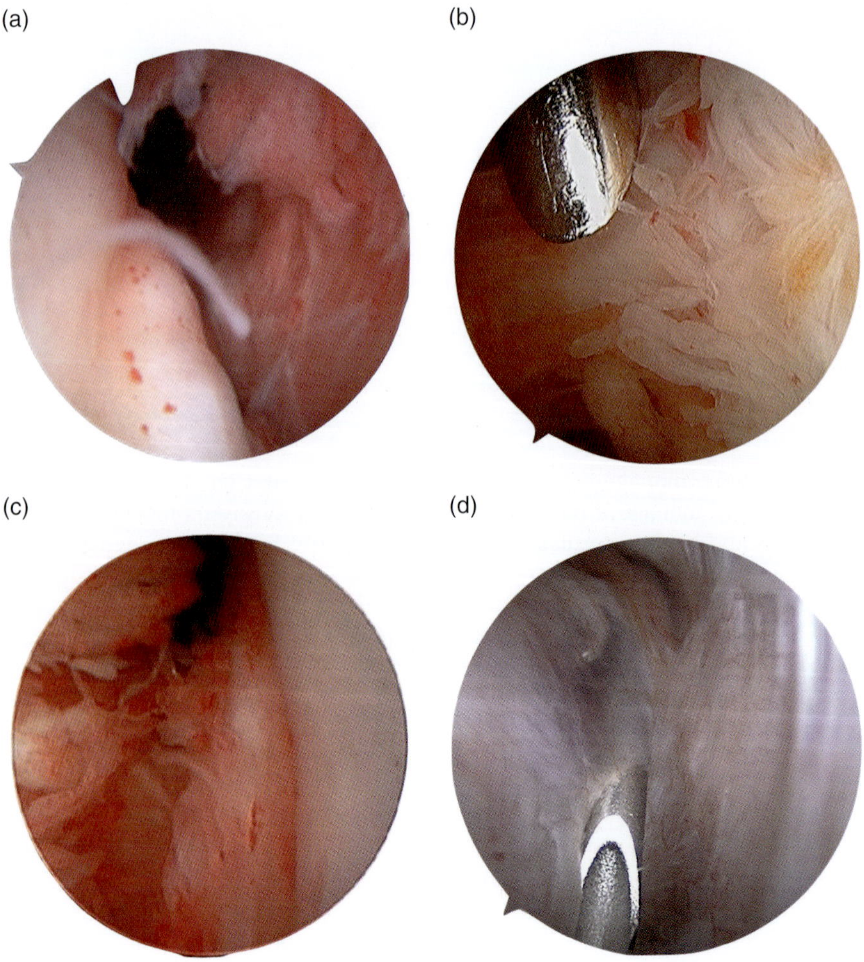

Figure 17.33 Chronic low-grade synovitis has been shown to occur commonly following previous TPLO surgery using second-look arthroscopy in most patients. Chronic synovitis is evident in these four patients as assessed by second-look arthroscopy 1–3 years following TPLO (a–c). Long-term management of synovitis may be prudent in order to inhibit the insidious progression of osteoarthritis. Normal synovium is pale pink and has a smooth surface (d).

evidence-based products may help reduce insidious osteoarthritis progression. Options for inhibiting long-term synovitis include nutritional supplements, injectable glycosaminoglycans, and oral antiinflammatory drugs. Selection of antiinflammatory products that have evidence-based outcome results and a high safety profile is recommended due to the need for long-term daily administration of the product to keep insidious inflammation under control [19, 20].

The goal of the surgeon should be to monitor published outcome data and carefully follow up on clinical patients to learn from their clinical experiences and make protocol changes to improve outcome and reduce complications [21].

References

1. Bottcher, P., Bruhschwein, A., Winkels, P. et al. (2010). Value of low-field magnetic resonance imaging in diagnosing meniscal tears in the canine stifle: a prospective study evaluating sensitivity and specificity in naturally occurring cranial cruciate ligament deficiency with arthroscopy as the gold standard. *Vet. Surg.* 39: 296–305.
2. de Lissovoy, G., Fraeman, K., Hutchins, V. et al. (2009). Surgical site infection: incidence and impact on hospital utilization and treatment costs. *Am. J. Infect. Control* 37: 387–397.
3. Whitney, W.O. (2003). Arthroscopically assisted surgery of the stifle joint. In: *Small Animal Arthroscopy* (eds. B. Beale, D. Hulse, K. Schulz and W. Whitney), 117–156. Philadelphia, PA: Elsevier Health Sciences.
4. Schulz, K., Holsworth, I.G., and Hornof, W.J. (2004). Self-retaining braces for canine arthroscopy. *Vet. Surg.* 33: 77–82.
5. Warnock, J.J., Nemanic, S., O'Donnell, M.D. et al. (2014). Comparison of 2 fluid ingress/egress systems for canine stifle arthroscopy using computed tomography. *Vet. Surg.* 43: 944–951.
6. Beale, B., Hulse, D.A., and Pozzi, A. (2018). Arthroscopy and arthrotomy of the stifle. In: *Advances in the Cranial Cruciate Ligament*, 2e (ed. P. Muir), 171–184. Hoboken NJ: Wiley Blackwell.
7. Rogatko, C.P., Warnock, J.J., Bobe, G., and Verpaalen, V.D. (2018). Comparison of iatrogenic articular cartilage injury in canine stifle arthroscopy versus medial parapatellar mini-arthrotomy in a cadaveric model. *Vet. Surg.* 47: O6–O14.
8. Cortés, I.I.I.I., Warnock, J.J., Ranganathan, B., and Bobe, G. (2019). Iatrogenic cartilage injury associated with the use of stainless-steel cannulas and silicone-guarded cannulas for canine stifle arthroscopy. *Vet. Surg.* 48: 1456–1465.
9. Beale, B. and Hulse, D.A. (2018). Arthroscopic follow-up after surgical stabilization of the stifle. In: *Advances in the Cranial Cruciate Ligament*, 2e (ed. P. Muir), 279–290. Hoboken, NJ: Wiley Blackell.
10. Pozzi, A., Hildreth, B.E., and Rajala-Schulz, P. (2008). Comparison of arthroscopy and arthrotomy for diagnosis of medial meniscal pathology: an ex vivo study. *Vet. Surg.* 37: 749–755.
11. Winkels, P., Pozzi, A., Cook, R. et al. (2016). Prospective evaluation of the Leipzig stifle distractor. *Vet. Surg.* 45: 631–635.
12. Fitzpatrick, N. and Solano, M.A. (2010). Predictive variables for complications after TPLO with stifle inspection by arthrotomy in 1000 consecutive dogs. *Vet. Surg.* 39: 460–474.
13. Hoezler, M.G., Millis, D.L., Francis, D.A. et al. (2004). Results of arthroscopic versus open arthrotomy for surgical. Management of cranial cruciate ligament deficiency in dogs. *Vet. Surg.* 33: 146–153.
14. Bohler, C., Dragana, M., Puchner, S. et al. (2016). Treatment of septic arthritis of the knee: a comparison between arthroscopy and arthrotomy. *Knee Surg. Sports Traumatol. Arthrosc.* 24: 3147–3154.
15. Hulse, D., Beale, B., and Kerwin, S. (2010). Second look arthroscopic findings after tibial plateau leveling osteotomy. *Vet. Surg.* 39: 350–354.
16. Vasquez, B., Hulse, D., Beale, B. et al. (2018). Second-look arthroscopic findings after CORA-based leveling osteotomy. *Vet. Surg.* 47: 261–266.
17. Daubs, B.M., Markel, M.D., and Manley, P.A. (2006). Histomorphometric analysis of articular cartilage, zone of calcified cartilage, and subchondral bone plate in femoral heads from clinically normal dogs and dogs with moderate or severe osteoarthritis. *Am. J. Vet. Res* 67 (10): 1719–1724.
18. Scanzello, C.R. and Glodring, S.R. (2012). The role of synovitis in osteoarthritis. *Bone* 51 (2): 249–257.
19. Vjarnson, M., Kwananocha, I., Kashemsant, N. et al. (2019). The effectiveness of marine based fatty acid compound (PCSO-524) and firocoxib in the treatment of canine osteoarthritis. *BMC Vet. Res.* 15: 349.
20. Kwananocha, I., Vijarnsorn, M., Kashemsant, N., and Lekcharoensuk, C. (2016). Effectiveness of disease modifying osteoarthritis agents and carprofen for treatment of canine osteoarthritis. *Thai J. Vet. Med.* 46 (3): 363–371.
21. Stine, S.L., Odum, S.M., Mertans, W.D. et al. (2018). Protocol changes to reduce implant-associated infection rate after tibial plateau leveling osteotomy: 703 dogs, 811 TPLO (2006–2014). *Vet. Surg.* 47: 481–489.

18 Complications Associated with the Meniscus and Decision Making

Stephen C. Jones, Selena Tinga, and Brian S. Beale

18.1 Introduction

There is a medial and a lateral meniscus within each stifle joint. The menisci are fibrocartilaginous semilunar discs, covered in a synovial membrane [1]. Both menisci are thin and concave axially and thick and convex abaxially; the lateral meniscus is slightly thicker with a slightly greater arc than the medial meniscus [1]. Each meniscus has a cranial and caudal meniscotibial ligament, and there is a cranial intermeniscal ligament [1, 2]. The lateral meniscus also has a meniscofemoral ligament running from the caudal horn to the caudo-lateral surface of the medial femoral condyle (Figure 18.1) [1]. The lateral meniscus is not attached to the joint capsule laterally due to the presence of the popliteal tendon of origin (Figures 18.1 and 18.2), in contrast to the medial meniscus which is attached to the joint capsule and medial collateral ligament via the coronary ligament [2]. The lateral meniscus is much more mobile due to these differences in ligamentous attachments (Figure 18.2) [2]. Vessels originate in the perimeniscal capsular and synovial tissues and penetrate the peripheral 25% of the menisci [3]. The functions of the menisci are complex and likely incompletely defined, but include load transmission, shock absorption, joint lubrication, and joint stability [4].

Meniscal pathology is most commonly seen secondary to cranial cruciate ligament (CCL) insufficiency [5]. The caudal pole of the medial meniscus is the most frequent location for damage because of its more intimate association with the tibia and joint capsule, which forces the medial meniscus to move with the tibia as it translates cranially and caudally in relation to the femur [5]. As the tibia is translating cranially and caudally, the caudal horn of the medial meniscus is crushed against the medial femoral condyle, leading to trauma and the development of tears [5]. The incidence of medial meniscal injury concurrent with CCL rupture is approximately 50% although the reported incidence ranges from 20% to 80% [6, 7]. In dogs with CCL insufficiency, risk factors for development of meniscal injury include those with complete or chronic CCL tears (versus partial or acute, respectively) and overweight dogs [7–9]. The added risk of a complete CCL tear is likely related to the increased instability that occurs with a complete versus a partial CCL tear [7].

Different types of meniscal tear morphology can develop, including vertical longitudinal ("bucket handle"), horizontal, radial, or

Complications in Canine Cranial Cruciate Ligament Surgery, First Edition. Edited by Ron Ben-Amotz and David L. Dycus.

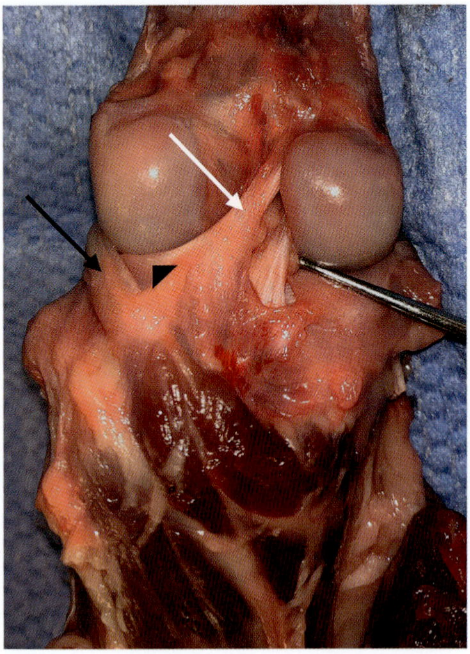

Figure 18.1 Caudal view of a dog's stifle joint. The caudal pole of the lateral meniscus (black arrowhead) is attached to the lateral surface of the medial femoral condyle of the femur via the meniscofemoral ligament (white arrow). Note the tendon of origin of the popliteus muscle (black arrow) immediately abaxial to the lateral meniscus. The meniscal probe is hooking the caudal cruciate ligament for reference.

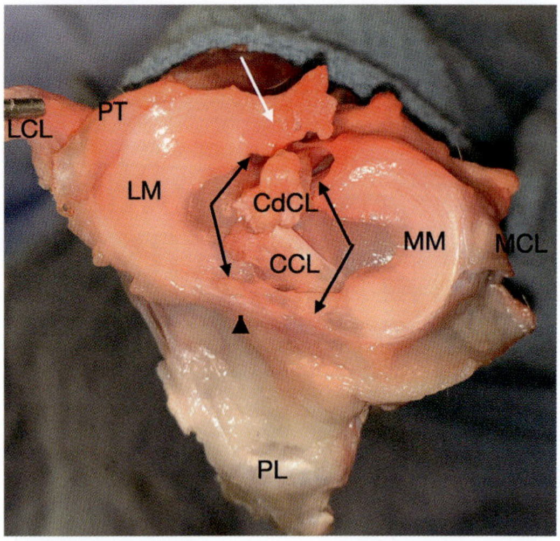

Figure 18.2 The structures associated with the proximal tibia have been exposed, including the patellar ligament (PL), medial (MM) and lateral (LM) menisci, the tibial portion of the cranial (CCL) and caudal (CdCL) cruciate ligaments, cranial and caudal meniscotibial ligaments (black arrows), meniscofemoral ligament (white arrow), intermeniscal ligament (arrowhead), medial collateral ligament (MCL), lateral collateral ligament (LCL), and popliteal tendon of origin (PT).

degenerative tears (Figure 18.3), or the intact meniscus can become detached from the joint capsule and the entire horn can become mobile and displaced [5]. The bucket handle tear is the most common morphology of medial meniscal tears, and is characterized by a medial to lateral tear that allows cranial and caudal motion of the axial border [8, 10].

18.2 Preoperative Meniscal Evaluation

Although it is impossible to definitively determine meniscal status based on the gait examination alone, one study found that dogs with CCL rupture and concurrent meniscal injury were significantly lamer (as denoted by a lower peak vertical force and vertical impulse) than dogs with CCL rupture without meniscal pathology [11]. During stifle manipulation, displacement of mobile meniscal tears can create a palpable or audible click [8, 10, 12]. It is believed that cranial tibial subluxation in the CCL-deficient stifle leads to impingement between the caudal pole of the meniscus and the femoral condyle, causing displacement of the torn portion of the meniscus and the resultant clicking that is heard and/or palpated.

When moving the stifle through a range of flexion-extension motion, two studies reported that detection of a meniscal click was highly specific (~95%) but had poor sensitivity (38–58%) for the presence of a meniscal tear, with a click being most commonly associated with a bucket handle tear compared to other tear morphologies [8, 10]. Additionally, palpation during anesthesia improved the sensitivity of detection of meniscal click as a test for meniscal pathology [8, 10]. Valen et al. tested multiple physical examination tests and found that performing the tibial compression test under axial loading through a range of motion (so-called "modified tibial compression test") had the highest sensitivity (63%) and performing the cranial drawer in extension had the highest specificity (97%) for detection of a meniscal

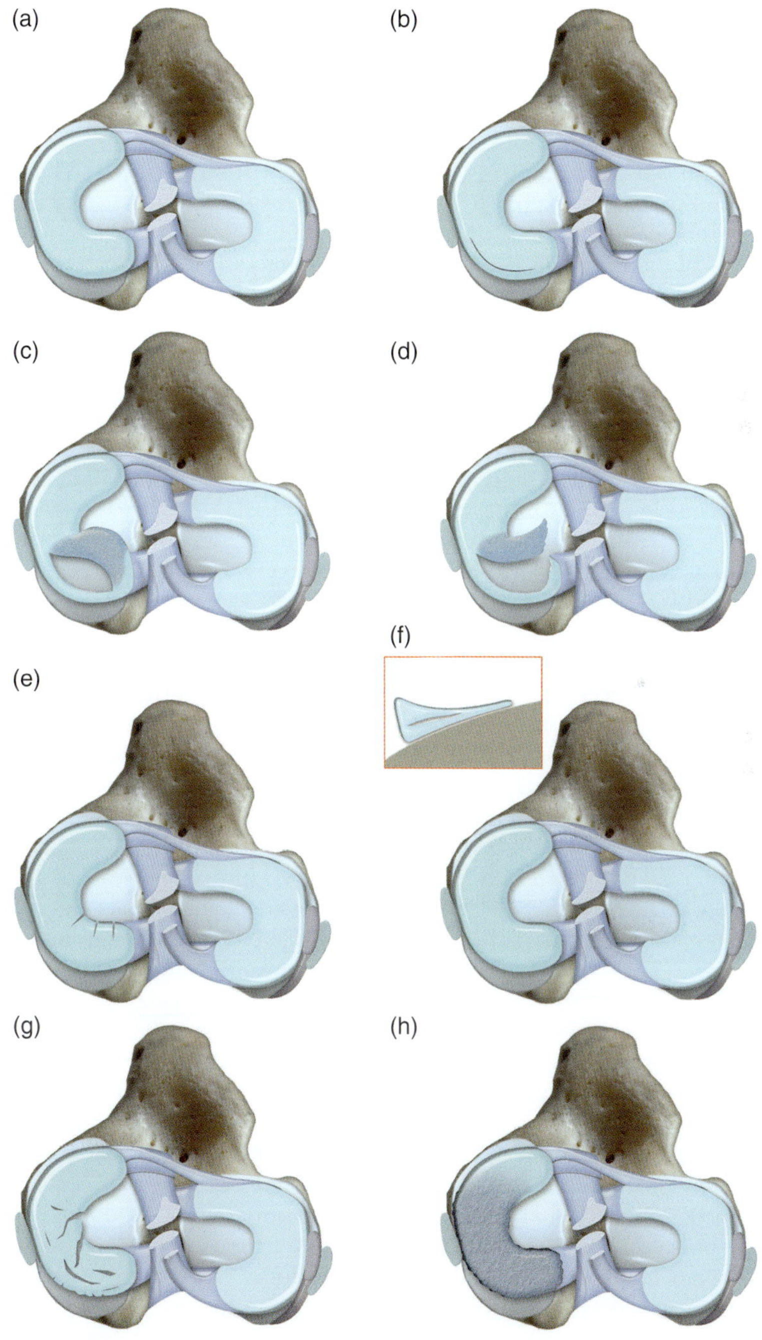

Figure 18.3 Illustration of the different medial meniscal tears that can be encountered. (a) Normal menisci. (b) Vertical longitudinal tear. (c) Displaced bucket handle tear. (d) Flap tear. (e) Radial tears. (f) Horizontal cleavage tear. (g) Complex tears. (h) Degenerative tears. Source: All images reprinted courtesy of Tim Vojt.

click as a diagnostic test for meniscal pathology [12]. Summarily, detection of a meniscal click is strongly indicative of the presence of a meniscal tear, specifically a bucket handle tear, but failure to detect a click does not necessarily mean that the meniscus is normal. This underpins the importance of a thorough meniscal evaluation at the time of surgical intervention, regardless of findings during the preoperative physical exam.

A number of diagnostic imaging modalities have been described for the assessment of menisci in dogs, including radiography, ultrasounography, computed tomography (CT), computed tomography arthrography (CTA), and magnetic resonance imaging (MRI). Although the status of the meniscus cannot be definitively determined by radiography, a study by Won et al. found a significant correlation between joint space narrowing on a standard mediolateral tibial plateau leveling osteotomy (TPLO) radiographic projection and the presence of a meniscal tear at surgery [13]. Ultrasound examination provides high sensitivity (90%) and specificity (93%) for diagnosis of medial meniscal tears [14]. Results, however, are highly dependent on the skill level of the ultrasonographer and the interpreter. CTA has shown a range of sensitivities (13–90%) and specificities (57–100%) for detecting simulated [15] and naturally occurring [16, 17] medial meniscal tears in dogs, highlighting the importance of the CTA protocol used and the skill level of the interpreter. In people, the use of dual-detector helical CTA technology was found to be similarly sensitive and specific to MRI in detecting meniscal pathology [18], but a study reassessing the sensitivity and specificity of CTA for detection of meniscal pathology using similar newer CT technology has not been performed in dogs.

Magnetic resonance imaging examination is considered the most appropriate first-line preoperative diagnostic for assessing meniscal pathology in people [19]. In veterinary studies using 1.5 T [20] or 3 T [21] MRI to detect meniscal pathology, sensitivity and specificity have ranged from 90% to 94% and 96 to 100%, respectively. Despite the utility of MRI for detecting meniscal pathology, it is not widely available in veterinary hospitals and its diagnostic utility in dogs is highly dependent on the magnetic strength, the size of the stifle joint, dog positioning, and the experience of the interpreter [12, 22].

Although MRI and CTA are noninvasive to minimally invasive methods of assessing the menisci preoperatively, both are associated with increased owner costs and require deep sedation or general anesthesia, with CTA also requiring an intraarticular injection, limiting their application for this purpose even in hospitals where the technology is available.

18.3 Exposure of the Meniscus and Diagnosis of Meniscal Tears

In animals with CCL disease undergoing surgical stifle stabilization, it is imperative that both the lateral and medial menisci are evaluated, as failure to identify a meniscal tear may contribute to a poorer outcome, resulting in a persistent or recurrent lameness, progressive osteoarthritis, and/or the need for additional surgical intervention. Although the caudal pole of the medial meniscus is the most commonly affected portion of the meniscus, the cranial pole, body, and caudal pole of both menisci should be examined. The joint examination can be performed via arthrotomy or arthroscopy.

Based on a cadaveric study using experimental models of various caudomedial meniscal lesions, it was found that the sensitivity and specificity of arthroscopy for detection of medial meniscal pathology were higher than those obtained using either a craniomedial or a caudomedial arthrotomy [23]. Importantly, the addition of a meniscal probe (Figure 18.4) improved diagnostic accuracy for detection of meniscal pathology, regardless of the approach used to examine the joint [23]. The odds ratio of correctly diagnosing the state of the medial meniscus when using a meniscal probe, when compared with observation alone, was 8.0 for arthroscopy, 2.1 for craniomedial arthrotomy, and 2.6 for caudomedial arthrotomy [23]. Another interesting finding of this study was the diagnostic superiority of a craniomedial arthrotomy over a caudomedial arthrotomy in CCL-deficient joints; conversely a caudomedial arthrotomy was more accurate at correctly diagnosing meniscal pathology than a craniomedial arthrotomy in dogs with an intact CCL.

The diagnostic superiority of arthroscopy has been corroborated in clinical studies [24, 25]. In a prospective study of 163 dogs with CCL rupture, meniscal pathology was 1.9 times more likely to be detected in stifles examined by arthroscopy than by an arthrotomy [24]. Similarly, a retrospective study of 531 dogs found that the rate of meniscal tear detection

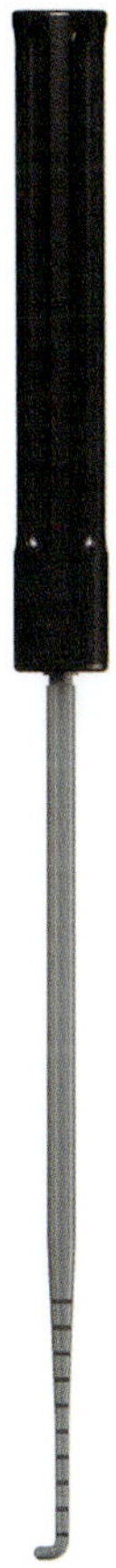

Figure 18.4 A typical meniscal probe. The right-angled tip helps the surgeon probe the femoral and tibial surfaces of the meniscus. The graduated marks on the probe are typically 1 mm apart and allow the surgeon to measure intraarticular structures.

was significantly higher with arthroscopy (odds ratio 1.5) compared to a craniomedial arthrotomy [25].

18.3.1 Meniscal Evaluation with an Arthrotomy

For the purposes of examining the stifle joint and performing meniscal evaluation, the joint is typically approached via a craniomedial, caudomedial or craniolateral arthrotomy. The surgical approach will be based on surgeon preference and which, if any, additional stifle stabilization procedures are being performed in that particular case.

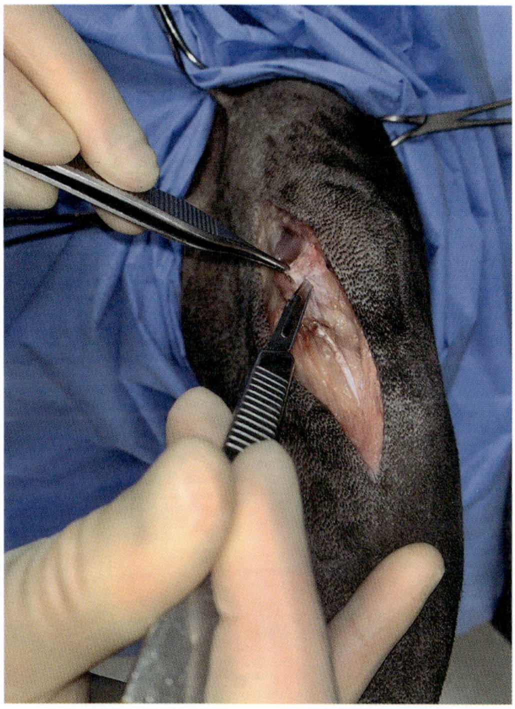

Figure 18.5 Performance of a craniomedial arthrotomy in a left stifle joint. After the medial fascia has been incised and reflected caudally, the joint capsule is grasped with thumb forceps at the level of the patellar apex, and tented to retract it from the underlying femoral cartilage. The arthrotomy is initiated with a scalpel blade, ensuring that the blade does not plunge too deep into the joint.

The surgeon must exercise caution when performing the arthrotomy, as inadvertent cartilage, meniscal, and/or patellar ligament damage is possible when entering the joint. Typically, to best protect intraarticular structures and allow correct tissue apposition during closure, it is recommended to incise the periarticular fascia and elevate this from the underlying joint capsule before performing the arthrotomy. The surgeon should then tent up the joint capsule with thumb forceps and make a small incision in the joint capsule, making sure not to penetrate the joint too deeply (Figure 18.5). The arthrotomy is then extended in a manner that protects the underlying cartilage and meniscus and neighboring patellar ligament, such as using a pair of Mayo scissors or incising over a mosquito hemostat placed within the joint (Figure 18.6). The surgeon should be especially careful not to cause iatrogenic

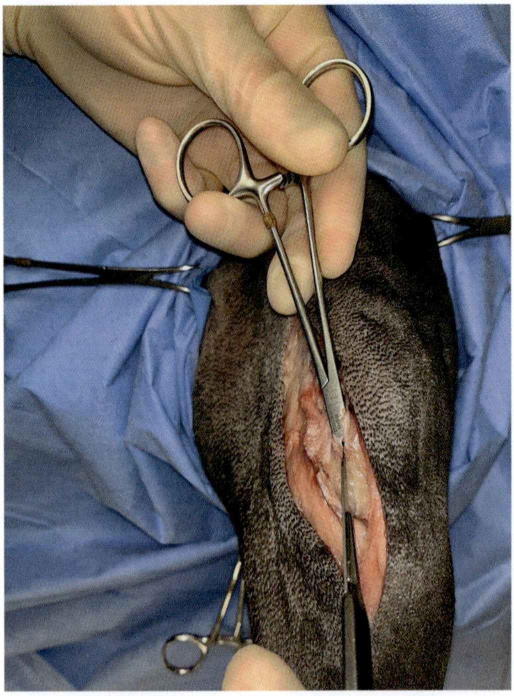

Figure 18.6 Performance of a craniomedial arthrotomy in a left stifle joint. A curved mosquito forceps has been advanced through the initial arthrotomy, positioned distally to the level of the patellar ligament insertion on the tibial tuberosity, and then "pulled" medially. This elevates the joint capsule away from the underlying articular cartilage, menisci, and ligaments. The arthrotomy is then continued distally by cutting over the mosquito forceps using a scalpel blade.

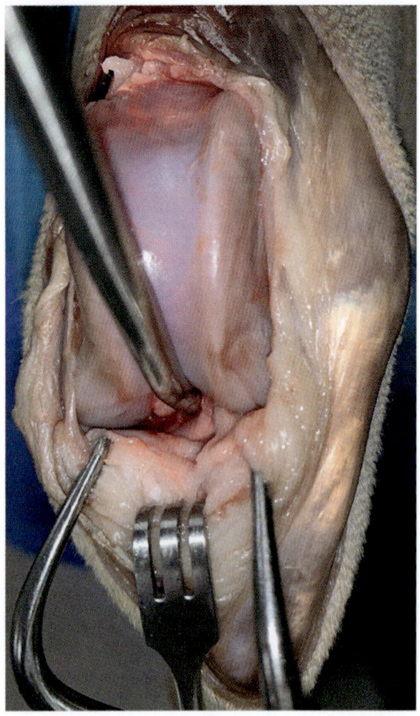

Figure 18.7 Full craniomedial arthrotomy with the patella luxated laterally. A Gelpi retractor is used to retract the infrapatellar fat pad abaxially and maintain retraction of the fascia and joint capsule. A Ventura stifle distractor, placed caudal to the tibial plateau, is levered against the trochlear groove to subluxate the tibia cranially. A cranially positioned Volkmann retractor further retracts the fat pad and also helps to translate the tibia cranially.

damage to the cranial pole of the meniscus and/or the intermeniscal ligament, as the joint capsule and fat pad are incised distally.

Improving exposure of the joint will improve diagnostic accuracy and reduce iatrogenic injury to intraarticular structures. Multiple techniques and instruments can aid in exposure of intraarticular structures. It is helpful to place a baby Gelpi to retract the infrapatellar fat pat abaxially (Figure 18.7). If an assistant is available, they can further retract the fat pad cranially using a sharp Senn/Volkmann retractor placed at the level of the intermeniscal ligament (Figure 18.7). The most challenging aspect of meniscal evaluation is the ability to visualize the caudal pole of the menisci. Many instruments have been used to help translate the tibial cranially, some developed specifically for this purpose, thus improving exposure of the caudal tibial plateau and caudal pole of the menisci. These include intraarticular devices such as levers (mosquito forceps, Hohmann retractor, various purpose-designed stifle distractors, etc.) or self-retaining devices (Gelpi retractor, Wallace stifle distractor, etc.), and extraarticular devices such as the Leipzig stifle distractor (extraarticular devices are discussed in the arthroscopy section of this chapter).

Intraarticularly placed lever devices are the simplest method of improving visualization of the caudal pole of the meniscus (Figure 18.7). The tip of the instrument is typically placed caudal to the tibial plateau and the instrument is levered against the trochlear groove of the femur (Figure 18.8). Although convenient, use of a lever instrument can result in multiple complications. The body of the lever can damage the cartilage of the trochlear groove (Figure 18.9). The tip of the lever instrument

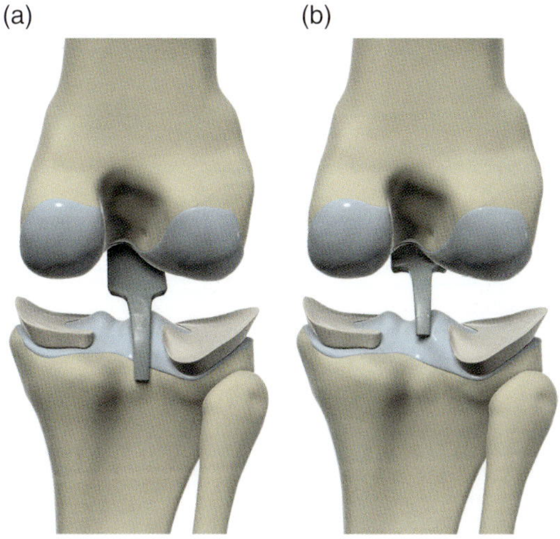

Figure 18.8 Illustration of the caudal aspect of the stifle joint. Note that ligamentous attachments are not depicted, to allow for visualization of the entire retractor. (a) When placing an instrument to lever the tibia cranially (Hohmann retractor illustrated here), the tip of the instrument should ideally be placed caudal to the tibial plateau. (b) Placing the tip of the instrument too proximally or cranially may not give sufficient purchase to distract the tibia cranially. Furthermore, the instrument may disengage when leverage is applied, leading to cartilage damage and/or a small iatrogenic fracture.

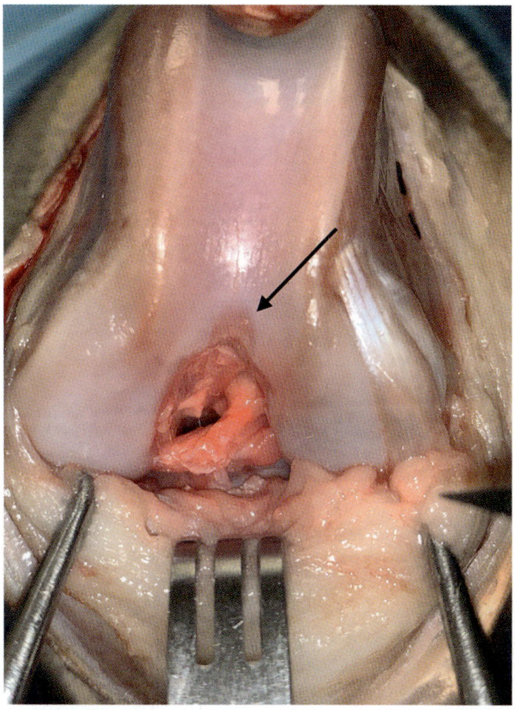

Figure 18.9 Cartilage damage (black arrow) created by a Ventura stifle distractor as it levered against the trochlear groove to subluxate the tibia cranially.

can be placed on (rather than caudal to) the tibial plateau, ideally between the caudal cruciate ligament and the caudal meniscotibial ligament of the medial meniscus. The advantage of placement at this location, over placing the tip caudal to the plateau, is that it may permit pushing the tibia distally in addition to generating cranial tibial subluxation. However, it is possible to create a small iatrogenic fracture when leverage is applied, if the instrument is not secured behind a ligamentous attachment, such as the caudal menisco-tibial ligament (Figure 18.10). Additionally, the tip of the lever instrument can slip cranially and damage the cartilage of the tibial plateau (Figure 18.11). Regardless of whether the tip of the lever instrument is placed on or caudal to the tibial plateau, it is advisable to place the tip of the instrument medial to the caudal cruciate ligament. This helps retract the caudal cruciate ligament laterally and improves exposure of the caudal pole of the medial meniscus and the caudal meniscotibial ligament (Figure 18.12).

One challenge with use of a lever device is that it can impede the surgeon's view of the lateral joint compartment when using a medial arthrotomy. Occasionally, the surgeon will have to remove the lever instrument and use a cranially positioned sharp Senn/Volkmann retractor or manually place the tibia in cranial drawer, to enable visualization of the caudal pole of the lateral meniscus. An additional limitation to the use of a lever instrument is the need for an assistant to maintain distraction as the surgeon examines the joint and treats any pathology. If sufficient assistance is not available, the use of a self-retaining retractor is a viable option. A sharp self-retaining retractor or distractor can be placed inside the joint, between the femur and tibia (Figure 18.13). The surgeon should ensure that the tips of the instrument are placed carefully; the proximal tip should not pierce the caudal cruciate ligament and the distal tip should be placed cranial to the intermeniscal ligament to protect the menisci and articular cartilage of the tibial plateau.

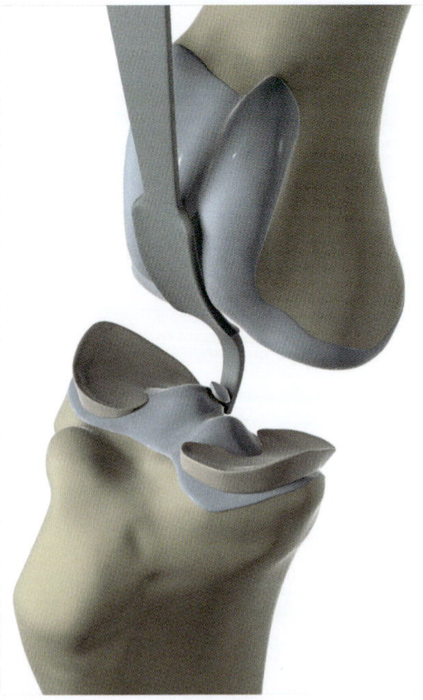

Figure 18.10 When the tip of the stifle distractor is not positioned sufficiently distal to the caudal aspect of the tibial plateau, it is possible to create a small iatrogenic articular fracture, as is illustrated on the lateral intercondylar eminence here. As this is not a surface in direct articulation with the femur, these chip fractures are generally left to heal without surgical intervention, with no known clinical consequence.

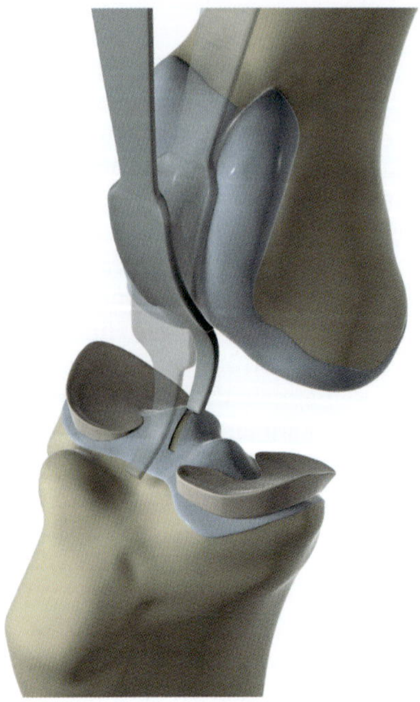

Figure 18.11 If the tip of the stifle lever distractor is placed on the tibial plateau (Hohmann retractor shown on the lateral intercondylar eminence here), the tip of the instrument can disengage when leverage is applied, causing damage to the articular cartilage.

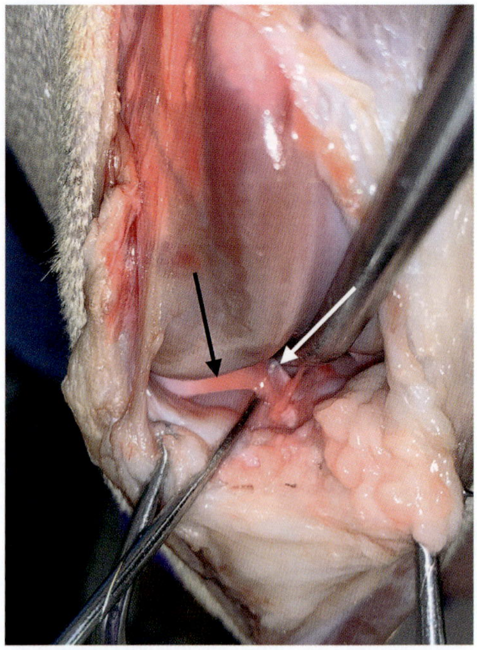

Figure 18.12 The tip of the stifle distractor is placed medial to the caudal cruciate ligament as it is positioned caudal and distal to the tibial plateau. This helps retract the caudal cruciate ligament laterally, thereby improving exposure of the caudal pole of the medial meniscus (black arrow) and the caudal meniscotibial ligament (white arrow), while also protecting the caudal cruciate ligament if any meniscal treatment is required.

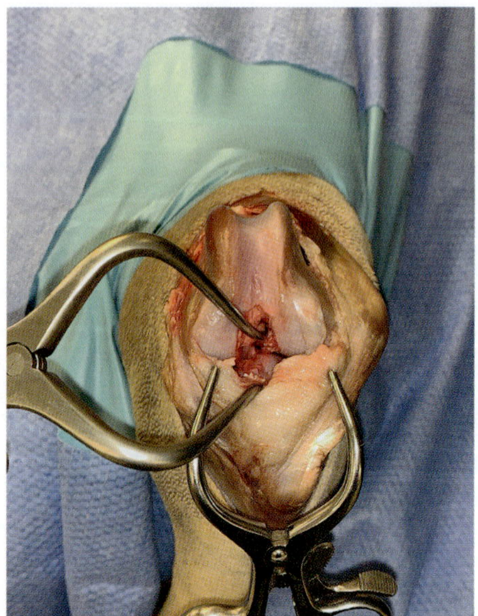

Figure 18.13 A Gelpi retractor has been placed intraarticularly to help distract the joint. The proximal tip of the Gelpi is placed in the intercondylar notch of the femur, lateral to the caudal cruciate ligament. The distal tip of the Gelpi is placed cranial to the intermeniscal ligament to prevent damage to the articular cartilage, menisci or meniscal ligaments.

18.3.2 Meniscal Evaluation with Arthroscopy

A comprehensive discussion of the complications of stifle arthroscopy is presented in Chapter 17 so the following discussion is limited to aspects of arthroscopy that relate directly to stifle examination, meniscal evaluation and treatment.

There is a steep learning curve associated with becoming proficient in stifle arthroscopy. Even in experienced hands, the stifle joint is considered one of the most challenging joints to examine and treat arthroscopically. While arthroscopy has many advantages over an arthrotomy, it has been shown in people that extensive experience and training are required to limit the number of complications encountered when performing specific challenging arthroscopic procedures [26]. The surgeon should pay careful attention when creating the arthroscopic ports, as cartilage, ligament, and/or meniscal damage can occur when entering the joint with a needle, scalpel blade or arthroscopic cannula [27]. Placement of the camera port slightly more proximal than the halfway point between the patellar apex and tibial tuberosity [14] can help the surgeon avoid the infrapatellar fat pad; however, this can make visualization of the caudal portion of the tibial plateau and caudal horns of the menisci more challenging. Conversely, if the camera is introduced more distally, the caudal tibial plateau is more readily viewed but debridement of the fat pad is typically required to facilitate accurate joint inspection.

One of the most common complications encountered with stifle arthroscopy is iatrogenic cartilage damage. A recent study found that stifle arthroscopy in dog cadavers resulted in an increased incidence, number, and overall surface area of iatrogenic cartilage damage, when compared with a medial parapatellar mini arthrotomy [28]. In an arthroscopic study of iatrogenic cartilage injury in dogs, incomplete healing of cartilage damage was noted 6 months after experimental creation of the cartilage defects [29]. Given that cartilage damage is a well-accepted osteoarthritis initiator [30], this study underpins the importance of preservation of the articular cartilage during all joint surgeries, including stifle arthroscopy.

Most cartilage damage tends to occur during meniscal treatment. The surgeon has a very focal view of the joint during arthroscopy at any point in time; as instruments are being introduced into the joint and during manipulation as part of the joint exploration and meniscal treatment, cartilage damage can occur outside the surgeon's field of view (Figure 18.14). The surgeon should therefore ensure that adequate stifle distraction is present, and that the introduction and manipulation of the arthroscopic instruments do not impinge on the articular cartilage. It is also important to use arthroscopic instruments of an appropriate size. In smaller dogs and cats, many of the commercially available instruments are too large and their use may cause unacceptable iatrogenic cartilage injury.

As with an arthrotomy, it is possible to utilize an intraarticular lever to translate the tibia cranially when performing stifle arthroscopy. This is typically placed via a separate arthroscopic port, but can also be placed through an enlarged instrument portal, and has been shown to significantly increase meniscal visualization and ease of probing of the medial meniscus [31]. One challenge with the use of a lever instrument is the potential to damage articular cartilage as the instrument is maneuvered past the scope into place. Additionally, the presence of a distractor can obscure comprehensive examination of parts of the joint and may require removal or repositioning of arthroscope and instruments to complete the arthroscopic examination. Use of extraarticular self-retaining stifle distractors has been described in the dog [32–34] and can help prevent some of the aforementioned limitations encountered when using a lever distractor. Extraarticular distractors involve placement of a medial-lateral wire/pin into the distal femur and proximal tibia. These pins are then connected to a distraction device which creates opening of the joint space (Figure 18.15). Their use permits improved visualization of the menisci [32, 34, 35], increased accuracy of detecting meniscal pathology [34, 35], improved ease of performing a meniscal release or meniscectomy and helps to prevent cartilage damage to the tibial plateau [36–38].

Despite the strong evidence supporting their use, complications can be encountered with the use of extraarticular stifle distractors. When describing the use of the Leipzig distractor, two cases of intraarticular placement of the tibial

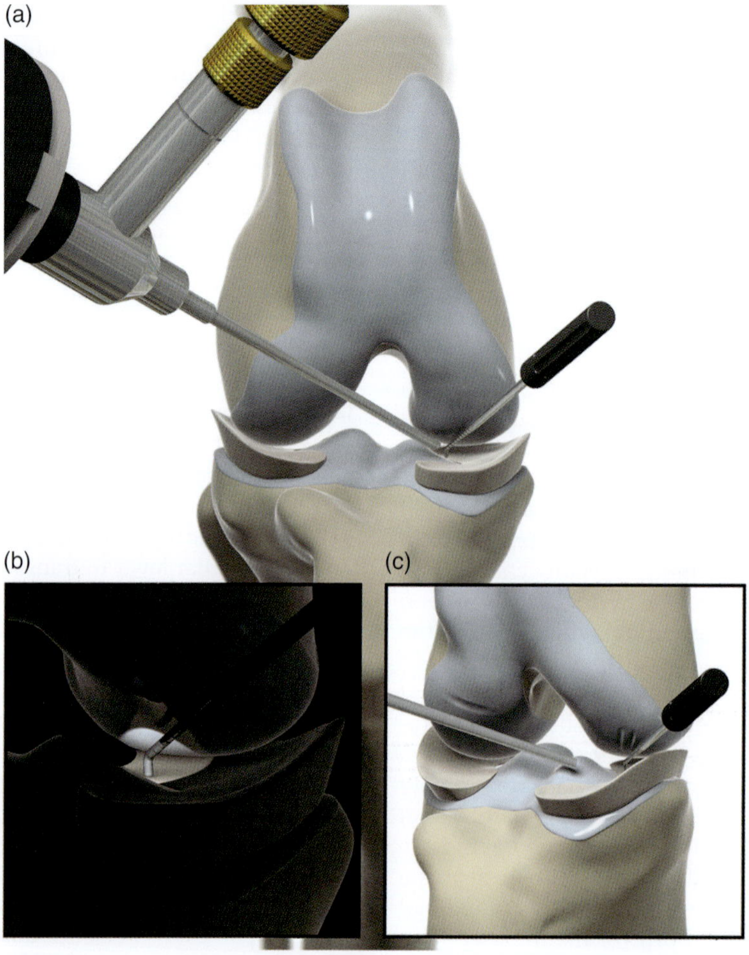

Figure 18.14 (a) In this illustration of arthroscopy of a right stifle, the arthroscope is placed through a craniolateral portal, with an instrument portal positioned craniomedially. (b) The surgeon's view of the intraarticular structures is limited to the area illuminated by the arthroscope. (c) During the process of joint evaluation and treatment, the surgeon must remain conscious of the position of the arthroscope and instruments outside the field of view, to prevent iatrogenic cartilage damage, as is illustrated on the femoral condyles here.

pin were documented [32]. In a later study on canine toy breed cadavers, utilizing pins placed in similar manner to the Leipzig, 20% of the femoral pins penetrated the joint capsule immediately cranial to the medial fabella [36]. In that same study, the authors also found that damage to the caudal cruciate ligament was more likely with use of a distractor and this is something that should be guarded against when performing meniscal release in conjunction with stifle distraction [36].

Although not explicitly documented in the literature, Böttcher et al. described the potential for collateral ligament strain when using the Leipzig distractor [32]. They advocate for the use of undersized rather than more rigid pins to allow pin bending and thus prevent overstretching of collateral ligaments during stifle distraction. The use of the Leipzig distractor can cause collapse of, and limit the evaluation of, the lateral stifle compartment [38]. It thus seems prudent to evaluate the lateral compartment first, before applying distraction to allow evaluation of the medial compartment. If additional access to the lateral stifle compartment is required (for example, to treat a lateral meniscal tear), the distractor can safely and successfully be placed laterally [38].

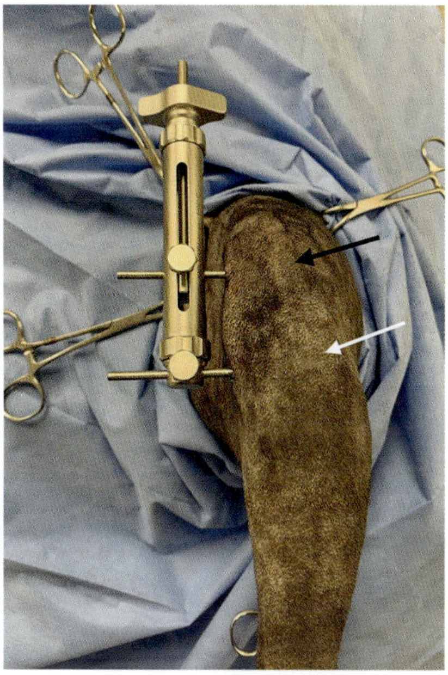

Figure 18.15 Leipzig stifle distractor. A negatively threaded pin (3 mm diameter) is percutaneously placed in the medial femoral condyle, perpendicular to the femoral long axis, halfway between the patellar apex (black arrow) and the medial fabella. A second similar pin is placed parallel to the first pin, at the most caudal aspect of the proximal tibia, at the level of the tibial tuberosity (white arrow). The distractor is placed over and secured to the pins before distraction is applied.

18.3.3 Detection of Meniscal Pathology

Regardless of the method of joint exploration (arthrotomy vs arthroscopy) or the technique used to distract the joint, the menisci must be thoroughly probed to evaluate for a meniscal tear. The most common meniscal tear diagnosed in dogs, the bucket handle tear [6], begins as a vertical longitudinal tear. The meniscus should be probed on both the femoral and tibial surfaces. It is inviting to probe the femoral side of the meniscus and move on if no pathology is detected, but an incomplete vertical longitudinal tear on the tibial side can easily be missed if that side of the meniscus is not probed (Figure 18.16). Despite the improve sensitivity of arthroscopy for detection of meniscal tears in experienced hands, incorrect classification of meniscal status is still a potential complication and the surgeon should be aware of all techniques to perform a thorough meniscal examination [23].

In addition to utilizing a probe during joint examination, positioning of the stifle during exploration is also important to enhance visualization and access to the caudal pole of the menisci. The surgeon should flex and extend the stifle throughout the examination as needed to improve visualization. The tibia can be manually manipulated into varus/valgus and internal/external rotation to improve access to the caudal joint surfaces. Typically, placing a valgus strain and external tibial rotation with the stifle in extension improves exposure of the medial meniscus. Conversely, internal rotation and varus strain with the stifle partially flexed helps improve exposure of the lateral meniscus. It is worth noting that manipulation of the tibia into cranial subluxation can be accomplished manually without the use of a distraction instrument, though it has been shown that visualization of the medial meniscus was significantly better when using a stifle distractor compared to manual manipulation [31]. Performance of the tibial thrust test can help displace bucket handle tears and is a useful maneuver to perform when examining the joint. Additionally, the authors have found that in cases where extraordinary difficulty in visualizing/probing the caudal meniscus is encountered, examining and treating the meniscus after TPLO (and thus potentially also after other leveling osteotomies) can sometimes be more rewarding and easier to perform.

18.4 Meniscal Treatment

18.4.1 Meniscal Release

During joint examination by arthrotomy or arthroscopy, the menisci should be classified as intact or torn, and this will dictate the need for further meniscal treatment. When the menisci are determined to be normal, the options are to perform no treatment or to complete a release of the caudal horn of the medial meniscus. Meniscal release allows the caudal pole of the meniscus to displace caudally, preventing its impingement between the femur and tibial plateau. The justification for performing a meniscal release on a normal meniscus is that there is an approximate 8–11% risk of postliminary meniscal tears after surgery for CCL rupture if a healthy meniscus is identified and no release is performed, and this risk is mitigated with a complete and accurate meniscal release [24, 39,

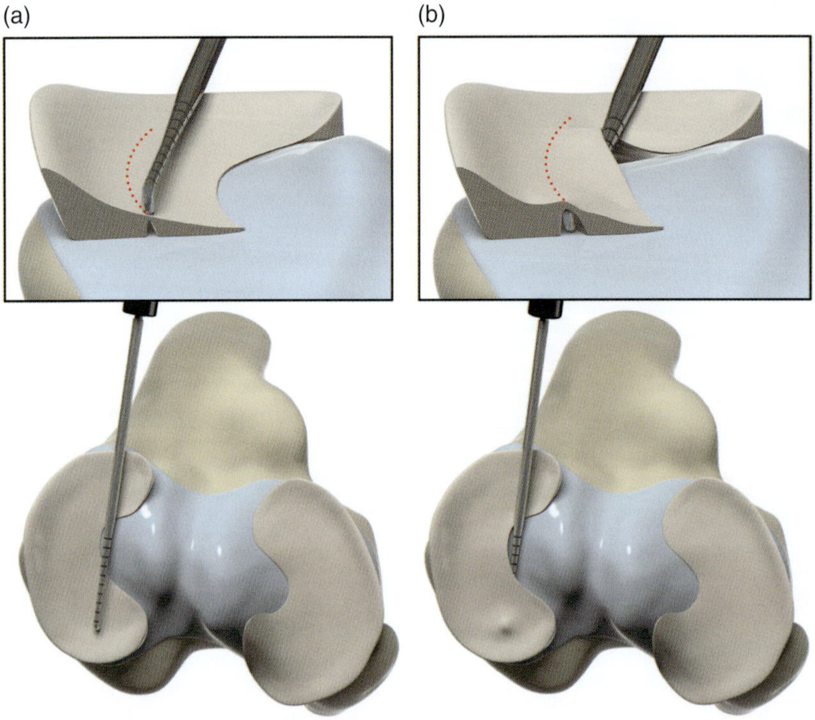

Figure 18.16 Probing the meniscus (via arthrotomy or arthroscopy). Both the femoral (a) and tibial (b) surfaces of each meniscus should be carefully probed to assess for any pathology. Note how an incomplete vertical longitudinal tear on the tibial surface of the medial meniscus can easily be missed if the surgeon only probes the femoral surface of the meniscus.

40]. Release of the caudal horn of the medial meniscus can be performed through the caudal medial meniscotibial ligament (or through the meniscus at its junction with the meniscotibial ligament) or at the midmeniscal body (immediately caudal to the medial collateral ligament).

The ligaments near the meniscal release site, specifically the caudal cruciate ligament for a meniscotibial desmotomy or the medial collateral ligament for a midbody release, are at risk of iatrogenic damage. Damage to these ligaments could result in abnormal joint mechanics which may result in pain and progressive osteoarthritis. The caudal cruciate ligament can be protected during a meniscotibial desmotomy by cutting away from the caudal cruciate ligament, and by placement of an intraarticular lever retractor medial to the caudal cruciate ligament, thus displacing the caudal cruciate ligament laterally (Figures 18.12 and 18.17). If performing a midbody meniscal release, damage to the medial collateral ligament can be prevented by performing the release at the appropriate location (caudal to medial collateral ligament) with the scalpel blade angled perpendicular to the tibial plateau (Figure 18.18).

The femoral or tibial articular cartilage in the region of the release may also be damaged during the procedure. Damage to the articular cartilage can be minimized during meniscal release by use of a stifle distractor to increase joint space [36] and by incising over an instrument (such as meniscal probe) (Figures 18.12 and 18.17) or using a meniscal knife (hook knife, push knife, meniscal cutter, etc.) rather than a standard scalpel blade. Importantly, meniscal knives can also create cartilage damage if forced into a small joint space or not used under direct visualization.

When performing a meniscal release, it is critical to ensure that a complete release is performed, as an incomplete meniscal release may, in effect, create a similar environment to a meniscal tear, resulting in pain and promoting the development of osteoarthritis (Figure 18.19). A cadaveric study comparing effectiveness of midbody meniscal release performed blind, via caudomedial arthrotomy, or via arthroscopy

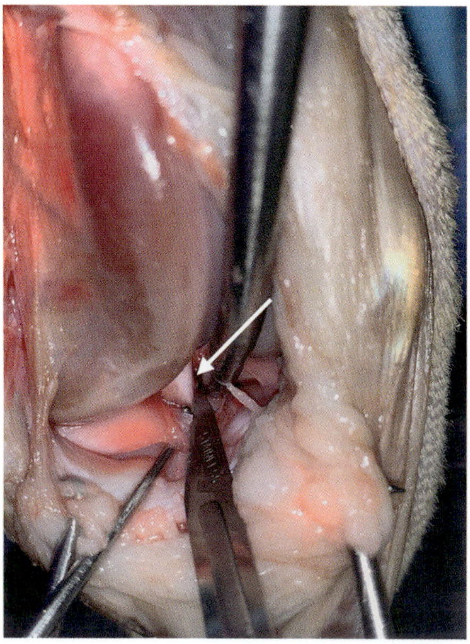

Figure 18.17 Performance of a caudal meniscotibial desmotomy of the medial meniscus. A meniscal probe has been placed under the cadual meniscotibial ligament to protect the articular cartilage of the tibial plateau during the desmotomy. The Ventura stifle distractor has been incorrectly placed (compare with Figure 18.12) lateral to the caudal cruciate ligament (white arrow), making it more vulnerable to damage from the scalpel blade during the desmotomy.

found that none of the approaches consistently resulted in complete and accurate meniscal release [41]. Importantly, the CCL was left intact and no joint distraction techniques were utilized in that study. A later study showed that the use of an extraarticular joint distractor increased the success rate of achieving complete meniscotibial desmotomy by 7.4 times in toy-breed dogs [36], and the benefit of using a joint distractor likely holds true in larger dogs as well.

Meniscal release is not a benign procedure, even when performed correctly (complete and accurate with no iatrogenic damage). Meniscal release has been shown to alter joint mechanics, decreasing contact area and increasing the peak contact pressure on the tibial plateau after TPLO in a cadaveric study [42]. These *ex vivo* results are supported by an experimental *in vivo* study which demonstrated that meniscal release resulted in lameness and medial compartment cartilage pathology within 12 weeks in dogs with otherwise normal stifle joints [43]. Therefore, the authors are of the opinion that meniscal release should not be performed routinely when a normal meniscus is identified. Rather, clients should be educated about the risk of postliminary meniscal pathology and be prepared for a second

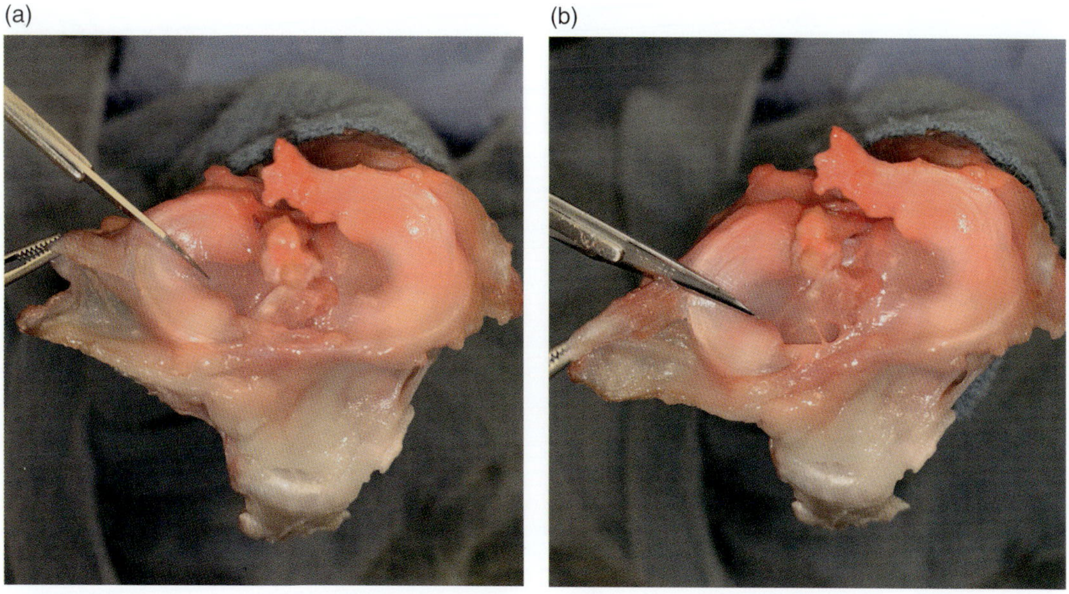

Figure 18.18 (a) Correct blade position for performance of a midbody meniscal release, caudal to the medial collateral ligament (held by Brown–Adson forceps). The blade is advanced through the meniscus perpendicular to the tibial plateau. (b) The scalpel blade is being directed cranially, which may result in a partial or complete medial collateral desmotomy.

procedure if a postliminary meniscal tear occurs, in lieu of meniscal release at the time of the original surgical procedure. However, if a client expresses the inability to pursue a follow-up procedure (for whatever reason) if a postliminary meniscal tear were to occur, meniscal release at the time of original surgery can be considered.

Another instance where release of a normal meniscus could be considered is when instability is incompletely resolved with the elected surgical procedure. However, the authors would encourage the surgeon to perform adjunctive stabilization procedures in an attempt to provide stifle stability over performing a meniscal release to mask secondary effects of residual instability in this instance. Finally, in some cases where complete debridement of damaged meniscal tissue is only possible with iatrogenic damage to the articular cartilage (for example, in a chronically affected joint with profound periarticular fibrosis), a meniscal release of residual tissue may be considered, thus allowing the damaged tissue to displace caudally and away from the weight-bearing portion of the joint.

18.4.2 Meniscal Repair or Debridement

When a meniscal tear is identified, the treatment of choice – meniscal repair, meniscal debridement (partial or hemimeniscectomy), or meniscal release – will depend on both the type of tear identified and the surgeon's preference. Displaced bucket handle tears, flap tears, and complex tears have been shown to generate >45% increases in peak joint contact pressure in experimental cadaveric models [44]. This is a clear indication that these specific types of tears definitively warrant treatment. Other tear morphologies may also warrant treatment, for example, if nonfunctional meniscal tissue is identified.

A study using a cadaveric model of a bucket handle meniscal tear showed that meniscal repair can reestablish joint contact mechanics that are not different from an intact meniscus [45]. Unfortunately, meniscal repair can only be recommended in very select clinical cases: acute, peripheral tears where the tissue remains healthy and the tear is located in the vascular zone of the meniscus (abaxial 25%) (Figure 18.20) [3]. Performing meniscal repair

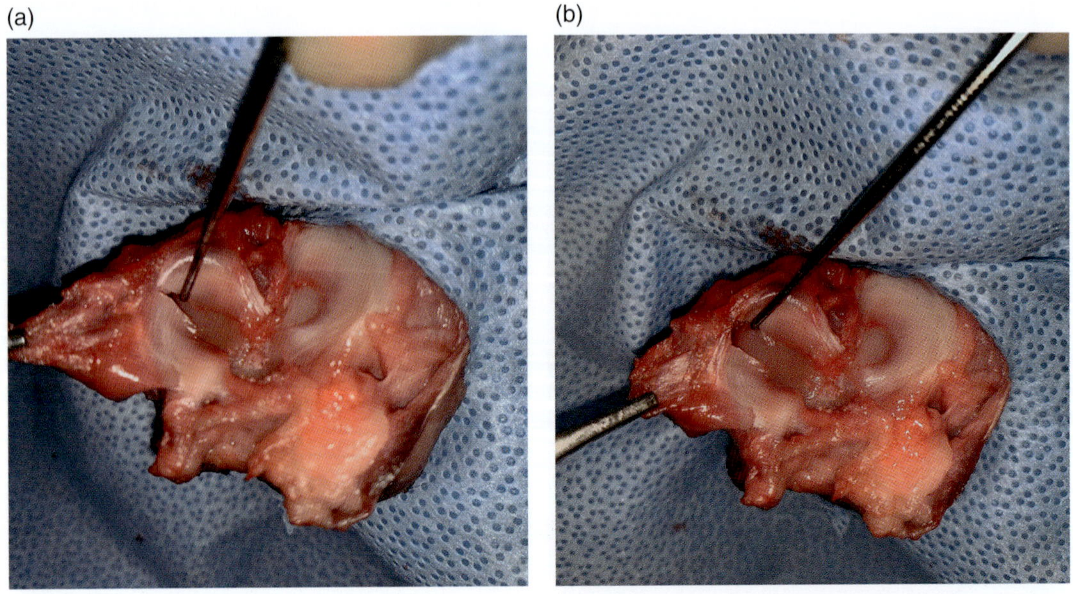

Figure 18.19 (a) An incomplete midbody medial meniscal release has been performed. The meniscus remains partially attached to the joint capsule abaxially, preventing displacement of the cadual pole of the meniscus. (b) The meniscal release has been completed. Note how the cadual pole of the meniscus displaces caudally when tensioned by the meniscal probe. The medial collateral ligament is being held by Brown–Adson forceps for reference.

on tears outside these parameters will likely result in continued meniscal pathology due to failure of adequate meniscal healing and ultimately failure of the repair. In a clinical study of 126 dogs with CCL rupture, medial meniscal tears eligible for repair were identified in 92 (14%) of 654 dogs with meniscal tears [46]. No complications of meniscal repair were encountered in this study, and the importance of appropriate case selection was stressed [46].

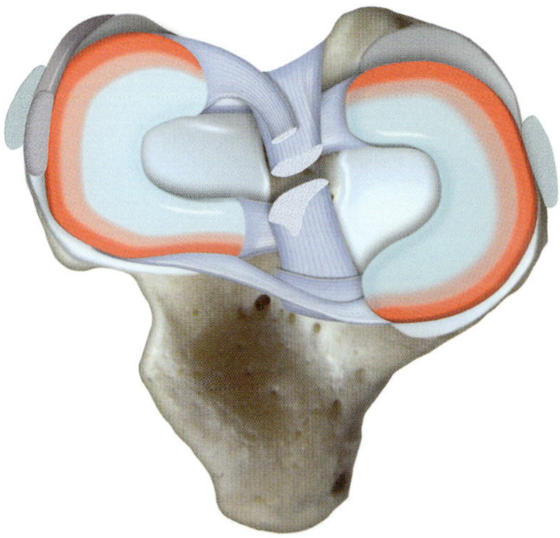

Figure 18.20 Illustration of the proximal aspect of the tibia. Meniscal blood supply is broken down into three zones: the red zone (abaxial ~25% of the meniscal width) receives the most robust blood supply; the middle red-white zone and the axial-most white-white zone occupy the remainder of the meniscus, with these zones receiving little (red-white) to no (white-white) blood supply. Source: Reprinted courtesy of Tim Vojt.

In the vast majority of medial meniscal tears, removal (Figure 18.21), rather than repair, of the damaged meniscal tissue will be necessary because most meniscal tears are chronic and/or are located in the inner, avascular portion of the meniscus. The clinical consequence of removal of damaged meniscal tissue varies depending on the amount of meniscal tissue excised. All functional meniscal tissue, including the meniscotibial ligaments and peripheral meniscal attachments, must be preserved to maximize meniscal function after debridement. Partial meniscectomy of 30% of the radial width does not change joint contact mechanics, whereas partial meniscectomy of 75% of the radial width increases peak contact pressure by 61% and caudal medial hemimeniscectomy increases peak contact pressure by 87% [47]. Therefore, tears encompassing the axial 30% of the meniscus can theoretically be treated by removing the damaged tissue without known adverse effects.

(a) (b) (c)

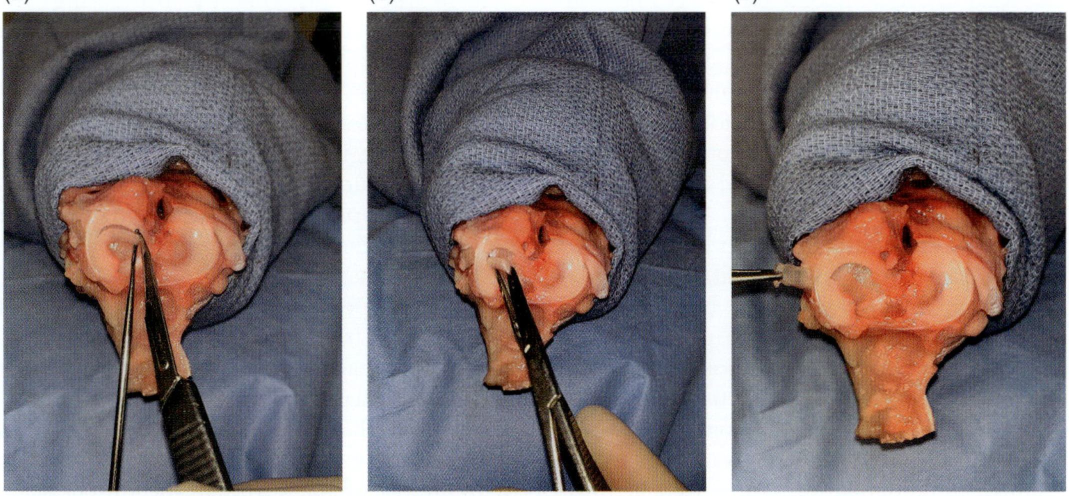

Figure 18.21 Simulated partial meniscectomy of a bucket handle tear of the caudal pole of the medial meniscus. (a) A meniscal probe hooks the axial portion of the tear and protects the underlying tibial plateau cartilage as a #11 blade is used to release the torn portion. (b) The axial portion of the tear has been released and is being retracted and elevated by a straight mosquito hemostat. A #11 blade is used to cut the abaxial portion of the tear. Note that the blade is cutting away from the tibial plateau, to protect the articular cartilage. (c) Completed partial meniscectomy.

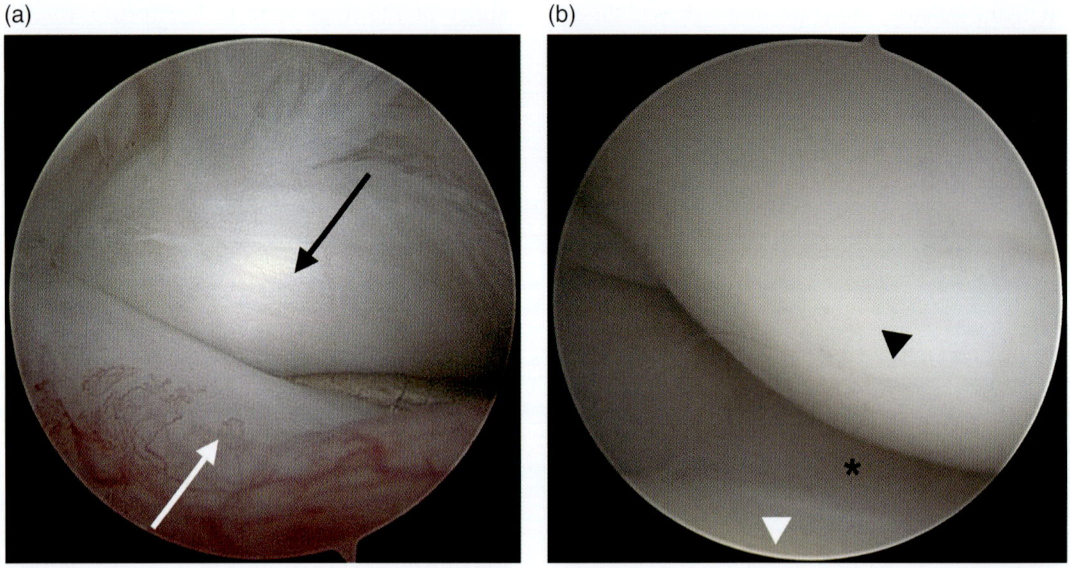

Figure 18.22 Arthroscopic view of the medial compartment of the stifle joint. (a) Peripheral tear of the caudal pole of the medial meniscus (black arrow) has displaced into the cranial joint compartment. Note the fold-line between the cranial pole (white arrow) and the caudal pole of the meniscus. (b) A meniscal probe was used to manipulate the caudal pole of the meniscus (*) back caudally. Note how the medial femoral condyle (black arrowhead) and medial tibial plateau (white arrowhead) are now visible.

Despite concern for alteration in contact mechanics with removal of torn meniscal tissue outside the axial 30%, damaged tissue must still be debrided and removed. There is no benefit to leaving nonfunctional tissue behind; in fact, this may lead to ongoing joint morbidity and contribute to patient discomfort, lameness, and progressive osteoarthritis. Debridement of meniscal tissue must continue until no further damaged tissue can be displaced during follow-up probing; it is not uncommon to encounter multiple bucket handle tears which often require multiple iterations of debridement. As mentioned previously, meniscal release can be considered for treatment of a meniscal tear if, for some reason, the meniscal tear cannot be completely debrided; this should not be a primary treatment of meniscal tears but should allow the remaining damaged meniscal tissue to move peripherally rather than becoming trapped within the weight-bearing portion of the joint.

During any meniscal treatment via arthrotomy or arthroscopy, the instruments (blades, forceps, punches, shavers, etc.) must be used cautiously, and should be under direct visualization in order to minimize damage to healthy intraarticular structures including ligaments, healthy portions of menisci, and articular cartilage. As previously noted, joint distraction should be employed to maximize working space and visibility within the joint, thereby protecting the structures within the joint. Additionally, if meniscal tissue (torn portion of caudal pole or entire caudal pole detached from the joint capsule) is displaced cranially into the near field of view, it may be beneficial to replace the tissue caudally into the normal anatomical position prior to debridement, in order to obtain orientation and improve working space (Figure 18.22).

Whenever possible, healthy structures should be protected from nonguarded blades by cutting the damaged meniscus over a probe or other instrument, or by angling the blade away from nearby healthy structures. The portion of the meniscus to be removed can be manipulated with an instrument such that the scalpel blade can be oriented parallel to cartilage surfaces to avoid damaging articular cartilage. Many alternatives to a scalpel blade have a guarded cutting surface, such as hook knives, push knives, meniscal cutters, punches, shavers, etc., but these instruments can also cause undesired damage if not used carefully and correctly under visualization and with joint distraction.

18.5 Lateral Meniscal Tears

The reported incidence of lateral meniscal tears is quite variable in the literature, which is likely primarily related to the methods (arthrotomy or arthroscopy) of joint examination. The lowest reported incidence of lateral meniscal pathology concurrent with CCL disease is 0%, examined by arthrotomy [6]. The highest reported incidence of lateral meniscal pathology concurrent with CCL disease in dogs is 77%, detected by arthroscopy [7]. Lateral meniscal tears have also rarely been reported in the face of a functional CCL, primarily in Boxers [48–50]. Pathology of the lateral meniscus is most commonly noted to be fibrillation or radial tearing of the axial edge, often primarily of the cranial horn [7], and the clinical implications of these tears are not known. However, vertical longitudinal tears, including progression to bucket handle and flap tears, and complex tears have also been reported [7, 49, 50]. Complete tears of the lateral meniscus have been shown to result in osteoarthritis and cartilage loss of the lateral compartment [50]. It is recommended to examine the lateral meniscus, in its entirety, in every dog with CCL disease, as described for the medial meniscus.

The guidelines for treatment of lateral meniscal tears follow those for treatment of medial meniscal tears, where unhealthy tissue must be debrided and removed. Response to debridement is variable [48, 49]. Similar precautions should be taken to protect the ligamentous structures, healthy portions of menisci, and articular cartilage during examination and treatment of the lateral meniscus as were discussed earlier with respect to the medial meniscus. Importantly, given the normal mobility of the lateral meniscus, it is unclear whether meniscal repair by suturing the meniscus to the joint capsule would be preferred over debridement of the tissue, even if the tissue is healthy and the damage is peripheral; no reports of lateral meniscal repairs or releases in dogs were identified during the writing of this chapter.

18.6 Postoperative Meniscal Complications

There are a few meniscus-related causes of postoperative lameness after surgery for CCL instability. A caudal medial meniscal tear can be diagnosed postoperatively in as many as 8–11% of cases where menisci were assessed as normal at the time of surgery and no meniscal treatment was performed [24, 39, 40]. These postoperative meniscal tears can be either latent or postliminary tears, where a latent tear is defined as a tear that was missed at the time of original surgery and a postliminary tear is one that forms after the original surgery. It is often difficult to determine whether a postoperative meniscal tear is latent or postliminary. It is theorized that medial meniscal tears occur secondary to the cranial-caudal instability found with CCL insufficiency. While in theory, surgical procedures performed to stabilize a CCL-deficient stifle joint, such as TPLO, should protect the meniscus from damage postoperatively, it has not been shown that there is any correlation with amount of postoperative instability and risk for development of a postliminary meniscal tear. The mean time between original surgery and diagnosis of postoperative meniscal tear ranges from 7.9 to 14.7 months between studies [24, 39]. Diagnosis and treatment of postoperative meniscal tears follow the same guidelines as those discussed for the original case work-up and treatment; joint exploration and meniscal surgery should be recommended when a meniscal tear is suspected.

Failure to address a meniscal tear may have a long-term impact on limb use, regardless of the success of the original surgery for CCL insufficiency, especially if there is significant advancement of osteoarthritis, as has been reported to occur with isolated meniscal pathology experimentally [43]. While treatment of meniscal pathology is usually relatively simple and efficacious, the need for additional surgery exposes the dog to the risks of anesthesia and surgery and requires additional financial and emotional investment from the owners.

References

1. Evans, H.E. and de Lahunta, A. (2013). *Miller's Anatomy of the Dog*, 4e, vol. 2013, 179–180. St Louis, MO: Elsevier Inc.
2. Carpenter, D.H. Jr. and Cooper, R.C. (2000). Mini review of canine stifle joint anatomy. *Anat. Histol. Embryol.* 29 (6): 321–329.
3. Arnoczky, S.P. and Warren, R.F. (1983). The microvasculature of the meniscus and its response to injury: an experimental study in the dog. *Am. J. Sports Med.* 11 (3): 131–141.
4. Flo, G.L. (1993). Meniscal injuries. *Vet. Clin. North Am. Small Anim. Pract.* 23 (4): 831–843.
5. Franklin, S.P., Gilley, R.S., and Palmer, R.H. (2010). Meniscal injury in dogs with cranial cruciate ligament rupture. *Compend. Contin. Educ. Vet.* 32 (10): E1–E10.
6. Bennett, D. and May, C. (1991). Meniscal damage associated with cruciate disease in the dog. *J. Small Anim. Pract.* 32 (3): 111–117.
7. Ralphs, S.C. and Whitney, W.O. (2002). Arthroscopic evaluation of menisci in dogs with cranial cruciate ligament injuries: 100 cases (1999–2000). *J. Am. Vet. Med. Assoc.* 221 (11): 1601–1604.
8. Neal, B.A., Ting, D., Bonczynski, J.J., and Yasuda, K. (2015). Evaluation of meniscal click for detecting meniscal tears in stifles with cranial cruciate ligament disease. *Vet. Surg.* 44 (2): 191–194.
9. Hayes, G.M., Langley-Hobbs, S.J., and Jeffery, N.D. (2010). Risk factors for medial meniscal injury in association with cranial cruciate ligament rupture. *J. Small Anim. Pract.* 51 (12): 630–634.
10. Gleason, H.E., Hudson, C.C., and Cerroni, B. (2020). Meniscal click in cranial cruciate deficient stifles as a predictor of specific meniscal pathology. *Vet. Surg.* 49 (1): 155–159.
11. Wustefeld-Janssens, B.G., Pettitt, R.A., Cowderoy, E.C. et al. (2016). Peak vertical force and vertical impulse in dogs with cranial cruciate ligament rupture and meniscal injury. *Vet. Surg.* 45 (1): 60–65.
12. Valen, S., McCabe, C., Maddock, E. et al. (2017). A modified tibial compression test for the detection of meniscal injury in dogs. *J. Small Anim. Pract.* 58 (2): 109–114.
13. Won, W.W., Lee, A.M., Butler, J.R. et al. (2020). Association of meniscal injury to joint space width on standard tibial plateau leveling osteotomy lateral radiographic projections of the canine stifle. *Vet. Radiol. Ultrasound* 61 (1): 16–24.
14. Mahn, M.M., Cook, J.L., Cook, C.R., and Balke, M.T. (2005). Arthroscopic verification of ultrasonographic diagnosis of meniscal pathology in dogs. *Vet. Surg.* 34 (4): 318–323.
15. Tivers, M.S., Mahoney, P., and Corr, S.A. (2008). Canine stifle positive contrast computed tomography arthrography for assessment of caudal horn meniscal injury: a cadaver study. *Vet. Surg.* 37 (3): 269–277.
16. Tivers, M.S., Mahoney, P.N., Baines, E.A., and Corr, S.A. (2009). Diagnostic accuracy of positive contrast computed tomography arthrography for the detection of injuries to the medial meniscus in dogs with naturally occurring cranial cruciate ligament insufficiency. *J. Small Anim. Pract.* 50 (7): 324–332.
17. Samii, V.F., Dyce, J., Pozzi, A. et al. (2009). Computed tomographic arthrography of the stifle for detection of cranial and caudal cruciate ligament and meniscal tears in dogs. *Vet. Radiol. Ultrasound* 50 (2): 144–150.
18. Berg, V.B., Lecouvet, F., Poilvache, P. et al. (2002). Spiral CT arthrography of the knee: technique and value in the assessment of internal derangement of the knee. *Eur. Radiol.* 12 (7): 1800–1810.
19. Crawford, R., Walley, G., Bridgman, S., and Maffulli, N. (2007). Magnetic resonance imaging versus arthroscopy in the diagnosis of knee pathology, concentrating on meniscal lesions and ACL tears: a systematic review. *Br. Med. Bull.* 84 (1): 5–23.
20. Barrett, E., Barr, F., Owen, M., and Bradley, K. (2009). A retrospective study of the MRI findings in 18 dogs with stifle injuries. 50 (9): 448–455.
21. Galindo-Zamora, V., Dziallas, P., Ludwig, D.C. et al. (2013). Diagnostic accuracy of a short-duration 3 Tesla magnetic resonance protocol for diagnosing stifle joint lesions in dogs with non-traumatic cranial cruciate ligament rupture. *BMC Vet. Res.* 9 (1): 40.
22. Przeworski, A., Adamiak, Z., and Glodek, J. (2016). Comparison of high-field and low-field magnetic resonance imaging of stifle joint disorders in dogs. *Pol. J. Vet. Sci.* 19 (3): 633–670.
23. Pozzi, A., Hildreth, B.E., and Rajala-Schultz, P.J. (2008). Comparison of arthroscopy and arthrotomy for diagnosis of medial meniscal pathology: an ex vivo study. *Vet. Surg.* 37 (8): 749–755.
24. Ritzo, M.E., Ritzo, B.A., Siddens, A.D. et al. (2014). Incidence and type of meniscal injury and associated long-term clinical outcomes in dogs treated surgically for cranial cruciate ligament disease. *Vet. Surg.* 43 (8): 952–958.
25. Plesman, R., Gilbert, P., and Campbell, J. (2013). Detection of meniscal tears by arthroscopy and arthrotomy in dogs with cranial cruciate ligament rupture. *Vet. Comp. Orthop. Traumatol.* 26 (01): 42–46.
26. Dietrich, F., Ries, C., Eiermann, C. et al. (2014). Complications in hip arthroscopy: necessity of supervision during the learning curve. *Knee Surg. Sports Traumatol. Arthrosc.* 22 (4): 953–958.
27. Cortés, I. III, Warnock, J.J., Ranganathan, B., and Bobe, G. (2019). Iatrogenic cartilage injury associated with the use of stainless-steel cannulas and

silicone-guarded cannulas for canine stifle arthroscopy. *Vet. Surg.* 48 (8): 1456–1465.
28. Rogatko, C.P., Warnock, J.J., Bobe, G., and Verpaalen, V.D. (2018). Comparison of iatrogenic articular cartilage injury in canine stifle arthroscopy versus medial parapatellar mini-arthrotomy in a cadaveric model. *Vet. Surg.* 47 (S1): O6–O14.
29. Klein, W. and Kurze, V. (1986). Arthroscopic arthropathy: iatrogenic arthroscopic joint lesions in animals. *Arthroscopy* 2 (3): 163–168.
30. Andriacchi, T.P., Mündermann, A., Smith, R.L. et al. (2004). A framework for the in vivo pathomechanics of osteoarthritis at the knee. *Ann. Biomed. Eng.* 32 (3): 447–457.
31. Park, J.Y., Jeong, B.S., Roh, Y.S. et al. (2018). Evaluation of an arthroscopic stifle lever for stifle joint distraction in toy breed dogs. *J. Vet. Sci.* 19 (5): 693–698.
32. Böttcher, P., Winkels, P., and Oechtering, G. (2009). A novel pin distraction device for arthroscopic assessment of the medial meniscus in dogs. *Vet. Surg.* 38 (5): 595–600.
33. Rovesti, G.L., Devesa-Garcia, V., Urrutia, P.G. et al. (2015). Evaluation of a distractor to increase joint space of the stifle joint in dogs: a cadaveric study. *Vet. Comp. Orthop. Traumatol.* 28 (03): 179–185.
34. Kim, J.H., Heo, S.Y., and Lee, H.B. (2017). Arthroscopic detection of medial meniscal injury with the use of a joint distractor in small-breed dogs. *J. Vet. Sci.* 18 (4): 515–520.
35. Winkels, P., Pozzi, A., Cook, R., and Böttcher, P. (2016). Prospective evaluation of the Leipzig stifle distractor. *Vet. Surg.* 45 (5): 631–635.
36. Kim, K., Lee, H., and Ragetly, G.R. (2016). Feasibility of stifle medial meniscal release in toy breed dogs with and without a joint distractor. *Vet. Surg.* 45 (5): 636–641.
37. Rovesti, G.L., Devesa, V., Bertorelli, L., and Rodriguez-Quiros, J. (2018). Facilitation of arthroscopic visualization and treatment of meniscal tears using a stifle joint distractor in the dog. *BMC Vet. Res.* 14 (1): 212.
38. Götzens, B., Medl, S.C., and Medl, N.S. (2019). ex vivo cadaveric study of a laterally placed Leipzig stifle distractor for arthroscopic evaluation of the lateral meniscus in dogs. *Vet. Surg.* 48 (S1): O25–O33.
39. Thieman, K.M., Tomlinson, J.L., Fox, D.B. et al. (2006). Effect of meniscal release on rate of subsequent meniscal tears and owner-assessed outcome in dogs with cruciate disease treated with tibial plateau leveling osteotomy. *Vet. Surg.* 35 (8): 705–710.
40. Costa, M., Craig, D., Cambridge, T. et al. (2017). Major complications of tibial tuberosity advancement in 1613 dogs. *Vet. Surg.* 46 (4): 494–500.
41. Austin, B., Montgomery, R.D., Wright, J. et al. (2007). Evaluation of three approaches to meniscal release. *Vet. Comp. Orthop. Traumatol.* 2 (02): 92–97.
42. Pozzi, A., Kim, S.E., and Lewis, D.D. (2010). Effect of transection of the caudal menisco-tibial ligament on medial femorotibial contact mechanics. *Vet. Surg.* 39 (4): 489–495.
43. Luther, J.K., Cook, C.R., and Cook, J.L. (2009). Meniscal release in cruciate ligament intact stifles causes lameness and medial compartment cartilage pathology in dogs 12 weeks postoperatively. *Vet. Surg.* 38 (4): 520–529.
44. Thieman, K.M., Pozzi, A., Ling, H.Y. et al. (2009). Contact mechanics of simulated meniscal tears in cadaveric canine stifles. *Vet. Surg.* 38 (7): 803–810.
45. Thieman, K.M., Pozzi, A., Ling, H.Y., and Lewis, D. (2010). Comparison of contact mechanics of three meniscal repair techniques and partial meniscectomy in cadaveric dog stifles. *Vet. Surg.* 39 (3): 355–362.
46. Moses, P.A. (2002). A technique for the surgical repair of caudal peripheral detachment and longitudinal peripheral tears of the medial meniscus in dogs. *Vet. Comp. Orthop. Traumatol.* 15 (02): 92–96.
47. Pozzi, A., Tonks, C.A., and Ling, H.Y. (2010). Femorotibial contact mechanics and meniscal strain after serial meniscectomy. *Vet. Surg.* 39 (4): 482–428.
48. Williams, R.A. (2010). Isolated lateral meniscus tear in a boxer. *Vet. Rec.* 167 (11): 419–420.
49. Langley-Hobbs, S.J. (2001). Lateral meniscal tears and stifle osteochondrosis in three dogs. *Vet. Rec.* 149 (19): 592–594.
50. Krier, E.M., Johnson, T.A., Breiteneicher, A.H. et al. (2018). Articular cartilage lesions associated with complete lateral meniscal tears in the dog. *Vet. Surg.* 47 (7): 958–962.

Index

Complications in Canine Cranial Cruciate Ligament Surgery, First Edition. Edited by Ron Ben-Amotz and David L. Dycus.